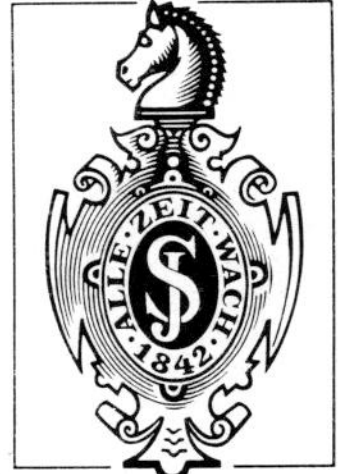

Neuroradiology

A Neuropathological Approach

R. Kautzky · K. J. Zülch
S. Wende · A. Tänzer

With 251 Figures

Springer-Verlag
Berlin Heidelberg New York 1982

Professor Dr. R. Kautzky
Em. Direktor der Neurochirurgischen Abteilung der Neurologischen
Universitätsklinik, Martinistraße 52, D-2000 Hamburg 20

Professor Dr. K.J. Zülch
Em. Direktor am Max-Planck-Institut für Hirnforschung, Abteilung für
Allgemeine Neurologie und der Neurologischen Klinik Köln-Merheim,
Ostmerheimer Straße 200, D-5000 Köln 91

Professor Dr. S. Wende
Neuroradiologische Abteilung der Neurochirurgischen Klinik der Universität
Mainz, Langenbeckstraße 1, D-6500 Mainz

Professor Dr. A. Tänzer †

Translator
Dr. W.M. Boehm
Neurosurgical Department, Erlanger Medical Center, Suite 202, 1010 East
Third Street, Chattanooga, TN 37403/USA

Translation of the German edition
Neuroradiologie auf neuropathologischer Grundlage, 2., neubearb. u. erw. Aufl.
© Springer-Verlag Berlin Heidelberg 1976

ISBN 3-540-10934-X Springer-Verlag Berlin Heidelberg New York
ISBN 0-387-10934-X Springer-Verlag New York Heidelberg Berlin

Library of Congress Cataloging in Publication Data. Neuroradiologie auf neuropathologischer Grundlage. English. Neuroradiology, a neuropathological approach. Rev. translation of: Neuroradiologie auf neuropathologischer Grundlage. Translated by W.M. Boehm and V.B. Kellett. Bibliography: p. Includes index.. 1. Central nervous system–Radiography. 2. Central nervous system–Diseases–Diagnosis. I. Kautzky, Rudolf, 1913–. II. Title. [DNLM: 1. Nervous system–Radiography. WL 141 N499] RC349.R3K3813 1982 .616.8′047572 .82–10791

Typesetting, printing, and bookbinding by Universitätsdruckerei H. Stürtz AG, Würzburg
2120/3130-543210

Preface to the English Edition

The warm reception of the German edition of this book in Germany and abroad stimulated us to have it translated into English. In this endeavor we were fortunate to enlist the able services of Dr. W.M. BOEHM and Dr. V.B. KELLETT, both of Chattanooga, as translators. Their combined efforts have produced a highly readable text which reflects excellently the original work. We are also very grateful for Dr. BOEHM's tireless efforts and close cooperation throughout this period, which greatly facilitated the progress of the work.

Neuroradiology has continued to evolve since the publication of the German edition and this has made minor changes and deviations from the German version necessary. In particular, the spectacular growth of computed tomography (CT) has necessitated some revision. By no means, however, has the evolution of computed tomography made the section on pneumoencephalography obsolete. On the contrary, a concise study of ventriculography and pneumoencephalography is most important in both understanding and correctly interpreting computed tomograms. In addition, since CTs are still not routinely available in many parts of the third world and in some rural districts of even the richest nations, conventional neuroradiologic procedures will remain important for some time to come and indications for their use must be given. Similarly, although the development of non-invasive angiography (digital enhanced angiography) promises to supplant conventional angiography in the not-too-distant future, the value of this procedure as a diagnostic tool and for comparative purposes will also remain for years to come.

Finally, the World Health Organization recently finished its work on the classification of tumors of the nervous system, a project which was initiated by and brought to fruition largely through the efforts of one of us (K.J. ZÜLCH). This new classification has necessitated some changes in terminology, which have been incorporated into the present translation.

More than 25 years have passed since the appearance of KAUTZKY and ZÜLCH's *Neurologisch-Neurochirurgische Röntgendiagnostik* (Diagnostic Radiology for Neurologists and Neurosurgeons), which has since become a German classic. The present translation is an updated version of the second, revised German edition of that work published in 1976.

It is hoped that this first American edition will not only provide the English-speaking community with the opportunity to read this outstanding contribution to the field of neuroradiology, but also fill a specific void in the current crop of neuroradiological reference works. With its special emphasis on neuropathology as the basis for neuroradiological change, it should prove invaluable both to the neuroradiologist and to the clinician specializing in neurology or neurosurgery. In addition, the detailed analysis of ventriculographic and pneumoencephalographic changes in response to tumors of various types and sites should serve as a useful tool in understanding and analyzing current computer tomograms.

This translation is a joint effort, undertaken at the request of Professor ZÜLCH, by Drs. W.M. BOEHM and V.B. KELLETT, both of Chattanooga, Tennessee. Dr. BOEHM is a neurosurgeon in a large group practice which also includes his father and brother. Dr. KELLETT was a distinguished educator with a doctorate in the Germanic languages who recently died after a long and fruitful career.

Special thanks are extended to MARY LYNN WILSON for her help in typing the English manuscript and to all those who contributed their time and energies to this project.

We regret that Professor Dr. A. TÄNZER, our coauthor, passed away during the preparation of the English edition.

Hamburg/Köln/Mainz, Autumn 1982

R. KAUTZKY K.J. ZÜLCH S. WENDE

Preface to the Second German Edition

The first edition of this book was well-received by the medical profession in Germany and elsewhere not only for its method of defining and describing alterations in the normal neuroradiological anatomy in response to brain disease, but also for its emphasis on the cause of such alterations. The book was so well-received, in fact, that many of its diagrams were subsequently incorporated into later texts and handbooks on the subject. In spite of this success, the passage of time and advances in the field of neuroradiology combined to make so much of the subject matter outdated or outmoded that a revision became a necessity.

In this endeavor the original authors, both practicing clinicians who have continued to work in the field of neuroradiology, were joined by two primary neuroradiologists in order to facilitate the expansion and revision of the text.

Two chapters in the first edition, which dealt with needle biopsy of tumors and CSF staining techniques, did not seem important enough to retain and were deleted. Some subjects – radioisotope brain scanning, cerebral blood flow measurements, and the rapidly evolving field of computed tomography – important as they are, seemed to us to exceed the frame of reference of this book and were therefore not covered in any detail.

In spite of many recommendations to further expand the work to include a section on normal and abnormal plain skull and vertebral X-rays, inclusion of this material did not seem appropriate in a textbook limiting its scope to special neuroradiological diagnostic procedures. On the other hand, myelography and the newly developed radiological pathology of cerebrovascular insufficiency did seem appropriate and were both added to the list of topics for discussion.

The remaining chapters from the first edition were updated to current standards and most of the X-ray pictures replaced with newer examples. The original concepts of the first edition were, however, retained.

In its present form this book should be considered an introduction to the art of diagnosing intracranial and intraspinal pathology by means of special neuroradiological procedures, with an emphasis on making the interpretation of these procedures understandable to the practicing clinician. To accomplish this goal, an attempt was made to closely correlate the radiographic contrast image obtained with the pathological morphology of the primary disease process. As in the first edition, the present revision begins with a discussion of intracranial mass displacements and the pathological morphology responsible for these displacements.

The expanded section on neuropathology will hopefully provide a broader basis for understanding and interpreting both the traditional neuroradiological diagnostic procedures and the newer computed tomograms.

As earlier, much emphasis is placed on normal variants and on the many sources of technical error which can contribute to false diagnoses. Only by understanding the limitations of a given procedure can its value as a diagnostic tool be realized.

In this way the book adapts itself particularly to the needs of the clinician, whether he be a neurologist, a neurosurgeon, or a psychiatrist. It is hoped, however, that it will also be well-received by radiologists and neuroradiologists alike since correlation of a specific radiographic contrast image with the underlying pathological process is essential to the proper interpretation of all neuroradiological diagnostic procedures, particularly those studies which are borderline abnormal. The method of presentation employed will hopefully guarantee that the neurosurgeon, the neurologist, and the neuroradiologist will all participate in the interpretive process. In this sense, the present work is a true communal effort by the authors, even though a given chapter may reflect the special interest of an individual author.

Special thanks are due to Doctor SCHMITZ-DRÄGER, chief radiologist at Köln-Merheim, for permission to copy numerous X-ray pictures.

The diagrams and illustrations used were prepared from drawings by medical student Mr. ANDRES, Miss INGRID VON MARCHTHALER, Dr. ILSE MÜLLER, Mr. HELMUTH MÜLLER-MOLO, Miss INGRID SCHAUMBURG, and Mr. HANS GÖLDNER, who also helped with the preparation of the X-ray pictures. We are also indebted to Mrs. MARGOT GÖLDNER for her secretarial work in preparing the manuscript for publication.

Finally, our thanks are extended to the publishers for their assistance and their patience in the publication of this work.

Hamburg/Köln/Mainz, Oktober 1976

R. KAUTZKY K.J. ZÜLCH S. WENDE A. TÄNZER

Contents

A. Intracranial Pressure and Mass Displacements of the Intracranial Contents

    I. Intracranial Anatomy and Mass Displacements 3
   II. Mass Displacements and Space-Occupying Lesions 6
      1. Etiology of Localized and Generalized Intracranial
        Pressure 6
      2. Herniation into the Cisterns 7
      3. Development of Occlusive Hydrocephalus 11
      4. Significance of Site and Type of Space-Occupying Lesions on
        the Type of Intracranial Mass Displacement 13
        a) The Hemispheric Processes 14
        b) The Paramedian, Especially Thalamic and Basal Ganglia
          Tumors 16
        c) Obstructions to the Ventricular Fluid Pathways in or Near
          the Midline 16
  III. Mass Displacements by Atrophic Processes 20

B. Special Neuropathology – Morphology and Biology of the Space-Occupying and Atrophic Processes with Their Related Neuroradiological Changes

    I. Space-Occupying Intracranial and Spinal Processes 25
      a) Predilections 25
      b) The Classification of Brain Tumors According to the
        World Health Organization 25
        1. Tumors of Neuroepithelial Tissue 27
        2. Tumors of Nerve Sheath Cells 37
        3. Tumors of Meningeal and Related Tissues 37
        4. Primary Malignant Lymphomas 39
        5. Tumors of Blood Vessel Origin 39
        6. Germ Cell Tumors 40
        7. Other Malformative Tumors and Tumor-Like Lesions 40
        8. Vascular Malformations 41
        9. The Tumors of the Anterior Pituitary 41
      10. Local Extensions from Regional Tumors 41
      11. Metastatic Tumors and Unclassified Tumors 41
      12. Less Common Tumors of the Base of the Skull . . . 41
      13. Space-Occupying Processes of the Spinal Canal . . . 42
      14. Space-Occupying Lesions Other than Neoplasms . . . 43
      15. Grading of Malignancy 44
   II. Atrophic Cerebral Processes 45
  III. Changes Following Trauma to the Skull and Brain 46
      1. Injuries Occurring as a Result of Falls or Secondary to Blunt
        Instruments (Flat Force, Circumscribed Force) 46

2. Traumatic Hemorrhages 46
3. Traumatic Cysts 46
4. Traumatic Brain Edema 46
5. Special, Rare Posttraumatic Events (Pneumocephaly, Carotid-Cavernous Fistula) 47
IV. Consequences of Craniocerebral Trauma as Revealed by Radiologic Contrast Procedures 48
V. The Pathogenesis of Infarcts 49
VI. Aneurysms and Arteriovenous Malformations 53
VII. Hypertensive Intracerebral Hemorrhage 53

C. Cerebral Angiography

I. History 57
II. Technique 58
1. Injection of the Contrast Medium 58
a) Puncture Methods 58
b) Catheter Techniques 59
c) Retrograde Injection Techniques 60
d) Catheter Techniques and Retrograde Angiography in Children 62
2. The Contrast Media 62
3. X-Ray Technique 63
a) Magnification Angiography 64
b) Subtraction 66
4. Dangers and Complications of Cerebral Angiography . . . 68
III. The Normal Cerebral Angiogram 70
a) The Arterial Phase of the Internal Carotid Artery Angiogram 70
b) The Capillary and Venous Phases of the Internal Carotid Artery Angiogram 81
c) The External Carotid Angiogram 84
d) The Arterial Phase of the Vertebral Angiogram 85
e) The Venous Phase of the Vertebral Angiogram 91
IV. The Pathological Intracranial Angiogram 94
1. Intracranial Space-Occupying Lesions 94
a) Displacement of Normal Blood Vessels 94
b) Pathological Vascularization in Space-Occupying Processes 113
2. The Angiogram in Head Injuries 118
3. The Diagnosis of Primary Intracranial Vascular Disease . . 127
a) Arterial Aneurysms 127
b) Arteriovenous Malformations 132
c) The Carotid-Cavernous Fistula 133
d) Vascular Stenoses and Vascular Occlusions 136
e) Intracerebral Hemorrhage 171
f) Disturbances in Venous Outflow 171
4. Cerebral Circulatory Standstill and Brain Death 173
V. Special Angiographic Procedures 174
1. Angiography of the Ophthalmic Artery 174
2. Orbital Venography 174
3. Direct Sinography 175
4. Angiography of the Jugular Vein 178

D. Pneumoencephalography

    I. History 183

   II. Injection Technique 184
      1. The Lumbar Pneumoencephalogram 184
      2. Suboccipital (Cisternal) Pneumoencephalography 186
      3. Ventriculography 187

  III. Radiologic Technique 190
      a) Recommended Standard Technique 190
      b) Positioning the Patient and Setting of the Apparatus for
         the Films 190
      c) The Causes of Nonfilling of the Ventricular System . . . 192
      d) Unilateral Filling 193
      e) The 24-h Pneumoencephalogram 193

  IV. Gas Resorption 193

   V. Autonomic Reactions 193

  VI. Complications 194

 VII. The Normal Pneumoencephalogram 197
      1. The Ventricular System 197
      2. The Subarachnoid Pathways 208

VIII. General Rules for the Interpretation of Pneumoencephalograms 216

  IX. The Pathological Pneumoencephalogram 219
      1. Space-Occupying Processes 219
      a) The Hemispheric Processes 220
      b) Tumors of the Lateral Ventricles, Basal Ganglia, and
         Thalamus 231
      c) Occlusion of the Midline Ventricular Pathways (Third
         Ventricle, Aqueduct, Fourth Ventricle) 233
      d) Cerebellopontine Angle Tumors 247
      e) The Normal Air Study in Space-Occupying Processes . . 250
      f) Multiple Tumors, Pseudotumor Cerebri 250
      g) Specific Diagnosis of Space-Occupying Processes from the
         Air Study 251
      2. Atrophic Processes 251
      a) Generalized Cerebral Atrophies 252
      b) Unilateral Atrophic Processes 256
      c) Atrophy of Lobes 256
      d) Local Circumscribed Atrophies 256
      3. Changes After Trauma to the Skull and Brain – Expert Legal
         Testimony 257
      4. Malformations 260
      a) The Septum Pellucidum Cyst 260
      b) Agenesis of the Corpus Callosum 261
      c) The Unpaired, Cyclops Ventricle 261
      d) Arachnoidal Cysts 261

   X. Indications and Contraindications for Angiography and
     Pneumoencephalography (or Ventriculography) in the Absence
     of CT 264

  XI. Comparison of the Indications for Conventional
     Neuroradiological Procedures and for CT 267

E. Myelography

  I. History 271
 II. Technique 272
     1. Myelography Using Water-Insoluble Positive Contrast Media 272
     2. Myelography Using Water-Soluble Positive Contrast Media 274
     3. Myelography With Negative Contrast Media 276
III. Complications and Errors 278
 IV. Indications 279
  V. The Normal Myelogram 280
 VI. The Pathological Myelogram 283
     1. Intramedullary Space-Occupying Lesions 283
     2. Intradural, Extramedullary Space-Occupying Lesions 284
     3. Extradural Space-Occupying Lesions 285
     4. The Spinal Arteriovenous Malformations 290
     5. Meningeal Adhesions and Arachnoiditis 291
     6. Posttraumatic Changes 292
     7. Spinal Cord Atrophy 292
     8. Congenital Malformations of the Spine and Its Contents . . 293

F. Spinal Angiography

  I. History 297
 II. Normal and Pathological Anatomy of the Spinal Cord Vessels 297
III. Examination Technique 299
     1. Demonstration of the Anterior Spinal Artery in the Cervical
        Region 299
     2. Demonstration of the Anterior Spinal Artery at the
        Thoracolumbar Junction 299
     3. Comparison of Various Methods Available for Spinal
        Angiography 299
 IV. Complications 301

G. Discography

  I. History 305
 II. Technique of Cervical Discography 305
III. The Normal Discogram 305
 IV. The Pathological Discogram 305
  V. Complications 306

H. Ossovenography and Epidural Venography

  I. History 309
 II. Anatomy 309
III. Technique 309
 IV. Results 309
  V. Complications and Contraindications 310

References 311

Subject Index 319

A. Intracranial Pressure and Mass Displacements of the Intracranial Contents

I. Intracranial Anatomy and Mass Displacements

The brain is completely surrounded by the bony skull and its closely adherent, tough, dural inner lining. This converts the enclosed space into a watertight chamber with the exception of the small, basally situated foramen magnum. In adults, these factors combine to prevent the skull from expanding. Consequently, the intracranial volume cannot fluctuate. In addition, the intracranial contents – blood, brain, and spinal fluid – are essentially noncompressible.

When these facts are considered in the light of another fact – that a great number of pathological states which affect the brain are mass-producing or space-occupying – it is apparent that certain secondary local displacements within the skull are inevitable in response to a mass lesion, and that a compensatory reduction in the mass of the normal intracranial contents equal to that of the pathological mass will be required to prevent increases in intracranial pressure. Conversely, when the pathological process leads to a reduction in the mass of the cerebral tissues – as occurs in the atrophic states – a compensatory increase in another intracranial component will be required to fill the void (Fig. 1).

Compensatory mass displacements of brain tissue in response to a space-occupying process occur in certain predictable patterns. The anatomy of the surrounding brain tissue, blood vessels, and spinal fluid spaces is thus distorted, but again in a predictable pattern. These predictable mass displacements can be visualized by various radiological diagnostic procedures using contrast media. These procedures, therefore, permit conclusions to be drawn about the underlying pathological process leading to the mass displacement.

Prior to describing the various radiologic diagnostic procedures themselves, it is essential that the fundamental rules of intracranial mass displacement caused by space-occupying lesions or atrophic processes be thoroughly understood.

Of the diagnostic procedures which are to be discussed, the common denominator and the factor of greatest importance is the mass displacement itself – rather than the precise pathological process causing it – since a distinction

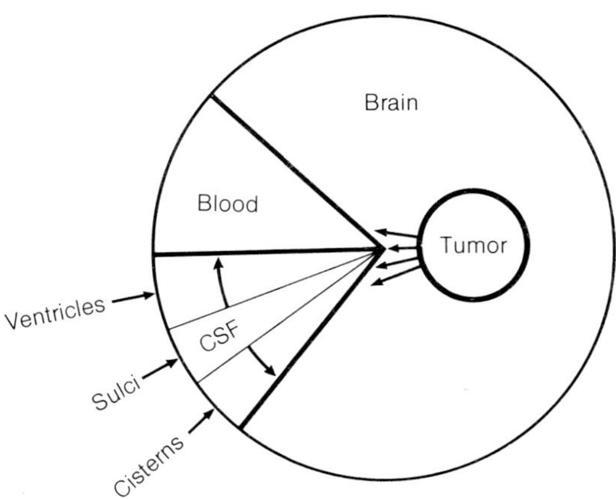

Fig. 1. The rigid, "watertight" skull is filled with brain, blood, and CSF. When a tumor growth begins, compensatory decrease in the volume of one of these components must occur to prevent a generalized increase in intracranial pressure. The first to do so is the CSF (the relationships with respect to volume are approximately correct)

cannot always be made between such mass lesions as tumors, abscesses, acute suppurations in association with meningitis, granulomas, parasitic processes, intracerebral or extracerebral hemorrhages, empyemas, arachnoidal cysts, radiation necrosis, hydrocephalic processes, or cerebral edema: all are space-occupying processes and can lead to mass displacements. Nor is the precise pathological process important to those mass displacements which accompany the cerebral atrophies, whether they follow trauma, inflammatory processes, infarcts, or other etiologies: the rules of mass displacement for all are fundamentally the same and vary only with the location, the size, and the rate of increase or decrease of the various lesions.

Of the cerebral contents mentioned earlier, the cerebrospinal fluid lends itself more readily to displacement. For this reason, pathological processes which are mass-producing or mass-decreasing will first be compensated for by changes in the volume of the spinal fluid spaces (Fig. 1). Fluctuations in the volume of blood within the skull are of lesser importance in the compensatory process, although loss of auto-regulatory mechanisms and dilation of the cerebral vessels can adversely contribute to the mass effect. The venous sinuses are incapable of much change, but other venous structures are easily compressed. Secondary atrophy of the cerebral tissues – as opposed to primary atrophies – follows longstanding compression as a result

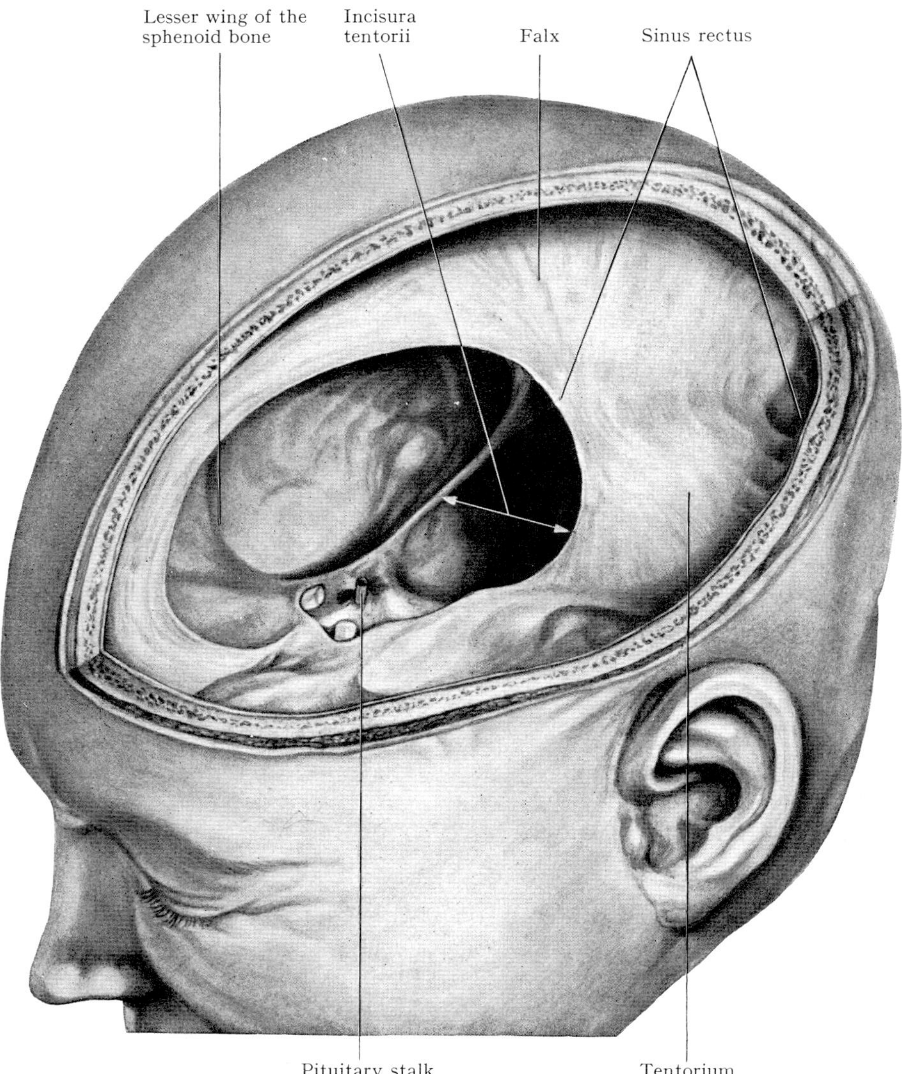

Fig. 2. The compartments of the skull with the falx and tentorium intact. The *arrow* indicates the tentorial hiatus

of extracellular fluid extravasations or any other cause of cell destruction.

As noted earlier, the rules of mass displacement are dependent upon the fixed volume of the adult skull. The situation in children is fundamentally different. Since the sutures of a child's skull are open, stretching of the dura and widening of the sutures can occur with a secondary increase in intracranial volume, often to grotesque proportions. Localized swelling of the skull can also occur, particularly in association with underlying arachnoidal cysts, but less frequently from other causes such as underlying tumors. On the other hand, since the normal infant skull expands in response to growth of the developing brain, underdevelopment of a part of the brain will lead to underexpansion of its overlying skull compared to the expected size. In fact, the normal size may even develop a compensatory expansion, thus increasing the skull deformity even further.

Let us now define the pathophysiology of the intracranial mass displacements. To begin with, every space-occupying process initially exerts evenly distributed excentric pressure on the surrounding tissues. Conversely, each atrophic process exerts an evenly distributed pull on its surrounding tissues. These forces, however, are opposed by other forces, the most significant of which is mechanical resistance caused by the structural adherence of the cerebral tissues and by points of fixation to the surrounding membranes. Another resisting force is the hydrodynamic resistance of the ventricular fluid, which is being actively produced and which can resist compression deformity of the ventricular spaces. A third force is likewise hydrodynamic and is caused by the influence of the blood pressure in maintaining the arteriovascular tree intracranially.

Of great significance in this latter effect is the fact that the three main cerebral arteries proceed in a wide curve against which the pressure wave acts, as it were, to stretch out the vessel. Because of the surrounding cerebral tissue, the vessel maintains its shape and in so doing forms a dynamic support for the brain tissue – a skeleton of sorts – which functions as long as the blood pressure is adequate to maintain it.

In addition, the brain is supported by the cerebrospinal fluid (CSF) channels and is suspended within the skull, attached to its dural lining by loose connections of blood vessels, nerves, and the pituitary stalk. Two thick dural sheets, the falx and the tentorium, partition the intracranial space into three large sections (Fig. 2). Since portions of the brain rest upon them, they also act as support structures and as a barrier to mass displacements; inferiorly, however, the brain rests upon the base of the skull itself. The falx bisects the supratentorial compartment into right and left, while the tentorium separates the infratentorial compartment – or posterior cranial fossa – from the supratentorial compartment (Fig. 2). The supratentorial compartment is further partitioned into anterior and middle cranial fossas, the dividing line being the edge of the lesser wing of the sphenoid. For the sake of the discussion which follows, it is worth mentioning that the dural partitions are of far greater significance than the division into anterior and middle cranial fossas.

To each side of the falx in the supratentorial compartment are found the two cerebral hemispheres, which are joined together below the edge of the falx (Fig. 2). The brain of the posterior fossa is connected with the cerebral hemispheres by means of the brain stem, which passes through the relatively small tentorial hiatus (Fig. 2). At this point the brain stem consists of the midbrain. Although it is usually small, the actual size of the tentorial hiatus can vary considerably.

These divisions of the intracranial space permit large mass displacements only in certain directions:
1) Within the confines of a hemisphere
2) From one hemisphere to the other beneath the falx
3) Through the tentorial hiatus in the direction of the brain stem
4) From the posterior cranial fossa through the tentorial hiatus superiorly

Even within the confines of these spaces, mass displacements are resisted and modified by means of the internal and external support structures of the brain. The external support structures hold the brain through attachments by means of veins, arteries, nerves, and the pituitary stalk to extracerebral structures, while the internal support structures consist mainly of the cerebral tissues themselves, particularly white matter pathways such as the internal capsule, corona radiata, association tracts, and cerebral peduncles. Although the CSF-producing ventricular system also acts as both a buttressing force and a safety valve in mass displacements, it is of much greater significance from the pathological standpoint when blockage of the various CSF pathways results in secondary hydrocephalus. This subject will be presented in greater detail in the following chapter.

II. Mass Displacements and Space-Occupying Lesions

1. Etiology of Localized and Generalized Intracranial Pressure

In the evolution of the space-occupying lesion, we can distinguish a definite temporal sequence.

Phase I

In the first phase a tumor squeezes spinal fluid from the subarachnoid spaces of the adjacent brain and flattens its convolutions against the inner surface of the skull. At the same time, it begins to distort the nearest ventricular cavity. A growing tumor, therefore, will begin to expand by expressing spinal fluid from the external subarachnoid spaces and by compressing and deforming the internal ventricular spaces. This leads to the characteristic changes of localized intracranial pressure increase, namely a circumscribed flattening of the convolutions, deformity of the adjacent ventricle, and initial displacement of the nearby arteries and veins (see upper part of Fig. 3).

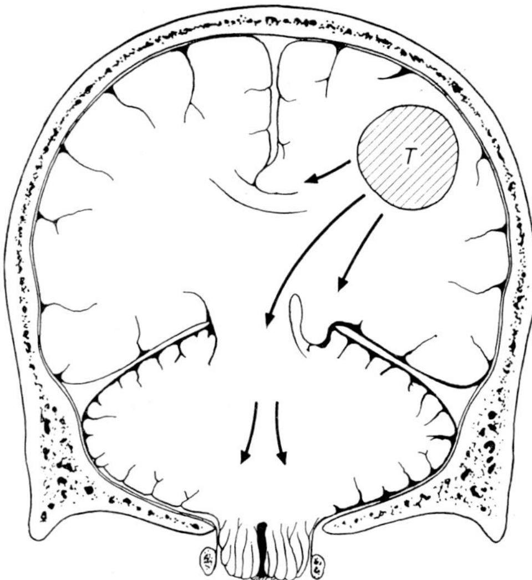

Fig. 3. Semischematic model of the mass displacements which accompany a parietal lobe tumor. *Above:* The gyrus cinguli is pushed to the opposite side. *Middle:* Medial portions of the temporal lobe are forced through the tentorial hiatus as a hernia displacing the midbrain. *Below:* The brain stem is forced caudally and the cerebellar tonsils herniate into the foramen magnum. In the vicinity of the tumor, the convolutions are flattened

Phase II

As the volume of the involved lobe increases further, a point is reached where spinal fluid shifts can no longer accommodate the expanding mass. In addition, localized cerebral edema will contribute to the space-occupying process causing the localized intracranial pressure effect to spread and to involve the entire hemisphere, which will attempt to accommodate it by expanding into the fissures, cisterns, and ventricles to the greatest possible degree (upper part of Fig. 3). Further compensation requires the shifting of increasing quantities of brain tissue from one anatomical compartment to the other. Thus, brain tissue will begin to herniate beneath the falx laterally, as well as in an axial direction through the tentorial hiatus (upper part of Fig. 3 and Fig. 9). Because of the strength of the falx, which is very tightly connected to the skull and is only movable at its lower edge to a minimal degree, lateral displacement must take place predominantly in the open space beneath the falx. The lower edge of the falx changes its position only in response to local pressure from a large space-occupying lesion in its immediate vicinity which has been producing intense pressures over a long period of time (Fig. 9). Exceptions to this rule are few, although they do occur. For example, an enormous infarct in the territory of supply of the anterior cerebral and middle cerebral arteries with extensive edema can cause acute lateral displacements with slanting of the falx within a few days.

Lateral mass displacements of the brain beneath the falx vary in a characteristic fashion depending upon the site of origin of the mass. Masses originating in the frontal areas are most readily associated with this kind of displacement since the falx is shorter anteriorly and the free space beneath is greater than posteriorly where the falx and splenium of the corpus callosum are in direct contact with one another (Fig. 4). The falx also supports the corpus callosum posteriorly and adjacent cerebral tissues including the septum by means of the bracing effect of the centrum semiovale in the median plane. Only if a space-occupying process first displaces the corpus callosum from the lower posterior edge of the falx is it possible for parietal lobe displacements to shift beneath the falx and across the midline. It is obvious from the foregoing discussion that lateral mass displace-

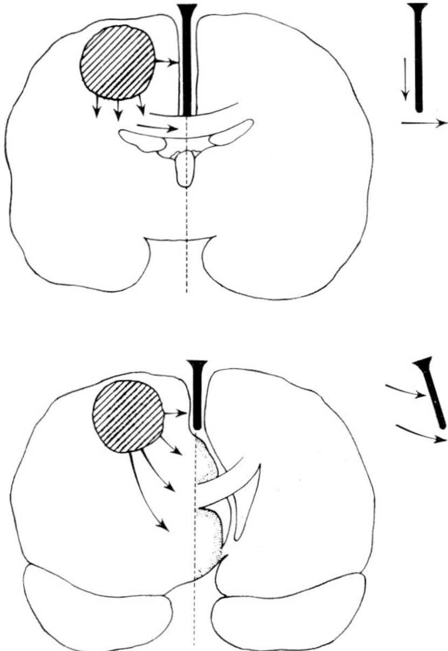

Fig. 4. Differences in mass displacement caused by space-occupying lesions in the parietal and frontal lobes. *Above:* In the parietal region the lower border of the falx lies in direct contact with the corpus callosum; thus, a lateral displacement is possible only when the corpus callosum is initially pushed downward since the falx itself, because of its attachment to the tentorium, will resist all but the most extreme degrees of pressure in this area. *Below:* A lateral displacement occurs much more easily in the frontal region where the distance between the free edge of the falx and the corpus callosum is greater. The falx can also be displaced laterally when the necessary pressure is present (see *diagrams,* right upper corner)

ment beneath the falx first requires axial displacement mediobasally in an anterior or posterior direction, at least as far as the inferior margin of the falx itself (Fig. 4). Lateral displacements initially involve the corpus callosum and gyrus cinguli, parts of the medial basal frontal lobe, as well as the deeper structures and vessels found in relationship to the third ventricle. These latter structures can undergo lateral displacement in parietal lesions without the aforementioned displacement of the corpus callosum away from the falx. This is significant because the deep veins which lie in this region are visible on angiograms.

Whenever lateral displacement of brain tissue crosses the midline, a secondary compression of the opposite hemisphere results. Simultaneously, axial herniations can also occur through the tentorial hiatus into the posterior cranial fossa (Figs. 3, 9). This is especially true in frontal space-occupying lesions where the ef-

fects of pressure are oriented more in a longitudinal direction. Axial herniations or transmissions of pressure can cause distortion and displacement of the midbrain, a process which can proceed by involving the brain stem in a rostrocaudal fashion, eventually pressing the hindbrain against the foramen magnum and spinal canal. In this case, the medulla oblongata and particularly the adjacent cerebral tonsils are wedged down into the spinal canal resulting in the so-called cerebellar or tonsillar pressure cone (Figs. 3, 9/II). Thus, a localized intracranial pressure effect may spread to become generalized and may result in axial displacements in the direction of the posterior cranial fossa (TÖNNIS 1938, 1959; ZÜLCH 1950, 1959; ZÜLCH et al. 1974a).

2. Herniation into the Cisterns

In the preceding section the various phases of growth of a space-occupying process were described. Local pressures spread to involve an entire hemisphere, are transmitted to the opposite hemisphere, and finally the posterior fossa is involved. In each phase the reserve spaces provided by the cisterns are systematically eliminated as brain tissue moves into them. These cisterns are portrayed in the conventional manner in Figs. 167, 168, and 173, while Figs. 5, 6, and 7 correspond better to the new computed tomograms. The mere presence of such a herniation is therefore clearly indicative of a mass displacement. By means of the radiological procedures of angiography and pneumoencephalography (Fig. 8) it is possible not only to determine the presence of herniations within the various cisterns, but also the approximate size of the space-occupying lesion itself. Reference is made in this regard to the study by RIESSNER and ZÜLCH (1939) describing the topography of herniations for each space-occupying process. This is particularly helpful when the mass displacement has not caused significant distortion of the ventricular system, but has caused herniation into the cisterns. A detailed description of the cisterns may be found on p. 208. At this point, however, consideration will be given to those herniations which are important in the analysis of pneumoencephalograms (LINDGREN 1948–1954; DiCHIRO 1967, 1971; ZÜLCH 1956b).

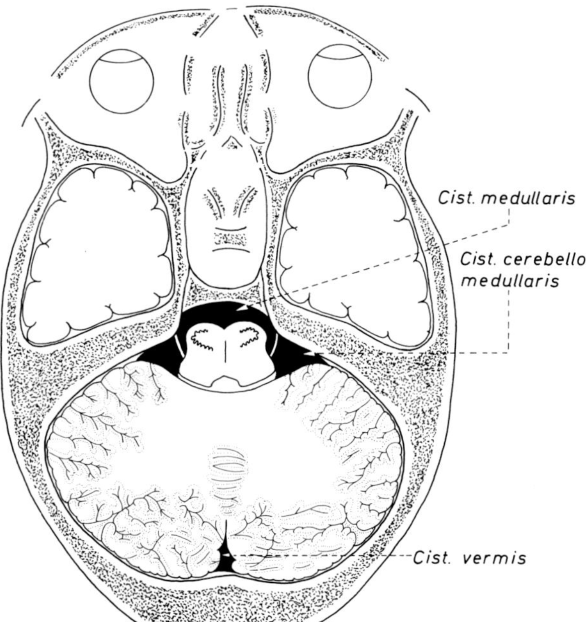

Fig. 5. The main cisterns of the brain in horizontal section
(to correspond with CT) near the base

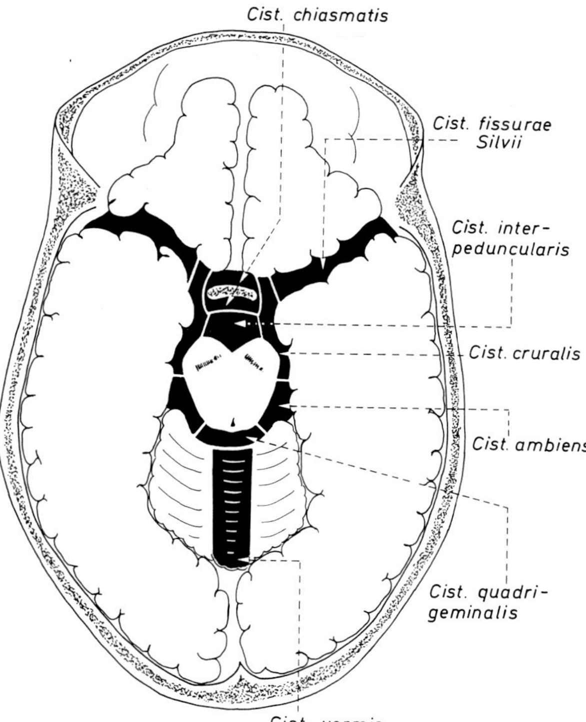

Fig. 6. Another horizontal section of the major cisterns at
a higher level than Fig. 5 (corresponds to CT)

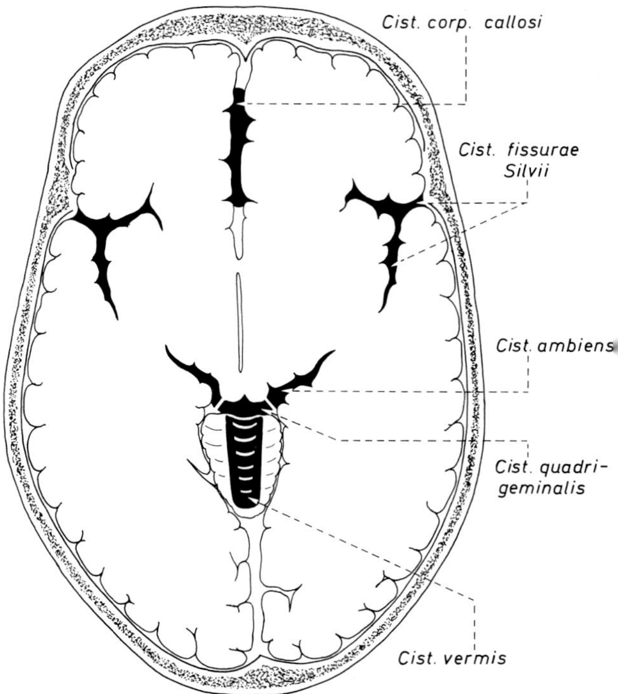

Fig. 7. Horizontal section of the cisterns above the level of
Fig. 6 (again, for comparison with CT)

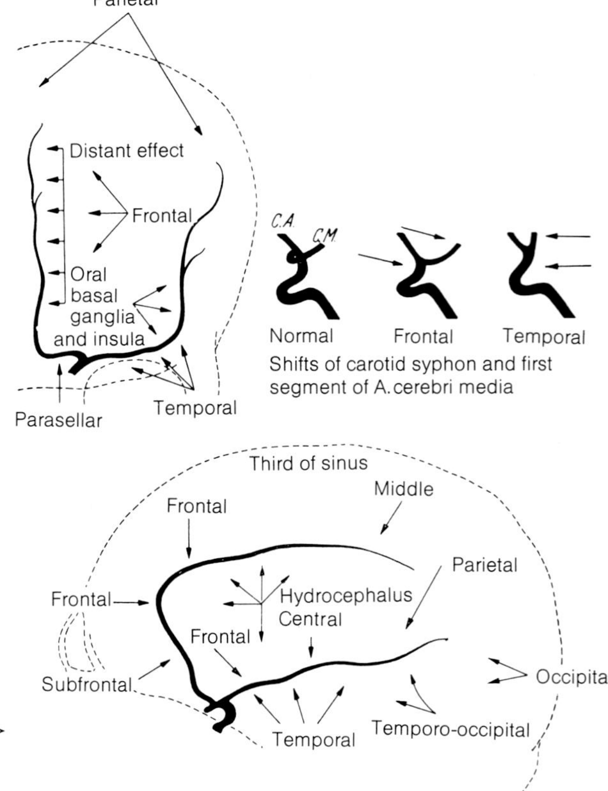

Fig. 8. Schematic representation of possible displacements ▷
of intracranial vessels due to mass-producing lesions in the
various areas

The following herniations are of significance:

a) Small hernias consisting of one or both *gyri recti* can be forced into the prechiasmatic portion of the chiasmatic cistern (frontobasilar tumors, hydrocephalic states) (Fig. 6).

b) The *uncus* of the *hippocampus* and neighboring tissues can be displaced laterally into the anterior portion of the crural cistern (temporal and parietal tumors). This leads to development of *anterior transtentorial (temporal) herniations* (Figs. 5, 6, 167, 168, 173).

c) Portions of the hippocampal gyrus and medial occipital cortex can be shifted into the posterior portion of the crural and ambient cisterns (temporal and parietal tumors). This leads to development of the so-called *posterior transtentorial (temporal) herniation*. In this manner the midbrain is displaced laterally and deformed and the aqueduct occluded resulting in a secondary hydrocephalus (Fig. 3).

d) The hippocampal uncus plus the hippocampal gyrus and the medial occipital cortex as a unit can also be displaced into the entire *interpeduncular* and *ambient cisterns* leading to a "total" temporal or transtentorial pressure cone (see pp. 10, 11, "herniation syndromes").

e) Anterior – seldom anterior *and* posterior – portions of the medial surface of the frontal and parietal lobes, especially the *gyrus cinguli*,

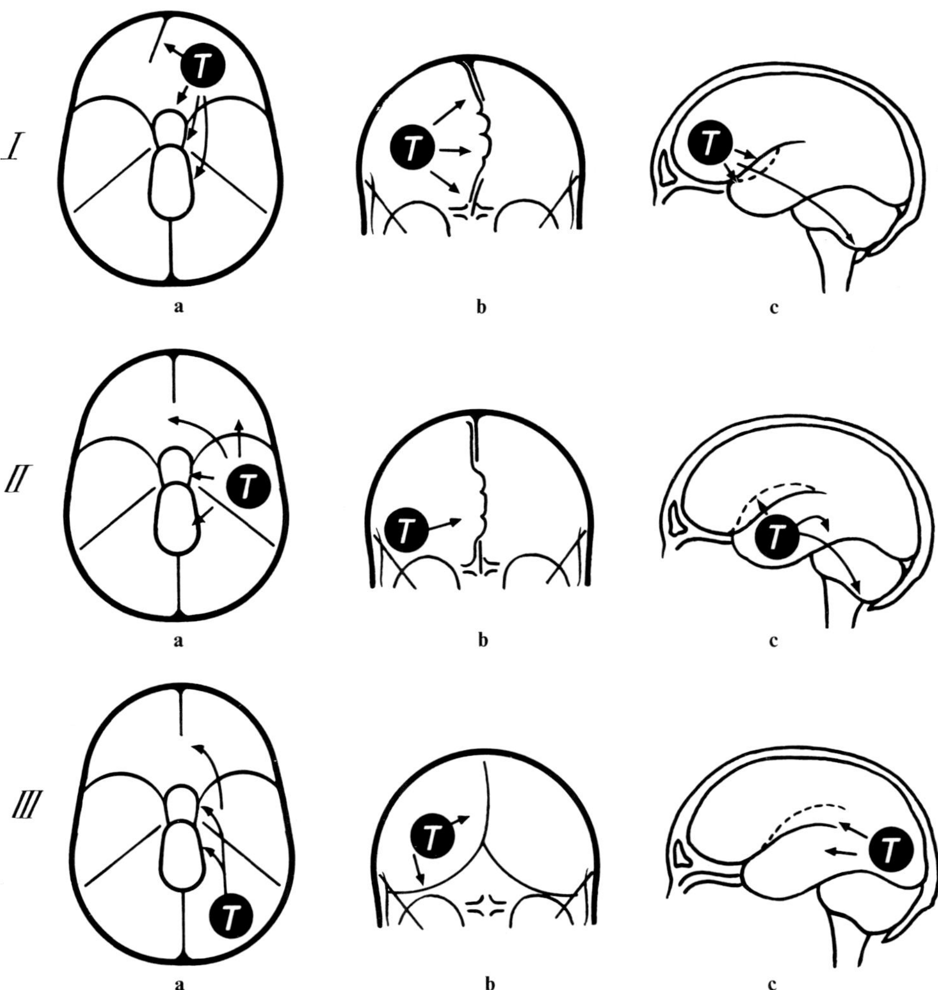

Fig. 9. Diagram of the important mass displacements caused by (*I*) frontal, (*II*) temporal, and (*III*) occipital tumors. (*I*) The mass effect of the frontal tumor displaces the falx obliquely, causes herniation of brain tissue over the sphenoid wing against the temporal lobe, and exerts pressure against the brain stem in an "axial" direction. (*II*) The temporal tumor causes herniations anteriorly toward the frontal lobe and elevates the Sylvian fissure. The uncus is forced medially and inferiorly into the tentorial hiatus. Note that the falx is not affected by tumors in this area. (*III*) The occipital tumor, surrounded by rigid dural sheets forming a cone-shaped enclosure, can only displace tissue anteriorly in the direction of the open end of the cone until a point is reached where lateral displacements can take place. Elevation of the posterior Sylvian fissure is also seen here

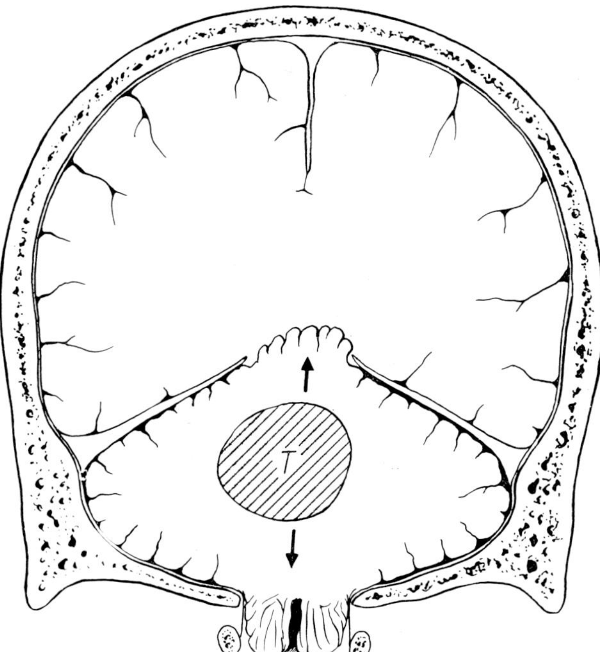

Fig. 10. Semischematic model showing mass displacement by a tumor in the posterior cranial fossa. Note the upward herniation through the tentorial hiatus and the downward herniation into the foramen magnum (cerebellar or tonsillar pressure cone)

are displaced with the adjacent corpus callosum under the falx to the opposite side in response to space-occupying processes (Figs. 3, 9/I + II). Of necessity, these herniations cause displacement of the anterior cerebral and callosomarginal arteries as well.

f) Space-occupying processes in the posterior cranial fossa can lead to an *upward herniation* of the anterior lobe of the cerebellum through the tentorial hiatus (upward cerebellar pressure cone). The midbrain is secondarily distorted and pushed forward and may even be displaced laterally, depending on the location of the space-occupying lesion (Fig. 10).

g) Also in response to a space-occupying process in the posterior cranial fossa, *tonsillar herniations* into the foramen magnum occur whereby compression of the medulla oblongata takes place (see also p. 11, "herniation syndromes"). Such tonsillar herniations are frequently asymmetrical.

Similar *tonsillar pressure cones* are frequently seen in *supra*tentorial mass-producing lesions, especially if they are situated close to the midline or within the *frontal lobes* or *basal ganglia* (Fig. 9/I). Such processes can cause a

marked "axial" displacement in the direction of the posterior cranial fossa.

h) Laterally situated cerebellopontine angle masses may occasionally cause cerebellar herniation into the *contralateral* cerebellopontine angle.

i) *Axial* displacements of the lower brain stem in either direction (upward or downward) are not sufficiently understood to explain their effect on the exiting *cranial nerves*. Space-occupying processes originating in the *supratentorial* compartments are known to crush the *third nerve* against the petroclinoid ligament with ipsilateral pupillary dilation. In generalized cerebral edema seen after sinus occlusions (particularly of the *right* transverse sinus) uni- or bilateral dysfunction of the *sixth nerves* often occurs. Paradoxically, the same effect on the sixth nerves may be seen in tumors of the posterior cranial fossa in children. The pathophysiology of this effect is not understood (see ZÜLCH 1964).

The various types of herniation just described may have dire consequences. In the first place, distortions of the CSF pathways can cause secondary occlusive hydrocephalus, particularly at the levels of the aqueduct of Sylvius (tentorial hiatus) and foramen of Magendie (foramen magnum). As a result of the developing hydrocephalus, a new mass-producing process begins, which will be discussed later.

A second consequence of mass displacements is seen in axial herniations through the tentorial hiatus (involving the *midbrain*), or through the foramen magnum (involving the *medulla oblongata*). Both areas of the brain stem contain vital centers which are easily damaged by the compressing and distorting effects of the herniated tissues. Damage to these vital brain stem centers can be life-threatening, a situation which makes clinical recognition of an evolving herniation syndrome essential (Figs. 3, 9, 10). The recognition of early herniations by means of angiography and pneumoencephalography, even before clinical symptoms develop, is therefore a most important diagnostic finding (see pp. 109 ff and 241 ff) (ZÜLCH 1950; PIA 1954; ECKER 1948; AZAMBUJA et al. 1956 a–d).

A third consequence of axial herniations occurs when the major brain stem arteries are so compressed and distorted as to produce a hemorrhagic infarct in their area of distribution – as, for example, occipital lobe infarcts due to strangulation of the posterior cerebral artery at the level of the tentorial hiatus with homonymous hemianopsia (see RIESSNER and ZÜLCH 1939). This occurs when the posterior cerebral artery within the tentorial hiatus is displaced medially and in a downward direction with the resultant traction acutely angulating the artery against the free edge of the tentorium.

The three major contributing arteries to the cerebral hemispheres proceed in three large cisternal systems: the anterior cerebral artery in the chiasmatic cistern and in the cisterns of the lamina terminalis and corpus callosum; the middle cerebral artery in the cistern of the Sylvian fissure; and the posterior cerebral artery in the interpeduncular, crural, and ambient cisterns.

Although hemorrhages also occur in the cerebellum and midbrain secondary to *axial herniations,* the diagnostic capacity of vertebrobasilar angiography is usually not sufficient to permit recognition of these prior to autopsy. However, if they are fairly large, they may be visualized on computed tomograms.

3. Development of Occlusive Hydrocephalus

The intracranial mass displacements described above have a profound effect upon the CSF pathways. It is well recognized that the major producer of CSF is the choroid plexus of the lateral ventricles, although additional contributions are made by the plexus in the 3rd and 4th ventricles. From each lateral ventricle the CSF flows through the foramina of Monro to the third ventricle, and then through the aqueduct to the fourth ventricle. From the fourth ventricle the CSF empties through the foramina of Luschka into both lateral recesses and through the foramen of Magendie into the cisterna magna and pontocerebellar cisterns. From the cisterna magna flow continues by way of the cisternal systems to the convexities, from whence it is reabsorbed by the arachnoidal granulations (Fig. 11). Although an additional quantity of CSF is probably formed from the vessels lying close to the ependymal and cortical surfaces, these contributions are of minor significance.

It is generally accepted that most of the CSF is reabsorbed by means of the arachnoid granulations. However, additional reabsorption takes place along the entire subarachnoid space and through the ventricular walls. That this is so is demonstrated by the absence of the arach-

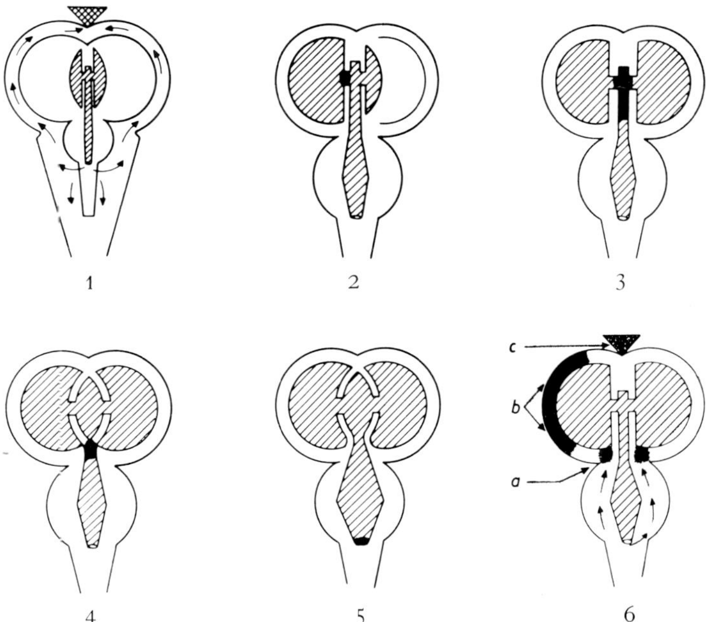

Fig. 11. The various forms of occlusive hydrocephalus and the typical sites for obstruction. *1,* schematic demonstration of the normal CSF circulation; *2,* unilateral obstruction of the foramen of Monro with asymmetrical hydrocephalus; *3,* bilateral obstruction of the foramina of Monro at the level of the third ventricle producing symmetrical hydrocephalus of both lateral ventricles; *4,* obstruction at the level of the aqueduct producing hydrocephalus of the lateral and third ventricles; *5,* obstruction at the level of the foramen of Magendie producing proximal hydrocephalus of all four ventricles; *6,* obstruction of the subarachnoid spaces at midbrain level and over the cerebral convexity. The latter is also called "communicating hydrocephalus." *a,* ambient cisterns; *b,* Sylvian fissure and subarachnoid spaces of the convexity; *c,* pacchionian granulations and sagittal sinus

1) At the trigone:	Tumors, such as the intraventricular plexus meningiomas
2) At the foramen of Monro, unilateral:	Ependymoma of the lateral ventricle

3) At the foramen of Monro, bilateral (Fig. 12)

a) The anterior group of third ventricular tumors	i) Ependymal or colloid cysts, choroid plexus papillomas, epidermoids ii) Meningiomas, gliomas of the septum pellucidum
b) The basal group of third ventricular tumors	i) Intraventricular craniopharyngiomas, large midline extraventricular craniopharyngiomas or pituitary adenomas pushing upwards, large pilocytic astrocytomas in the hypothalamus or chiasmatic area, gangliocytomas (rare), ii) CSF metastases
4) At the aqueduct (posterior group of third ventricular tumors)	i) Pineocytomas, germinomas, and other pineal cell tumors; teratomas ependymomas ependymal or arachnoid cysts (rare) ii) Gliomas of the quadrigeminal plate iii) Primary aqueductal stenosis (through scarring, congenital maldevelopment, or gliomas)
5) Tumors within or adjacent to the fourth ventricle	i) Pilocytic astrocytomas of the vermis and floor of the fourth ventricle medulloblastomas ependymomas choroid plexus papillomas hemangioblastomas (Lindau) ii) Extracerebral processes of the posterior cranial fossa as neurilemmomas, meningiomas, epidermoids, glomus tumors, chrondromas, etc.

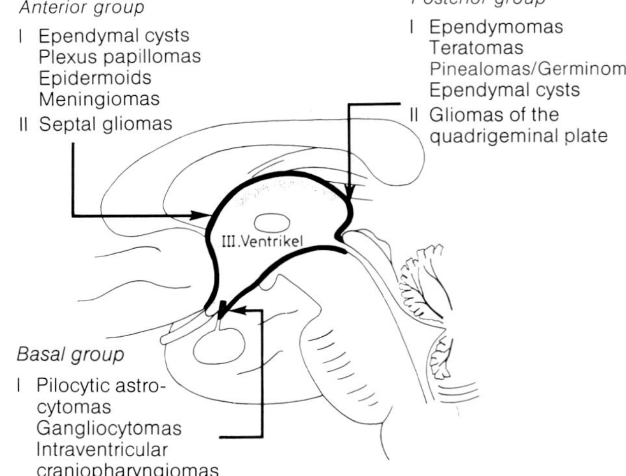

Fig. 12. Tumors of the third ventricle, divided according to their localization – anterior, posterior, and basal groups

noid granulations in newborn infants, in whom they are not yet developed, yet the accompanying hydrocephalus is usually mild and of no clinical significance.

Regardless of the precise manner of reabsorption of the CSF, which is still debated, of greater significance to the present discussion is the fact that obstructions to the flow of spinal fluid from the ventricular system to its major point of reabsorption – the subarachnoid space over the cerebral convexities – can occur through mass displacements and can in turn be mass-producing when hydrocephalus ensues. This situation may also result from scarring within the ventricular system itself as long as the isolated portion of the ventricular system itself contains the choroid plexus. Depending on the site of obstruction, the hydrocephalus may be quite asymmetrical (Fig. 11). For example, a mass which causes obstruction at the level of the trigone of the lateral ventricle leads to hydrocephalus of the temporal and posterior horns, while an occlusion at the level of the foramen of Monro will lead to hydrocephalic enlargement of the entire lateral ventricle. When the occlusion is in the midline, however, the hydrocephalus becomes symmetrical. Occlusions of both foramina of Monro will lead to hydrocephalic enlargement of both lateral ventricles, while an occlusion at the level of the aqueduct will include the third ventricle as well. When the foramina of Magendie and Luschka are obstructed, the resultant hydrocephalus will also involve the fourth ventricle (Fig. 11).

Additional sites of obstruction to the flow of spinal fluid can occur outside the ventricular system within the subarachnoid spaces, thus blocking the progress of the spinal fluid to its ultimate point of reabsorption in the arachnoid granulations. Especially typical of this condition is the obliteration of the cisternal ring around the midbrain seen as a side effect of basilar meningitis, particularly the heavy scarring which may follow medically treated tuberculous meningitis. Meningitis of other types, as well as subarachnoid bleeding, can also cause obliteration of the subarachnoid pathways (Fig. 11).

The hydrocephalus resulting from obstruction outside the ventricular system has been designated nonobstructive or "communicating" hydrocephalus, in contrast to the "obstructive" type caused by a block within the ventricular system proper. Logically, however, both conditions should be considered obstructive in etiology.

Consideration will now be given to a comparison of the various sites of obstruction with the major tumor "groups" or other processes causing them (Fig. 12).

If an obstructive process occurs *within* the ventricular system, or immediately adjacent to it, the resultant obstructive hydrocephalus may be quite intense, much more so than that caused by obstructions which occur *outside the ventricular system* itself. Acoustic neurilemmomas of the cerebellopontine angle, for instance, cause a less intense degree of hydrocephalus; however, even remote space-occupying processes may cause a significant degree of secondary hydro-

cephalus when mass herniations of brain tissue distort and obstruct the ventricular pathways at the level of the aqueduct or foramen of Magendie.

One or both of the foramina of Monro can become occluded when a mass in the cerebral hemisphere of sufficient size (glioblastoma, metastasis, abscess with significant brain edema) causes herniation beneath the falx and distortion of the contralateral hemisphere. In this fashion, spinal fluid accumulates proximal to the foramina of Monro, resulting in symmetrical enlargement of the lateral ventricles. In fact, however, the ipsilateral ventricle is frequently incapable of expansion due to adjacent tumor pressure. Consequently, only the contralateral ventricle may enlarge, and its enlargement may only be moderate since the obstruction is usually not complete. Nonetheless, whatever degree of hydrocephalus develops, the addition of a new space-occupying process in the supratentorial compartment causes further increase in intracranial pressure with further mass herniations, particularly in the axial direction, with considerable danger of a herniation syndrome developing.

4. Significance of Site and Type of Space-Occupying Lesions on the Type of Intracranial Mass Displacement

The type and size of a mass displacement depend to a great extent on the site of the space-occupying process. There are three major sites to be considered in this regard:

a) Those involving the *cerebral hemispheres,* which are further subdivided into *midline* (median) lesions (located directly in the path of the midline ventricular system between the foramina of Monro and Magendie) and the *paramedian* processes which lie directly adjacent to the *ventricular system,*

b) The paramedian tumors of the *thalamus and basal ganglia,*

c) Other lesions in or close to the midline which may cause obstruction to the flow of spinal fluid.

In the first group mass displacements occur during the evolution of a space-occupying process in the manner described earlier. In the third group there is a rapid development of a hydrocephalic state which then dominates the entire picture. The second group occupies a middle position between both. In some the mass effect is more significant, while in others the hydrocephalus appears most significant.

The type of space-occupying lesion can also influence the subsequent mass displacement. Whether a tumor is *rapidly* growing or *slow* growing and whether it is *infiltrating* or *displacing* tissue can be quite significant. An infiltrating tumor, for instance, takes up less space than a tumor which displaces tissue. However, in the malignant infiltrating type of glioma, which also causes tissue destruction, this advantage is far outweighed by the magnitude of associated cerebral edema. On the other hand, a slow growing meningioma which displaces tissue may give the brain more time to adjust and adapt itself than a faster growing infiltrating tumor with its associated cerebral edema (intracellular and extracellular). Thus, many "malignant" processes (such as glioblastomas and metastases, as well as some abscesses) are especially prone to further development of a considerable mass effect and rapid increase in intracranial pressure.

a) The Hemispheric Processes

Frontal Tumors

In space-occupying processes of the frontal lobe, mass displacements take place in a lateral direction under the anterior edge of the falx toward the opposite side (Fig. 9/I). Moreover, the anterior free ridge of the falx can itself yield

to the pressure of large tumors which are immediately adjacent to it, especially if the tumor is slow growing. This displacement is of necessity diagonal since one end of the falx always remains attached to the skull. In a similar fashion portions of the frontal lobe and blood vessels immediately adjacent to the falx are also displaced over the midline to the opposite side, in contrast with more remotely situated tumors in which the anterior free edge of the falx and its associated structures are both midline (Fig. 13). This type of displacement is characterized radiologically as a "near" sign. These will be considered in greater detail later (see p. 108 ff and Fig. 9/I b, II b). As noted this sign is usually seen only in slow growing tumor processes, but may also occur acutely in massive space-occupying lesions (such as complete infarction in the distribution of the anterior and middle cerebral arteries).

In addition to subfalceal herniations in frontal mass lesions, the basal parts of the frontal lobe may be displaced posteriorly and inferiorly over the sphenoid wing into the *middle* cranial fossa, displacing the "sphenoid portion" of the middle cerebral artery in a posterior inferior direction (for angiographic changes see p. 108 and Fig. 60).

Because of its closeness to the "central axis" of the brain, the frontal lobe tumor is especially prone to "axial" herniations affecting the posterior cranial fossa (Fig. 9/I c). This explains the sudden and frequent development of a tonsillar pressure cone in frontal lobe processes, an observation which was made earlier.

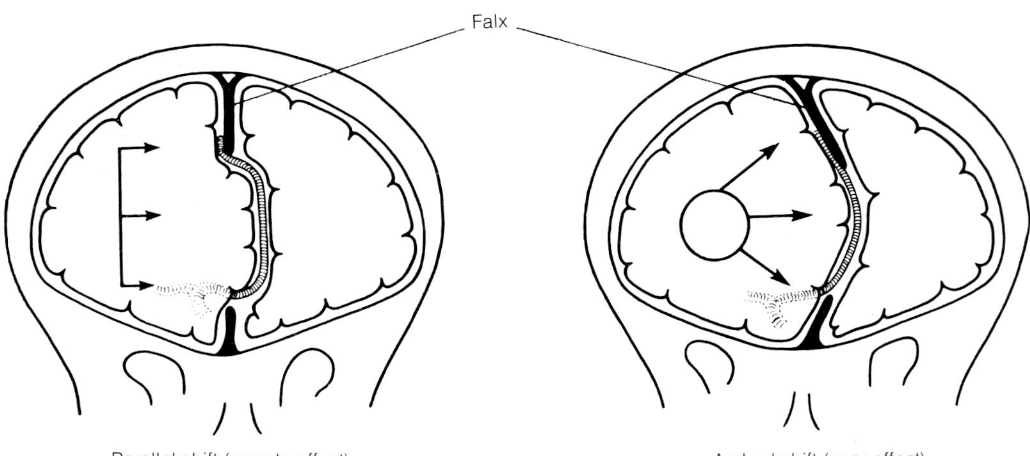

Fig. 13. The various lateral displacements of the frontal lobe, depending upon tumor position ("near" lobe (right) and "far" (left) signs)

Parietal Tumors

Parietal space-occupying processes cause displacement of the cerebral gyri above the corpus callosum initially in an anterior direction and produce more of an anterior subfalceal herniation (Fig. 4). The reason for this is that despite the relatively posterior placement of the tumor, the adjacent posterior edge of the falx is so close to the splenium of the corpus callosum that herniation here meets with greater resistance than the described alternative. It is very characteristic of parietal space-occupying process that the medial portion of the temporal lobe herniates through the tentorial hiatus into the crural and ambient cisterns and produces a "temporal" pressure cone similar to that produced by temporal tumors (see p. 6 and Fig. 3). Infrequently, the described herniation is incomplete and involves both compartments so that it cannot be characterized as belonging to either the anterior or posterior types (see p. 10).

Temporal Tumors

In space-occupying lesions within the temporal lobe the resultant mass displacement causes herniations in an upward and anterior direction as well as laterally to the opposite side (Fig. 9/II). Because of this the entire Sylvian fissure, including its resident vessels, is displaced upward and anteriorly against the frontal lobe (Fig. 9/IIa, c). Simultaneously the cerebral tissues lying adjacent to the third ventricle, including the "internal cerebral veins", are also shifted laterally and to a greater degree than the more distally situated frontal horn and septum pellucidum, which are only involved later (see Fig. 14 and p. 222ff). Comparison of the relative displacement of the septum versus the third ventricle on anteroposterior air studies is of particular significance in this regard (Fig. 14).

As a consequence of these lateral displacements, both foramina of Monro may be constricted by the mass of the thalamus, while the aqueduct is distorted and compressed by the temporal pressure cone. This results in obstruction of the flow of the spinal fluid with contralateral hydrocephalus – contralateral because the ipsilateral ventricle is already compressed by the expanding temporal mass.

It is also characteristic of displacements in temporal tumors that the corpus callosum is

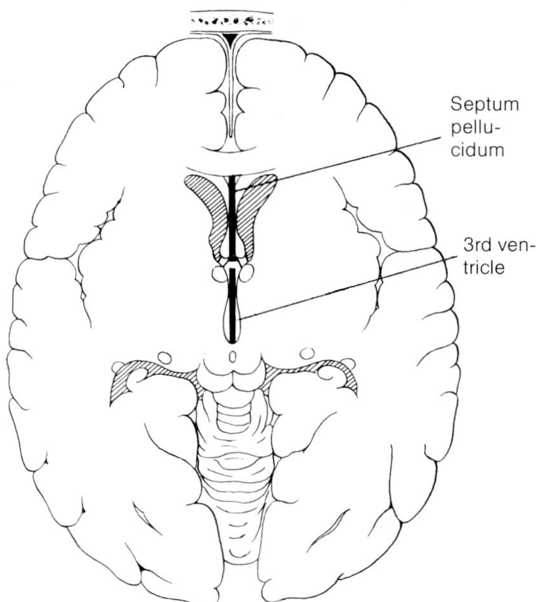

Fig. 14. Schematic representation of the respective midline positions of the septum pellucidum and the third ventricle in line with one another on this horizontal brain section. In the anteroposterior view of the pneumoencephalogram they are also normally in a midline position, one on top of the other. Because mass-producing lesions rarely affect both of them in a similar manner, varying "dissociations" of these structures on the pneumoencephalogram can be used to localize frontal, temporal, or parietal tumors

not depressed but remains almost horizontal (Fig. 15). This permits the distinction to be made between temporal tumors and the previously described frontal and parietal lobe tumors. As has been noted, the more anteriorly and superiorly lying tumors lead to an "anterior" type (uncal) herniation into the interpeduncular cistern. In the more posteriorly and superiorly situated tumors the herniation is more "posterior" into the crural and ambient cisterns. Tumors of enormous size may cause a combined frontal and posterior herniation. In frontal herniations the cerebral peduncle alone is displaced, while in posterior herniations the cerebral peduncle and quadrigeminal plate are both displaced laterally, inferiorly, and posteriorly. In this type of herniation the posterior communicating and posterior cerebral arteries, which lie within the cistern, are also displaced medially and downward by the advancing tissue mass (see p. 10). The displacements of these vessels can be seen in anteroposterior and lateral arteriograms, as well as in the anteroposterior air study (see Fig. 60 and p. 220ff).

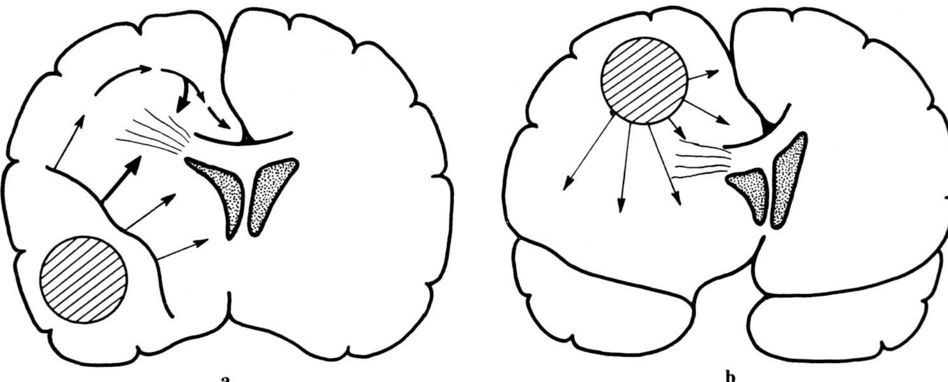

a   b

Fig. 15a, b. Variations in the displacement of the corpus callosum in temporal and frontal tumors are explained by the different pressure forces in operation. **a** In temporal tumors the forces are distributed in such a manner that the pressure on the corpus callosum from below is balanced by that from above, and the corpus callosum remains level. **b** In posterior frontal lobe tumors, the forces combine to depress the involved corpus callosum in the manner shown

Occipital Tumors

The occipital lobe lies within a cone-shaped chamber formed by the skull and the junction of two dural membranes (the falx and tentorium) which yield slightly and only to prolonged and persistent local pressure (Fig. 9/III b). In order to compensate for a space-occupying process in this area, the displaced brain tissue is forced anteriorly in the direction of the parietal and temporal lobes. At this point herniations beneath the falx to the opposite side may occur just as with lesions originating in the parietal and temporal areas. Larger occipital tumors cause anterior displacement of the trigone and occipital horn of the ventricle (Fig. 9/III c), whereas smaller lesions in this area may cause only local indentations into the horn. In common with the temporal lobe lesion, the third ventricle is displaced more laterally than the septum pellucidum (see Fig. 14 and p. 222).

b) The Paramedian, Especially Thalamic and Basal Ganglia Tumors

Tumors of the Basal Ganglia

Space-occupying processes in these deep nuclei (especially in the thalamus) are an intermediate group between the aforementioned cerebral hemisphere lesions and those lesions which block the midline ventricular pathways (to be considered later). The distended thalamus pushes laterally and superiorly against the trigone and causes it to arch like a bow. It also displaces the corpus callosum superiorly and pushes the third ventricle medially and to the opposite side in such a fashion that the ventricle forms a shell around the tumor. As a result of the displacement and distortion of the third ventricle and aqueduct, a secondary hydrocephalus develops involving both lateral ventricles as well as the anterior third ventricle.

Tumors of the Lateral Ventricles

Tumors of the lateral ventricles are in a special category. They may enlarge for considerable periods of time within the ventricular system and cause obstruction to spinal fluid pathways only when they distort and displace the third ventricle or aqueduct – as in tumors of the trigone and temporal horn – or when they obstruct the foramen of Monro (Fig. 11), as in frontal horn tumors. In either event a partial or total, but usually asymmetrical, hydrocephalus follows (see p. 231 ff).

c) Obstructions to the Ventricular Fluid Pathways in or Near the Midline

Locally situated primary obstructions to the flow of spinal fluid occurring between the foramen of Monro and the foramen of Magendie (see p. 233 ff) lead to a symmetrical hydrocephalus of the proximal ventricles (Fig. 11). Initially the obstruction may be only "partial" or "valve-like" which permits development of the hydrocephalus over a long period of time. When, however, a *total occlusion* occurs acutely, marked ventricular enlargement can follow within a *short period* of time. In such cases the ventricles can "blow up" like a balloon, compressing the overlying brain and emptying the subarachnoid spaces. Removal of the obstruction will often lead to a rapid resumption of the normal ventricular shape and size as well as a reopening of subarachnoid spaces – a tribute to the elasticity of the cerebral tissue. This point is particularly apparent in a comparison of air studies (p. 235) done *before* and *after* removal of a lesion causing hydrocephalus. Similarly, autopsies done in the late postoperative period frequently show little evidence of the preoperative hydrocephalus.

Certain variations in the development of a symmetrical, as opposed to asymmetrical, hydrocephalic occlusion deserve special comment. As the lateral ventricles enlarge they push their "roof", namely the corpus callosum, superiorly until it is shoved against the lower edge of the falx. This occurs much earlier to the parietal splenium of the corpus callosum than to the frontal rostrum (see Fig. 4 and p. 6ff). As in the atrophic processes, the frontal horns enlarge more rapidly than the rest of the ventricular system and the corpus callosum is rapidly displaced upward. At this point the bowing of the anterior cerebral artery (particularly its pericallosal branch as seen in the lateral angiograms) follows the contour of the lower edge of the falx (Fig. 58a). As the hydrocephalus progresses, however, the lateral ventricles continue to expand and rise above the inferior edge of the falx on either side. This is clearly visible in the air study as seen from the anteroposterior view. With the ventricles moderately dilated, the angle of the corpus callosum between the frontal horns is blunt (Fig. 211). As the hydrocephalus progresses, the angle of the corpus callosum between the frontal horns becomes increasingly more acute and finally reaches zero degrees. In the course of this process, the septum pellucidum is usually torn so that in the final phases of a marked hydrocephalus there is communication between both lateral ventricles.

If the third ventricle is also involved in the hydrocephalic process, *it balloons out in an anterior and inferior direction* and forms a paperthin bubble which presses downward against the *chiasm* and *sella* like a tumor and produces a clinical syndrome appropriate to its location (chiasmatic/hypothalamic/pituitary syndrome).

When hydrocephalus develops as a result of a primary closure of the aqueduct and involves the third ventricle in its entirety, posterior expansion can occur with enlargement of the *suprapineal recess* to the size of a chestnut. It then drapes over the quadrigeminal plate into the posterior tentorial hiatus, compresses the *superior vermis* of the cerebellum, and leaves a corresponding indentation. There are also associated clinical symptoms appropriate to involvement of the quadrigeminal plate and cerebellum. With cerebellar tumors this is not possible because upward herniation of the anterior lobe (Fig. 10) prevents downward entry of the distended suprapineal recess into the tentorial hiatus.

Occasionally, a saclike outpocketing of arachnoid occurs in the pineal region having the characteristics of an open arachnoidal cyst. This compresses the quadrigeminal plate in a manner similar to a mass lesion. Such cysts can be seen in children in the longstanding hydrocephalus of aqueductal stenosis and are caused by perforation of the ventricular wall in the region of the medial trigone with cyst formation.

Obstructions in the Third Ventricle

Space-occupying processes primary to the *anterior* third ventricle cause blockage of the foramina of Monro. Such occlusions are most typically caused by a cherry-sized ependymal (colloid) cyst which is situated between both foramina of Monro and beneath the fornix (Fig. 11). Actual tumors occurring in this region tend to be larger than the cysts and tend to distort the shape of the third ventricle more (see p. 235ff). Distinction is made between three large groups of tumors of the third ventricle: anterior, posterior, and basal (see Fig. 12, pp. 237, 238). Large growing tumors originating beneath the third ventricle and above the sella turcica constitute the "basal" group and can secondarily block the foramen of Monro. The major tumors in this group are pituitary adenomas and craniopharyngiomas which often break into the third ventricle from below where they continue to grow. Individual craniopharyngiomas may sometimes originate within the lumen of of the third ventricle, which tends to persist as a narrow CSF pathway along the upper rim of its earlier location. A similar picture is seen with all extracerebral tumors of the sella region when they break into the third ventricle. Tumors of the third ventricle bend the internal cerebral vein upward and out and, when they are sufficiently enlarged, may even displace the basal vein of Rosenthal out and downward. Basal third ventricular tumors rising from the vicinity of the sella tend to elevate the horizontal A-1 segment of the anterior cerebral artery (Fig. 52), which permits them to be clearly distinguished from those tumors which originate within the third ventricle.

Occlusions of the Aqueduct

Tumors of the midbrain tectum, for example, pineal or posterior third ventricular tumors, compress and obstruct the aqueduct (see pp. 11, 12, 238). These can be grouped together as "quadrigeminal plate tumors" because practically all affect this structure in a similar fashion and all cause "secondary" occlusion of the aqueduct. They displace the vein of Galen upward (or laterally and upward) and the basilar artery anteriorly against the clivus, which is apparent on the arteriogram. "Quadrigeminal plate tumors" also displace the pineal depending on the point of maximal effect of the space-occupying process. Because it is usually calcified, the pineal may be seen on the plain films.

"Primary" aqueductal stenosis, however, causes mostly obstruction of the spinal fluid pathways without a significant local mass effect (Fig. 11). Small tumors, ependymal membranes, and inflammatory scars can all lead to primary aqueductal stenosis. Unfortunately, the location and shape of the blockage on the ventriculogram, in our experience, does not give definite information about the obstructing process. As a generalization, the club-shaped aqueductal closure tends to be caused more frequently by membrane formation, while closures which are cone-shaped tend rather to be inflammatory or neoplastic in origin.

Occlusions Within the Fourth Ventricle at the Foramen of Magendie or in the Lateral Recesses

All space-occupying processes in the posterior cranial fossa lead sooner or later to occlusions of the spinal fluid pathways and cause considerable enlargement of the third and lateral ventricles. It is characteristic for all space-occupying processes of the posterior cranial fossa to cause distortion of the aqueduct. This can vary from either a simple posterior displacement to a typical "kinked" deformity. When the space-occu-

pying process originates in the upper vermis, the anterior lobe of the cerebellum will herniate upward through the tentorial hiatus and compress the midbrain aqueduct causing the most marked "kinking" effect. In contrast, tumors lying in the posterior portion of the fourth ventricle cause only a moderate distortion of the aqueduct. The rule of thumb is as follows: the closer the space-occupying process is to the tentorium, the greater the bend in the aqueduct. Similarly, the nearer the space-occupying process is to the foramen of Magendie, the softer will be the bend in the aqueduct. The aqueduct is also subject to distortion and occlusion shortly after the bend occurs in tumors of the vermis (pilocytic astrocytoma, medulloblastoma), while in tumors of the posterior portion of the fourth ventricle (ependymoma) the anterior portion of the fourth ventricle is still tumor-free and will therefore develop a hydrocephalic enlargement along with the third and lateral ventricles. The more lateral the space-occupying lesion lies, the less will be the bend in the aqueduct and the better the anterior portion of the fourth ventricle will be visualized. In this case, the pressure against the midbrain and aqueduct is effected primarily in an angular direction. Thus the aqueduct and fourth ventricle are displaced to the opposite side by these various situations, which is readily apparent on the ventriculogram. Tumors of the "lateral" recess of the posterior cranial fossa will cause greater posterior displacement of the ipsilateral tonsil than the opposite tonsil. This is known as the "tonsillar" sign and is apparent both at surgery and on the pneumoencephalogram.

Pontine tumors displace the aqueduct uniformly in a posterior direction and convert the fourth ventricle into a narrow plate. The aqueduct thus displaced forms a gentle, arching curve. The posterior portion of the third ventricle is also occasionally displaced somewhat superiorly and forward. It is possible to distinguish extrapontine tumors of the clivus from intrapontine tumors by the position of the basilar artery in the pontine cistern on the pneumoencephalogram: the artery is either displaced away from the clivus or pressed against it. In all other space-occupying lesions of the posterior cranial fossa of significant size, the basilar artery is pressed against the clivus.

As a consequence of herniation of the cerebellum through the tentorial hiatus in the "upward direction", the posterior cerebral and/or superior cerebellar arteries are, under certain conditions, trapped and displaced superiorly. In the posterior direction tonsillar herniation results in the familiar cerebellar pressure cone which often pushes the posterior inferior cerebellar artery into the cisterna magna and even into the spinal canal, a situation which is readily apparent on the lateral vertebral arteriograms.

When the mass lesion lies in the *cerebello-pontine angle,* distortion of the aqueduct and fourth ventricles through basolaterally applied pressure is only moderate. Also the occlusion is usually incomplete although the neighboring vessels in this area, namely the basilar, superior cerebellar, and anterior inferior cerebellar arteries, are frequently displaced (Fig. 63) and the pontocerebellar cistern filled (see p. 241).

A summary of the major influences of space-occupying processes on individual segments of the intracranial arteries can be seen in Fig. 8.

III. Mass Displacements by Atrophic Processes

The cerebral atrophic processes comprise all of those disease processes which cause loss of brain substance. Only occasionally can radiographic techniques utilizing contrast media demonstrate the manner in which the loss of tissue has occurred. Tissue loss from trauma, from primary vascular disturbances (mostly arteriosclerotic narrowing or thrombosis), as well as from inflammatory processes all have a similar radiological appearance in their later stages. The predilection for site and the manner of extension of damaged areas may, however, give some hint as to the pathological process occurring (Fig. 16, p. 252ff). These processes also tend to pass through a variety of phases. Many begin with a space-occupying effect caused by extracellular or intracellular edema, hyperemia, or hemorrhage. During this phase, the rules of mass displacement in *space-occupying processes* given in the preceding chapter are in effect (see p. 6ff).

After resolution of the mass effect and after breakdown and removal of damaged tissue, there occurs a "net loss" of cerebral mass — the common denominator in all atrophic processes. The time interval between onset of damage and atrophy is usually of the order of several weeks.

As in space-occupying processes where there is a "net addition" of tissue, atrophic processes characterized by a "net loss" of tissue also require some compensatory adjustments in view of the fixed volume within the skull. This occurs through expansion of the ventricular system and subarachnoid spaces. Whether the major compensatory process is ventricular expansion or expansion of the subarachnoid spaces depends upon the type and the site of the offending process. In "open" head injuries and less commonly in "closed" head injuries, a meningocerebral cicatrix develops with adhesions between the meningeal coverings. When such adhesions occur, a loss of cerebral tissue can only be compensated for through dilation of the adjacent portion of the ventricle. It is also possible that the contracting scar can result in a local pulling on the ventricular wall. After extensive areas of brain tissue destruction have occurred, for example, after acute carotid oc-clusion, a migration of the entire ventricular system in the direction of the resolved infarct can occur in the later stages (Figs. 16, 216) regardless of whether meningocerebral cicatrix has fixed the brain surface to the dura. Another group includes those cases in which the brain tissue is not bound to the dura by a scar, as in injuries caused by forceps deliveries, by trauma in which the area of destruction does not include the arachnoid, and by less extensive local infarcts. In these cases, a cyst develops at the site of injury which may communicate widely with the cisterns. This is the rule after vessel occlusions in children in whom the cysts are called porencephalic cysts (see pp. 256, 263). Abnormalities of cellular metabolism from any cause, as for example, senile atrophy or even arteriosclerosis, lead to a generalized enlargement of the ventricular system as well as the subarachnoid spaces. Depending upon the precise disease process operative, there may be a predilection for cortical atrophy or for white matter atrophy (see p. 252ff). Tissue shrinkage which follows diffuse cerebral edema or compression from any self-limiting mass lesion will cause rather pronounced ventricular enlargement.

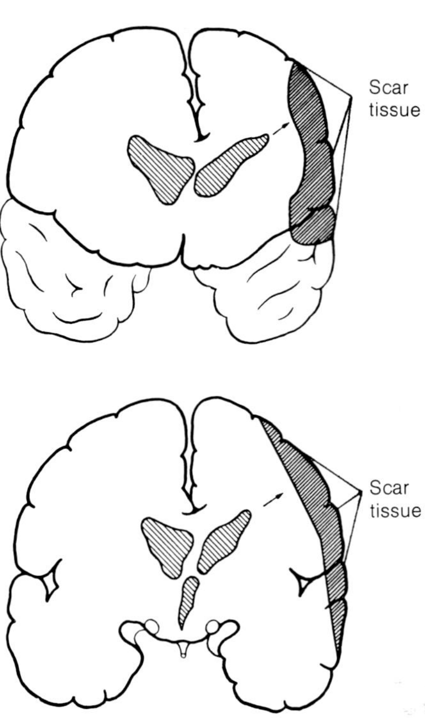

Fig. 16. Semischematic representation of brains with a diffuse cortical contusion (*shaded area*) which have undergone resolution and atrophy, leading to ventricular "migration." A similar process follows vascular occlusions with infarcts

When a space-occupying process begins to develop in a brain which has already undergone atrophic changes from another cause, the compensatory process may be so facilitated because of the enlarged subarachnoid spaces that recognition of the lesion can be significantly delayed (see p. 250). In addition, false localizing signs are commonly seen in such cases. Both factors are likely to be operative in cases where a frontal lobe tumor develops in the elderly individual. Here the diagnosis can be quite difficult.

Experiences with many cases of pathologically verified brain atrophy permit the following conclusions regarding enlargement of the CSF pathways to be drawn:

There is a rather pronounced enlargement of the ventricular system after *trauma,* most likely as a result of shrinkage of the white matter from edema damage, while the subarachnoid spaces are involved only to a lesser extent. Local changes, however, can be quite pronounced (see Figs. 218, 219). *Brain damage in infancy and early childhood* also produces a rather marked *ventricular expansion,* quite frequently with a local emphasis. This is especially true of patients with focal neurological deficit; however, when severe emotional disturbances predominate, there is a pronounced enlargement of the subarachnoid spaces in comparison to the ventricles, a condition which has been called the "cock's-comb" cortex (see Fig. 215, p. 256). In seizures of undetermined etiology there is an almost even involvement of the ventricles and the subarachnoid spaces in the hydrocephalic process. In *intoxications* and *metabolic disturbances,* white matter damage predominates secondary to the edematous process and accordingly leads to rather marked ventricular changes. *Senile* and *pre-senile* dementias affect mainly the gray matter but also the white matter to a significant extent, characteristically causing severe hydrocephalus with substantial enlargement of the subarachnoid spaces as well. Occasionally the ventricular enlargement is of lesser consequence. *Multiple sclerosis* as well as the encephalitides can also lead to enlargement of the ventricles and subarachnoid spaces. *Meningitis* during both the acute and chronic phases causes predominantly ventricular enlargement. *Vascular occlusions in later life* as opposed to those of early childhood lead to a local retraction of brain substance of considerable dimensions, which tends to manifest itself by enlargement of the adjacent ventricular chamber rather than the overlying subarachnoid space. With acute infarcts secondary to carotid occlusion, this effect can be striking. When such an infarct has occurred, the opposite hemisphere can also show atrophic changes as a result of a vascular "steal" syndrome (see pp. 166, 256ff). On the other hand, *chronic changes* caused by arteriosclerotic narrowing of a major feeding vessel affects the gray and white matter more evenly, and accordingly shows a comparatively equal involvement of the ventricles and subarachnoid spaces. Chronic alcoholism may also result in early atrophy of substantial proportions, with the subarachnoid spaces being sometimes more involved than the ventricles.

For literature, see: Azambuja et al. (1956a–d), Di Chiro (1971), Ecker (1948), Fischer (1939, 1940), Pia (1954), Riessner and Zülch (1939), Tönnis (1959), Zülch (1958, 1959, see references, 1965, 1968, 1971b, 1975), Zülch et al. (1974, see references).

B. Special Neuropathology – Morphology and Biology of the Space-Occupying and Atrophic Processes with Their Related Neuroradiological Changes

Site and expansion of the space-occupying and atrophic processes are to a certain degree type-specific. The neuroradiologist must therefore familiarize himself with the various kinds of disease processes.

I. Space-Occupying Intracranial and Spinal Processes

a) Predilections

There are sites of predilection not only for the meningiomas, which are well-known, but also for those tumors originating from the neuroectoderm – the "gliomas" in the broadest sense (see Fig. 18). This will be better demonstrated in the following paragraphs. In addition, the various tumors show a certain age preference for the onset of symptoms; many malignant and benign tumors also show a sexual preference (Fig. 17a–n). From these generalizations there is only one exception – the sarcoma. It follows no rules.

In the following, a short schematic summary of the site, shape, and pattern of spread of the most common intracranial tumors will be given as well as a review chart of the segmental distribution of the most common spinal tumors. Finally, observations on the rate of growth of the various tumor types will also be given inasmuch as this information too is of importance to the neuroradiologist. Sources for the preceding discussions are from the atlases of ZÜLCH (Springer-Verlag, 1971 b, 1975), which can also be used as sources for the following section. However, the new *World Health Organization Publication* No. 21 on the *International Histological Classification of Tumours* will be used here and should be used in the future as the standard reference source for tumor nomenclature.

b) The Classification of Brain Tumors According to the World Health Organization

This recently completed WHO study was undertaken in order to avoid misunderstandings between the involved clinical, pathological, and radiological neurospeciality groups which might result solely from differences in terminology. Neither epidemiological nor prognostic studies are relevant unless the terminology employed is equally understood by all groups. In addition to old disagreements in terminology

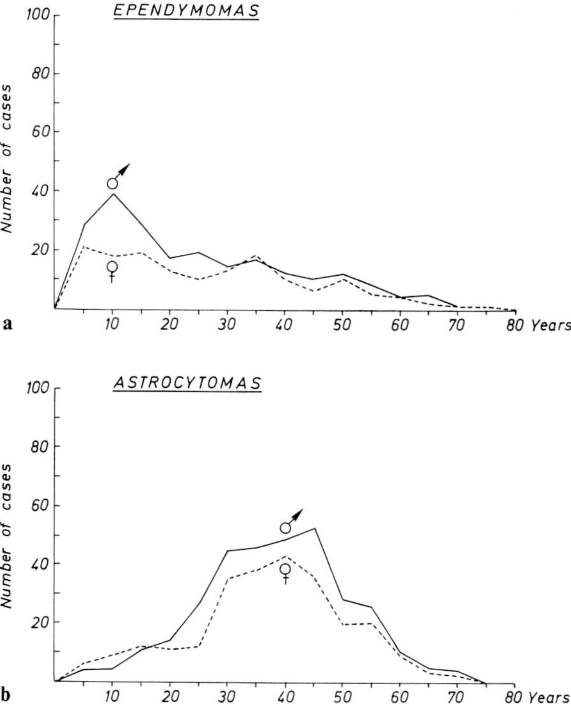

Fig. 17. **a–n** Frequency of different tumor types for the various age groups (according to sex). **n** Block diagram depicting the correlation between brain tumors of all types and patient age (according to sex)

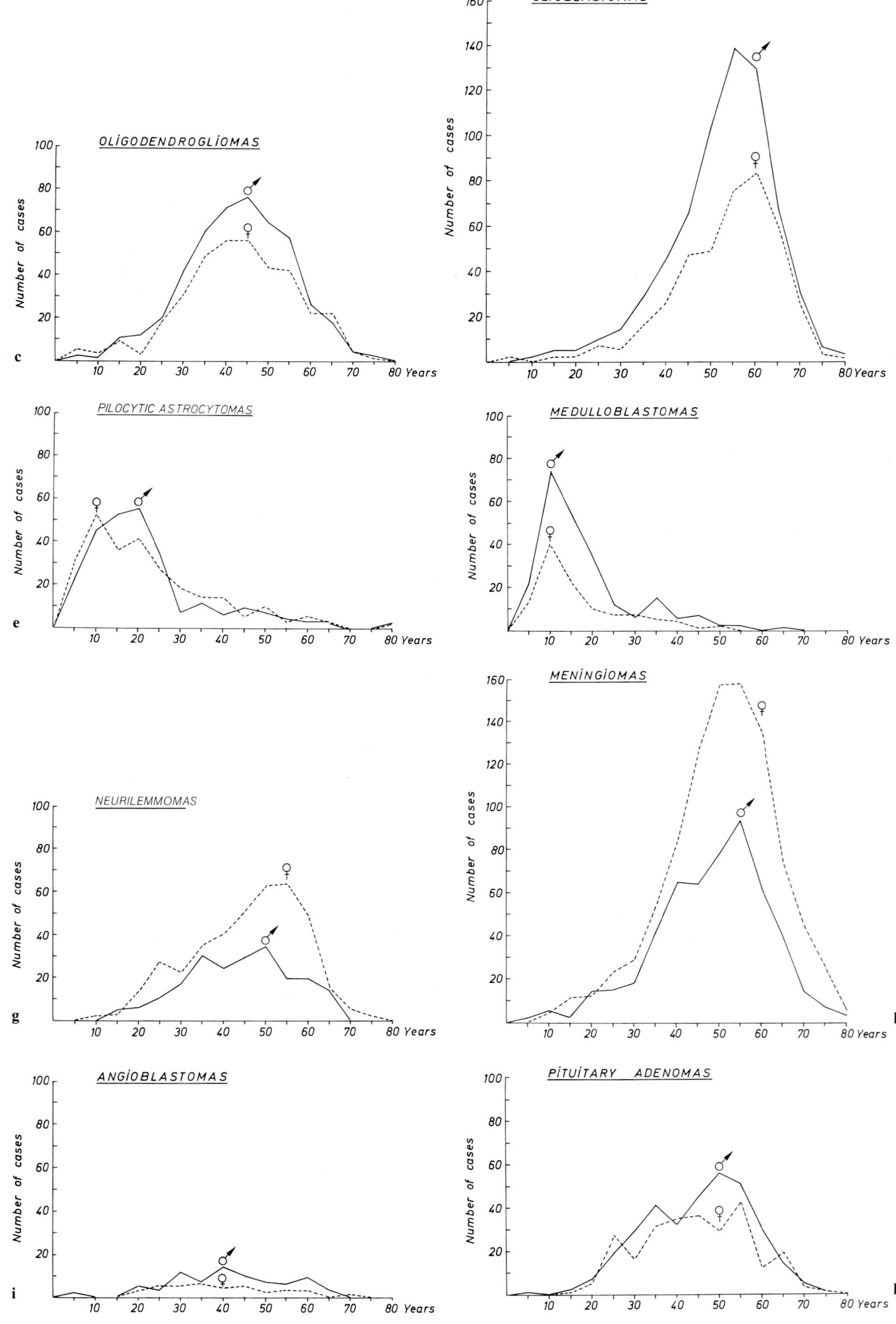

OLIGODENDROGLIOMAS
Number of cases
100
80
60
40
20
10 20 30 40 50 60 70 80 Years
c

GLIOBLASTOMAS
Number of cases
160
140
120
100
80
60
40
20
10 20 30 40 50 60 70 80 Years
d

PILOCYTIC ASTROCYTOMAS
Number of cases
100
80
60
40
20
10 20 30 40 50 60 70 80 Years
e

MEDULLOBLASTOMAS
Number of cases
100
80
60
40
20
10 20 30 40 50 60 70 80 Years
f

NEURILEMMOMAS
Number of cases
100
80
60
40
20
10 20 30 40 50 60 70 80 Years
g

MENINGIOMAS
Number of cases
160
140
120
100
80
60
40
20
10 20 30 40 50 60 70 80 Years
h

ANGIOBLASTOMAS
Number of cases
100
80
60
40
20
10 20 30 40 50 60 70 80 Years
i

PITUITARY ADENOMAS
Number of cases
100
80
60
40
20
10 20 30 40 50 60 70 80 Years
k

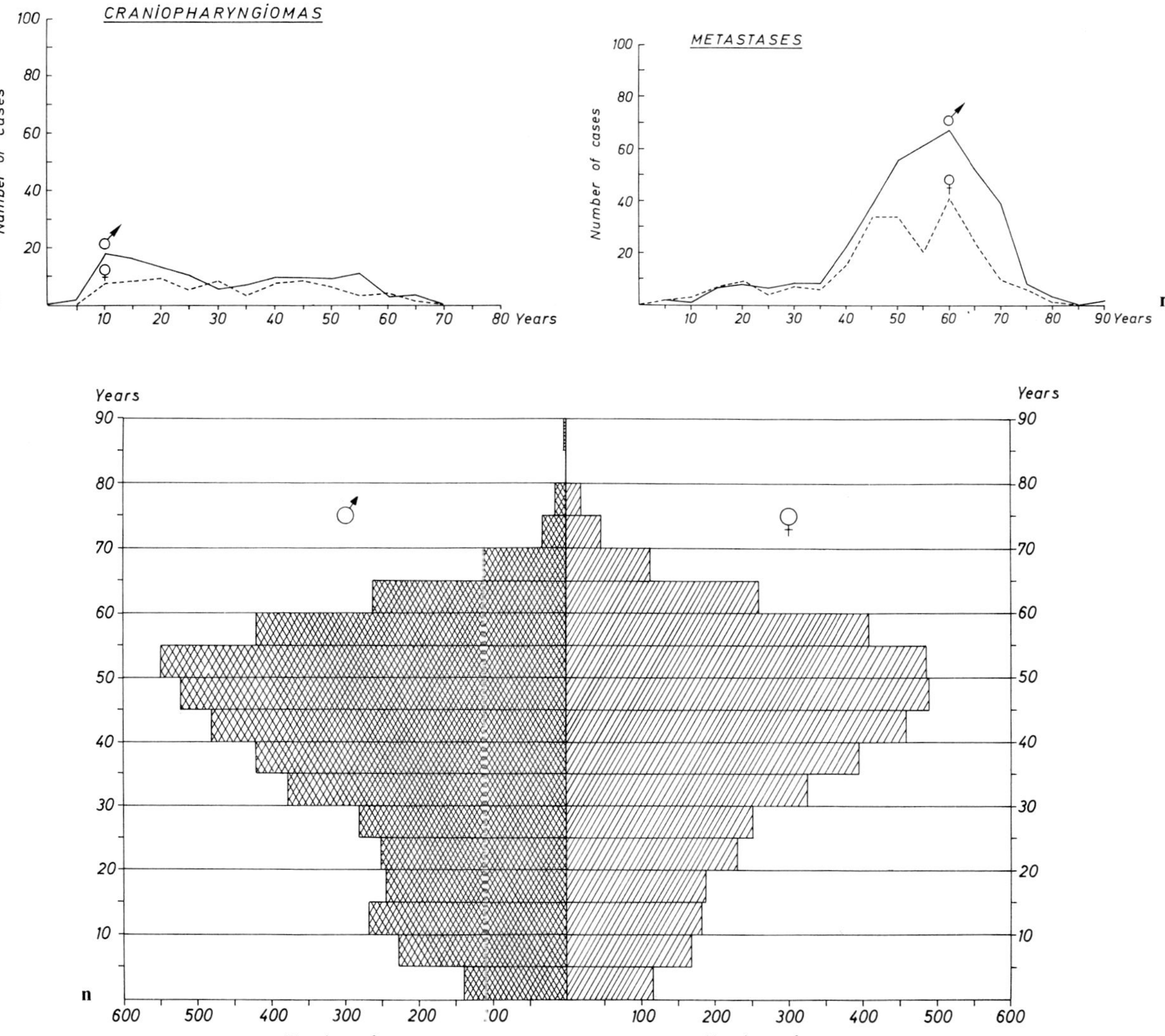

within the neuropathological ranks, new problems have arisen since the advent of computed
tomography (CT). For example, attempts have
been made to grade tumors on the basis of the
CT alone. This has led to a discrepancy between
the morphological and the CT grading of gliomas (WENDE et al. 1977).

Under the new WHO system of classification, the old pathological designation of grade I
astrocytoma has been rather severely restricted
since its most representative member – the so-
called pilocytic astrocytoma – did not usually
conform to this grading in its entirety. Consequently, the bulk of grade I astrocytomas diagnosed under the old system will actually belong
to grade II under the new WHO classification.

In previous publications we have emphasized differences in the various neuropathological nomenclatures in use (BAILEY and CUSHING
1926, 1930; PENFIELD 1931; ROUSSY and OBER-
LING 1931; DEL RIO HORTEGA 1945; KERNOHAN
et al. 1949) in the hope that a common histological classification agreeable to all parties would
eventually be adopted. It is hoped that the new
WHO classification will meet this need.

1. Tumors of Neuroepithelial Tissue

(A) Astrocytic Tumors (see Fig. 18)

Astrocytomas are subdivided into the well-
known fibrillary, protoplasmic, and gemisto-
cytic tumor subgroups. All are grade II and
have a frequency of occurrence of 7%–9%.

There is a predilection for the frontodorsal (No. 2), frontomedial (No. 12), and frontolateral (No. 9) as well as parietal regions (mostly the precentral or postcentral gyrus, No. 20). They are also found in the thalamus (No. 5), midbrain, aqueduct, pons (No. 74), and spinal cord. Most involve the cortex and are less frequently found in the white matter, where they grow diffusely and constantly infiltrate the adjacent brain (No. 47). Metastases are unknown. Astrocytomas are semibenign (grade II). Malignant degeneration of the "anaplastic" forms (grade III) – approximately 10% – leads in the direction of the glioblastomas. With the exception of these malignant types, the vascularization is otherwise slight with no pathological or large vessels. Cystic degeneration is frequent. There is no tendency to calcification and no sex preference.

The adoption of a separate subgroup to include *pilocytic astrocytoma* is new. This tumor corresponds to the older "polar spongioblastoma" of BAILEY and CUSHING (1926) and of our own former classification. However, it is separated in the WHO classification from the aforementioned three groups of astrocytomas because of its better biological behavior (grade I!). With a frequency of 7%–8%, these are benign, well-delineated gliomas with a predilection for the "midline". They are one of the two most common cerebellar tumors (Nos. 67, 68), and are also found in the hypothalamus and chiasm (No. 39), as well as in the optic tracts and rarely in an "extraventricular cerebral" location (similar in this regard to the ependymoma). They may be found in the aqueduct, quadrigeminal plate (No. 58) and also in the spinal cord as "pencil gliomas". In the cerebellar location they are cystic and rarely calcified with only minimal necrosis. They are benign with rare malignant degeneration. Vascularization is not marked and is capillary in type. They are more common among young females than young males, and are the most frequent brain tumors affecting children.

The ventricular tumor of tuberous sclerosis is also included in the astrocytic series and is termed *subependymal giant cell astrocytoma.*

The term *astroblastoma* is still controversial. The diagnosis should be restricted to growths with astrocytic cells arranged in a perivascular pattern with thick processes radiating toward a central blood vessel. Since a similar pattern of processes may occur with glioblastomas and other groups, the term "astroblastoma" would be used only in the above-defined sense and with great reluctance.

The malignant form of astrocytoma has long been accepted and is to be designated the *anaplastic astrocytoma* (grade III).

(B) Oligodendroglial Tumors (see Fig. 18)

The typical histological pattern of the *oligodendroglioma* is easily recognized. Frequency is 8%–12%. Regional predilection is for the frontolateral areas in F-2 and F-3 (No. 8). Often, the parietal (No. 17), temporal (No. 24), temporo-occipital, and frontomedial (No. 13) areas, as well as the thalamus (No. 49) and corpus callosum (No. 43) are also involved. There is a tendency to calcification and small cysts are occasionally seen, but necrosis is rare. Oligodendrogliomas of the thalamus (No. 49) are usually seen in children. There is diffuse infiltrating growth which gives a knotty appearance to the cortex ("cortical warts"). The vascular network is often thick with a diffuse blush in the capillary phase of the angiogram. When malignant degeneration has occurred – *"anaplastic"* (polymorphic) *oligodendroglioma* – there is a marked increase in the variety and number of vessels, and a tendency to necrosis. Oligodendrogliomas are semibenign (grade II); when anaplastic, grade III. There is no sexual preference.

Not infrequently a conspicuous mixture of oligodendroglial cells and astrocytes occurs. In such cases the term *mixed oligoastrocytoma* is employed (grade II).

Fig. 18. Schematic representation of the most common intracranial tumors: ▷

Frontal tumors

1 Meningioma of the anterior third of the sagittal sinus – frontodorsal meningioma. *2* Frontodorsal astrocytoma. *3* Frontodorsal glioblastoma. *4* Meningioma of the anterior third of the sagittal sinus (bilateral). *5* Falx meningioma (frontomedial meningioma). *6* Bilateral falx meningioma. *7* Frontolateral glioblastoma. *8* Frontolateral oligodendroglioma. *9* Frontolateral astrocytoma. *10* Frontolateral (F 3) meningioma. *11* Frontolateral meningioma (also known as the convexity meningioma). *12* Frontomedial astrocytoma. *13* Frontomedial oligodendroglioma (parasagittal oligodendroglioma). *14* Olfactory groove meningioma (frontobasal meningioma). *15* Frontobasal glioblastoma

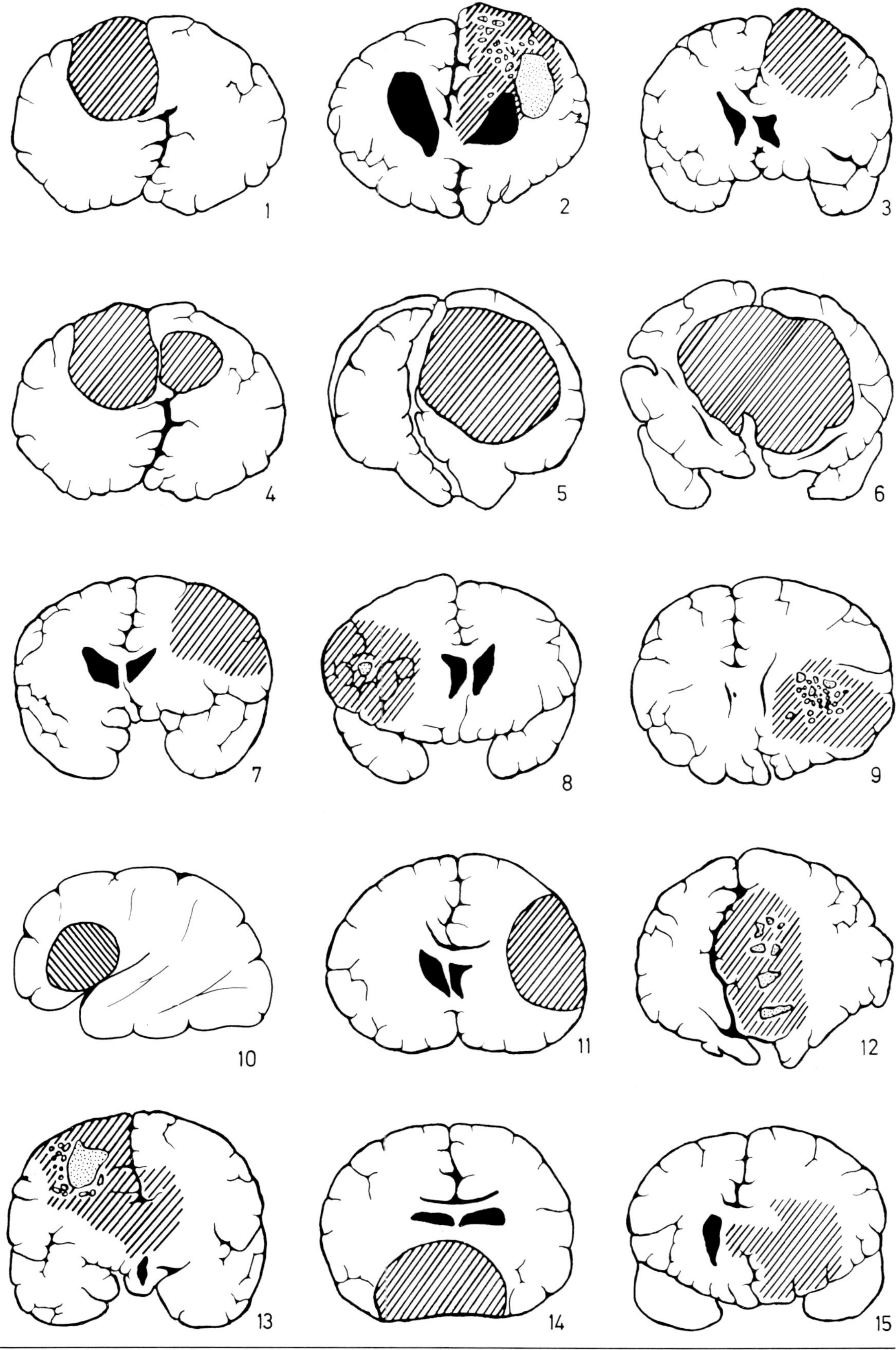

Fig. 18 (continued)

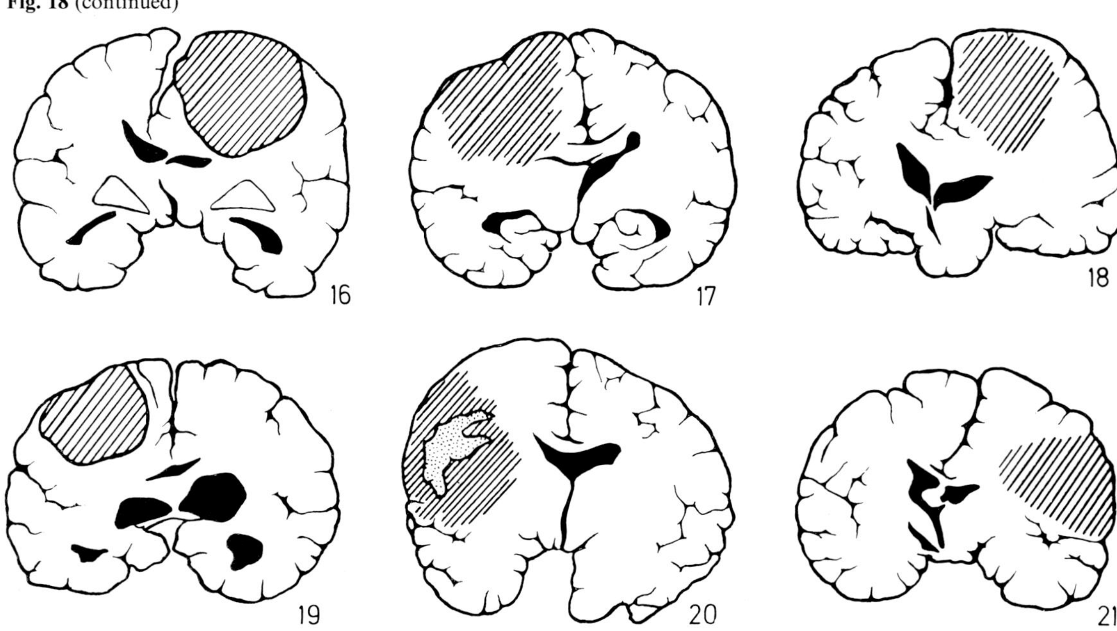

Parietal tumors

16 Parietodorsal meningioma (meningioma of the middle third of the sagittal sinus). *17* Parietodorsal oligodendroglioma. *18* Parietodorsal glioblastoma. *19* Meningioma of the convexity. *20* Parietolateral astrocytoma. *21* Parietolateral glioblastoma

(C) Ependymal and Choroid Plexus Tumors (see Fig. 18)

The ependymal tumors most typically found *within* the ventricles consist of true ependymal rosettes, perivascular rosettes, blepharoplasts and ependymal canals and are usually grade I, while the extraventricular tumors of the younger age groups may be anaplastic (grades II and III).

With a frequency of 4%–5%, these are situated in all parts of the central nervous system. The "extraventricular" ependymomas of children are the most common supratentorial gliomas occurring in this age group and are situated adjacent to the outer wall of the lateral ventricle (No. 30). The "intraventricular" type can be seen in the lateral ventricles adjacent to the foramina of Monro, within the third ventricle, or in front of the quadrigeminal plate (No. 56); in the aqueduct (less often), commonly on the caudal floor of the fourth ventricle (No. 71), or the central canal of the spinal cord (No. 78), or they are typically seen involving the cauda equina and filum terminale. The "extraventricular cerebral ependymomas of children" (No. 30) have large cysts and a predilection for the area where the parietal, temporal, and occipital lobes join together. They are frequently cystic and occasionally also calcified in this region. All ependymomas grow by displacement rather than infiltration, and infrequently metastasize within the CSF pathways except when tumor particles have broken free during surgery. Vascularization is by way of diffuse small capillaries.

The rare form of *anaplastic ependymoma* may resemble glioblastoma or medulloblastoma, but features of ependymal differentiation are present (grades III and IV).

Subependymoma is a small or large intraventricular tumor composed of nests of uniform ependymal cells, situated in a stroma of dense acellular glial fibers. These tumors have also been termed *subependymal glomerate astrocytomas*.

Growing out of the ependymal lining between the foramina of Monro in the anterior portion of the third ventricle are the pea to cherry-sized benign "colloid cysts" of the foramina of Monro (ependymal cysts, No. 40). These are non-neoplastic true cysts and are lined only by a membrane.

Choroid plexuspapillomas consist of a papillary pattern of low columnar or cuboidal cells covering a delicate vascular connective tissue

Fig. 18 (continued)

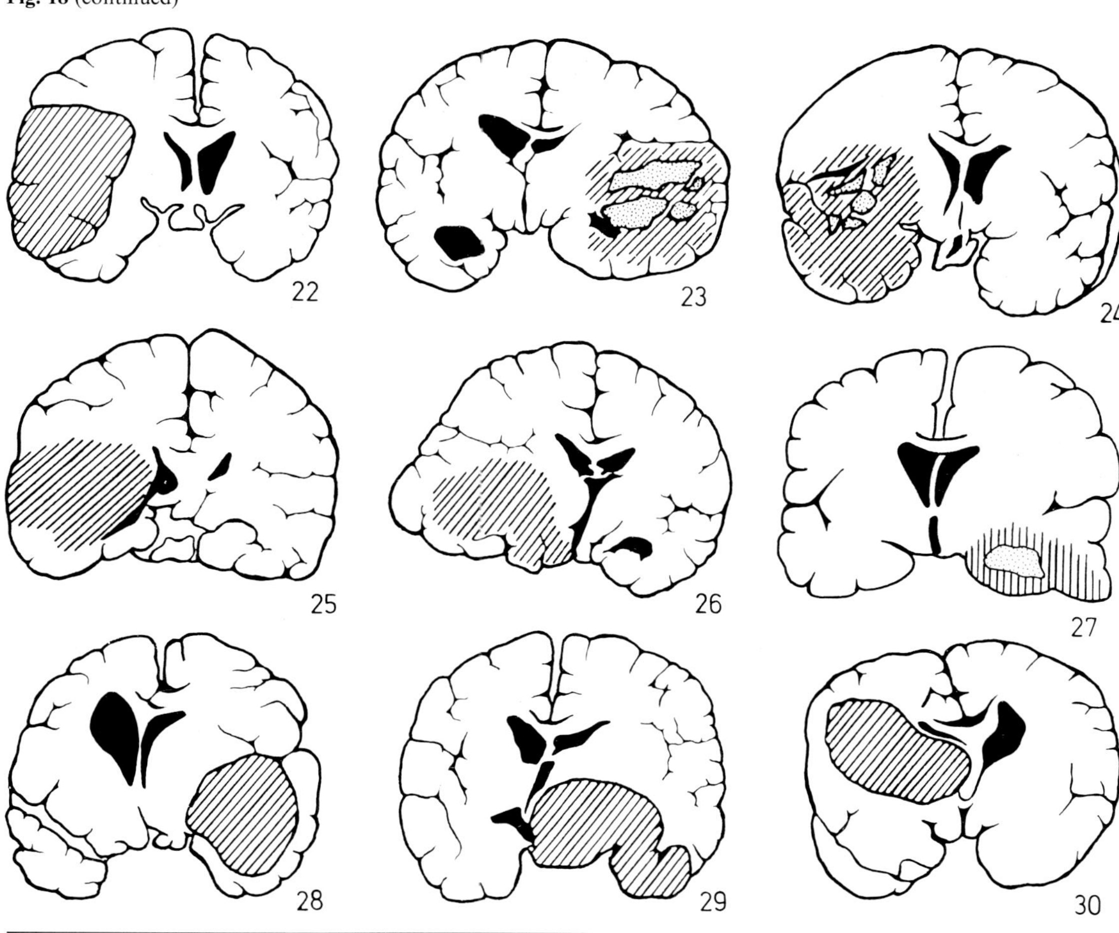

Temporal tumors

22 Meningioma of the Sylvian fissure. *23* Temporal astrocytoma. *24* Temporal oligodendroglioma. *25* Temporolateral glioblastoma. *26* Temporomedial glioblastoma. *27* Temporobasal gangliocytoma. *28* Sphenoid wing meningioma. *29* Meningioma-en-plaque of the sphenoid wing. *30* Ependymoma of the cerebral hemisphere (cerebral ependymoma)

core (grade I). Some of these tumors are heavily calcified (usually in the temporal horn). With a frequency of 0.5%–1%, these arise in the fourth ventricle as well as in the lateral ventricles with a predilection for the trigone; also in the third ventricle; rare in the lateral recesses. They grow by displacement and are benign. They are not cystic and are not infrequently seen in the newborn. Occasionally cysts will form in the adjacent tissues surrounding the tumor. CSF seeding is observed in some cases. Anaplastic choroid plexus tumors are very rare (grades III and IV).

(D) Pineal Cell Tumors (see Fig. 18)

These are rare tumors and include the *pineocytoma,* an isomorphous tumor with uniform cy-

tology and processes radiating toward the vascular stroma (grades I–III), and the *pineoblastoma,* a highly cellular malignant pineal tumor, very closely resembling the medulloblastoma (grade IV). Frequency is 0.5%. The usual site is the region of the quadrigeminal plate (Nos. 55, 59).

There is still controversy about the origin of pineal tumors in that some investigators believe that the "two cell pineal tumor" in fact consists of two entities: (a) a genuine tumor of pineal parenchymal cells which has the typical cell processes with clublike expansions at their tips described by del Rio Hortega (1945); (b) the germinoma, a more common tumor at this site. For comparison, the germinoma is described below even though it is not included among the neuroepithelial tumors in the WHO classification (see Riverson and Zülch 1979).

Germinomas are tumors composed of large primitive spheroidal cells indistinguishable

Fig. 18 (continued)

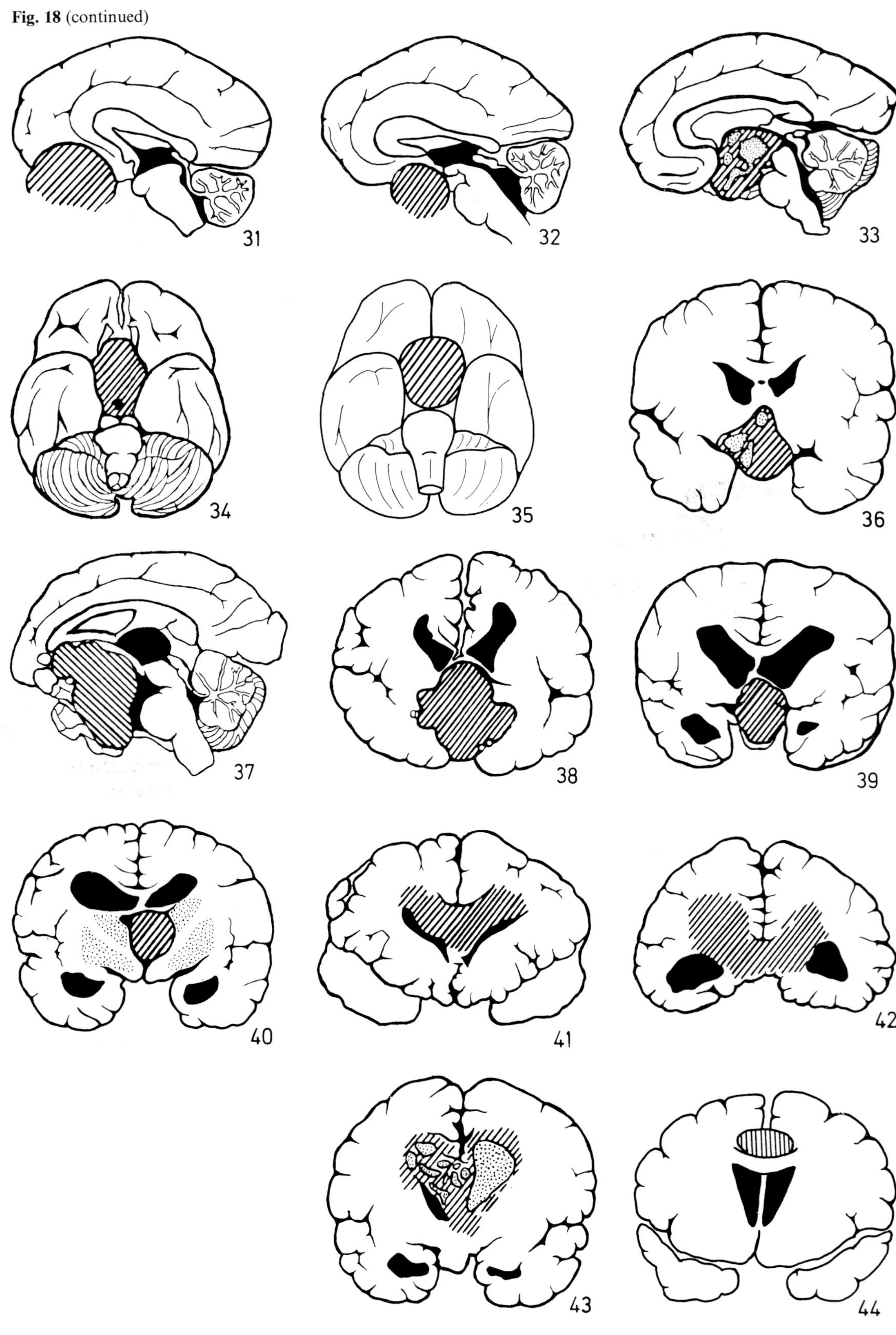

Fig. 18 (continued)

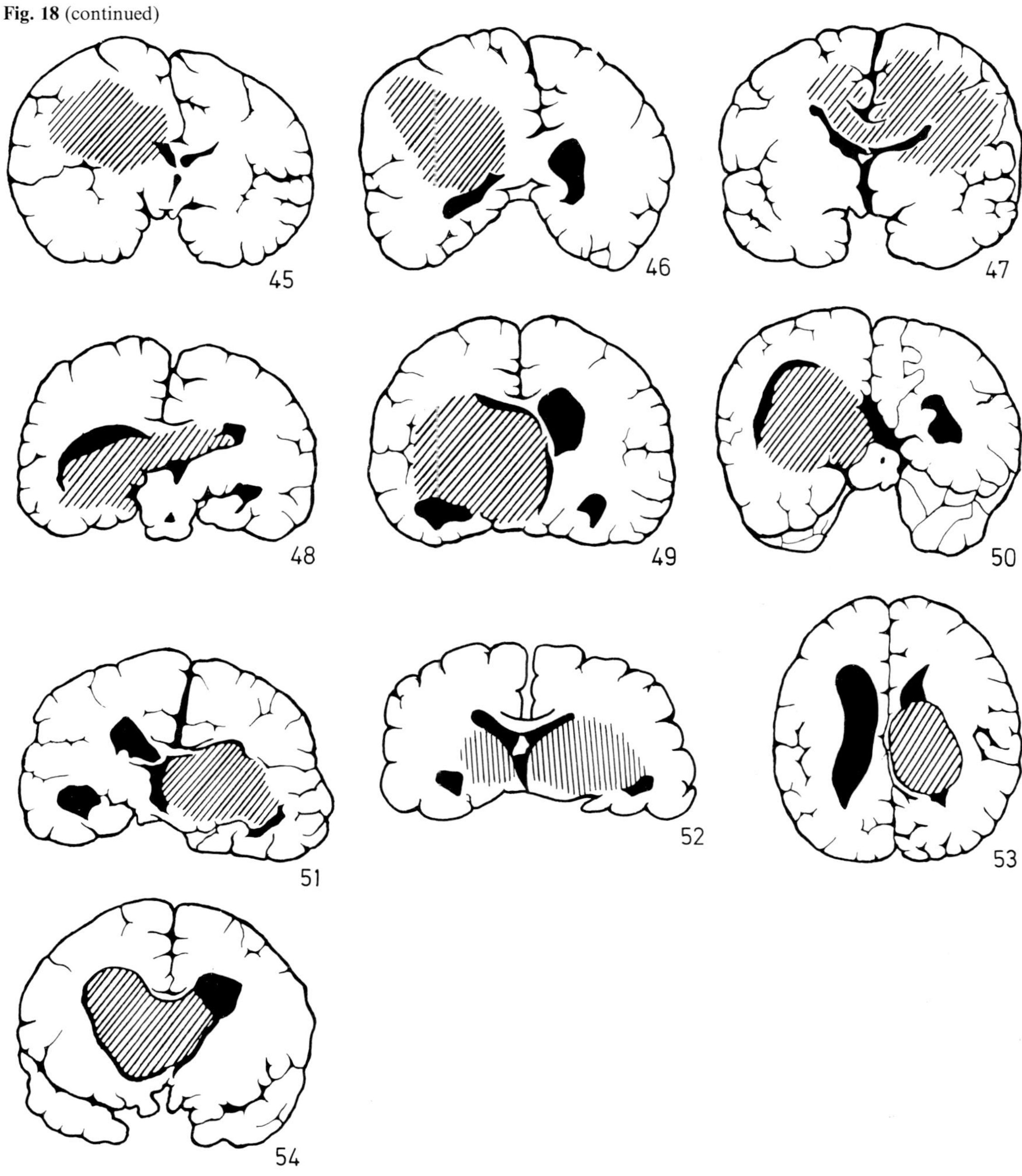

Paramedian tumors of the cerebral hemisphere

45 Glioblastoma of the rostral radiation of the corpus callosum. *46* Glioblastoma of the caudal corpus callosum. *47* Diffuse astrocytoma. *48* Glioblastoma of the fornix. *49* Oligodendroglioma of the thalamus. *50* Glioblastoma of the thalamus. *51* Astrocytoma of the thalamus. *52* Glioblastoma of the thalamus (bilateral). *53* Meningioma of the lateral ventricle. *54* Ependymoma of the lateral ventricle (at the foramen of Monro)

◁ *Midline tumors of the cerebral hemisphere*

31 Olfactory groove meningioma. *32* Tuberculum sellae meningioma. *33* Craniopharyngioma. *34* Cranipharyngioma. *35* Tuberculum sellae meningioma. *36* Craniopharyngioma. *37* Pituitary adenoma. *38* Pituitary adenoma. *39* Pilocytic astrocytoma of the chiasm. *40* Ependymal (colloid) cyst of the foramen of Monro. *41* Glioblastoma of the rostral corpus callosum. *42* Glioblastoma of the caudal corpus callosum. *43* Oligodendroglioma of the corpus callosum. *44* Lipoma of the corpus callosum

Fig. 18 (continued)

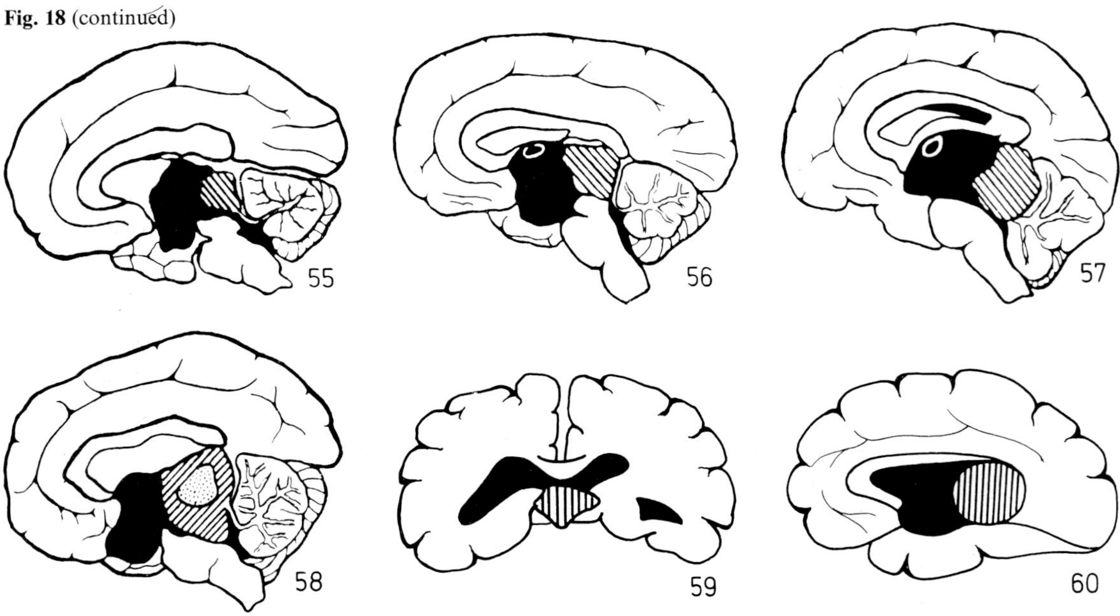

Midline tumors (mesencephalic)

55 Pinealoma – germinoma. *56* Ependymoma of the posterior third ventricle (quadrigeminal plate region). *57* Glioblastoma of the midbrain. *58* Pilocytic astrocytoma of the midbrain. *59* Pinealoma – germinoma. *60* Meningioma of the quadrigeminal plate (of the tentorial hiatus)

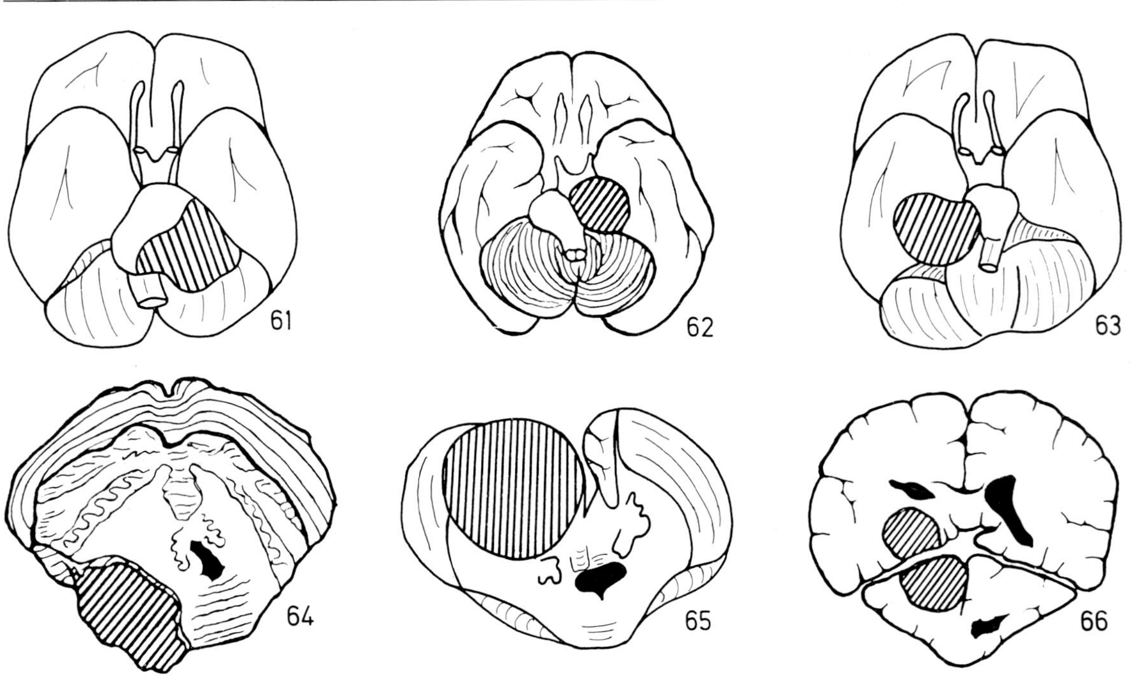

Parmedian tumors of the posterior fossa

61 Epidermoid of the cerebellopontine angle. *62* Meningioma of the tip of the petrous pyramid (cerebellopontine angle). *63* Neurilemmoma of the cerebellopontine angle. *64* Neurilemmoma of the cerebellopontine angle. *65* Peritorcular meningioma. *66* Meningioma of the tentorium

Fig. 18 (continued)

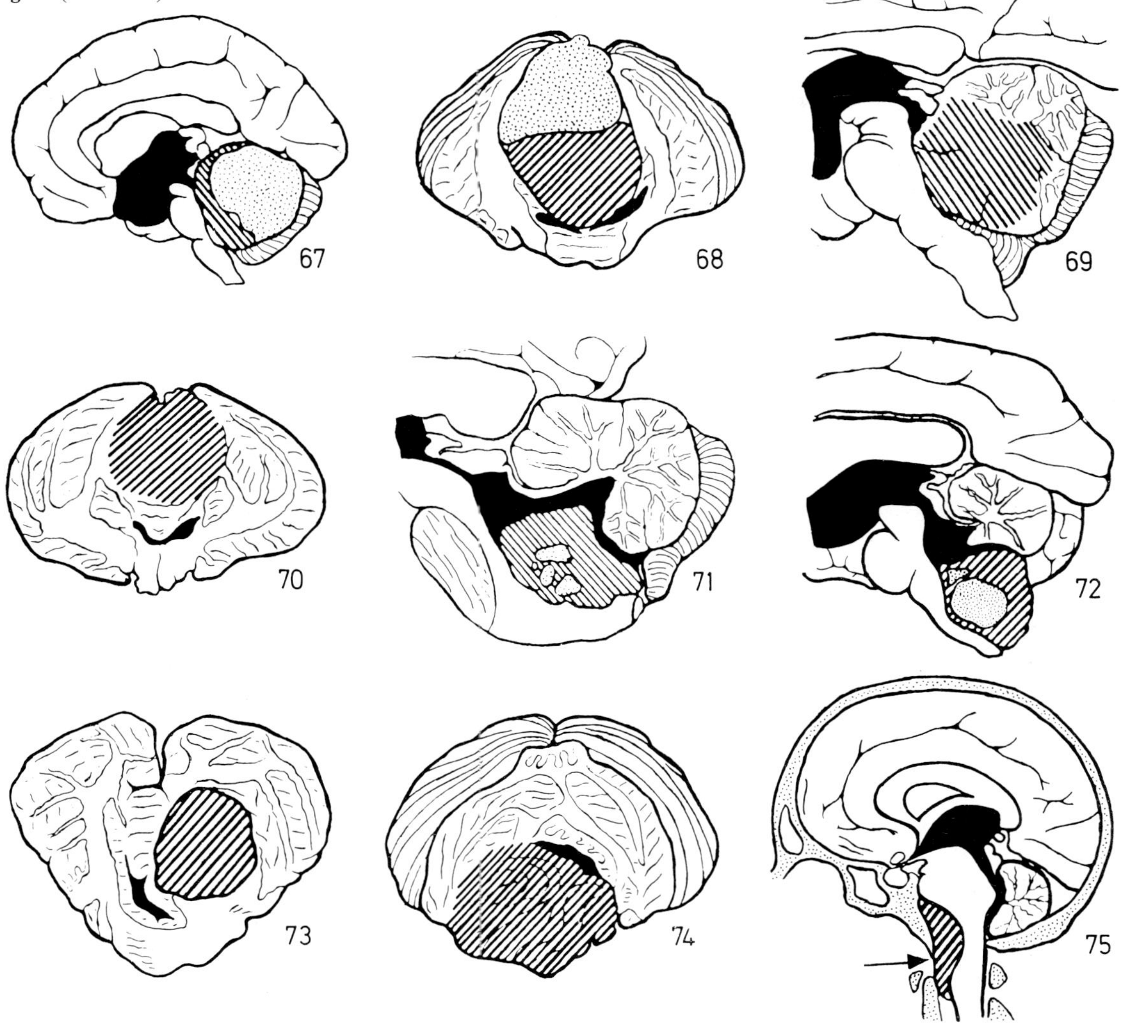

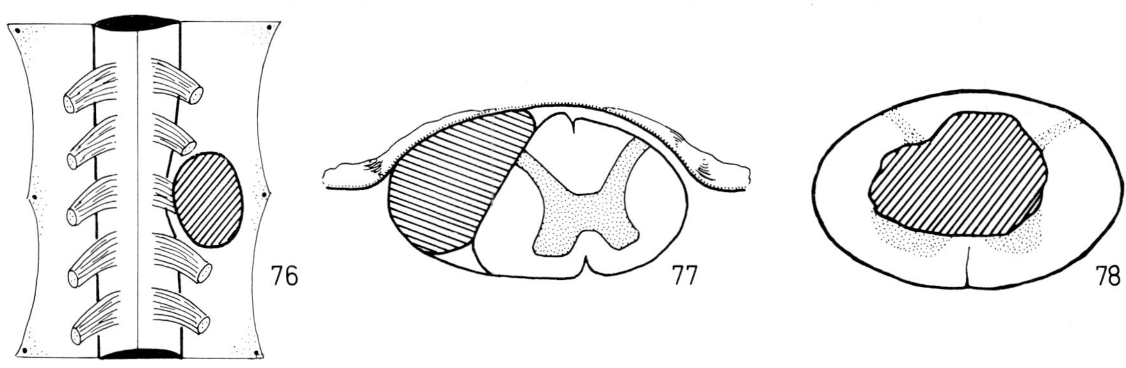

Midline tumors of the posterior cranial fossa

67 Pilocytic astrocytoma of the cerebellum. *68* Pilocytic astrocytoma of the cerebellum. *69* Medulloblastoma of the cerebellum. *70* Medulloblastoma of the cerebellum. *71* Ependymoma of the fourth ventricle. *72* Hemangioblastoma of the fourth ventricle. *73* Hemangioblastoma of the cerebellar hemisphere. *74* Astrocytoma of the pons. *75* Meningioma of the clivus (craniospinal meningioma)

Spinal tumors

76 Spinal neurilemmoma. *77* Spinal meningioma. *78* Spinal ependymoma/pilocytic astrocytoma

from the testicular seminoma and the ovarian dysgerminoma. The "two cell type", consisting of large epithelial and many lymphoid cells in its stroma, predominates. Multinuclear giant cells may be found. According to prominent authorities, germinomas are not only the most frequent tumors of the pineal region, but are also encountered in the hypothalamic region as the formerly so-called *ectopic pinealoma*. They are very sensitive to radiation (grades II and III).

"Ectopic" forms found in the infundibulum (genuine or aberrant metastases) are often larger than the primary tumor.

They grow by infiltration. There is a significant tendency to calcification, but rarely to necrosis or cystic degeneration. There is also a tendency to metastasize diffusely in the spinal fluid pathways, similar to the medulloblastoma. They are predominantly found in males and among children and young adults.

(E) Neuronal Tumors (see Fig. 18)

Gangliocytomas consist of mature ganglion cells and are well-circumscribed; a dysplastic variant of this tumor occurs in the cerebellum (grade I).

The gangliocytoma containing neoplastic glial cells as well as mature ganglion cells is to be classified as *ganglioglioma* (grades I and II).

If the spectrum of neuronal cells is larger and immature neuroblasts occur in addition to ganglion cells, the term *ganglioneuroblastoma* (grade III) is employed.

There are rare *anaplastic gangliocytomas* and *gangliogliomas* (grades II–IV) in which malignant characteristics are more prominent.

Neuroblastoma is a cerebral tumor composed of small, darkly staining, poorly differentiated cells with slender processes and a tendency to form pseudorosettes (grade IV). It is closely related to the retinoblastoma and sympathoblastoma.

The *gangliocytomas* of various subtypes (see above) occur with a frequency of only 0.4% and are thus an uncommon group of neuroepithelial tumors. They most frequently lie in the medial basal temporal lobe, as well as on the floor of the third ventricle and in the region of the tuber cinereum, in the medulla oblongata, in the spinal cord, and in the cerebellum. They are plum to apple-sized, often cystic or solid tumors, often extending into the arachnoid. Most are relatively benign, the malignant types being quite rare. The temporobasal variant is often calcified and cystic (No. 27) and very benign (grade I).

(F) Poorly Differentiated and Embryonal Tumors – Glioblastoma Multiforme and Medulloblastoma (see Fig. 18)

The dominant member of this group is the *glioblastoma multiforme* with its variegated architecture of necrosis, pseudopalisading, fistulous vessels, vascular endothelial proliferation, and old and fresh hemorrhages (grade IV).

If the connective tissue stroma appears to consist of elements which have undergone malignant transformation, the tumor may be classified as a *glioblastoma with sarcomatous component,* or a mixed glioblastoma and sarcoma (grade IV). If, on the other hand, the glioblastoma has a predominance of bizarre, highly multinucleated (monstrous) giant cells, the term *giant cell glioblastoma* may be appropriate (grade IV). These tumors have also been considered sarcomas (monstrocellular sarcomas; see p. 38) by some investigators.

The frequency of the glioblastoma multiforme is approximately 12%–20%. There is a predilection for the frontolateral (No. 7), frontobasal (No. 15), and frontodorsal (No. 3) areas; also the parietolateral (No. 21) and parietodorsal (No. 18), as well as the temporolateral (No. 25) and temporomedial (No. 26) areas. Quite typical is the "butterfly" glioblastoma, which is seen in the anterior (No. 41) or posterior (No. 42) regions of the corpus callosum. Occasionally this is limited to one side and extends from corpus callosum anteriorly or posteriorly into the corona radiata and farther peripherally. Rare are glioblastomas of the thalamus (Nos. 50, 52), of the quadrigeminal plate (No. 57), or the pons, and only exceptionally do they occur in the spinal cord. They are not known to occur in a cerebellar location. Glioblastomas grow by infiltration and are destructive. They are characterized by a significant degree of necrosis and also by fresh or old bleeding. There is usually marked cerebral edema as well as marked vascularization with many fistulous connections. Metastases are spontaneous within the ventricular system and lead to small warts and knots. They are highly malignant (grade IV). There is a predilection for the male sex, as with the medulloblastomas. This is a tumor of the middle-aged and elderly.

The second, also very common, neoplasm in this group of the undifferentiated neuroepithelial tumors is the *medulloblastoma* (grade IV), which is characterized by poorly differentiated cells and a tendency to form pseudorosettes. The frequency of occurrence is approximately 4%. Most are seen in the midline of the cerebellum where they lie in the roof of the fourth ventricle (Nos. 69, 70) and extend into the inferior vermis. They are seldom seen in the pons, are diffusely infiltrating, and frequently metastasize throughout the spinal fluid pathways. Knotty metastases can be found in the lateral ventricles, hypothalamus, and cauda equina. There are no cysts, and rarely small areas of necrosis. They are more common in boys than girls, and are predominantly seen in children and young adults.

"Desmoplastic" forms are occasionally seen with an excessive amount of connective tissue proliferation.

This *desmoplastic* variant of the *medulloblastoma* (also called "circumscribed cerebellar arachnoidal sarcoma" by some authors) is supposed to occur in older patients and to have a somewhat better prognosis than the other, more typical medulloblastomas.

2. Tumors of Nerve Sheath Cells
(see Fig. 18)

Neurilemmoma is the designated name under the new WHO classification for those well-known tumors composed of Schwann cells (grade I), earlier known as neurinomas or schwannomas.

Anaplastic neurilemmomas rarely occur (grade III).

Neurofibromas are localized or diffuse tumors consisting of a mixture of Schwann cells and fibroblasts with abundant collagen fibers, usually occurring as a component of von Recklinghausen's disease (grade I).

Anaplastic malignant neurofibroma is the malignant counterpart of the neurofibroma (grades III and IV). This malignant transformation has also been called "neurosarcoma".

The term *neuroma* is not used for the above entities because a neuroma is a non-neoplastic overgrowth of nerve fibers, Schwann cells, and other components of scar tissue.

The frequency of the *neurilemmomas* (neurinomas) is 7%–8%. There is a predilection for the 8th cranial nerve (Nos. 63, 64), less commonly for the 5th cranial nerve. They are also commonly found on the posterior roots of the spinal cord (No. 76) or in the cauda equina. In the thoracic area they commonly take a dumbbell shape, which permits further growth to occur outside the spinal canal. They are benign (grade I). They usually occur in middle age and are more common among women. In the spinal dumbbell or peripheral tumors, malignant degeneration ("anaplasia") is known but is not common (see above). The acoustic tumors may reach the size of a chestnut but when diagnosis is made earlier they may be much smaller and they may lie within the auditory canal. They compress the pons medially, the medulla oblongata caudally, and the cerebellum with the pons dorsally and dorsolaterally. They never calcify. The posterior fossa growths are not usually cystic, while the spinal growths can have impressive cysts. On the caudal end of the tumor in the cerebellopontine angle, single or multiple arachnoidal cysts are occasionally found. Bilateral cerebellopontine angle neurilemmomas are known and thought perhaps to be a "forme fruste" of "neurofibromatosis". They are occasionally seen together with other tumors in von Recklinghausen's disease. Neurilemmomas show a predilection for women and are more common in middle age.

3. Tumors of Meningeal and Related Tissues (see Fig. 18)

(A) Meningiomas

According to the WHO classification meningiomas are subdivided into nine varieties composed of both traditional and new categories (see Table 1).

The *meningotheliomatous, fibrous, transitional,* and *psammomatous* subgroups are well-established histological entities. Rare entities include the *angiomatous meningioma,* in which vascular channels predominate; the *hemangioblastic,* similar in tissue to the cerebellar form; the *hemangiopericytic,* which is encapsulated and indistinguishable from hemangiopericytomas elsewhere in the body; and the *anaplastic meningioma,* which is the malignant variant. Except for the *hemangiopericytic* meningiomas, which may have a poorer prognosis than the others, and the *anaplastic forms,* meningiomas are benign (grade I).

Meningiomas occur with a frequency of 14%–15% and are the most common extracerebral intracranial tumors. They are also commonly seen in the spinal canal and share the distinction (with neurilemmomas) of being one of the two most common extramedullary growths (No. 77). Predilection sites for meningiomas are as follows: parasagittal meningioma (No. 1); meningioma of the falx (Nos. 5, 6); meningioma of the convexities, especially fronto-laterally in the third frontal gyrus (Nos. 10, 11); on the sphenoid wing and in the temporal fossa (Nos. 28, 29); in the Sylvian fissure (No. 22); region of the olfactory groove (Nos. 14, 31); on the tuberculum sellae (Nos.32, 35) (suprasellar meningioma); in the region of the quadrigeminal plate (No. 60); and in the region of the tentorium (No. 65) (peritorcular meningioma), which often takes the shape of an hourglass (No. 66). Meningiomas are also found in the cerebellopontine angle (No. 62), in the choroid plexus of the lateral ventricles (No. 53), seldom in the fourth ventricle, velum interpositum of the third ventricle, or on the clivus (No. 75) (craniospinal meningioma), lower down (spinocranial), and finally within the spinal canal (No. 77). Extracranial meningiomas are seen in the orbit, especially on the optic sheath, and may also be extradural within the spinal canal. They are more frequent among women. They are well-encapsulated with varying degrees of hardness and are often calcified, seldom cystic tumors. They either erode bone (erosion in association with increased vascularization) or incite bony overgrowth (hyperostosis). Hyperostosis is especially marked in the region of the sphenoid wing. Bony involvement of the sella and skull can take the form of spicules. Arterial and venous channels are likewise considerably enlarged on the plain films (middle meningeal artery, sphenoparietal sinus, diploic veins). Meningiomas vary in size between a pea and a fist. Strangulation of the larger intracranial arteries (the siphon in sphenoid wing meningiomas) is possible, which may lead to a secondary cerebral infarct. There is commonly perifocal edema. The arterial supply to these tumors is often double, originating from both the internal carotid and external carotid. Metastasis to other parts of the body is quite rare, but has been reported. Multiple meningiomas are not so rare, but diffuse meningiomatosis is not common.

Meningiomas in common with neurilemmomas, ependymomas, pilocytic astrocytomas and neurofibromas are all frequent accompaniments of von Recklinghausen's disease. The malignancy rating is usually benign (grade I), but recurrent forms are occasionally grades III or IV (as in the fibrosarcomas). They occur most commonly in the middle and older age groups. The spinal meningiomas are seen later, in the 5th and 6th decades, predominantly in women in the thoracic region and usually calcified with high-grade psammoma formation. In exceptional cases meningiomas may also be found in children and in young adults.

The *anaplastic meningioma* (grades II or III) can occur in many of the subgroups and displays anaplastic features, but its anaplastic changes are not yet so far developed as in the primary fibrosarcoma of the dura.

(B) Meningeal Sarcomas

The *primary fibrosarcoma* of the dura mater is histologically well-differentiated and fairly well-circumscribed, yet primarily invasive (grades III or IV).

The rare *polymorphic cell sarcoma* is less well differentiated with a greater variation in size and shape of the cells (grades III or IV).

Primary *meningeal sarcomatosis* is a diffuse sarcomatous infiltration of the subarachnoid space (grade IV).

The frequency of all sarcomas involving the CNS is 2%–3%. There are many varied growth types and sites of occurrence. They may grow diffusely in the blood vessel sheath or in cerebral tissue. Of the circumscribed forms one has been called "arachnoidal cell sarcoma of the cerebellum", which is a well-delineated hard growth similar to the "desmoplastic medulloblastoma" and virtually identified as such by others. This category also includes the "monstrocellular sarcoma", a tumor similar (or identical?) to the giant cell glioblastoma; it shows necrosis and/or cystic degeneration, but hardly any fistulous tumor vessels. Also in the circumscribed category are reticulum cell sarcomas in the various parts of the cerebral and cerebellar hemispheres, as well as epidurally in the spinal canal. These tumors show secondary invasive tumor growth in the surrounding vertebrae and can be thought of as a special form of "malignant lymphoma". Necrosis is common and is not associated with hemorrhage. Sarcomas have no age, sex, or site predilection.

The "monstrocellular sarcoma" will be discussed below in more detail.

Table 1. Correlation of the various brain tumors with their corresponding malignancy grading[a]

Degree of malignancy	Prognosis after "total" removal	Tumors	
		Extracerebral	Intracerebral
Grade I benign *	Cure or at least survival time of 5 and more years	Neurilemmoma Meningioma Craniopharyngioma Pituitary adenoma Others	Astrocytoma, pilocytic Ependymoma of the ventricles Choroid plexus papilloma Gangliocytoma (temporobasal) Hemangioblastoma
Grade II semibenign **	Postoperative survival time: 3–5 years	Neurilemmoma, anaplastic Meningioma, anaplastic	Astrocytoma Oligodendroglioma Ependymoma (cerebral, extraventricular) Choroid plexus papilloma Ganglioglioma
Grade III relatively malignant ***	Postoperative survival time: 2–3 years	Pituitary adenocarcinoma Meningioma, anaplastic, "Neurosarcoma"	Astrocytoma, anaplastic Oligodendroglioma, anaplastic Ependymoma, anaplastic Gangliocytoma, anaplastic Germinoma
Grade IV highly malignant ****	Postoperative survival time: 6–15 months	Sarcomas and other highly malignant local extensions	Glioblastoma Medulloblastoma Sarcoma, primary

[a] The data reflect biological behavior without radiation and chemotherapy.

(C) Xanthomatous Tumors

The *fibroxanthomas* and their malignant variants are all quite rare. Histologically, the xanthomatous component predominates.

(D) Primary Melanotic Tumors

Primary melanomas as well as *meningeal melanomatosis* rarely occur in the central nervous system.

(E) Others

All kinds of fibromas, chondromas, chondrosarcomas, etc., are included in this group.

4. Primary Malignant Lymphomas

This category includes reticulum cell sarcoma, microglioma, microgliomatosis, reticulosarcoma, periadventitial diffuse sarcoma and all other types of lymphoma which occur primarily in the central nervous system.

The spinal *epidural* reticulosarcoma (or lymphosarcoma), familiar to the neurosurgeon and neuroradiologist, responds well to radiation treatment and therefore has a more favorable prognosis.

5. Tumors of Blood Vessel Origin
(see Fig. 18)

Included in this category are the well-known *hemangioblastomas* of Lindau. These have a frequency of 1%–2%. They tend to involve the cerebellum (No. 73) and are less commonly seen at the outlets of the 4th ventricle (No. 72) or within the cerebral hemispheres. In the spinal cord they are usually pencil-shaped tumors and are cyst builders. Multiple hemangioblastomas may be found in the vicinity of the foramen magnum. They grow by infiltration and can be differentiated from the angioblastic meningioma by the lack of a capsule and the lack of a connection to the dura. There is a pronounced tendency to cystic degeneration especially in the cerebellum. There is no calcification and no necrosis. They are benign (grade I). Multiple hemangioblastomas are not uncommon and the "recurrent" tumor may well be only a second tumor in the vicinity. Malignant degeneration has not been reliably described. Distinguishing this tumor from the hemangiopericytoma is occasionally difficult. It is a tumor of middle age.

The *"Lindau syndrome"* occurs when there is a *combination* of retinal and cerebellar tumors; *von Hippel-Lindau's disease* is an inherited form of this syndrome.

Monstrocellular sarcoma: This group has already been mentioned above (p. 38). These tumors seem to be relatively well demarcated, involve any age group and both sexes equally, contain abundant reticulin stroma, and are characterized by monstrous cells of enormous size and with many nuclei and inclusions. Although they are malignant (grade IV), the above characteristics distinguish them from the glioblastoma.

6. Germ Cell Tumors

Embryonal carcinomas and *choriocarcinomas* are rare malignant tumors easily recognized by the general pathologist. The *germinoma* was described earlier in the section on pineal tumors (p. 31). *Teratomas,* by definition, contain tissue from more than one germinal layer and occur in many regions of the CNS. They are benign (grade I) and will be more fully described below.

7. Other Malformative Tumors and Tumor-Like Lesions (see Fig. 18)

The craniopharyngioma is the most common tumor of childhood in the sellar region. This is an extracerebral tumor with a frequency between 2%–5%. The majority can be broken down into three categories:
a) Intrasellar (No. 36) with enlargement and destruction of the sella.
b) Suprasellar (Nos. 33, 34) with and without sellar widening and destruction.
c) Rarely intraventricular in the third ventricle.

There is a tendency toward cystic degeneration. Calcification is frequent, necrosis uncommon. The mode of extension is similar to the pituitary adenoma which is described below. Craniopharyngiomas are more common in young men.

The Rathke's cleft cyst is intrasellar whereas the *epidermoid* and *dermoid* – familiar tumors in general pathology – usually occur in the cleft lines.

The epidermoid and dermoid cyst in combination with the teratoma (see Fig. 18) are all extracerebral tumors with a frequency as follows: epidermoid 0.6%–1.5%, dermoid 0.1% and teratoma approximately 0.3%.

Epidermoid cysts: These have a predilection for the pons ("parapontine", No. 61), for the chiasm (parapituitary), quadrigeminal plate, posterior corpus callosum, Sylvian fissure, lateral ventricles, third ventricle, fourth ventricle, longitudinal fissure (anterior corpus callosum), spinal cord, and within the diploë of the skull. In the large intraventricular epidermoids, the fine capsule is often torn permitting entrance of air during an air study. These tumors may be associated with a spinal fluid pattern which is frequently characterized as "chronic lymphocytic meningitis". They are occasionally calcified.

Dermoid cysts: These have a predilection for the parapituitary and parapontine areas; also for the midline of the posterior cranial fossa and the sacrum. In addition, they are found in the maxillo-orbital closing line and grow in the direction of the orbit. They are frequently calcified with hair and grisly material present.

Teratoma: Teratomas are especially frequent in the pineal region (approximately 50%), the pituitary region (16%), the white matter (16%), the lateral ventricle, and other locations. The size varies from a pin-head to a child's fist. Teratomas are knotty and well-encapsulated, bony hard, occasionally calcified, or interspersed with bone, cartilage, hair, and teeth islands. These are rarely anaplastic and malignant. The male sex is predominantly affected.

The *colloid cyst* of the third ventricle is a true cyst, most commonly found at the foramen of Monro (synonyms: *paraphysial* or *neuroepithelial* cyst).

The *enterogenous* cyst, lined by mucin-secreting epithelium, may occur intraspinally.

Other cysts include the arachnoid or ependymal-lined cysts. The *lipomas,* although benign, have a dangerous tendency to grow into the stromal septa, as in the region of the spinal cord or corpus callosum. They are more commonly found just above, rather than within, the corpus callosum, but also involve the chiasm, the pons, and the spinal cord as well as the cauda equina. They are benign. The overlying leptomeninges are calcified and may therefore be visible on plain skull films.

The *choristoma (pituicytoma* or *granular cell myoblastoma)* is found in the pars nervosa of the pituitary gland. Hypothalamic *neuronal hamartomas* are rare and are malformations, but may also grow and take on the features of a space-occupying lesion. They are usually associated with precocious puberty. The *nasal glial heterotopias* (or nasal gliomas) are extremely rare, benign lesions.

8. Vascular Malformations

Vascular malformations include the following well-known entities: *capillary (teleangiectasia)* or *cavernous angiomas, arteriovenous malformations, venous malformations* and *Sturge-Weber's* disease.

9. The Tumors of the Anterior Pituitary (see Fig. 18)

The *pituitary adenomas* are extracerebral tumors with a frequency of occurrence somewhere between 8% and 12%. The most common type (see below) is the chromophobe with the eosinophilic type being less frequent, and the basophilic type being rare. Growth begins in the sella turcica and extends by bulging the diaphragma sella into the suprasellar region (Nos. 37, 38). With it there is often a rupture of the dura. The anterior cerebral artery and the chiasm are displaced upward and laterally by the expanding growth. The eosinophilic tumors remain in an intrasellar location for a long time. The chromophobe adenoma is frequently larger and has associated cysts, but rarely necrosis. Occasionally bleeding into the tumor occurs, but calcification is very rare. Chromophobe adenomas have been known to reach a large size by extending upward into the third ventricle, laterally in the direction of the temporal lobe, anteriorly into the frontal lobe, or into both frontal and temporal areas. Malignancy rating is grade I, with malignant degeneration occurring only as a rarity. These are most commonly seen in middle age. There is no sex predilection.

In recent decades a finer subclassification of endocrine tumors has been achieved, particularly in the "microadenomas".

These subgroups are primarily defined by their endocrine function (for instances prolactin-secreting adenomas) and secondary clinical sequelae, may be microscopic in size, and will not be discussed here in any detail.

The more traditional *acidophil, basophil, mixed acidophil-basophil,* and the *chromophobe* subgroups will suffice for this volume. The malignant variant is known as the *pituitary adenocarcinoma.*

10. Local Extensions from Regional Tumors

Among the regional tumors which may extend locally into the cranial cavity are the glomus jugulare tumor (chemodectoma), the chordoma, the chondroma and chondrosarcoma, the rare olfactory neuroblastoma, and the not infrequent adenoid cystic carcinoma (cylindroma). In addition to these rather unique entities, a number of other tumors – such as the nasopharyngeal carcinoma – may involve the brain and/or spinal cord.

11. Metastatic Tumors and Unclassified Tumors

Metastatic tumors retain the histological characteristics of the primary neoplasm and are malignant by definition.

Some intracranial tumors may still remain *unclassified* and, if they cannot be fitted into any of the above categories with sufficient certainty, are listed in a separate grouping – *Unclassified Tumor* – which is the final category of the WHO classification.

12. Less Common Tumors of the Base of the Skull

For predilection sites see the diagram (Fig. 19) which excludes the more common pituitary adenomas, sphenoid wing meningiomas, and craniopharyngiomas. Of importance are the "cylindromatous" epitheliomas of the base of the skull ("adenoid cystic carcinomas") as well as other carcinomas of the adjacent sinuses. Chordomas are mostly posterior to the sella. The large extradural aneurysms of the carotid

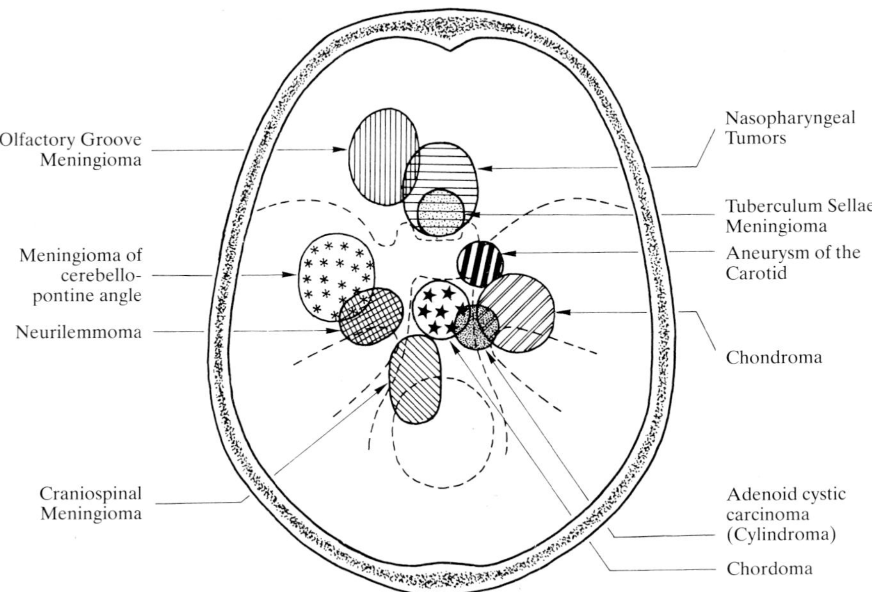

Fig. 19. Schematic representation of the position of the less common tumors involving the base of the skull (excluding pituitary adenomas, craniopharyngiomas, and sphenoid wing meningiomas)

artery are found in a *parasellar* location. Additional tumors include the teratomas, epidermoids, and temporal meningiomas of the base of the skull. Occurring on the apex of the petrous pyramid are chondromas, which are often calcified, meningiomas, and intracranial glomus tumors (chemodectomas). Glomus tumors are treacherous vascular tumors which can also be found in the external acoustic meatus or in the foramen magnum. On the outer side of the *petrous pyramid* are found the trigeminal neurilemmomas, while the craniospinal meningiomas are met at the level of the foramen magnum on the lower end of the clivus. Finally, there are the parasellar teratomas and epidermoids, the latter also occurring in the cerebellopontine angle.

13. Space-Occupying Processes of the Spinal Canal (see Fig. 20)

Intramedullary: Most common are the ependymomas, followed by the pilocytic astrocytomas and the hemangioblastomas of Lindau. There are also gliomas of other types. Large space-occupying cysts extending over many segments should be classified as "syringomyelia" only

with the greatest reluctance since they probably represent long cysts in tumors or ischemic lesions.

Extramedullary: Spinal meningiomas and neurilemmomas are most common. Lipomas are primarily found on the dorsal surface of the spinal cord or cauda equina, firmly established within the white matter and infiltrating the mesodermal septa. Spinal teratomas and dermoids are often seen together with fusion defects or cutaneous anomalies (for example, rippling of the skin and pathological hairgrowth). Extramedullary intraspinal tumors include the meningiomas of the dura, more common in the thoracic area; the dorsal root neurilemmomas; also meningiomas, occasionally associated with cysts, in the spinal canal. Less commonly seen are dumbbell-shaped neurilemmomas which extend out through the intervertebral foramen into the adjacent body cavity. Occasionally, arachnoiditis is found within the spinal canal. Epidural tumors, particularly reticulum cell sarcomas or other "lymphomas", are especially common to the thoracic area and very often cause destruction of adjacent vertebral bodies. Frequently, metastases and other malignant processes are also found involving the vertebral bodies. Arteriovenous malformations are not that uncommon, while encapsulated aneurysms are unheard of.

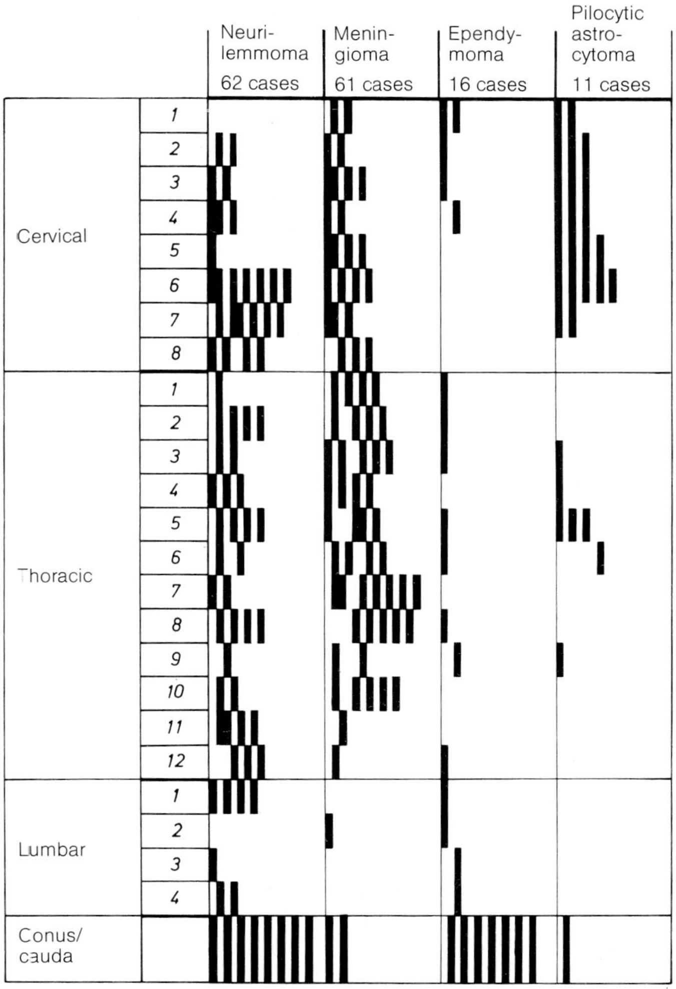

Fig. 20. Distribution of the most common spinal tumors and their sites of preference

		Neurilemmoma 62 cases	Meningioma 61 cases	Ependymoma 16 cases	Pilocytic astrocytoma 11 cases
Cervical	1				
	2				
	3				
	4				
	5				
	6				
	7				
	8				
Thoracic	1				
	2				
	3				
	4				
	5				
	6				
	7				
	8				
	9				
	10				
	11				
	12				
Lumbar	1				
	2				
	3				
	4				
Conus/cauda					

14. Space-Occupying Lesions Other than Neoplasms

Although the following entities are not represented in the WHO Classification, a short morphological description is given because of their importance in neurosurgery and neuroradiology.

Parasites: In most parts of the USA and Europe there are only isolated cases of *cysticercosis* or genuine *echinococcosis*. The cysts of *cysticercus* are bean-shaped or larger, with much of the lesion infesting the brain and spinal fluid systems tending to take a "racemose" form lying in clusters on top of one another within the cisterns. In later stages calcification is apparent on the skull films. Intracranial cysticercosis is frequently not calcified at a time when muscular lesions are already heavily calcified.

The *echinococcus* is a much larger parasite ranging in size from a pigeon egg to an orange. It is not uncommonly seen in the intracranial spaces, but is often multilocular when present. In the spinal canal it is occasionally multiple and extends along the spinal roots from the thoracic cage into the extradural spaces of the vertebral canal.

Granulomas: Now extremely rare (lues, tuberculosis) in many parts of the world.

Arachnoiditis may function as a space-occupying process by obstructing the flow of spinal fluid within the cisterns. The sites of predilection are the cisterna magna, the chiasmatic and peripeduncular cisterns, and the spinal canal. There are often compartmentalized cysts.

Arachnoidal cysts (see above): These are frequently congenital in etiology, mostly involving the Sylvian fissure but also found above the corpus callosum. They may be fist-sized with corresponding mass displacement of adjacent arteries and local bulging of the overlying (temporal) skull.

For quick reference, a number of graphs and drawings have been included which summarize much of the information provided earlier (see Figs. 17, 18). The series of schematic drawings in Fig. 18 ff. represent typical sites and shapes of various intracranial and intraspinal tumors in order to provide the reader with a mental image of what secondary neuroradiological changes to look for and to emphasize the possibility of reaching a type-specific diagnosis from site and shape alone. This format is necessarily limited to show only the main tumor types involving each region.

15. Grading of Malignancy

Finally, the following table has been added to correlate most of the intracranial tumors with an approximate malignancy grading. Although this table and Figs. 17 and 18 are not part of the official WHO publication cited above, they generally reflect the data given in the publication.

For literature see: BAILEY and CUSHING (1926, 1930), PENFIELD (1931), ROUSSY and OBERLING (1931), BAILEY (1932), DEL RIO-HORTEGA (1945), KERNOHAN et al. (1949), OBRADOR ALCALDE and SANZ IBANEZ (1955), ZÜLCH (1956), UICC (1965), RUSSELL and RUBINSTEIN (1971), ZÜLCH (1971), RUBINSTEIN (1972), ZÜLCH (1975), WENDE et al. (1977), ZÜLCH (1965, 3rd edition in press; 1978, 1979).

II. Atrophic Cerebral Processes

*Topographical Peculiarities of the
Atrophic Processes (see p. 251 ff.)*

Atrophic processes, i.e., processes associated with progressive tissue loss, can have many etiologies. The brain in such cases as a whole or in part is reduced in size and is underweight. In comparative autopsy studies, it is recognized that a "physiological" atrophy of the brain has already begun by the 25th year of life, accompanied by enlargement of the spinal fluid pathways (see Fig. 180). In association with this physiological atrophy of old age is enlargement of the frontal horns of the ventricles, followed later by enlargement of the region of the trigone, and finally of the temporal horns as well. The subarachnoid pathways show enlargement especially in the frontal areas, followed by the parietal and temporal lobes in the vicinity of the Sylvian fissure. The basal convolutions do not take part in this atrophy of old age. Thus, the atrophy of old age has a distinct topographical predilection.

Besides the physiological atrophy of old age, there are premature processes of aging known as the presenile dementias, which in individual cases can occur especially early and can be particularly marked. Alzheimer's disease leads to a generalized cortical and white matter atrophy occasionally with a predilection for the temporal lobe. Pick's disease varies according to type from a predominantly frontal to a predominantly temporal atrophy. It can also involve both areas equally and may also be especially marked in the parietal lobe. In Pick's disease the marked ventricular enlargement in association with marked enlargement of the overlying subarachnoid spaces results in a cock's-comb appearance to the convolutions which macroscopically appears to resemble the edible portion of a walnut. Characteristic of Pick's disease and in contrast to all the other forms of atrophy is the marked involvement of the basal convolutions in the atrophic process. Huntington's chorea is associated with atrophic involvement of the basal ganglia as well as both frontal lobes, with marked enlargement of the frontal horns and overlying subarachnoid spaces. In multiple sclerosis, and following other less common encephalitides, there is a predominant involvement of the white matter. Corresponding to this one mainly finds ventricular enlargement. With most of the intoxications there is also a diffuse ventricular enlargement. Alcoholism differs by its equal involvement of both white matter and cortex. In protein deficiencies and in starvation there is involvement of the white matter with the cortex suffering little damage. In the systemic atrophies of the cerebellum there is a cortical atrophy, which leads to widening of the fissures between the lobes and a preferential involvement of the vermis with enlargement of the adjacent fourth ventricle. In olivopontocerebellar atrophy the pons is also involved. With reference to posttraumatic changes, see p. 256.

The pathologic etiology of the atrophic process is important for radiological diagnosis only insofar as it influences the shape and size of the ventricles and the subarachnoid pathways. From the site and degree of the secondary enlargement of the spinal fluid pathways it is possible, with a certain probability, to arrive at a specific diagnosis. The diagnosis is implied by virtue of the fact that individual pathological processes have a characteristic localization and intensity of tissue loss.

III. Changes Following Trauma to the Skull and Brain

(see also p. 257)

With the increase in the number of "acceleration" type injuries, the after-effects of trauma to the brain and skull have become quite diverse. Prior to this development, it was usually possible to predict the type of injury occurring in association with a fall, or a blow from an instrument, with a certain degree of accuracy based on the direction of the blow. Today – and this is particularly true of injuries sustained in car accidents – there is so much jarring of the body that the corresponding forces at work cannot be localized with any degree of predictability. By consulting the literature on this subject, however, it is possible to put together certain patterns of injury as follows:

1. Injuries Occurring as a Result of Falls or Secondary to Blunt Instruments

a) As a Result of a Broad, Flat Force

When the blow is light and undirected, a *concussion (commotio)* results which gives a reversible disturbance of brain stem function with a secondary disturbance of blood flow, transient cerebral edema, and a tendency toward subsequent hydrocephalus. When the force is stronger, *contusion* of the brain stem may ensue. With a known direction of the blow, frontal/temporal/parietal originating *coup* and *contrecoup* injuries may be expected. Especially typical in this regard is the *contrecoup* fronto-orbital injury from an occipital blow.

b) As a Result of a Circumscribed Force

Cerebral Contusion

In association with a corresponding contrecoup injury
    with the skull intact
    with the skull fractured or crushed.

2. Traumatic Hemorrhages

a) Acute epidural:
through a tear in the branch of the middle meningeal artery
through a tear in a sinus.
(Differences in the site of the bleeding vary according to what portion of the frontal/temporal/occipital arterial branch is involved.)
b) Acute subdural: through laceration of a cortical vessel; most of these occur in the temporal, parietal, or frontal regions.
c) Intracerebral: under a contusion or laceration involving the white matter (especially in the frontobasal regions), rarely also "delayed".
d) Deep white matter bleeding in older individuals occurring in a variety of locations.
e) The late appearing chronic subdural hematoma, which is encapsulated.
f) Brain abscesses: these occur as frequently in brain contusions and lacerations as in intracerebral hemorrhages whenever there is a communication to the outside permitting introduction of infection and the subsequent development of an abscess. In civilian injuries, however, these are not very common.

3. Traumatic Cysts

These occur through removal of contused tissue in the subcortical location. They may occasionally communicate with the ventricular system.

4. Traumatic Brain Edema

a) Diffuse after a concussion (commotio): 3–4 days.
b) Perifocal in association with *contusion* and particularly with *bleeding*: 1–4 days.
c) With a posttraumatic thrombotic occlusion of the carotid artery in the neck, or in association with a dissecting aneurysm of the middle cerebral artery at the level of the sphenoid wing, with secondary infarcts.
d) Edema in association with a thrombotic occlusion of a large venous sinus or a large cortical vein.

5. Special, Rare Posttraumatic Events

a) Pneumocephaly

This occurs when air enters the ventricular system or intracranial cavity by communication with an adjacent nasal cavity or one of the adjacent air-filled sinuses.

b) Carotid-Cavernous Fistula

Secondary to a traumatic tear of the carotid artery in the cavernous sinus leading to development of a fistula with corresponding changes in the pattern of vascular flow.

IV. Consequences of Cranio-cerebral Trauma as Revealed by Radiologic Contrast Procedures

In the acute and subacute phases of brain injury (see p. 257), diagnostic contrast techniques are of value in the demonstration of hemorrhages, of space-occupying cerebral contusions with edema, of blood vessel injuries, and of acute traumatic brain abscesses. Similarly, in the later phases of injury they may reveal posttraumatic brain atrophy, chronic subdural hematomas, posttraumatic hydrocephalus, spinal fluid fistulas, and chronic traumatic brain abscesses. However, the need for these procedures in trauma has been largely supplanted in recent years by the advent of computed tomography. Since this is not yet uniformly available, indications for the older contrast techniques will be given below.

In the *early* phase of brain injury, cerebral angiography is the procedure of choice when CT is not available. This procedure readily permits the diagnosis of an *extracerebral hematoma* to be made since it demonstrates the separation of the peripheral vessels on the brain surface from the inner table of the skull caused by the presence of the hematoma. It is, however, necessary to keep in mind that additional exposures – the oblique views – may be required to demonstrate hematomas of the frontal or occipital poles. In spite of these maneuvers, small temporal hematomas may not be recognized. In addition, bilateral hematomas may leave the anterior cerebral artery in the midline. Frequently, epidural and subdural hematomas cannot be differentiated from each other. In rare cases the epidural hematoma may be localized over the superior sagittal sinus in which case the sinus will be separated from the inner table of the skull by the presence of the hematoma, facilitating the diagnosis. Also, the site of predilection of the subdural hematoma (extending over the frontal/temporal/occipital regions) helps to differentiate it from the epidural hematoma, which is more localized.

With angiography, intracerebral hematomas usually give the picture of avascular space-occupying processes. They often cannot be differentiated from a localized cerebral contusion or from more generalized brain swelling. These differences are, however, readily resolved by computed tomography. It should not be forgotten that intra- and extracerebral hematomas can also occur in the posterior cranial fossa, though rarely. Occasionally it is possible to demonstrate *escape of the contrast medium* from vessels into either an intracerebral or an epidural hematoma. That the contrast is extravascular in location is suggested by the fact that it remains visible longer in this location than in the adjacent damaged vessel. When, on the other hand, the contrast medium remains within the circulation but demonstrates a temporary external stain at the level of the hematoma, this is suggestive of a traumatic false aneurysm.

Blood vessel injuries are more readily demonstrable on angiography than with the CT scan, particularly the internal carotid artery tear within the cavernous sinus which produces an arteriovenous fistula. This problem can also make its appearance in delayed fashion some time after the traumatic event has occurred (see p. 133). The venous phase will also permit the diagnosis of a traumatic *thrombosis* of a *sinus* or a *large vein* to be made.

Acute traumatic brain abscesses will present as avascular space-occupying processes on the angiogram and are thus difficult to distinguish from other post-traumatic mass lesions. In the absence of CT, the diagnosis can only be suggested by the clinical situation. This is also true to a certain extent for the chronic abscess, although in this case there is sometimes a fine vascularization apparent within the surrounding capsule.

Posttraumatic disturbances of the spinal fluid pathways in later stages of injury may be demonstrated by computed tomography, pneumoencephalography, or with a radioactive tagging technique such as rhisacisternography. Angiographic findings characteristic of hydrocephalus will be described in another section (see p. 106).

V. The Pathogenesis of Infarcts

The consequence of stenosis or occlusion of a large or a small artery is mainly a disturbance in blood flow. This usually results in a complete or incomplete infarct in the territory of supply of the affected vessel, which could not be prevented by anastomoses and collateral circulation. Anastomoses are common, but circulatory disturbances are the rule for the end arteries of the brain, i.e., the relatively large median and paramedian deep perforating and brain stem arteries (including the recurrent artery of Heubner, the pontine arteries, and especially the arteries to the medulla oblongata). After perforating the brain substance these arteries, as well as all other small branches from the larger brain arteries, are functionally considered "end arteries" since their anastomoses consist only of capillaries and these small capillaries are not sufficient to re-establish adequate blood flow to the affected territory.

For other arteries, anastomoses are common in the presence of angiographically demonstrated vessel occlusions; thus it is important to consider whether a sufficient anastomotic network is available to re-establish blood flow to the affected area. Because of this, it is impossible to predict the hemodynamic and morphological consequences of a demonstrated occlusion in the absence of other information suggesting that an infarct or ischemic episode has, in fact, occurred. On the other hand, when the clinical neurological evaluation is compatible with a major disturbance in blood flow secondary to a stenosis or an occlusion, particularly when these disturbances can be demonstrated by CT or by other diagnostic methods, the diagnosis of infarct becomes secure.

With these considerations of pathogenesis in mind, the known rules for the development of regional disturbances play a more decisive role. In association with the appropriate hemodynamic alterations, certain anatomical configurations lend themselves to blood flow disturbances. These include the terminal ramifications to a single maintenance territory from a small end artery, or the *border zone* between two such territories (see Fig. 21). Similar disturbances in flow can also arise in the *watershed* zone between two major arteries. On the surface of the brain one finds such zones in the periphery of the territory of supply of the three large arteries, or in the depths of the brain between a territory of one of the surface vessels and that of one of the deeper perforating arterial systems, for example between the striatum and the insula. By considering these special hemodynamic facts when one is confronted with a localized narrowing of the blood vessel wall capable of affecting blood flow, and by considering other more general hemodynamic factors (cardiac output, blood pressure, oxygenation, viscosity, etc.), it is possible to correlate the *site,* the *size,* and ultimately the *severity* of a particular disturbance in blood flow with the observed lesion. The most frequent sites for disturbances of flow in the cerebral hemispheres are shown on the diagram (see Fig. 22a, b). Their relative frequency is also well known (see Fig. 23, data from 700 infarcts).

A particularly dramatic example of such blood flow disturbances with regional peculiarities can be seen in the example of an occlusion of the vertebral artery in which infarcts in seven distinct levels of territorial maintenance were found (see Fig. 24). These were situated in the medulla oblongata, in the pons, midbrain, and thalamus; in the mediobasal temporal and occipital lobes, as well as in the ventral and dorsal

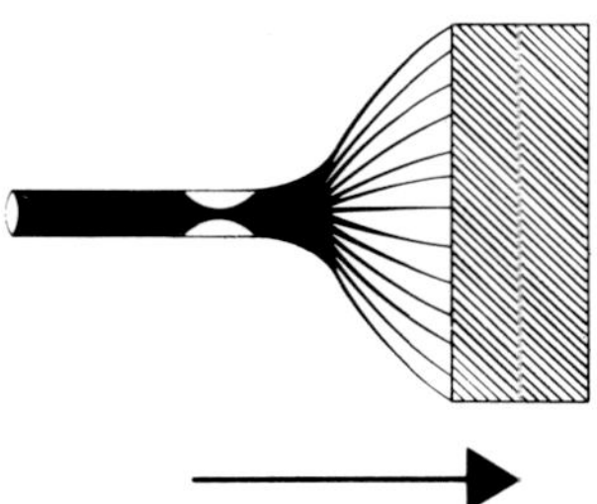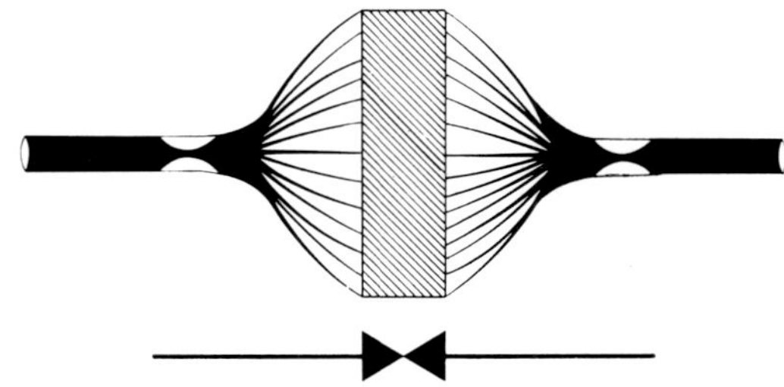

Fig. 21. Hemodynamics of cerebral insufficiency. The first diagram shows flow disturbances at the margin of a territory of supply ("last meadow"). The second diagram shows flow disturbances in the "watershed" zone between two territories of supply

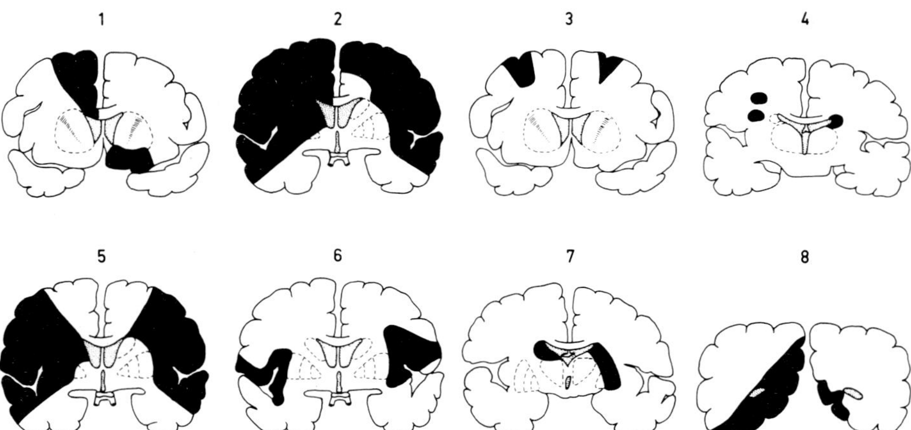

Fig. 22. a Topography of the most common types of cerebral infarcts: *1*, anterior cerebral artery; *2*, anterior and middle cerebral arteries, with (*left*) and without (*right*) participation of the lenticulostriate vessels; *3*, watershed zone infarcts; *4*, cystic infarcts in the centrum semiovale (*left*) and caudate (*right*); *5*, and *6*, infarcts in the territory of supply of the middle cerebral artery: *5*, total (*left*), cortical (*right*) and *6*, minimal (*left*), wedge-shaped (*right*); *7*, end-artery and border zone infarcts of the perforating branches of the middle cerebral artery; *8*, occipital infarcts of the posterior cerebral artery (maximal and minimal)

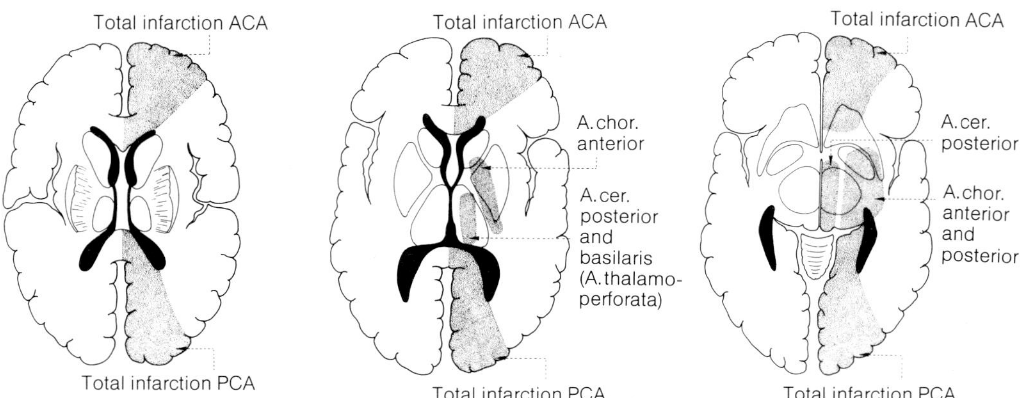

Fig. 22 b. Horizontal sections (as would be seen on computed tomograms) of maximal infarcts following occlusion of selected cerebral arteries

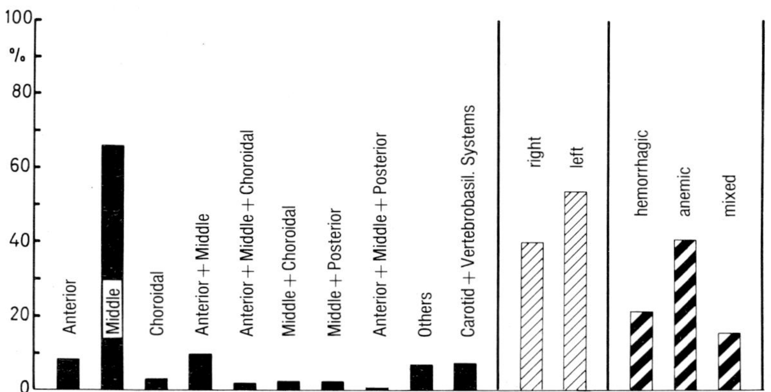

Fig. 23. Average frequency of cerebral infarcts (from computed tomograms)

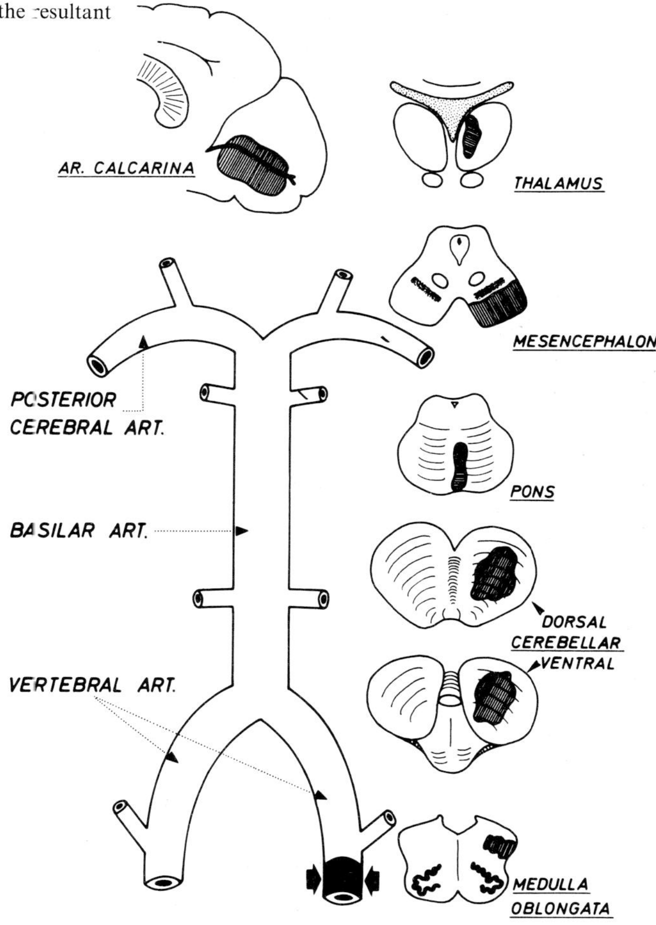

Fig. 24. Occlusion of a single vertebral artery with the resultant infarct pattern in seven different susceptible zones

cerebellum. Although these were only "partial infarcts" in each territory, the example does demonstrate the unique unilateral distribution of blood in the vertebrobasilar system. Infarcts can vary in size within an individual territory, as with the middle cerebral artery where an infarct may be either "total", "medium large", "wedge shaped", or "minimal". These variations undoubtedly vary with the effectiveness of the collateral circulation reaching the middle cerebral territory from the anterior cerebral and posterior cerebral arteries (see Fig. 25). Finally, it should also be pointed out that an infarct can also occur directly adjacent to an occluded vessel or, in some incomplete stenotic lesions, directly in the middle of the major area of supply of the affected vessel. It should be emphasized that the latter situation is seen only in stenotic lesions and not in occlusions. It should also be emphasized that an irreversible infarct can be found in the presence of "open" (radio-graphically patent) small arteries. How to distinguish a *red* (hemorrhagic) as opposed to a *white* (anemic) infarct on an angiographic basis remains undecided, whereas the distinction is easily made on computed tomograms. The hyperemia of many such infarct zones is "reactive", that is to say, caused by local metabolism. In these cases there is mostly the finding of "early" venous filling. Both situations – early venous filling and hyperemia – do not necessarily occur simultaneously however. The reason for this dissociation is not known.

A last phenomenon has recently generated some special interest: occasionally neurological and electrophysiological evidence of symptoms from the "false" side will be found, for example, in the opposite hemisphere from an occluded internal carotid artery. In this situation the blood flow disturbance arises when the "healthy" hemisphere is deprived of blood to supply the occluded side (steal syndrome). The

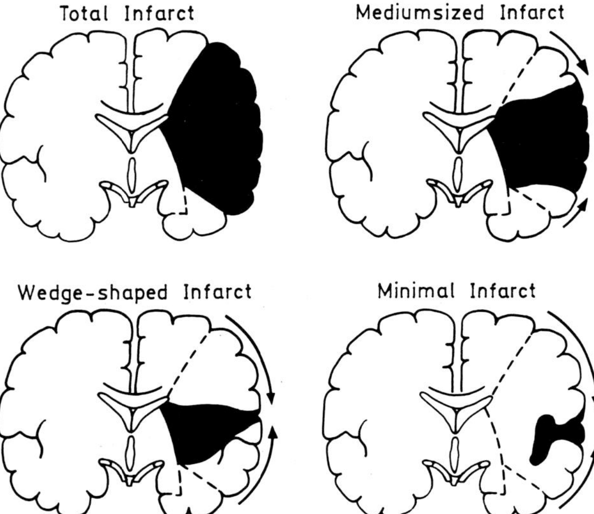

Fig. 25. Various sizes of middle cerebral artery infarcts shown in coronal section. These vary according to the effectiveness of meningeal anastomoses from the anterior and posterior cerebral arteries

explanation for this hemodynamic arrangement, which occurs at the expense of the nonoccluded hemisphere, is not known (Fig. 130). It is apparent that in such cases an angiographic study limited to the symptomatic hemisphere will not reveal the true pathology.

Cerebral infarcts in newborn or in younger children have their peculiarities. Porencephaly in general is a reflection of cyst formation within a middle cerebral infarct occurring at birth, and is indicative of the tendency of the developing brain to cyst formation. In "spastic" children (Little's syndrome), there is predominantly ischemic damage and atrophy in the convolutions near the midline. In the presence of unilateral hyperkinesia, the basal ganglia are also involved in the atrophy. Extensive scar formation after ischemic damage during childhood is termed ulegyria. These changes can occur in "lobar" fashion (lobar sclerosis), but also can be more generalized and involve an entire hemisphere as after a post-ischemic (usually asphyxiation) phenomenon.

With these rules it is possible to derive from the neuroradiological procedures the greatest amount of information about disturbances of blood flow. Since it is not possible to diagnose with certainty *from the angiogram alone* even such a radical disturbance in blood flow as an infarct, it is necessary to deduce what has happened from the information available. On the other hand, areas of infarct can be easily demonstrated on the CT scan and even the isotope scan when they are unequivocally positive. This is unfortunately not always the case with the latter since there is a limited time frame in which positive studies may be obtained.

VI. Aneurysms and Arteriovenous Malformations

The arterial aneurysm and arteriovenous malformation will not be described in great detail here. Only four points will be outlined which are of significance for neuroradiology:

1) An arteriovenous malformation can lead to considerable local brain atrophy since the increased blood flow through the lesion occurs at the expense of adjacent areas, which are then deprived of their required allotment of blood.

2) There is a definite predilection for the formation of a berry aneurysm at the bifurcation of certain vessels in a frequency which is statistically computed (see the Table from McDonald and Korb (1939), and in many later works).

3) When one of these berry aneurysms bleeds into the neighboring brain tissue, the three most common sites for the hemorrhage are as follows:
   a) between the basal frontal lobes from the anterior communicating aneurysm
   b) in the temporal lobe entering from a mediobasal direction from a ruptured posterior communicating aneurysm
   c) in the basolateral frontal lobe or medial temporal lobe entering from the Sylvian fissure from the aneurysm of the middle cerebral artery.

4. Even if the aneurysm itself is not visualized, segmental arterial spasm can be used to demonstrate the location of extravasated blood and the probable site of the lesion.

VII. Hypertensive Intracerebral Hemorrhage

The majority of intracerebral hemorrhages in hypertensive patients are found in the putaminal region and are secondary to rupture of one of the striate arteries. Arteriosclerosis (arteriolosclerosis, hyalinosis) is thought to play a role in this process, but "micro-aneurysms" have also been incriminated in the literature. Other sites of involvement include the thalamus, the pons, the dentate region of the cerebellum, and the subcortical layers of the cerebral hemispheres (the "atypical" hypertensive hemorrhages).

For literature, see: Bailey (1951), Bailey and Cushing (1926, 1930), Courville (1967), Henschen (1955), Kernohan and Sayre (1952), Meyer et al. (1957, 1960a, b), Penfield (1927), Rubinstein (1972), Russell and Rubinstein (1971), Tönnis (1938), Zülch (1956b – see references, 1958, 1965, 1971b, 1975), Zülch and Mennel (1974 – see references).

C. Cerebral Angiography

I. History

In 1927 EGAS MONIZ reported a new investigative technique by means of which one could inject a contrast medium into the cranial arteries and then demonstrate them radiographically. In his original description, EGAZ MONIZ called his technique "arterial encephalography", but later changed the name himself to "cerebral arteriography" (for the cerebral arteries) and "cerebral phlebography" or venography (for the veins). "Cerebral angiography" became the general term MONIZ chose to include both the venous and arterial phases. In the more than 50-year history of cerebral angiography, continuous attempts have been made to perfect this technique so that the discomforts and risks to the patient have been minimized, while the diagnostic results have been maximized. Improvements in cerebral angiography have occurred as a result of advances in three areas: the contrast medium, the injection techniques, and the X-ray technique.

Moniz's first successful angiogram was performed with a 25% sodium iodide solution which was injected into the exposed carotid artery. The use of sodium iodide, however, was discontinued after a series of bad side effects.

In 1931 Thorotrast was introduced, a 25% colloidal solution of thorium dioxide. It was notable for its high contrast and the lack of any complications during the injection. It was soon demonstrated, however, that Thorotrast could lead to capillary damage and thrombosis. An especially bad delayed side effect occurred because Thorotrast was not excreted, but was instead stored in the reticuloendothelial system where its radioactivity made it a potent carcinogenic agent. Malignant tumors of various organs began appearing from 10 to 15 years after the use of this contrast agent. For this reason Thorotrast as a contrast medium was discarded and was replaced by iodinated compounds in organic binding. The first of these to make their appearance were the di-iodinated compounds followed by tri-iodinated compounds which, because of their high content of iodine, led to a more intensive contrast.

Moniz exposed the carotid artery for the injection of the contrast agent. LOMAN and MYERSON were the first, in 1936, to inject contrast medium through a percutaneous puncture of the carotid artery. In Germany, this method was advocated by WOLFF and SCHALTENBRAND (1939).

The approach to the vertebral artery did not prove to be so simple. In 1933 MONIZ and his associates exposed the subclavian artery and injected Thorotrast in retrograde fashion to demonstrate the vertebral artery (see 1940). In 1937 SHIMIDZU achieved the same objective by percutaneous puncture of the subclavian artery. In 1940 Takahashi introduced percutaneous puncture of the vertebral artery itself as a routine method in the angiographic process.

In the 1940's, the catheter method made its appearance. RADNER described the possibility in 1947 of a catheter being inserted into the radial artery and passed to the arch of the aorta in order to demonstrate the vessels which arise there. LINDGREN (1956) devised such a procedure opacifying the vertebral artery after an injection of a contrast medium through a catheter in the femoral artery. This was made possible by the contributions of SELDINGER, who in 1953 had developed the technique named after him by inserting a percutaneous catheter into the femoral artery with the help of a guide wire.

The technique of retrograde angiography is based upon the experiences of CASTELLANOS and PEREIRAS (1939) who were able to fill the aorta with contrast medium injected in retrograde fashion through the brachial artery of a child. The technique of retrograde angiography has contributed greatly to our knowledge of pathological changes in the four major cerebral arteries and of the resultant disturbances in circulation caused by these changes.

In recent years, selective catheterization of the external carotid artery and supraselective catheterization of its branches have won wide recognition, as have embolization techniques for treatment of arteriovenous malformations and for highly vascular tumors (DJINDJIAN et al. 1969, 1970).

The contrast study of certain venous systems was the subject of interest in the 1950s. In 1951 DEJEAN and BOUDET introduced orbital venography and Fischgold and his associates in 1953 direct sinus punctures. In 1960, GEJROT and LINDBLOM described the technique of retrograde demonstration of the jugular vein.

Specialization in angiographic diagnostic techniques of the cerebral vessels from a radiological standpoint has taken place only in the last 20 years through construction of special equipment and through utilization of special radiological techniques. The significance of two-plane serial angiography was known to Moniz. Today, this area is technically as advanced as X-ray cinematography. Stereo-angiography, which was introduced as a diagnostic technique in the late 1930s, has not been widely accepted. On the other hand, after the industry had demonstrated the technical feasibility of the technique, angiotomography and magnification methods have both found many adherents (see p. 64).

One important improvement came in 1934 when ZIEDSES DES PLANTES (see 1961) described the photographic technique of subtraction (see p. 66).

II. Technique

1. Injection of the Contrast Medium

Injection of the contrast medium can take place in various ways and by various methods: through *direct puncture* of the carotid artery or of the vertebral artery, through *catheterization* of one of the four major cerebral arteries, or through *retrograde high pressure injection* into the brachial artery, known as *retrograde angiography*.

a) Puncture Methods

The Puncture of the Carotid Artery

The percutaneous puncture of the carotid artery takes place in adults under local or under general anesthesia. In children, as also in very nervous or agitated adult patients, general anesthesia is usually necessary. For the puncture, a site is chosen approximately halfway between the lower border of the mandible and the clavicle. At this level the best palpations of the distal common carotid artery are found along the medial edge of the sternocleidomastoid muscle.

The puncture itself can be difficult if the carotid artery is covered by a goiter. Goiter tissue, especially its capsule, offers considerable resistance to the cannula. In such cases, it is often necessary to go above the goiter in order to puncture the vessel. If the vessel lies further medially, that is, adjacent to the larynx, it is advisable to first inject several cc's of local anesthesia medial and dorsal to the artery. By this means the vessel is displaced laterally and anteriorly and is thus brought to a more favorable position for the puncture. An additional laterodorsal and lateral injection, as well as a subcutaneous ventral injection of anesthetic provides excellent anesthesia.

A variety of cannulas have been employed for the puncture; in Germany one developed by BUCHTALA and GERLACH (1954) has passed the test of time in that variations on its design continue to be used. It consists of a needle with a sharp and a blunt stylette. Depending on the age of the patient, different diameter needles are employed from 1 to 1.4 mm.

The puncture takes place with the neck slightly extended, as a result of which the pulsations of the carotid artery are better felt. Marked extension of the neck is not recommended since the taut platysma muscle will then interfere with palpations of the carotid artery. The index and middle finger of the left hand softly palpate the vessel in order not to compromise or irritate the carotid sinus; this is especially important in older patients. The skin is entered in an oblique direction at an angle of approximately 60° and the point of the cannula is advanced to the anterior wall of the carotid artery; the direct transfer of pulsations of the vessel points to a correct position of the needle. Then, by means of a bold forward thrust, the needle perforates the anterior wall of the carotid artery. If the needle point lies correctly within the lumen of the vessel, pulsating arterial blood will issue forth after removal of the sharp stylette. Then the blunt stylette is placed into the cannula and both are twisted so that the oblique cut of the needle point is nearly parallel to the posterior wall of the artery. In this position the tip of the needle will not rub against the vessel wall. The outer end of the needle is then lowered so that the inner end will be raised slightly within the vessel lumen and the entire cannula is advanced in a cranial direction. This maneuver may fail if the tip of the cannula has already pierced the posterior wall of the artery. If this occurs, one should withdraw the needle with the outer end still lowered until the point "pops" free into the open lumen. Then it is advanced as before. For confirmation of the correct position of the needle within the lumen, 2–3 ml of contrast medium may be injected under fluoroscopy or with a single X-ray exposure. If simultaneous demonstration of the internal carotid and external carotid arteries is desired, then the point of the cannula is left in the distal common carotid artery. If the cannula is advanced further, selective injections of either the internal carotid artery or the external carotid artery are possible.

Confirmation of a successful selective catheterization of the internal carotid artery or external carotid artery can be accomplished by again injecting small amounts of contrast. Another method is to inject 5–10 ml of Ringer's lactate rapidly. If the cannula lies within the internal carotid artery, blanching is seen in a circumscribed area of skin in the medial supraorbital territory of supply of the ophthalmic artery shortly after the injection. This is then usually followed by a transient reddening of the same area (the "frontalis test"). If the needle lies instead in the external carotid artery, the patient experiences a cold feeling in the mucous membrane of the cheek or a blanching of the cheek.

Puncture of the Vertebral Artery

Direct puncture of the vertebral artery has been largely replaced by the catheter technique. When direct puncture is used, Lindgren's method is most frequently employed. The patient's head is slightly extended so that entry to the intervertebral foramina and its resident vertebral artery is facilitated. The index and middle finger of the left hand first push the common carotid artery laterally under the sternocleidomastoid muscle. The cannula is then introduced in an oblique direction lateral to the vertebral bodies and between the costotransverse processes of C-3 and C-4 or C-4 and C-5. A pulsatile flow of blood confirms that a successful puncture has been made. Because of the anatomical position of this vessel the needle cannot be advanced further, so that the danger of an intramural or a para-arterial injection is proportionally greater. Each movement of the head will increase this danger, yet the head must be moved for the subsequent X-ray exposures. A possible complication with this method is the introduction of the cannula into the subarachnoid space with subsequent intrathecal injection of contrast medium and all its unfavorable consequences. A lightning-like pain in the neck or one radiating into the shoulder implies that the needle point has penetrated too deep and has irritated a cervical root.

An alternative method described by MASLOWSKI (1955) recommends vertebral artery puncture above the level of the atlas. The puncture site lies directly behind the mastoid process. In spite of the better possibility of advancing the needle into the artery, this procedure offers no real advantage over the method of LINDGREN (1950).

A problem which not infrequently arises to complicate the direct puncture of the vertebral artery is unilateral hypoplasia of the vessel. This more frequently affects the right vertebral artery than the left. In some cases the diameter of the vessel may not exceed 2–3 mm. Under such conditions a direct puncture of the hypoplastic vessel is not possible.

For literature, see: BUCHTALA and GERLACH (1954), LINDGREN (1950), NEWTON and POTTS (1974).

b) Catheter Techniques

Direct catheterization of the four major cerebral arteries is carried out most frequently by way of a femoral catheter. The contrast demonstration of the vertebral artery and the right carotid artery can also be accomplished through a single catheter introduced into the axillary artery. This latter method is usually employed only if the femoral catheter technique is not successful.

The Technique of Femoral Artery Catheterization

The described percutaneous introduction of a catheter into the femoral artery will follow the method of SELDINGER (1953). Under local anesthesia the femoral artery (in most cases the right) is punctured beneath the inguinal ligament with a Potts-Courmond or similar cannula. Through this cannula one inserts a twisted-spiral guide wire with a flexible end, over which the cannula is removed and the catheter introduced into the artery. After withdrawal of the guide wire, the catheter is first aspirated to remove air bubbles, then immediately irrigated with a 1:1,000 heparin solution. It is then carefully advanced under fluoroscopic control through the aortic arch to the origin of the cerebral vessels.

At present there are a variety of catheters available made from a number of different materials. One of the oldest types is the Oedman/Ledin catheter made from polyethylene tubing which is, however, comparatively stiff. Thus, it is somewhat more likely to produce an intimal tear if it encounters a vascular irregularity along the way. In recent years catheters of softer material have come onto the market. The outer surface is quite smooth with the result that the danger of thrombus formation has been dramatically reduced. These catheters may be ordered already preformed – that is, of special design for probing the individual branches of the aortic arch – or unformed, in which case the tip must be individually shaped to the desired curvature under steam heat. The preformed catheters are, as a rule, obtained in sterile packages. Otherwise, the sterilization of the catheter requires an appropriate disinfecting solution.

The catheterization of the left vertebral artery is achieved relatively easily in children and in young patients with a straight catheter, because the descending aorta and the origins of the subclavian and the vertebral arteries form almost a straight line. It is recommended, however, that the tip of the catheter be very slightly curved, for this permits a certain maneuverability through twisting to facilitate its introduction into the subclavian artery and subsequently into the vertebral artery. If the introduction of the catheter into the subclavian artery/vertebral artery does not succeed after a number of attempts, it is recommended that the exact origin of this vessel be determined under fluoroscopic control or by means of film exposure through injections of 3–4 ml of contrast medium. This determination should facilitate introduction of the catheter. Should the left vertebral artery prove to be hypoplastic, no further attempts should be made to inject it. Rather, an attempt should be made to introduce the catheter into the brachiocephalic trunk and then into the right vertebral artery for demonstration of the vertebrobasilar system. In most cases, it is first necessary to change the catheter to one with a greater bend to the tip, or to introduce into the catheter a wire probe with a bent tip, so that the catheter does not slide into the left subclavian artery but rather takes the route of the brachiocephalic trunk to the right. It is necessary to proceed in a similar fashion (contrast injections) when one is attempting to identify the left or the right common carotid arteries, as well as when one is attempting to selectively catheterize the internal carotid or the external carotid arteries. It is also possible to accomplish superselective catheterization of the branches of the external carotid by this method, when a correspondingly thin and soft catheter must be used.

In older patients, arteriosclerotic changes are found quite often on the larger vessels so that the catheters must be advanced with the greatest care in order not to break off fragments from the plaques. Occlusions of the abdominal aorta, or the iliac artery, or the femoral artery can present insurmountable obstacles.

The Technique of Axillary Artery Catheterization

If the catheterization of the vertebral artery is not successful with a femoral catheter, one may still attempt to demonstrate this vessel by means of a percutaneous catheter introduced through the axillary artery. This procedure is most successful on the right side when the tip of the catheter has a rather accentuated curve. It is successful on the left side only if the vertebral artery originates in the region of the bend of the subclavian artery. An acute origin of the left vertebral from the ascending part of the subclavian artery does not permit introduction of the catheter as a general rule.

For literature, see: NEWTON and POTTS (1974).

c) Retrograde Injection Techniques

Attempts by Moniz and Shimidzu to demonstrate the cranial vessels through contrast injections into the subclavian artery were the first indirect methods of cranial angiography. BARBIERI and VERDECCHIA (1957) first described the supraclavicular puncture, while POUYANNE et al. (1960) chose the infraclavicular route. WEIBEL and FIELDS (1963) chose a modification of the infraclavicular puncture of the subclavian artery as follows: they introduced bilateral catheters and simultaneously injected the contrast medium through a y-shaped connecting tube into both vessels. The tip of the left catheter lay in the subclavian artery, the right catheter in the brachiocephalic trunk. Approximately 30 ml of contrast medium was injected rapidly. In this fashion, very good demonstration of the right carotid artery and both vertebral arteries was accomplished. This method was, however, superseded by retrograde injection of the brachial artery.

In *retrograde angiography* by way of the brachial artery, it is desirable to perform the puncture where the pulsations of the artery are best felt. In most cases this is at the margin of the biceps muscle in the distal third of the upper arm. Here the vessel runs very superficially and is fixed by the lacertus fibrosus. This point is also distal to the origin of a number of vessels and provides for an adequate collateral circulation in case the vessel becomes occluded at the puncture site.

After sterilization of the skin and injection of a local anesthetic, the vessel is punctured with a trocar needle. The size of the lumen must be sufficient to permit rapid injection of the contrast medium. If both walls of the vessel have been perforated, then the stylette is removed and the needle pulled back until its tip lies within the lumen of the vessel. That this is so is recognized by the pulsatile flow of the arterial blood. A dull stylette is then inserted into the needle which is longer than the needle itself and so protects the wall of the vessel from

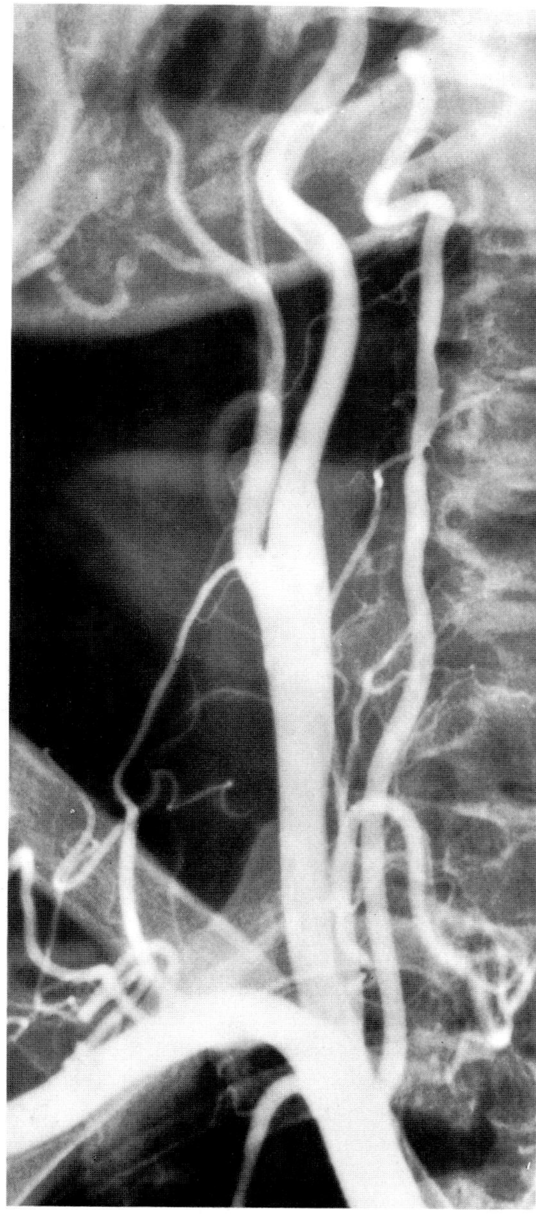

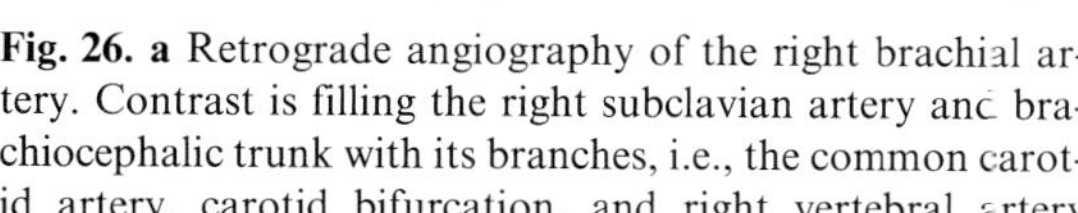

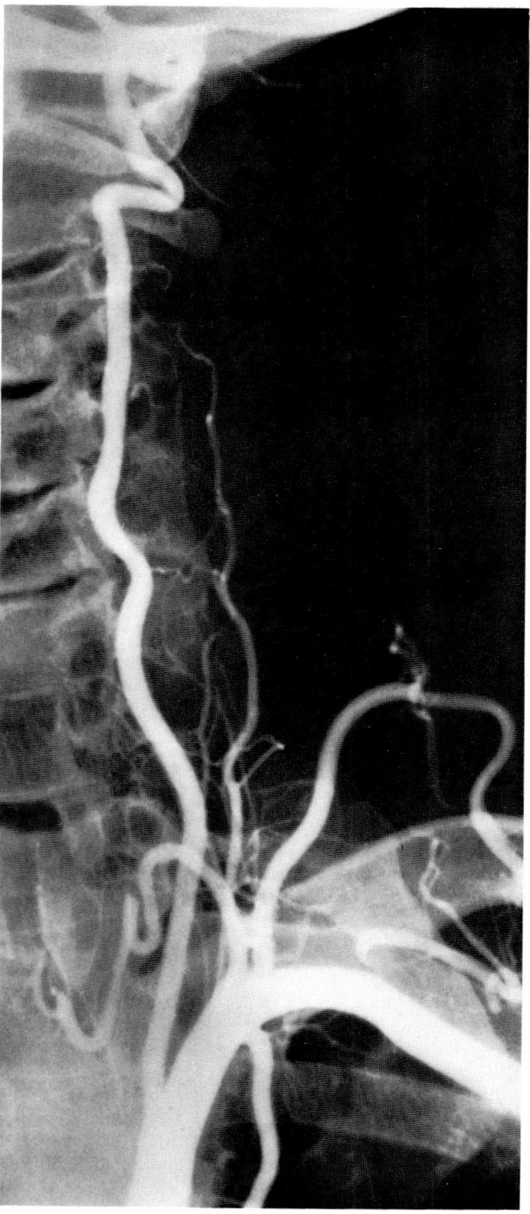

Fig. 26. a Retrograde angiography of the right brachial artery. Contrast is filling the right subclavian artery and brachiocephalic trunk with its branches, i.e., the common carotid artery, carotid bifurcation, and right vertebral artery (with two slight stenoses). **b** Retrograde angiography of the left brachial artery. Contrast is filling the left subclavian artery and its branches, including the left vertebral artery. The kinking is due to an osteophytic spur

further damage as the cannula is advanced into the brachial artery. Before the contrast medium is injected with the help of an automatic pressure injection, the peripheral brachial circulation is cut off by means of a blood pressure cuff which is pumped up to a pressure exceeding the systolic blood pressure.

The quantity of the contrast medium injected generally amounts to about 25–30 ml. The injection pressure lies between 4 and 6 atm.

Shortly after the beginning of the injection a series of X-ray exposures in the lateral and sagittal (anteroposterior) planes begins with the help of an automatic film changer.

With injections into *the right brachial artery*, the contrast medium extends back into the right subclavian artery and then into the brachiocephalic trunk. From the subclavian artery the vertebral artery may be visualized, and from the brachiocephalic trunk the common carotid artery may be visualized (Fig. 26a). By simultaneously compressing the left carotid artery, it is also possible to obtain a retrograde filling of the left-sided anterior intracranial circulation.

If, on the other hand, the route of injection is by way of the *left brachial artery,* it is only possible to demonstrate the left vertebral artery since the carotid artery on the left side rises directly from the arch of the aorta (Fig. 26b). Should the left vertebral artery not be demonstrated in this fashion, a direct origin of this vessel from the arch of the aorta may be presumed (5% of cases).

The radiographic demonstration of intracranial flow through the major vessels as well as through the smallest intracranial vessels by this method is outstanding. Similarly, a direct percutaneous contrast injection into the carotid artery or the vertebral artery is equally rewarding. Irregularities in contour of the cerebral vessels in the region of the neck are better demonstrated by the catheter technique and are more readily diagnosed as pathological changes than with the direct puncture technique and its needle artifact.

For literature, see: GOULD et al. (1955).

d) Catheter Techniques and Retrograde Angiography in Children

It is also possible in infants and children to obtain cerebral angiograms by way of the femoral catheter technique, as well as by retrograde brachial injections. Percutaneous puncture of the femoral artery is almost always successful in children after the second to third year, while it is often necessary to expose the vessel during the first year of life. Percutaneous puncture of the brachial artery in children older than three is rarely difficult, while in the first two years of life – and particularly in the first few months – it is rarely successful. It is then necessary to resort to exposure of the brachial artery in the biceps fold in the distal third of the upper arm. Following the exposure an opening is made in the vessel with an injection needle, through which a thin polyethylene catheter is inserted for a distance of 5–10 cm. In infants and young children 10–15 ml contrast medium under a pressure of 2–3 atm is injected. Upon completion of the procedure, the skin incision is closed with sutures and a pressure bandage applied over the vessel. Several complications from the angiographic study have been described, but only in children who already had brain damage. A certain percentage of cases may be complicated by thrombosis of the vessel; however, circulatory disturbances do not result from this occlusion because of the existence of a good collateral circulation.

2. The Contrast Media

For cerebral angiography at this time, the non-ionic contrast media are clearly the agents of choice. In addition to low toxicity, contrast media in cerebral angiography should be painless, should not damage the endothelium of blood vessels or penetrate the blood brain barrier, and should be well tolerated by the nervous system. The meglumine salts of iodine (at concentrations up to about 300 mg/ml) which were previously in use in Europe – and continue to be employed in the United States – fulfilled these requirements satisfactorily, but have been largely supplanted in Europe by new non-ionic contrast media. These newer agents are superior to the meglumine salts in that they are painless, the resultant endothelial injury is reduced due to the lower osmotic pressure, and neural tolerance greatly increased because of the lack of electrical charge and ions. It is hoped that these agents will also be approved for use in the United States in the not-too-distant future.

For the demonstration of the carotid system, no more than 10 ml of contrast medium is needed for a single injection. For the contrast demonstration of the vertebrobasilar system, the injection should not exceed 6–7 ml. When the contrast medium has to be injected more than once, it is advisable to pause between individual injections in order to afford the brain an adequate recovery period. The total dose of contrast medium should not exceed 40 ml in any carotid study, should be limited to 14–16 ml with a vertebral study, and should not exceed 150 ml in retrograde brachial studies.

All contrast agents result in a sensation of warmth shortly after the injection, similar to a hot flash. After introduction of the contrast medium into the ophthalmic artery, the patient may experience a sensation of light. Upon introduction of the contrast medium into the external carotid artery, the corresponding half of the face first pales and then in a few seconds turns red.

Hypersensitivity reactions after injections of a contrast medium do occur, so means for the treatment of an allergic reaction must be at hand with each study. Iodine allergy does not necessarily mean that an individual patient will react to the contrast medium itself. Since the iodine complex is bound, the hypersensitivity reaction must be directed against the entire molecular complex. The value of pretesting for sensitivity with a small amount of contrast medium is open to question, so it is not necessary that this measure be routinely employed.

3. X-Ray Technique

It is the object of cerebral angiography to give the most accurate picture possible of the cerebral arteries, capillaries, and veins, as well as their relative positions, and to provide information about their circulation time.

This objective is most satisfactorily accomplished by *two-plane serial angiography* in which laterally and sagittally (anteroposterior) directed X-ray beams are employed. Under certain conditions this study can be supplemented by axial projections. Oblique views may also be necessary in order to answer special questions.

The most effective apparatus for the production of serial angiograms has proven to be the rapid film changer. In certain situations, for example, to confirm a sinus thrombosis or an interference with the cerebral blood flow, the rate of change of the machine can be prolonged. It is recommended that alternative exposures in the corresponding sagittal and lateral frames be employed, rather than simultaneous exposure. In this fashion, two-plane angiography can be achieved with a single contrast injection in a manner which reduces the effects of scattered radiation from each beam.

To achieve the *proper position* of the head, it is practical to place the patient on height-adjustable examination table. By raising the table it is possible to extend the neck to a position which is best suited for the carotid puncture. By lowering the table after puncture with the cannula in place, it is possible to assume the position best suited for the X-ray exposures without any awkward movements. In this respect it is essential that the alignment of the head be symmetrical, for even a slight tilting of the head makes determination of the midline position of the vascular structures most difficult. In addition, the head must be fixed in this exact *symmetrical* position in order to prevent adventitious movements during the period of injection and film exposure. The simplest and most practical method of fixing the head is by means of a tape around the forehead which is fastened on either side. This mechanical device permits improvements to be made as necessary.

The X-ray beam for the *sagittal* (anteroposterior) exposure is inclined toward the feet so that the line of the beam makes an angle of 12°–15° with the German horizontal (orbitomeatal line). In this fashion, the upper margins of the petrous pyramids are projected on the roofs of the orbit or at least the upper quarter of each orbit. In older patients, flexion of the neck is more difficult, so the angle of incidence of the beams must be correspondingly increased.

In posterior fossa angiography of the vertebrobasilar system, it is necessary to assure that the vascular structures are not superimposed on the base of the skull. In order to accomplish this, the angle of the beam must be increased so that a 25° angle is made with the orbitomeatal line.

The employment of *axial* projections in cerebral angiography is only rarely indicated. It is usually for the demonstration of aneurysms which are not distinctly shown on the sagittal or lateral exposures because of superimposition of other structures. The head of the patient is maximally extended and the X-ray beam so inclined toward the head that the central beam makes an angle with the orbitomeatal line of approximately 65°–80°. For the demonstration of the vertebrobasilar system, a lesser angle is chosen than for demonstration of the carotid system.

For the angiographic clarification of anatomical relationships in the vicinity of the anterior communicating artery, as well as the region of the carotid bifurcation and origin of the ophthalmic artery, *oblique views* are frequently needed (LOEFSTEDT 1950). The head is turned about 30° to the contralateral side and the X-ray beam inclined 20° toward the feet. Should elucidation of the region of the posterior communicating artery or individual branches of the middle cerebral artery be needed, the head must be inclined 20° to the side to be studied and extended slightly (the opposite of the LOEF-STEDT position).

Cinematographic techniques in cerebral angiography are particularly useful in the study of circulatory relationships of the carotid and vertebrobasilar systems. In addition, this technique may permit demonstration of a small aneurysm superimposed on other structures by turning the head during injection of the contrast medium.

In recent years, a new technique utilizing *angiotomography* has been developed. It also has as its objective the elimination of superimposition of other structures on the desired area. Its most important application lies in the diagnosis of aneurysms, particularly the demonstration of the neck of the aneurysm. In order to demonstrate contiguous areas tomographically with a single contrast injection, simultaneous cassettes are employed. These are so constructed that several films are exposed at the same time arranged at distances of 2.5–5 mm from each other so that correspondingly different depths can be studied.

For literature, see: GOULD et al. (1955), LANG (1963), SCOTT et al. (1963), WEIBEL and FIELDS (1963).

a) Magnification Angiography

For some years now the magnification technique for cerebral angiography has been employed with great success.

A *geometric enlargement* occurs when the patient is placed in the plane of the film in the direction of the X-ray beams with the focal length to the film held constant. In this setting, the distance between the film and the head of the patient can be varied and will result in different degrees of enlargement, which can be predicted according to a magnification factor. The resulting enlargement by this technique enhances, rather than diminishes, the resolution of finer details. At the same time, there is an enhancement in terms of the contrast medium itself which results from the considerably reduced diffusion of volume. As a result of geometric magnification techniques, objects which are poorly demonstrated in the conventional films because of their small size, or because of poor resolution, can now be readily recognized on the magnification film.

With the use of a 0.3 mm focus tube, a magnification factor of 2.25 is optimum. Vessels with a lumen as small as 120 μ diameter are here clearly portrayed; however, a further increase in the magnification factor with this focus tube is not possible, since the degree of resolution diminishes abruptly beyond this point and the resulting X-ray pictures are no longer sharp. On the other hand, it is possible to increase both the resolution and the magnification factor by changing the focus tube to a 0.1 mm tube, which is the smallest available. Under these conditions a magnification factor of 4 is possible, with vessels having a lumen of 80 μ becoming clearly visible.

In addition to the geometric magnification technique described, *photographic enlargement* of the exposed film is also possible. With this photographic enlargement technique, it is also possible to obtain a definite contrast enhancement under certain circumstances as long as the films being copied show distinct contrast. Improvement in the resolution, on the other hand, cannot be achieved by this technique; nor does photographic enlargement or survey with a magnification glass offer the advantages of geometric enlargement because the grain of the film and the lines in the cassette are likewise enlarged and thus hamper recognition of detail. The geometric magnification technique is therefore clearly superior to photographic enlargement techniques.

Magnification Films in the Lateral Projection

Initially, a normal angiographic series in two planes is carried out. After evaluation of the films, the magnification technique is employed. For this, the 0.3 mm focus tube on the lateral film changer is set up at a distance of 55 cm from the vessel plane of the patient. With the X-ray tube set up at a distance of 45 cm from the same vessel plane, a magnification factor of 2.25 is achieved.

With the 0.1 mm finest focus tube, the distance between the film changer and the vessel plane is 65 cm, and the distance between the X-ray tube and the vessel plane, 35 cm. Under these conditions a magnification factor of 3 is achieved.

Since with this magnification technique only a portion of the angiogram will be visible, it is necessary to insure that the desired area is being visualized. Consequently, a preliminary

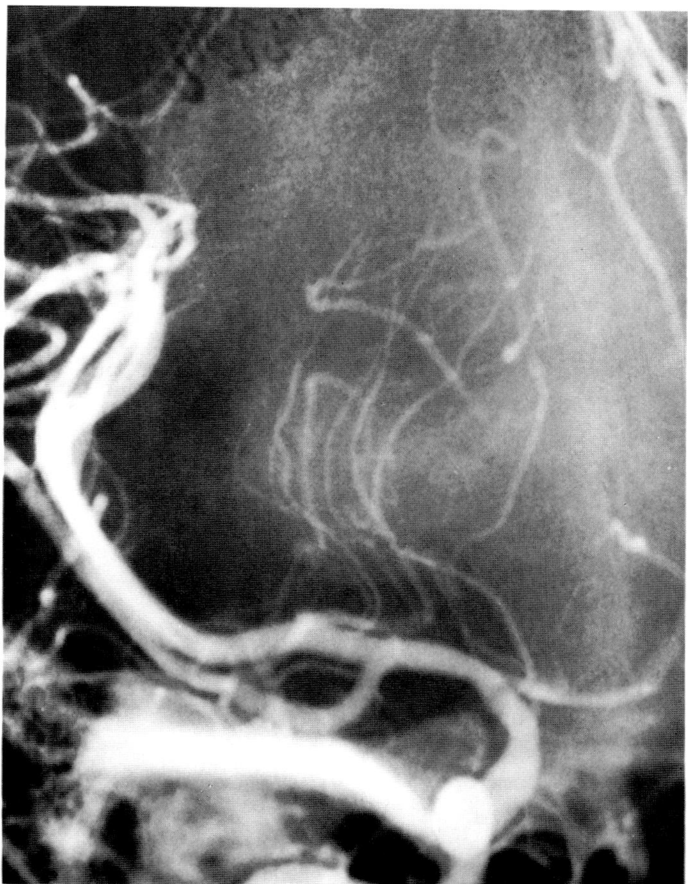

Fig. 27. Sagittal magnification angiography demonstrating microaneurysms of the lenticulostriate arteries

X-ray exposure is carried out. The preliminary exposure also permits one to estimate the optimum exposure time. Some overexposure is acceptable since this does not result in a worsening of the picture quality. Underexposure, on the other hand, results in a loss of contrast sharpness and diminishes resolution and should be avoided. It is important to insure that the magnification technique takes place without a grid.

Magnification Technique in the Anteroposterior Projection

Magnification films in the anteroposterior projection are especially valuable from a diagnostic standpoint. Successful employment of this technique, however, is dependent upon proper instrumentation to achieve a magnification factor of 3.5. A height-adjustable table is essential, as is an adjustable anteroposterior film changer. This movable changer should permit distances up to 30 cm between the vessel plane and the films to be realized. For the magnification technique, the patient table is raised in comparison to the routine angiogram, while the anteroposterior film changer is lowered. The distance between the X-ray tube (0.3 mm focus or 0.1 mm fine focus) and the vessel plane should be kept in the same relationship as in the aforementioned lateral exposures. This also goes for the distance between the vessel plane and the film changer.

What advantages result from the magnification technique?

a) Brain tumors: There is a better demonstration of pathological vessel changes, vascular lakes, and vessel fistulas (so-called arteriovenous fistulas). When there is better recognition of the details of tumor vessels, the radiographic estimate of tumor pathology is more reliable. Small tumor vessels on routine angiograms are very often hidden or not recognizable. This technique has proven to be particularly valuable with respect to proof of tumor recurrence.

b) Vessel changes: The ability to demonstrate brain vessels with a lumen of 120–300 μ by means of magnification technique is particularly advantageous. In patients with cerebral arteriosclerosis the magnification technique offers precise information about vessel irregularities, clearly distinguishing between plaques and intimal tears. In the anteroposterior view, the magnification technique shows the lenticulostriate arteries particularly clearly and permits a detailed analysis of their course which was never before possible.

The magnification technique has also proven useful in the demonstration of microaneurysms and microangiomata (Fig. 27). Through the determination of displacements in the internal auditory artery and contrast blushes in its area of supply, the diagnosis of tumors in the cerebellopontine angle has been greatly facilitated. This technique has also provided information about the vascular supply to the inner ear in patients with hearing difficulties.

Magnification Angiography Under Conditions of Hypocapnia and Hypertension

Through forced hyperventilation it is possible to lower the PCO_2 from its normal value of 38 mmHg to a value of 10–15 mmHg, which results in vasoconstriction. This vasoconstriction can be enhanced if a simultaneous induced elevation in blood pressure of 50 mmHg is brought about through intravenous infusion of a pressor agent. Vessel constriction will not occur in the pathological vessels of a tumor and these vessels stand out particularly clearly in relation to the normal constricted vessels (Fig. 28 a–c).

This modification of the magnification technique permits a more exact determination of tumor size and also allows one to more easily distinguish multiple tumors occurring in the same area (such as metastases). In any case the possibility of arriving at a pathological diagnosis of the brain tumor is enhanced. The magnification technique under hypocapnia and hypertension can effectively bring out a tumor blush which was not previously apparent, thus aiding the differential diagnosis between a brain tumor and a brain infarct. It should be emphasized, however, that the assumption essential to such a differentiation is that vessels in the region of an infarct do not lose their autoregulatory mechanisms which, however, is not true in a significant number of cases.

For Literature, see: WENDE et al. (1974).

b) Subtraction

The interpretation of the cerebral angiogram presents difficulties when the denser parts of the skull are superimposed upon the contrast-filled vessels. It is possible in these situations, by means of a subtraction technique, to obtain better demonstration of these vessels.

The subtraction technique was introduced to the field of roentgenology in 1934 by ZIEDSES DES PLANTES (see 1961). The principle of this technique is to erase, as it were, the bony structure of the skull by projecting two films on top of each other – one taken *prior* to the injection and the other *during* the actual injection of the vessels. This procedure involves reversing a positive to a negative image and can be carried out by photographic as well as by electronic means.

The Technique of Photographic Subtraction

First, a plain skull X-ray is made in the projections desired. This reference film, however, should not be taken until after the vessel has been punctured and the head fixed in position since it is essential that the position of the skull be unchanged in both the contrasted and non-contrasted films. In place of the reference film, it is also possible to use the first picture of the angiographic series itself. Following this, a reversal of the plain X-rays is produced as follows: the plain film together with a special film is fixed in a copier and is exposed to bright light. This results in the creation of a so-called complementary diapositive. This complementary diapositive must precisely overlie the bony structure of the selected picture from the angiographic series and it too is placed in the copier with a special film.

If the bony structures on the plain X-ray are too dense, the subtraction pictures will not be optimal. In such cases another secondary diapositive copy is prepared. In this situation the plain X-ray and the original complementary diapositive are copied overlying each other. The resulting double diapositive is placed together with the original diapositive and with the film containing the injected vessels, each superimposed on the other. This combination, when copied with the proper film, results in the desired subtracted film.

It is also possible to use a later phase of the angiogram instead of a plain X-ray for subtraction purposes, so that the arterial phase can be contrasted with the venous phase in the same film. In this situation the vessels are represented in opposite black and white tones, whereas the

Fig. 28 a–c. Frontal metastatic carcinoma: **a** routine lateral angiogram; **b** the same patient with magnification technique (normal ventilation); **c** magnification angiography of the same patient with hyperventilation

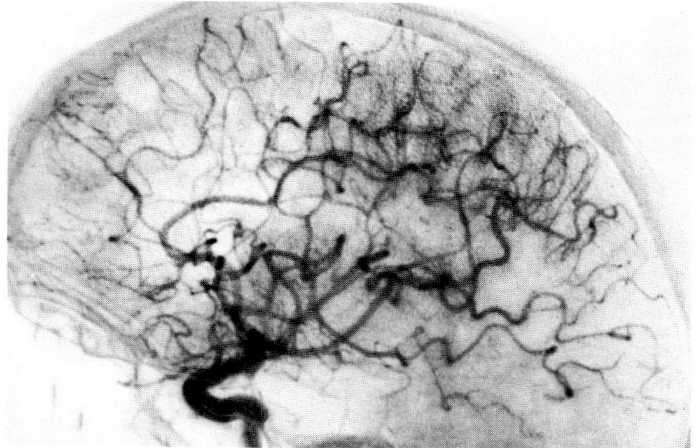

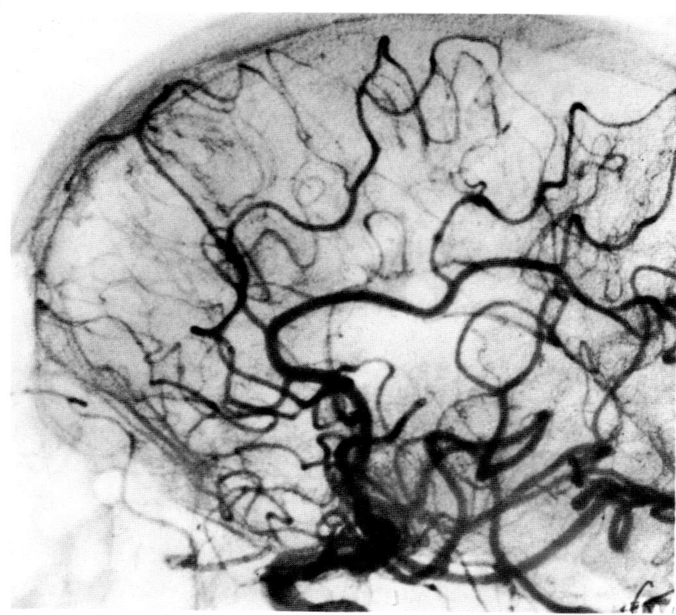

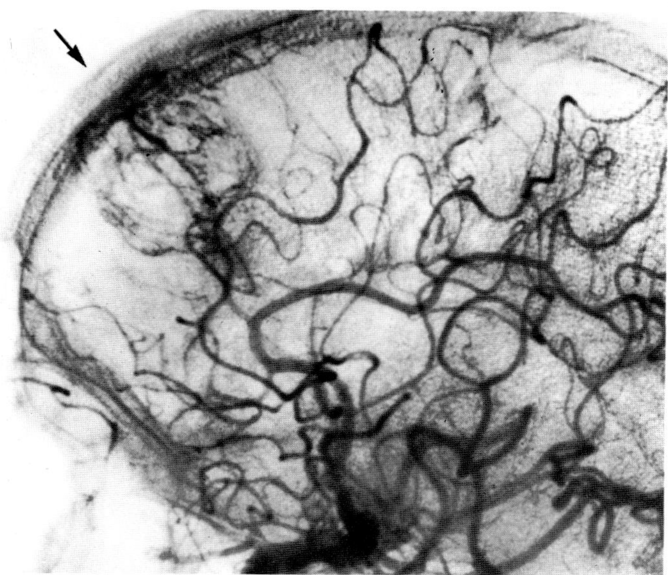

bony structures are erased as with the earlier techniques.

A rapid subtraction is also possible electronically with a supplementary technical display panel. Here the subtraction technique is performed electronically with the machine, using a regular copy of one picture and a reversed copy of the contrasted image of the other in order to produce the subtraction picture on the monitor. After the image has been obtained, it can be photographed by means of a Polaroid camera for preservation as a permanent document if this is desired.

Advantages of This Technique

All vessel segments which are ordinarily superimposed over bony structures can be better demonstrated with the subtraction technique, especially the sinus structures and smaller arteries in the posterior cranial fossa, arteriovenous malformations at the base of the brain, carotid-cavernous fistulae, tumors of the base of the skull, orbital tumors, details of the intraosseus siphon segment of the internal carotid artery, the vertebral arteries, the basilar artery, collateral circulation in association with occlusion of the internal carotid artery, and so on.

For literature, see: ZIEDSES DES PLANTES (1961).

Digital Vascular Imaging

Recently a new angiographic method using computers has been developed which does not require arterial puncture or direct arterial injection of the contrast agent. Instead, a simple intravenous injection of contrast medium is carried out and the ill-defined contrast images of the vessels to be studied enhanced with a computer so that differences in density of 1% can be detected. This technique, called Digital Vascular Imaging (DVI) or Digital Enhanced Angiography, is dependent upon subtraction of non-contrasted structures as well as computer-assisted enhancement of the contrasted images, all of which have been converted to electrical signals by a photoelectric receiver. Thus, the subtraction and the enhancement are both carried out electronically and the need to develop and superimpose X-ray films is eliminated.

The procedure is carried out simply by first exposing the desired area prior to contrast injection, and then by obtaining additional exposures after contrast injection. The computer subtracts all but the contrasted images and enhances subtle differences in contrast concentration so that excellent resolution is achieved.

With this technique, both extracranial and intracranial vessels as small as 1 mm in diameter may be visualized. It has been particularly valuable in the study of the extracranial cerebral vasculature in the neck (arteriosclerotic stenoses and ulcerations), but may also be of benefit in demonstrating intracranial vascular occlusions, aneurysms, AVMs, and vascular tumors.

The need to avoid any form of motion (such as swallowing) for prolonged periods is a minor disadvantage, but is clearly outweighed by the numerous advantages of this technique, particularly reduction in risk to the patient in comparison to standard angiography. In fact, Digital Vascular Imaging can be performed on an outpatient basis with no premedication or followup care necessary.

4. Dangers and Complications of Cerebral Angiography

Cerebral angiography is not entirely without risk, so each patient should be informed about possible complications for medicolegal purposes. The incidence of complications in the literature varies from 0.2% to 4.5%. This not insignificant variation in side effects may be ascribed in part to the fact that the statistical samples were dissimilar (some patients being more at risk than others) and in part to variations in the skill and experience of the physician performing the procedures. For example, patients with disturbances of cerebral blood flow are more at risk than those with normal circulatory relationships, assuming both are being studied for a similar disease process (see p. 136).

Complications can result from the *anesthetic agents,* from the *puncture* and *injection process,* and from the *contrast medium* itself. Pains at the puncture site or radiating into the jaw should not be considered as a complication, nor should a slight swallowing difficulty, a transient hoarseness, or temporary enlargement of the pupil.

Anesthetic complications will not be discussed in great detail here; however, it must be emphasized that the *injection* of even small amounts of *local anesthetic* into the *carotid artery* can result in a seizure. In such situations, the study must be terminated immediately. Instances of this kind can be avoided if aspiration is carried out before each injection of local anesthetic to verify that the needle does not lie within the lumen of the carotid artery.

In patients with a *hypersensitive carotid sinus* reflex even minimal manipulation of the carotid sinus can result in signs and symptoms of circulatory collapse. With older patients in particular, attempts should be made to limit palpation of the carotid artery to a minimum.

Of far greater consequence than the complications cited above are those which may follow incorrect puncture of the carotid artery or the vertebral artery. If the intima of the rear wall of the artery has been damaged or torn by the point of the cannula, a dissecting aneurysm may well follow. If the point of the cannula has penetrated the intima, a subintimal deposition of injected contrast medium or irrigating solution may follow, which can result in an arterial occlusion. Such an intramural injection may cause transient signs and symptoms, but may also result in permanent paralysis. This complication can be avoided if the cannula has a short polished end and is advanced only after a blunt stylette has been inserted. Intimal injuries can also be caused by the advancing tip of an intravascular catheter, especially if this is made of rigid material. It is, therefore, recommended that only flexible disposable catheters be used of the sort which have come on the market in the last few years. Similarly, the tip of the wire probe should also be flexible.

Both the puncturing cannula and the intravascular catheter can dislodge fragments of the arteriosclerotic plaque and can disperse these throughout the bloodstream.

The *para-arterial contrast injection* is less important since there is no danger of interruption of the carotid artery blood flow. Nonetheless, it is quite painful.

To verify the *correct position* of the injection cannula as well as the catheter, test injections of 2–3 ml contrast medium are often employed.

Both the cannula and the catheter act as sites for *thrombus* formation, particularly when either of them remains for a long time within the artery. The danger of dissemination of thrombus material is increased when multiple injections of contrast are necessary. As a precaution the cannula or catheter should be irrigated at frequent intervals with a heparinized solution.

If a relatively thick catheter is introduced into a narrow artery, the lumen of the artery may be partially or totally occluded. As a consequence, circulatory disturbances in the territory of supply of this artery may result. A relatively thick catheter, as well as a proportionately stiff cannula, can result in *spasm* of the artery under examination (see Fig. 109).

Complications, and particularly permanent injuries resulting from the *contrast medium,* have become much less frequent in comparison to earlier years because of advances in the contrast media available, particularly the newer nonionic agents which are much less dangerous than the sodium salts formerly employed. Injuries which have occurred result from disturbances in the permeability of the blood brain barrier, which is based upon changes in the permeability of the endothelium and in the acid-base balance. Edema and punctate hemorrhages in the brain have been described. Hypersensitivity reactions are rare but must be dealt with promptly when they occur. Medication for treatment of shock should be available at all times. When there is a marked slowing in the circulation, the amount of contrast medium used should be significantly reduced since the possibility exists that a larger bolus of contrast medium would worsen the cellular hypoxia which is presumed to be present and could lead to further injury.

After *vertebral angiography* transient blindness has been reported lasting up to 24 h. The incidence of this complication is reduced if the catheter is withdrawn immediately from the artery at the end of the injection of contrast medium, which permits a rapid clearing of the contrast substance from the vertebrobasilar system by replacing it with normal blood. It has become accepted that this complication is entirely due to effects of the contrast agent on the visual cortex itself.

Transient blindness has also been reported after retrograde brachial artery angiography. This technique has been known to result in transient irritation of the median nerve as well. A more important side effect, however, is the loss of the radial pulse for a period of hours following the procedure which may indicate the presence of a thrombus at the puncture site, an indication for surgical intervention. A similar situation can exist at the puncture site into the femoral artery as well as into the axillary artery for catheter studies, and is again indicated by the loss of the distal pulse in the hours immediately following the procedure. For literature, see: WENDE et al. (1974).

III. The Normal Cerebral Angiogram

The circle of Willis forms a ringlike series of anastomoses between the vertebrobasilar system and both internal carotid systems. Nonetheless, each internal carotid artery generally maintains its own half of the brain. Under normal conditions the circle of Willis is only a potential source of anastomoses.

Serial angiography (Fig. 29, 30) not only provides information about the anatomical relationships of the cerebral vessels, but also permits conclusions to be drawn about the flow of blood through them. An important measurement in this regard is the estimation of the circulation time which in the pathological state can be significantly impaired. Such changes may be seen locally or more generally. The most precise estimate of circulation requires the use of radioisotopes, but cerebral angiography can be used as an acceptable alternative if certain parameters affecting circulation time are held constant. According to GREITZ (1956), the normal circulation time measured with ^{131}I is 4.13 s. Values estimated from the angiogram are less accurate since they depend on the size of the bolus and concentration of the contrast medium, and on the accuracy of the starting point and endpoint of the measurement, which can be affected by the time required for injection of the contrast medium. Some authors estimate the circulation time as the interval between the beginning of the injection and the end of the venous phase, while others use the interval between the entrance of contrast medium into the carotid siphon and its disappearance from the veins. On average, these values fall in the range of 7–8 s. In these evaluations, the program selector which fixes the frequency of film exposures should be used to facilitate the determinations (see p. 63).

In children, the circulation time is faster than in later years. Slowing of the circulation – that is, a prolongation of the circulation time – is found in association with increased intracranial pressure. A local increase in circulation occurs in all forms of arteriovenous shunts regardless of whether they are caused by tumors or by arteriovenous malformations. The danger presented by the contrast medium itself, in the presence of localized changes in the circulation time caused by cerebrovascular disease, has been discussed on p. 139.

In order to facilitate interpretation of the films, it is important to project the various planes beside each other and in every case to determine which vessel segments in the anterior and the lateral views correspond. In this regard the original nomenclature of individual vessel branches proposed by FISCHER (1938, 1939; later called FISCHER-BRÜGGE) can be used to great advantage. Even if these designations are not always those employed by the skilled diagnostician, they will undoubtedly help the beginner to gain a general understanding of the angiogram as a whole and to facilitate the analysis of the pictures in a systematic fashion. In the following pages, these designations will be extensively employed in the interpretation of the normal cerebral angiogram.

a) The Arterial Phase of the Internal Carotid Artery Angiogram

With injection of a contrast medium into the internal carotid artery, not only is the internal carotid artery itself visualized but also the ophthalmic artery, the anterior choroidal artery, the anterior cerebral artery, and the middle cerebral artery on the same side. It is dependent on the anatomical arrangement of the circle of Willis and on the hemodynamic conditions in effect at the time of the injection whether the anterior communicating artery (with the anterior cerebral artery of the opposite side) and the posterior communicating artery (with the posterior cerebral artery of the same side) are filled in addition (Fig. 31a and b). A totally closed circle of Willis appears in about 20%–30% of cases. In approximately 70%–80%, individual segments of the circle of Willis are hypoplastic or even aplastic. This can affect the anterior and posterior communicating arteries, as well as the pars circularis of the anterior cerebral artery, and the posterior cerebral artery (see p. 140). For this reason, the anterior cerebral artery is occasionally not visualized, a situation which should not lead one to erroneously assume it is occluded. Contrast viewing of the anterior cerebral artery by way of a hypoplastic pars circularis can be demonstrated in most cases through compression of the opposite carotid artery. In a similar manner, visualization of the anterior communicating artery can also be frequently achieved (Fig. 32).

Lateral Projections

In the lateral projections (Fig. 33) the internal carotid artery can be seen in the region of the neck as a broad band. In some variants it is stretched taut and in others twisting and winding to such an extent that definite loops are sometimes formed as it makes its way to the base of the skull. Here it turns horizontally and enters the carotid canal of the temporal bone. This segment of the internal carotid artery is known as the "canal segment". At this point the carotid artery rises superiorly to the body of the sphenoid (C-5). This portion of the artery is, for the most part, covered laterally by the Gasserian ganglion, for which reason it has been designated the "ganglion segment". At the end of this segment the artery bends again in horizontal fashion into the cavernous sinus (C-4) and then penetrates the dura, reversing its course and turning sharply in an occipital direction. It then proceeds posteriorly and horizontally, or with a slight incline, as it passes over the dorsum sellae. This portion of the internal carotid artery which describes a tight curve and projects itself at about the level of the sella (C-4 to C-2) is called the "carotid siphon segment". This segment can also be broken down into an infraclinoid or *"cavernous segment"* (C-4), a *"carotid knee"* (C-3) and a supraclinoid or *"cisternal segment"* (C-2). The siphon segment can show rather impressive variations.

While in the neck the internal carotid artery gives off no branches, in the cavernous sinus there are usually some small twigs to the Gasserian ganglion and to the hypophysis. These are usually so fine that they are seen only on subtraction views. From this segment the thin meningeal branches to the tentorium also arise and become clearly visible when there is a tumor on the tentorium or lying adjacent to the tentorium. Tumors and AVMs in this region lead to hypertrophy of these arteries, which have been named after BERNASCONI and CASSINARI (Fig. 34).

There are variants which depend upon the persistence of embryonic vessels, such as *anastomoses* between the internal carotid artery and the basilar artery. The *primitive trigeminal artery* connects the cavernous segment of the internal carotid artery and the basilar artery (Fig. 35). It lies for the most part in an extradural location and enters the intracranial space through the dura only at the clivus. The *primitive acoustic artery* connects the canal segment of the internal carotid artery with the basilar artery, while the *primitive hypoglossal artery* runs from the cervical portion of the internal carotid through the canal of the hypoglossal nerve and then empties into the basilar artery.

After the siphon, the internal carotid artery ends in its terminal segment (C-1), which runs superiorly and finally divides into the anterior cerebral (A-1) and middle cerebral (M-1) arteries. These vessel segments – C-1, A-1, and M-1 – comprise the carotid bifurcation or *carotid fork,* a literal designation of its appearance on the anteroposterior projection.

The first regularly visible side branch of the internal carotid artery is the *ophthalmic artery.* It arises from the upper portion of the knee of the carotid siphon and projects itself on the anterior clinoid process. It is between 1.8 and 2.2 mm in diameter. It enters the orbit through the optic foramen where it is initially found under the optic nerve. In its further course, it runs laterally and superiorly to the optic nerve until it reaches the medial upper quadrant of the orbit. In the lateral projection, it is possible to distinguish a proximal, a middle, and a distal segment. The middle segment extends from the origin of the first branches of the ophthalmic artery to the choroid layer of the eye, which in 80% of cases is visible as a delicate curvilinear layer of contrast. An accurate study of the distal ramifications of the ophthalmic artery is only possible on subtraction views.

The *posterior communicating artery* arises from the next portion of the internal carotid artery, as it proceeds posteriorly (near the junction with the terminal segment). The length and caliber of this vessel vary significantly. It forms a basal convex curve but is only demonstrated in approximately 20%–30% of the cases, depending upon anatomical relationships and flow dynamics. Its caliber is, for the most part, smaller than the posterior cerebral artery. It can, however, also be similar in size to the posterior cerebral artery when this latter artery originates directly from the internal carotid artery (embryonal origin – approx. 20%–30% of cases). The common infundibular dilatation of the posterior communicating artery at its origin from the internal carotid should not be confused with an aneurysm. There are also a number of other fine branches which supply

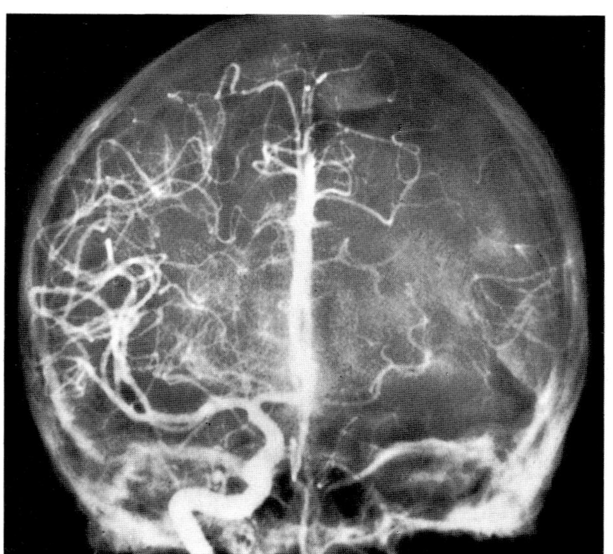

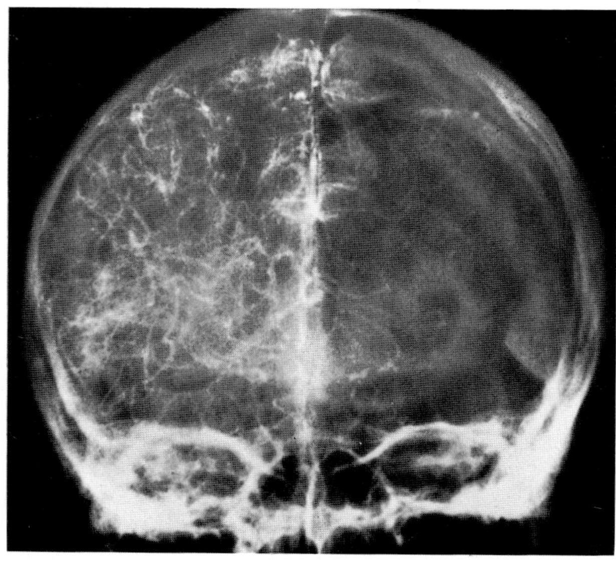

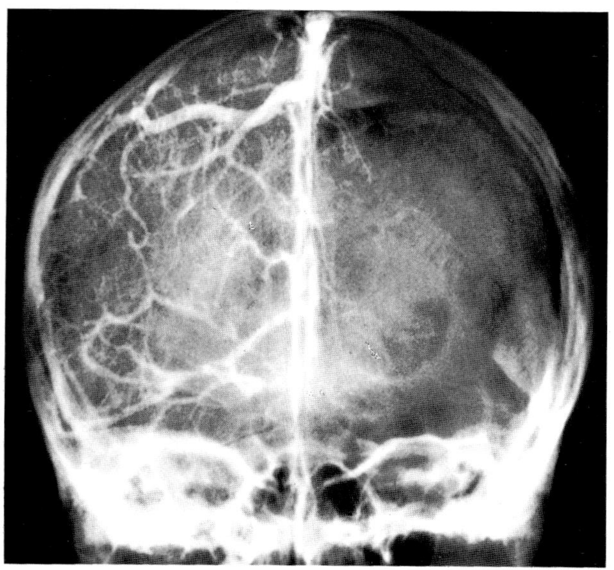

Fig. 29a–c. Normal anteroposterior view of a serial angiogram of the right internal carotid artery: **a** arterial phase; **b** capillary phase; **c** venous phase

Fig. 30a–c. Lateral views of the sequence in Fig. 29a–c

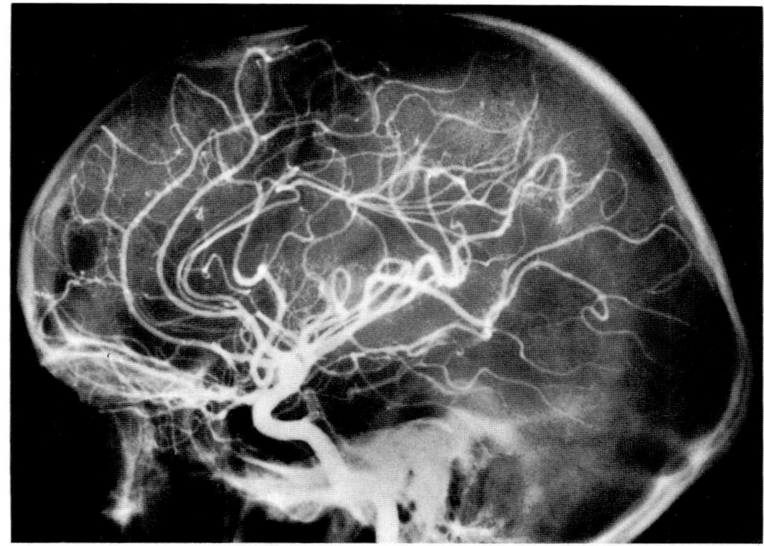

a

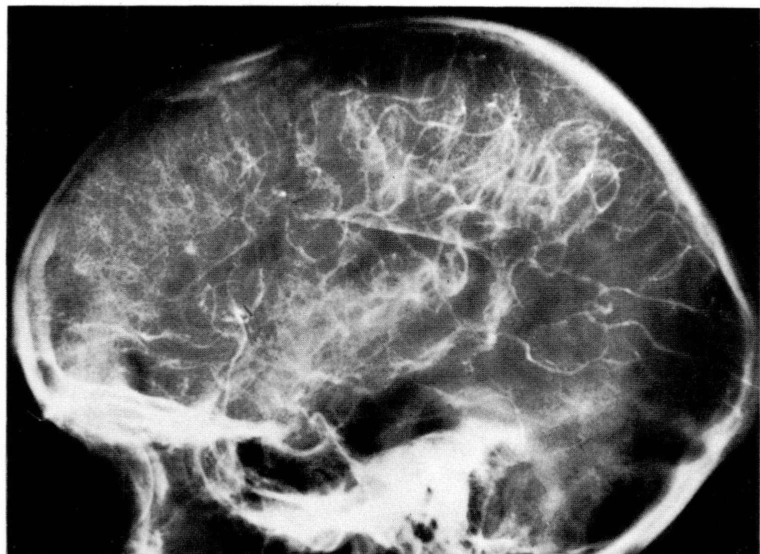

b

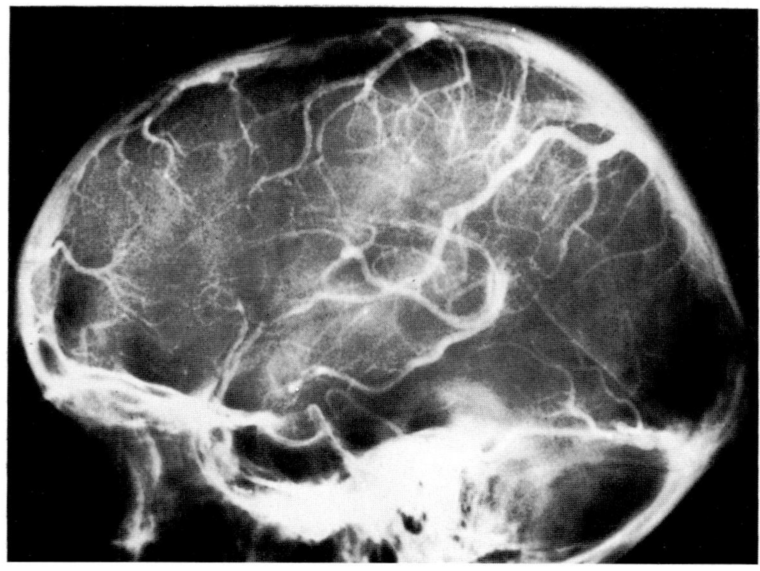

c

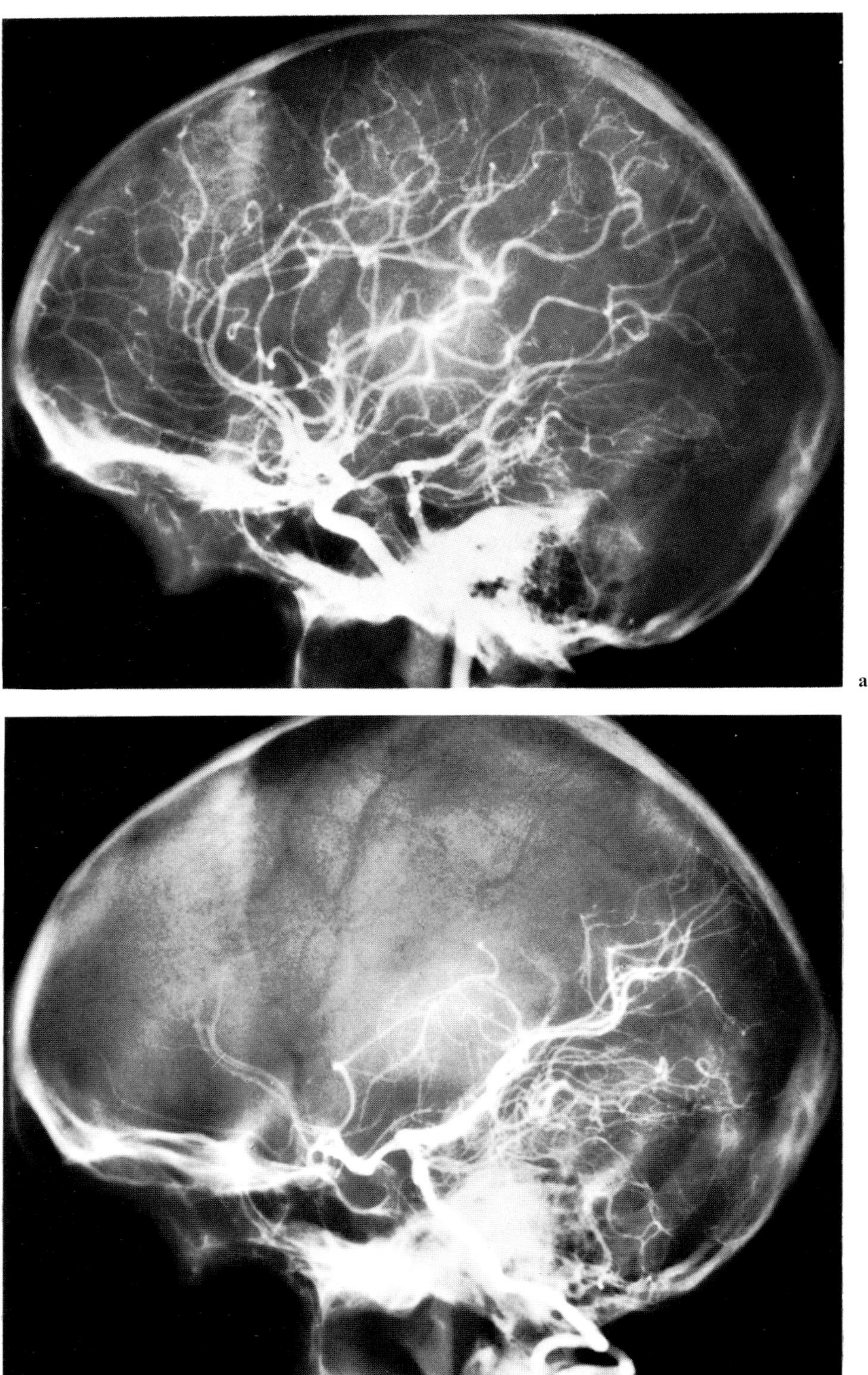

Fig. 31 a, b. Angiography of the right internal carotid artery (**a**) and vertebral artery (**b**) in the same patient. The posterior communicating artery will fill with contrast medium from either side, depending upon the effective pressure gradient within the internal carotid artery system or the vertebrobasilar system at the time of the study period

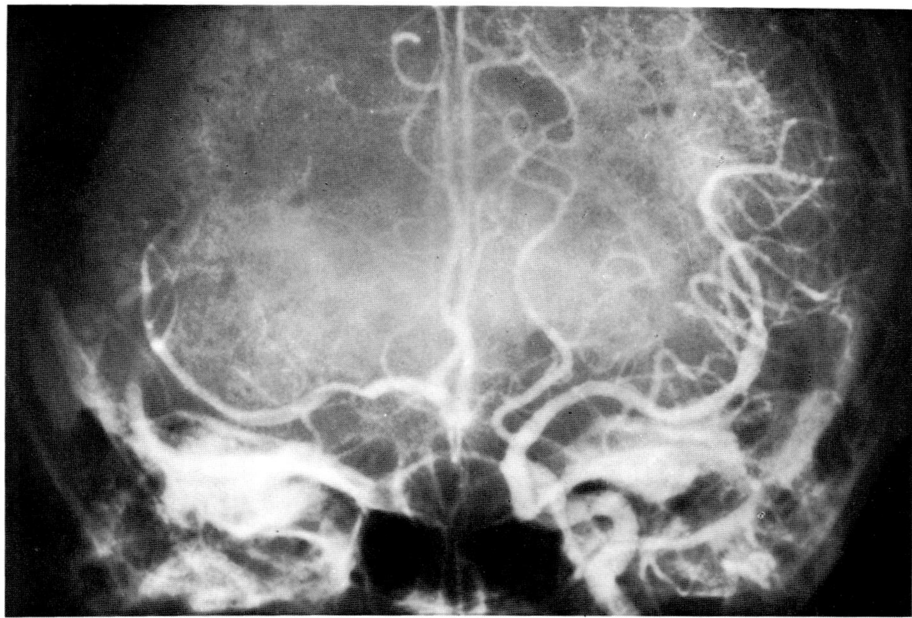

Fig. 32. Despite hypoplasia of the pars circularis of the left anterior cerebral artery, the right carotid system (because of right internal carotid occlusion) is filling via the anterior communicating ramus

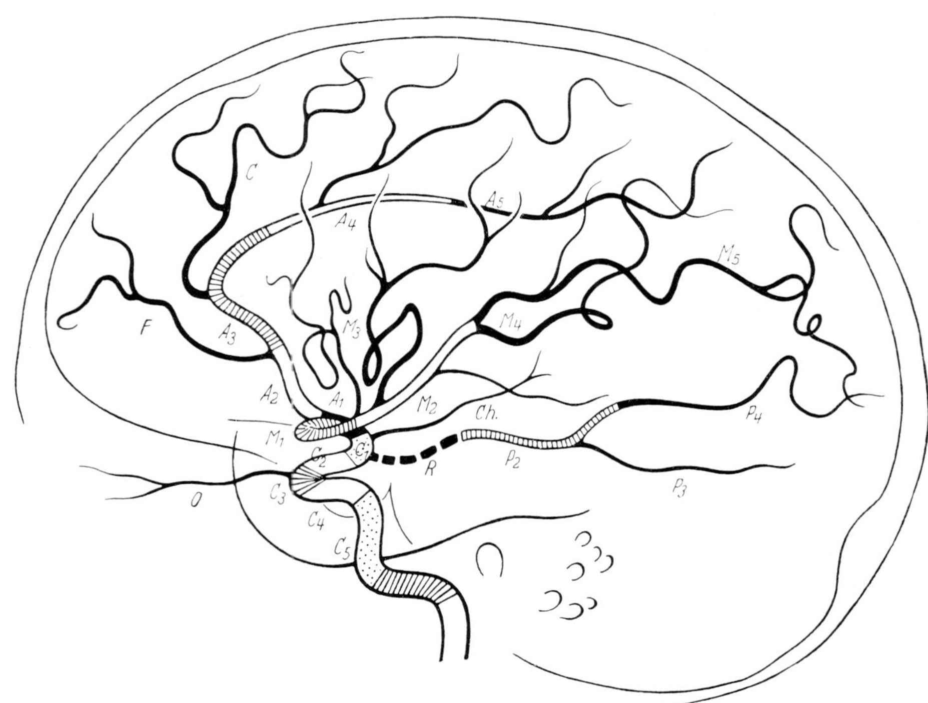

Fig. 33. Schematic representation of the internal carotid arteriogram from the lateral view (see also Fig. 30a–c)

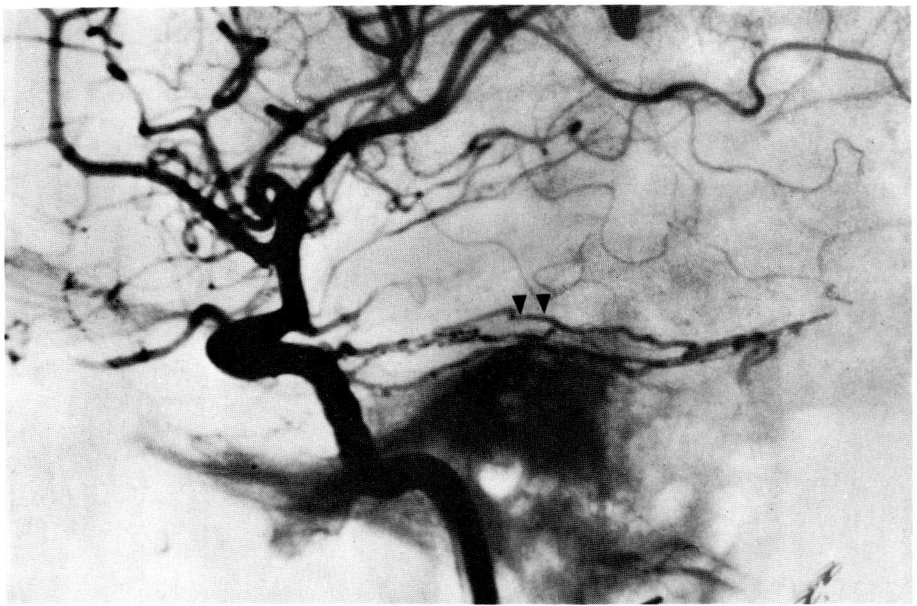

Fig. 34. Hypertrophy of the artery of Bernasconi and Cassinari (*arrows*) with an AVM in the tentorial region (postoperative state)

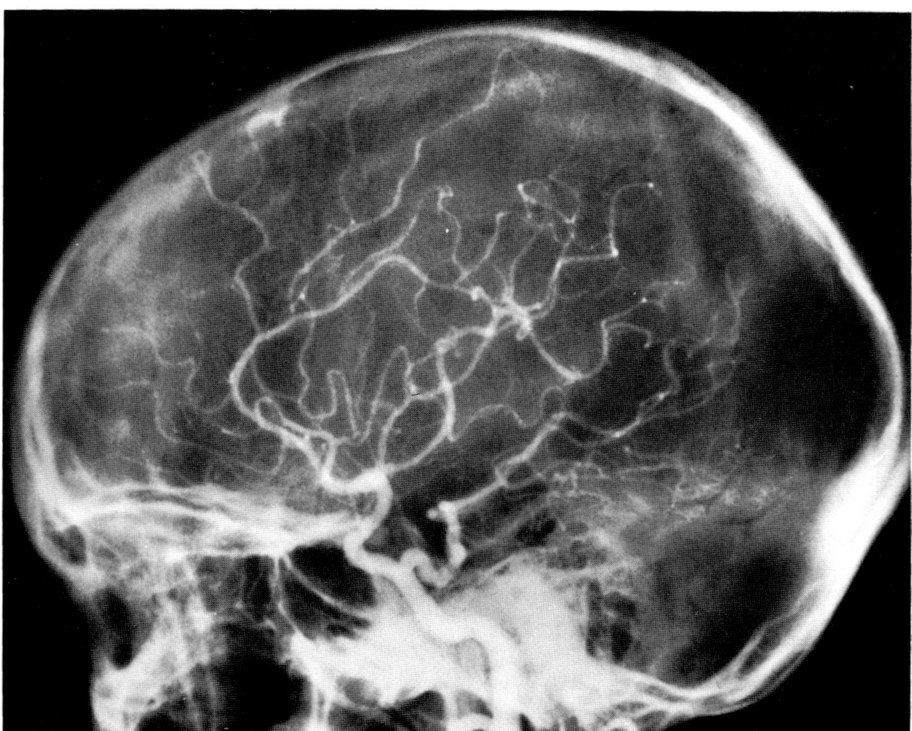

Fig. 35. Primitive trigeminal artery

the chiasm, the oculomotor nerves, the hypothalamus, and the deep nuclei.

A few millimeters beyond the origin of the posterior communicating artery is the next branch of the internal carotid, the *anterior choroidal artery*. It may also originate from the most distal portion of the internal carotid, or from the initial segment of the middle cerebral artery. It runs initially in a basal direction and then in a shallow, upwardly concave curve in the direction of the choroid glomus where it rises rapidly, becoming less visible in the process. Anastomoses are common with branches of the posterior choroidal artery as it supplies portions of the internal capsule, the basal ganglia and thalamus, and the choroid plexus of the temporal horn.

The carotid bifurcation into the anterior cerebral and middle cerebral arteries is not apparent on the lateral projection of the carotid arteriogram because of superimposition of the initial segment of the middle cerebral artery. An "open" bifurcation alleviates this problem and is seen in association with pathological mass displacements or in cases of poor positioning of the head.

After the *anterior cerebral artery* arises from the internal carotid artery, it initially continues in a medial, horizontal, and slightly rostral direction. This segment is known as the "chiasmal segment" of the anterior cerebral artery, or the *pars circularis* (A-1). In the lateral projections, portions of the anterior cerebral artery are usually superimposed upon the origin of the middle cerebral artery. Next, the anterior cerebral artery describes a mildly S-shaped curve which is known as the "orbital segment". Initially it runs in a basal convex and then basal concave (A-2) fashion following the rostrum of the corpus callosum, and then turns sharply in an occipital direction (A-3). This is known as the knee of the pericallosal artery, or the epicallosal artery, or the artery of the corpus callosum. The further course of this artery on the surface of the corpus callosum is known as the "callosal segment" (A-4).

The frontobasal artery arises in the region of the *orbital segment* of the anterior cerebral artery and supplies the medial basal surface of the frontal lobe. Further distally, usually proximal to the knee of the pericallosal artery, are found two larger branches – the frontopolar artery and the callosomarginal artery. The first runs to the frontal pole; the second, whose ori-

gin is variable, runs initially parallel to the dorsal segment of the pericallosal artery in the cingulate sulcus in an occipital direction, and then rises to the margin of the cortical surface. After giving off several variable branches, it loses itself in the parietal region as the terminal segment of the anterior cerebral artery (A-5) Heubner's recurrent artery is not visible. The terminal segment of the pericallosal artery sometimes appears displaced because it runs occipitally in an inferior direction. Such a course should not suggest vascular displacement. If the anterior cerebral artery of the other side is also visible, both vessels should run side by side, albeit superimposed upon one another.

The lateral exposure of the *middle cerebral artery* is intelligible only if one keeps the anatomical course of this vessel in mind (refer to Figs. 33, 36, and 37). After its origin from the internal carotid artery, the middle cerebral artery (which is the lateral branch of the carotid fork), runs laterally and horizontally in the Sylvian fissure with a slight posterior curve behind the sphenoid wing. This is the "sphenoid wing segment". As it progresses further into the depths of the Sylvian fissure, it takes a more posterior and superior course and rises toward the parietal cortex. This is called the "insular segment". Finally, it divides in the posterior portion of the insula or on the temporoparietal surface into its terminal branches.

On the lateral angiogram the sphenoid wing segment of the middle cerebral artery (M-1) runs in an anterograde fashion. Because of this, the vessel appears to form a blind loop running from the carotid bifurcation anteriorly and somewhat posteriorly. The delusion of the "blind" loop is achieved as the vessel forms a curve, the superior portion of which represents the proximal sphenoid wing segment. The picture is complicated still further by the fact that the sphenoid wing segment is also superimposed on the pars circularis of the anterior cerebral artery (A-1). Clearly visible on the lateral projection is the insular segment (M-2) and the terminal branches of the middle cerebral artery (M-3, M-4, and M-5). The *insular segment* consists of two or three, and occasionally many more, branches which run as a bundle in the parietal direction. This group of vessels is referred to as the *Sylvian vessel group*. The axis of this vessel group is usually represented by a line connecting the foramen incisivum of the maxilla with the anterior clinoid process. This

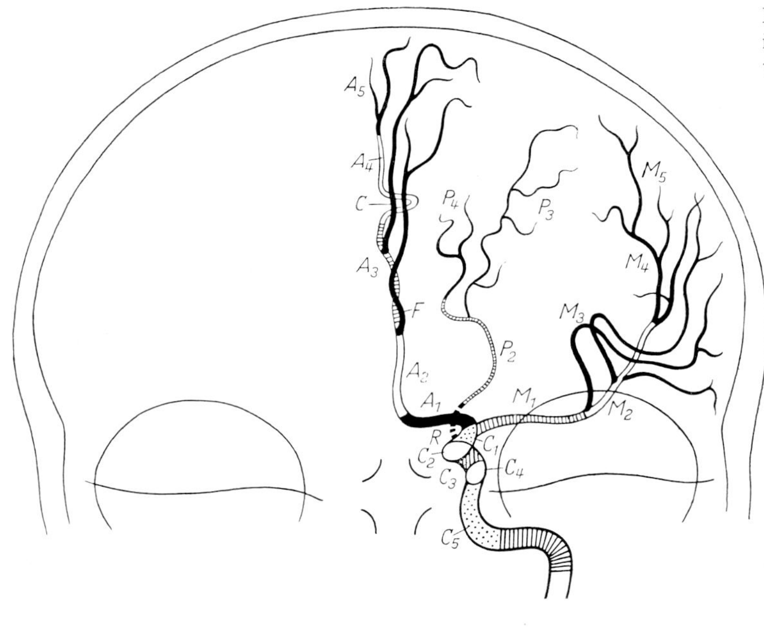

Fig. 36. Schematic representation of the internal carotid arteriogram from the anteroposterior view (see also Fig. 29a–c)

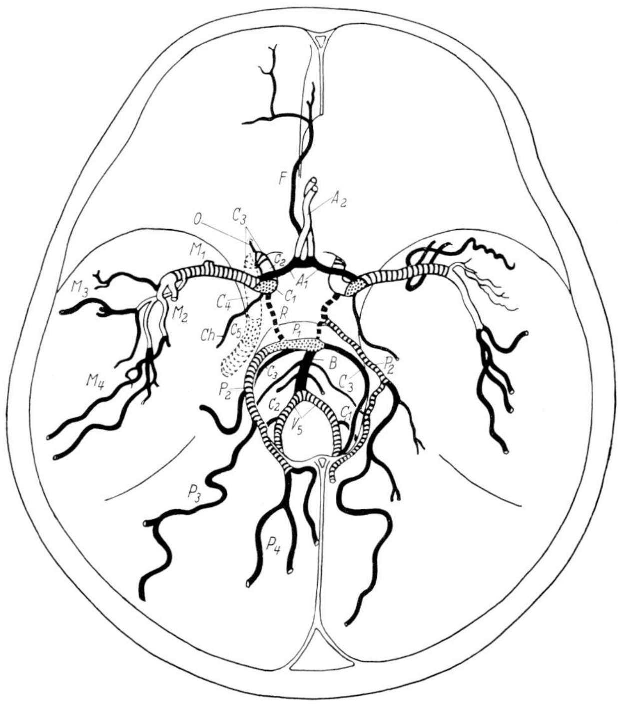

Fig. 37. Schematic demonstration of the blood vessels at the base of the brain. Each vessel is numbered as in Figs. 33, 36, 42, 43, and 44 (because of the combined presence of both carotid and vertebral branches, the letter *C* is used here to depict the "carotid" as well as the "cerebellar" arteries)

line ordinarily forms an angle of approximately 60° with the axis of the base of the skull.

The *terminal ramifications* of the middle cerebral artery vary considerably from individual to individual. With relative frequency, it is possible to differentiate three major branches: The most superior is the posterior parietal artery, the middle is the artery of the angular gyrus, and the inferior is the posterior temporal branch. Even more variable are the branches to the frontal and parietal operculum (the ascending arteries of the M-3 segment). These are known as the orbital artery, the frontal artery, and the parietal arteries. The branches running inferiorly out of the Sylvian fissure are the temporal arteries (anterior and middle), while the fine branches to the deep nuclei (basal ganglia and thalamus) arising from the sphenoid wing segment (the medial and lateral lenticulostriate arteries) are mostly hidden on the lateral exposure by the insular segment of the middle cerebral artery. Only when this insular segment is displaced or occluded are the lenticulostriate branches clearly visible.

The Anterior Projection

On the anteroposterior view (Fig. 36) the *internal carotid artery* appears in the *neck* initially as a more or less vertical band which then turns in a medial direction and runs horizontally until the *carotid canal* is reached. In the next segment, known as the *ganglion segment* (C-5), it rises vertically to the cavernous sinus. The next few centimeters form the siphon segment (C-4 to C-2). Since this segment is also usually vertical and in the direction of the X-ray beams, it appears foreshortened and is recognizable only as a slight curvature or thickening of the band of contrast (this should not be confused with an aneurysm). The ophthalmic artery, which projects anteriorly in a sagittal plane and runs only slightly in a lateral direction, is poorly evaluated in this projection. It is, however, possible to demonstrate it quite well by means of an orbital projection with the head gently reclined so that the upper edge of the petrous pyramid projects on the lower rim of the orbit. *The terminal segment* of the internal carotid artery (C-1) runs for 1–2 cm in a posterior direction, although with a slightly lateral tendency, to end by dividing into the initial segments of the anterior cerebral and middle cerebral arteries (A-1 and M-1). The sudden divergence of these two vessels medially and laterally in a different plane from the sagittal meanderings of the internal carotid artery is striking and is aptly described in the German literature as the *carotid fork* (carotid bifurcation).

The first segment of the *anterior cerebral artery* – the *pars circularis* or the *chiasmal segment* – runs horizontally but may ascend or descend slightly as it proceeds medially to the interhemispheric fissure. It gives off a series of delicate branches, the perforating arteries, which are only partially visible on the angiogram. From the medial third of the pars circularis, a branch arises which is fairly constant in size and course and which is usually readily apparent on the arteriogram. This is the recur-

rent *artery of Heubner* which first runs laterally and then turns superiorly and posteriorly somewhat above the carotid bifurcation. In the interhemispheric fissure the anterior cerebral artery makes a 90° turn in the parietal direction and remains in the median plane as it makes its way posteriorly. In this course it does not ordinarily overstep the midline. This portion comprises the *orbital segment,* the *knee,* and the *callosal segments* (A-1, A-3, and A-4). In this section of vessel the anterior cerebral and the pericallosal artery as well give off many irregularly arranged branches which initially also keep to the median plane, but which spread out laterally when they rise over the edge of the interhemispheric fissure. Arising from the first third of the anterior cerebral artery is the frontopolar artery, which can sometimes be very well demonstrated. On the anteroposterior view, as has already been stated, it is not infrequently possible to demonstrate the filling of the opposite anterior cerebral artery.

The *middle cerebral artery* runs from its origin at the carotid bifurcation in a lateral direction. Its course is initially horizontal – the *sphenoidal segment* – and gives rise to many small branches. These form clusters which initially course in a medial direction and then turn laterally and posteriorly in an outwardly convex curve. These are the medial and lateral lenticulostriate arteries, which supply parts of the basal ganglia, as well as the internal capsule and external capsule. For demonstration of these arteries, the sagittal (anteroposterior) magnification technique is particularly valuable.

Having arrived approximately at the lateral half of the orbit, the middle cerebral artery turns superiorly and posterolaterally at an angle of approximately 60°. This portion of the middle cerebral artery corresponds in its course to the area of the insula, for which reason it has been designated the *insular segment* (M-2). From here originate the ascending branches (M-3) which include the orbital artery, the frontal arteries, and the parietal arteries. They form peculiar slings as they span the operculum and endeavor to reach the convexity. They are superimposed upon themselves and upon the true end branches of the middle cerebral artery (M-4 and M-5), so that it is difficult to analyze any one of this maze of vessels. At the convexity of the brain, the terminal branches of the middle cerebral and anterior cerebral arteries form a netlike web of *meningeal anastomoses*. Some descending branches (temporal arteries) project themselves over the temporal lobe.

The *posterior cerebral artery* on the anteroposterior view can also be demonstrated, but naturally only distal to the posterior communicating artery by means of which it is filled on the carotid study. This is filled in retrograde fashion for the most part and is superimposed in its further course by the carotid bifurcation. If the head of the patient is not correctly aligned for the study, the branches of the posterior cerebral artery are so superimposed that they cannot be differentiated one from the other. With further tilting of the central beam the posterior communicating artery appears medially and beneath the carotid bifurcation. The portion of the posterior cerebral artery that runs in the ambient cistern bends laterally over the bifurcation and forms a medially concave curve outlining the midbrain, finally returning to the midline. This is the P-2 segment of the posterior cerebral artery (see vertebral angiogram, p. 85 ff.), which ultimately arrives in the vicinity of the pineal gland. Of the terminal branches of this artery, those to the occipital lobes running peripherally within the interhemispheric space are markedly foreshortened as a result of the unfavorable projection. The terminal branches to the temporal lobe, on the other hand, run from the pineal region obliquely in a lateral direction. When the anterior cerebral artery is not filled with contrast it is important not to mistake the posterior cerebral artery for a displaced anterior cerebral artery.

The *anterior choroidal artery* is recognized on the anteroposterior view only with great difficulty. It originates as a fine branch – again markedly foreshortened because of the projection – lateral to the posterior cerebral artery from the region of the carotid bifurcation.

The Half-Axial, Axial, and Oblique Views

For filming in the half-axial projection, the X-ray tube should be angled approximately 10° more than with the conventional view, the central beam forming an angle of about 20° with the orbitomeatal line. This projection approximates that used for the sagittal view on the vertebral angiogram. In this projection the carotid bifurcation is pictured correspondingly higher and the anterior cerebral and middle cerebral arteries are generally drawn out in the

long axis. The posterior cerebral artery is more distinctly demonstrated in this projection.

The *axial* projection (for technique, see p. 63, 91) can supplement the anterior and lateral views particularly with respect to those segments of the internal carotid, anterior cerebral, and middle cerebral vessels which run near the base of the skull, as well as providing further details about the ophthalmic artery. The cervical segment and the ascending portion of the canal segment of the internal carotid artery are so foreshortened in this projection that they cannot be judged accurately. Very clearly portrayed are the horizontal segment in the carotid canal, the intracavernous segment (C-5), and the carotid siphon (C-4 to C-2); however, the intracavernous segment and the terminal portion of the internal carotid artery including its bifurcation tend to be superimposed. The axial view is occasionally quite informative with regard to localization of aneurysms and also gives excellent portrayal of the initial segments of both the anterior cerebral and middle cerebral arteries (A-1 and M-1) (Fig. 37). *Oblique projections* after LOEFSTEDT (for technique, see p. 63) are employed to better demonstrate the anterior communicating artery, the carotid bifurcation, and also the lateral segment of the middle cerebral artery. For the most part this projection is used to outline the neck of an aneurysm more distinctly.

Peculiarities of the Internal Carotid Arteriogram in Early Childhood

The lateral view and also the anteroposterior view of the arterial phase of the carotid arteriogram in early childhood show differences from the adult arteriogram peculiar to early childhood which must be considered in order to interpret the films correctly. In early infancy the angiogram still resembles the fetal vascular architecture. In the anteroposterior view the pars circularis of the anterior cerebral artery ascends as it passes medially, a course which suggests the presence of a suprasellar space-occupying process. The initial segment of the middle cerebral artery also ascends slightly as it moves laterally. On the lateral exposure, it appears as though the siphon is less folded than in the adult and that the middle cerebral artery sits higher (Fig. 38). This course of the middle cerebral artery should not be mistaken for displacement secondary to a temporal tumor.

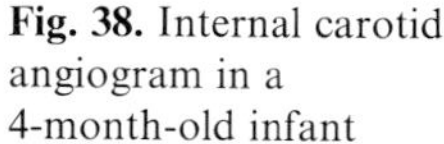

Fig. 38. Internal carotid angiogram in a 4-month-old infant

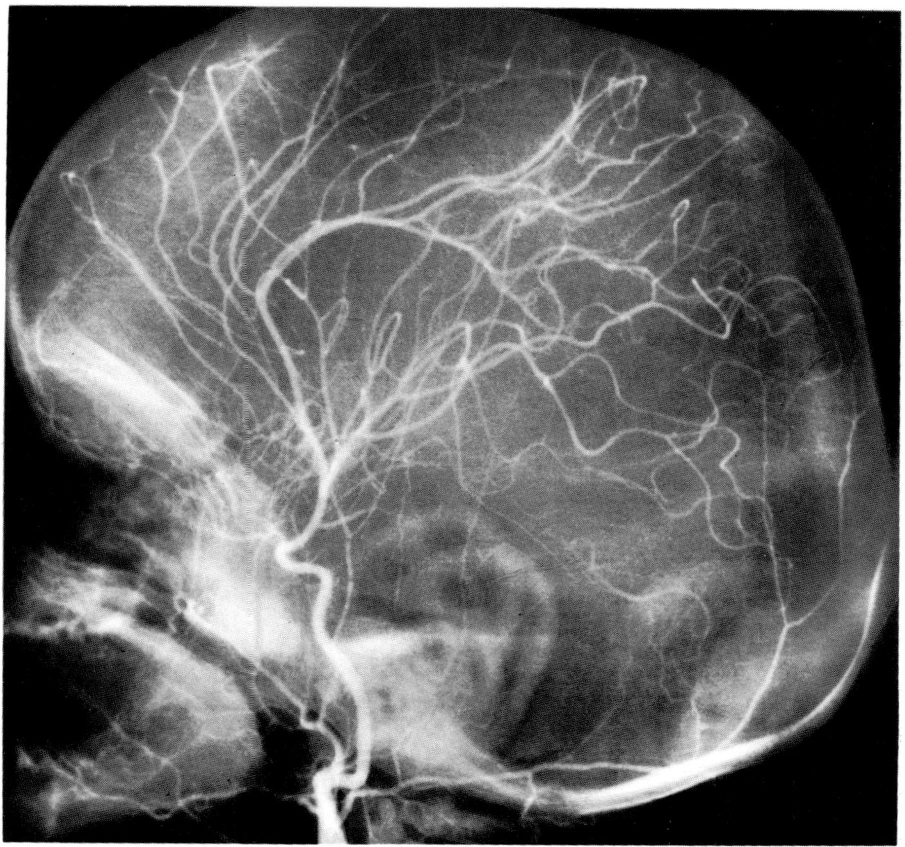

b) The Capillary and Venous Phases of the Internal Carotid Artery Angiogram

The capillary phase of the carotid angiogram lasts only about 0.5 sec, so that the film corresponding to this phase as a rule shows only the last small arteries and the earliest veins together. The capillary phase, in comparison to the arterial and venous phases, plays a distinctly subordinate role. With regard to the significance of the venous phase on the arteriogram, reference is made to the work of Moniz; however, only after the development of serial angiography was it possible to recognize normal variations with respect to the venous phase, and thus to permit deviations from the normal to be recognized and employed in the diagnostic evaluation.

The cerebral veins can be divided into *external (cortical)* and *internal (central)* groups (compare Fig. 29, 30, 40, 41, and 64).

The external cerebral veins, whose shape and course vary markedly, may be divided into two systems depending on the direction of their flow: the *ascending veins* and the *descending veins*. This grouping and the oblique interconnections (anastomoses) between them are best understood by referring to the embryonic cerebral vasculature.

The number and caliber of the ascending veins vary considerably. Two veins stand out in general because of their large size. These are the *precentral vein* of Trolard and the *parietal vein* of Rolandi. The ascending veins initially run along the cerebral cortex somewhat vertically in the direction of the superior sagittal sinus, but turn sharply in an anterior direction just before joining up with the sinus. Thus, the flow through this section is parallel to, but in the opposite direction of flow in the superior sagittal sinus. The terminal branches of these veins rising to the superior sagittal sinus are called *bridging* veins.

The descending veins, known for their large caliber, are the *middle cerebral veins* (veins of the Sylvian fissure) and the *temporal occipital vein* (vein of Labbé). The middle cerebral vein coming out of the Sylvian fissure courses in a posterosuperior to anteroinferior direction and empties either into the sphenoparietal sinus or directly into the cavernous sinus. The vein of Labbé is a continuation of the veins of the temporal lobe and courses horizontally or in a flat curve from anterosuperior to posteroinferior. It forms anastomoses with the vein of Trolard and also with the Sylvian veins and eventually empties into the transverse sinus.

The *basal veins* of the frontal lobe can be divided into two groups. The *medial group* arises on the medial surface of the frontal lobe and empties into the anterior portion of the superior sagittal sinus. The *lateral group* empties into the veins of the Sylvian fossa or into the lateral part of the sphenoparietal sinus.

The position and the course of the *deep cerebral veins* distinguishes them from the cortical veins in that they are more constant and less variable, for which reason their importance to angiographic diagnosis is significantly greater. The most important of these are the *internal cerebral veins,* the *basal vein of Rosenthal,* and the *great vein of Galen.*

The *internal cerebral veins* are paired and run side by side in the roof of the third ventricle from the foramen of Monro to the suprapineal recess. At the foramen of Monro, the thalamostriate vein empties into the internal cerebral vein, forming a rather acute angle between the two vessels. The shape and the position of this angle – known as the venous angle – are important factors in the evaluation of the venous phase. The venous angle is formed from the acute angular passage of the *thalamostriate* vein into the internal cerebral vein and has a relatively fixed topographical location with respect to the foramen of Monro.

The expected location of the venous angle can be calculated by the following method: on a lateral exposure of the venous phase a line is drawn connecting the two reference points: endobregma to posterior clinoid process, and endolambda to the junction of the floor of the frontal fossa with the frontal bone. The venous angle normally lies in the region of the crossing of these two lines.

The thalamostriate vein receives its blood, as its name suggests, from the thalamus and from the striatum, but also from the internal capsule. It runs on the lateral and inferior wall of the cella media of the lateral ventricle and best outlines the lateral wall of the ventricle in the sagittal (anteroposterior) exposure. An enlarged curve of this vein suggests ventricular enlargement (see Fig. 58 b).

Occasionally, however, the thalamostriate vein enters the internal cerebral vein well posterior to the foramen of Monro. At the foramen of Monro, both the *vein* of the *septum pellucidum* and the *choroidal veins* also empty into the internal cerebral vein. The vein of the septum pellucidum runs from anterosuperior to posteroinferior while forming a slightly convex inferior curve. It drains the blood from the septum pellucidum, from the anterior corpus callosum, and from the head of the caudate nucleus. It can also occasionally empty directly into the thalamostriate vein. The choroidal vein receives its blood from the choroid plexus of the lateral ventricle and is only visible in the venous phase of the vertebral angiogram. The internal cerebral vein exhibits a harmonious swinging course similar to a sine curve. In its anterior two-thirds it is convex superior and in its posterior third convex inferior. At the top of the suprapineal recess both internal cerebral veins join to form the *great vein of Galen,* which curves around the splenium of the corpus callosum and after a short course empties into the sinus rectus. Nearby, the small branches which form the *basal veins of Rosenthal* are identified. These come from either side of the suprasellar region, form a bend around the brain stem through the ambient cistern, and then empty into the great vein of Galen. Occasionally, they may enter the posterior portions of the internal cerebral veins or directly into the sinus rectus. They bilaterally drain the small veins of the anterior and posterior perforated substances, the veins of the hypothalamus, of the mamillary bodies, and also of the gyrus hippocampus and interpeduncular fossa.

Certain infratentorial veins also empty into the internal cerebral veins which, however, are only visible in the venous phase of the vertebral angiogram. The anterior pontomesencephalic veins, as well as the anterior medullary vein and the anterior spinal vein, all empty as a rule into the basal vein of Rosenthal, while the precentral cerebellar vein routinely drains into the great vein of Galen (for details see pp. 92 and 112). For the temporal sequence of contrast filling of the cerebral veins, the following rules apply: first the frontal veins appear, then the parietal ascending veins, and finally the deep cerebral veins.

The Veins of the Orbit

The arterial supply of the orbit comes essentially from the ophthalmic artery; however, the following branches of the external carotid also supply the orbit: the orbital ramus of the middle meningeal artery, the orbital ramus of the deep temporal artery, and the infraorbital artery. All three are branches of the maxillary artery. In spite of this rich arterial supply, the orbital veins on the carotid arteriogram are only rarely portrayed well enough that they can be demonstrated without subtraction views. The reason for this may well lie in the fact that the venous outflow from the orbit can take several paths, with the result that no one path is sharply outlined. Venous drainage can occur by way of the *angular vein,* by way of the *superior ophthalmic vein,* or the *inferior ophthalmic vein.* Both ophthalmic veins empty into the cavernous sinus, but the inferior ophthalmic vein also communicates with the pterygoid venous plexus. These veins possess no valves, as a result of which reversal of flow is fairly common. The superior ophthalmic vein is rather densely opacified in cases of thrombosis of the sagittal sinus and in the later phases of a circulatory standstill. In order to evaluate the course of the ophthalmic veins properly for diagnostic purposes, direct orbital venography is necessary (see p. 174).

The Dural Sinuses

Anatomically, these are divided into two groups: a *superior* and an *inferior* group of venous sinuses. The superior group consists of the *superior sagittal sinus,* the *inferior sagittal sinus,* the *sinus rectus,* the *transverse sinuses,* and the *sigmoid sinuses.* To the inferior group belong the *sphenoparietal sinuses,* the *cavernous sinus,* and the *superior and inferior petrosal sinuses* (Figs. 29, 30, 40, 41, 64).

The *superior sagittal sinus* has its origin anteriorly at the crista frontalis and follows the sagittal sulcus posteriorly to the internal occipital protuberance, increasing in size as it does so. Through the addition of noncontrasted blood entering the sinus from ascending veins of the opposite side, the density of contrast within the superior sagittal sinus is frequently poor or laminated. Not infrequently the anterior third of the superior sagittal sinus is aplastic. In this situation the frontal ascending veins flow posteriorly in a paramedian direction to enter the superior sagittal sinus at a point which is generally just posterior to the coronal suture. This anatomical variant should not be mistaken for a thrombosis of the sinus itself. In the lateral projection bony structures can simulate the superior sagittal sinus so that subtraction views may be necessary.

In the sagittal (anteroposterior) projection, the anterior and posterior segments of the superior sagittal sinus are superimposed on one another. If one wishes to better outline the entire sinus it is necessary to turn the head somewhat to the right or left (see also the chapter entitled "Direct Sinography"). The posterior third of the superior sagittal sinus can deviate from the midline to the right or to the left, most commonly to the right (see below).

The *inferior sagittal sinus* runs along the inferior edge of the falx and receives veins from this structure as well as from the corpus callosum. It is not always visible in the carotid angiogram. At the point where the falx joins the tentorium the inferior sagittal sinus passes into the sinus rectus, which is generally visible on the carotid study. The sinus rectus also receives blood from the great vein of Galen.

The superior sagittal sinus and the sinus rectus join together to form the *confluence of sinuses* at the level of the internal occipital protuberance. From here blood passes to the *transverse sinuses,* then to the *sigmoid sinuses,* and finally to the *jugular veins* on either side. Whenever the posterior third of the superior sagittal sinus deviates from the midline to a paramedian position, its blood generally flows only into the transverse sinus on the side to which it is deviating. In approximately two-thirds of the cases, flow from the superior sagittal sinus goes entirely or predominantly into the right transverse sinus, whereas in approximately one-third of the cases it goes predominantly or entirely to the left. In approximately 10% of cases it is evenly distributed to both sides. These relationships are emphasized and must be considered carefully when the possibility of a sinus occlusion exists through tumor growth or thrombosis. The *occipital veins* and the *superior cerebellar veins* also empty into the transverse sinus and are plainly visible in the venous phase of the vertebral angiogram. In a particularly good vertebral study the *occipital sinus* is occasionally visualized running along the posterior margin of the falx cerebelli against the inner table of the skull from the vicinity of the posterior rim

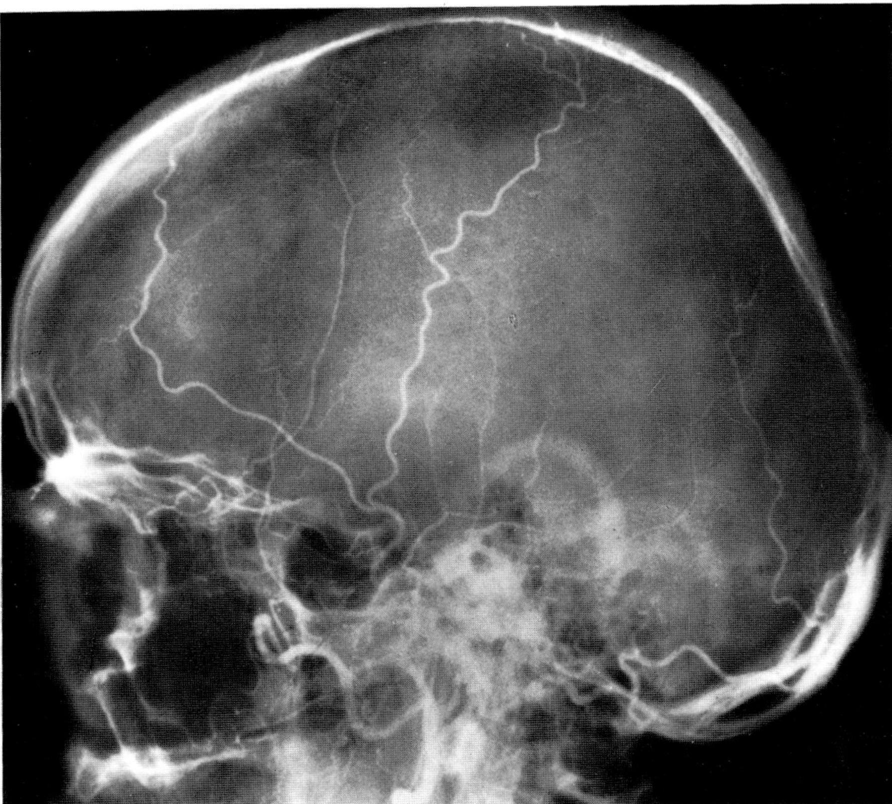

Fig.39. External carotid angiogram. Lateral view in the arterial phase

of the foramen magnum to the confluent sinus. The *sigmoid sinus* passes into the bulb of the jugular vein at the approximate level of the jugular foramen.

The *sphenoparietal sinus* runs in a dural fold on the posterior edge of the lesser wing of the sphenoid and empties beneath the anterior clinoid process into the *cavernous sinus,* which also receives the greatest part of the blood from the orbital veins. As a result of superimposition of bony structures, it can usually be seen well only in subtraction views. The anterior and posterior intercavernous sinuses form cross connections between the right and left cavernous sinuses. The cavernous sinus is primarily drained by the *superior* and *inferior petrosal sinuses* as well as by the *basilar plexus.*

The direct contrast injection into the superior sagittal sinus is described in the section on "Direct Sinography" (see p. 175). Retrograde contrast filling of the sigmoid and transverse sinuses, as well as the cavernous sinus, by means of the jugular vein is described in the chapter entitled "Jugular Venography" or "Retrograde Sinography" (see p. 178).

c) The External Carotid Angiogram

In neuroradiology the following branches of the external carotid artery have particular importance (Fig. 39):

The *ascending pharyngeal artery* originates from the proximal portion of the external carotid artery and rises as a long thin vessel medial to the internal carotid artery as far as the base of the skull.

The *occipital artery* rises from the dorsal aspect of the external carotid artery, crosses the transverse process of the atlas, and climbs on the medial side of the mastoid process to the occiput where it divides into many branches in the scalp. It forms anastomoses with branches of the superficial temporal artery, with the posterior auricular artery, and with the occipital artery of the opposite side, as well as with muscular branches of the vertebral artery. A direct anastomosis goes to the main stem of the vertebral artery at the level of the foramen magnum.

The *middle meningeal artery* is the most important branch of the maxillary artery and enters the intracranial fossa through the foramen spinosum. It is seen on the arteriogram in the vicinity of the wing of the sphenoid and takes a curvilinear course in an occipital direction, crossing the ascending branch of the superficial temporal artery in its further course. This vessel and its branches are thin and lie in vascular channels of the skull so that they can be readily identified by comparing the angiogram and the plain skull X-rays with its vascular markings.

The *superficial temporal artery* arises anterior to the tragus of the ear and divides into its frontal and parietal terminal branches on top of the temporalis fascia. It is important not to mistake the superficial temporal artery for the middle meningeal artery. In this regard the superficial temporal artery is usually thicker and as a rule rather tortuous. From this vessel an anastomotic branch runs to the frontalis artery, which serves a collateral function in the case of an internal carotid occlusion (see Fig. 126).

The *angular artery* is the end branch of the facial artery. It supplies the outer nose on which it runs and anastomoses with the dorsal nasal artery, a branch of the ophthalmic artery.

The external carotid study is especially important in determining the blood supply of meningiomas and glomus tumors, as well as arteriovenous malformations in the distribution of the external carotid artery. To demonstrate tumors and angiomas supplied by individual branches of the external carotid artery, a superselective catheterization of these branches has been quite successful in recent years. The external carotid system is particularly important from both a clinical and neuroradiological standpoint in occlusions of the internal carotid artery. The possibilities for development of collateral circulation from the external carotid artery to the internal carotid system are discussed on p. 159.

d) The Arterial Phase of the Vertebral Angiogram

Preliminary Anatomical Comments

The vertebral artery is the major branch of the subclavian artery. Its initial segment lies in the vertebral-scalene triangle where it is covered by the vertebral vein. At the level of the 6th cervical vertebra it enters the costotransverse foramina of the six upper cervical vertebrae, in which position it crosses the ventral cervical roots as they exit from the intervertebral foramina. To prevent distortion by rotation of the neck at the level of the atlas, the artery forms a wide lateral curve going to and from the transverse foramen of the atlas, which is situated further laterally than the other foramina. The upper limb of the curve then bends in a medial direction and passes dorsal to the lateral mass of the atlas in the sulcus for the vertebral artery along its posterior arch. This sulcus in many cases forms a short canal which is called the arcuate foramen of the atlas. Finally, the vertebral artery bends anteriorly and passes through the posterior atlanto-occipital membrane to the foramen magnum where it pierces the dura and the arachnoid membranes. Here it gives off the posterior inferior cerebellar artery and joins the vertebral artery from the opposite side on the clivus to form the basilar artery. After entering the dura, both vertebral arteries also give off fine branches to form the *anterior spinal artery*.

Positioning Techniques

As with the carotid angiogram, routine serial films in the lateral and anteroposterior projections are made (Figs. 40, 41). For the anteroposterior projection, however, the angle of the beam is tilted more caudally (see p. 63). The axial projection brings both vertebral arteries and the basilar artery with its proximal branches clearly into view (Fig. 44).

The Lateral Projection

Within the costotransverse foramina of the upper six cervical vertebra the vertebral artery takes a more or less linear course to the level of the axis (V-1 segment). Just above this vertebra it forms a short posteriorly convex loop (V-2 segment) which becomes increasingly larger and, at the level of the atlas, changes to an anteriorly convex curve. The upper limb of this curve lies in the vertebral artery sulcus on the posterior rim of the atlas (V-4 segment). The artery then bends anteriorly and superiorly in the direction of the clivus (V-5 segment) until it joins the opposite vertebral artery at the approximate level of the midclivus (Fig. 41, 42).

In the upper cervical region the vertebral artery gives off muscular and spinal branches. The muscular branches supply the paravertebral neck musculature and anastomose with

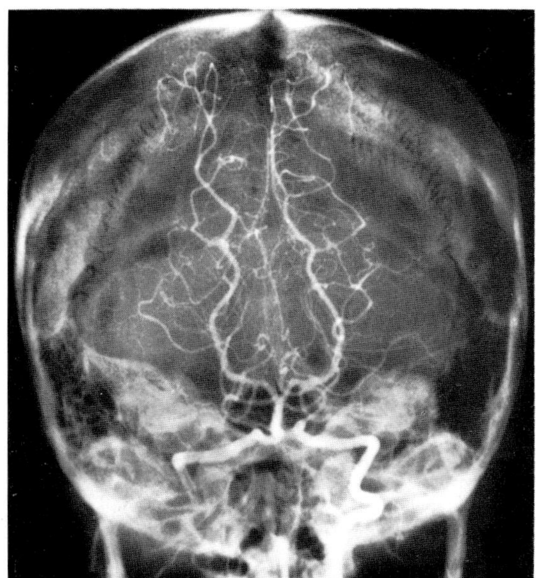

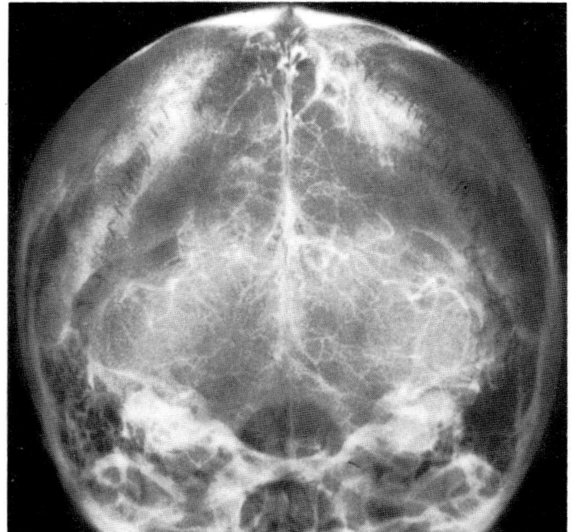

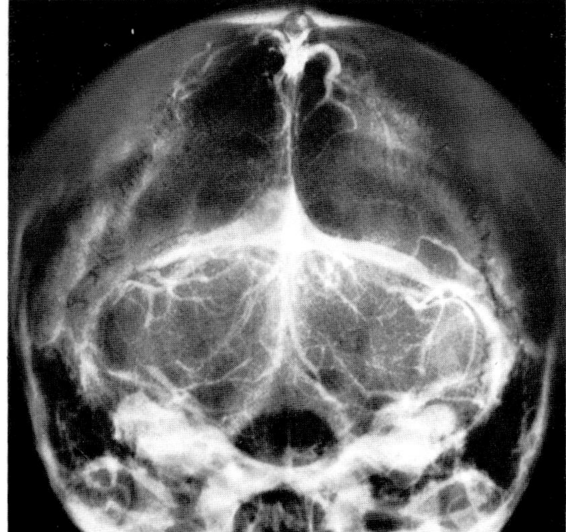

Fig. 40a–c. Normal serial angiogram of the vertebral artery (anteroposterior view)

Fig. 41 a–c. Lateral view of the same sequence as Fig. 40

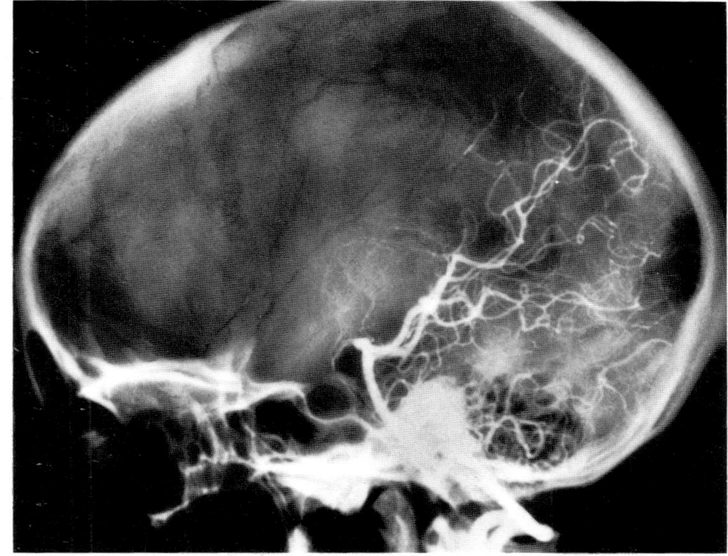

a

b

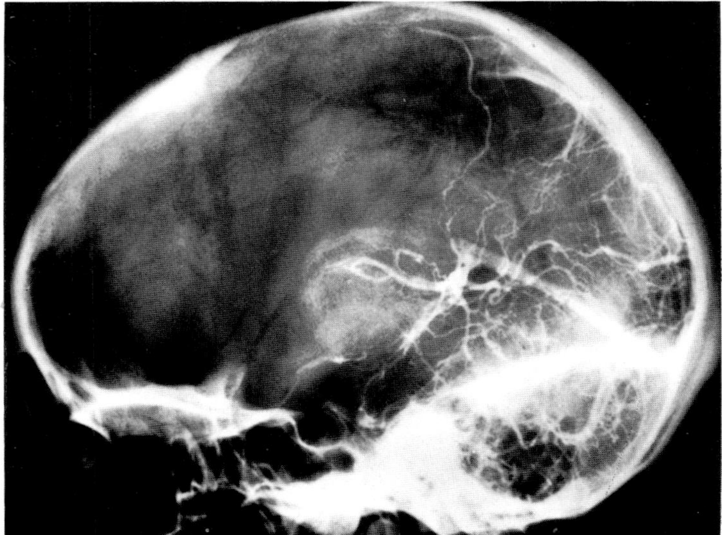

c

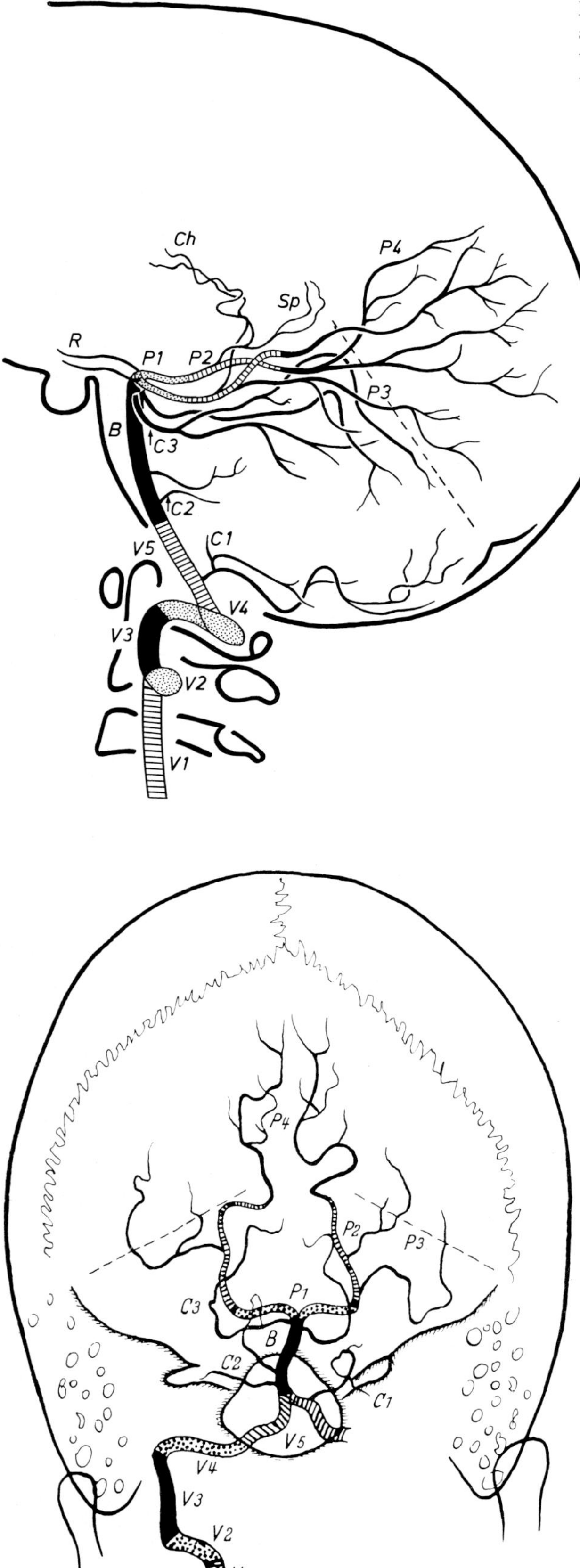

Fig. 42. Schematic demonstration of the lateral view of a vertebral arteriogram. The *dotted line* represents the tentorium. For the appropriate letter designations, see text

Fig. 43. Schematic demonstration of the normal vertebral arteriogram: half-axial sagittal view, arterial phase. The *dotted line* again represents the tentorium. Letter designations are explained in the text

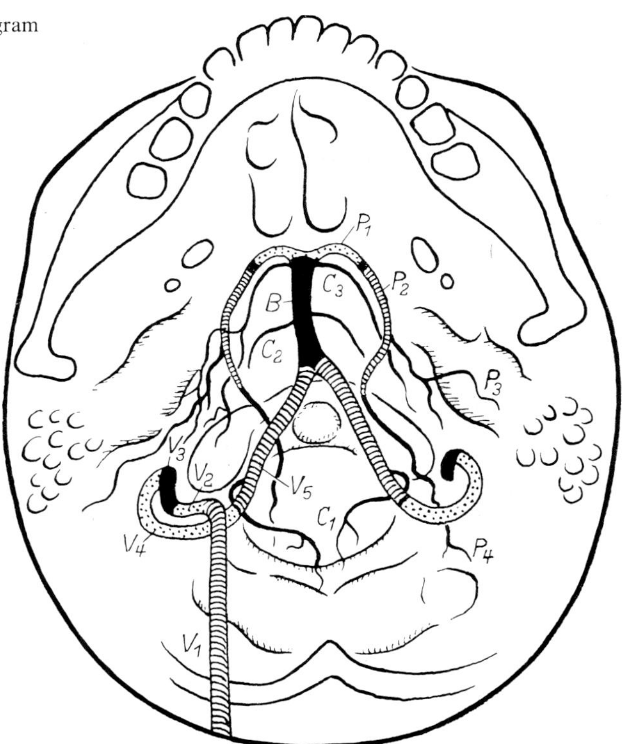

Fig. 44. Schematic demonstration of a vertebral arteriogram in the axial view

branches of the occipital artery and the ascending pharyngeal artery.

After the vertebral artery has passed through the foramen magnum, it gives off its first branch of major size and importance, the *posterior inferior cerebellar artery* (C-1), also known as "Wallenberg's artery". On the lateral projection this forms an S-shaped loop which lies above the level of the foramen magnum. The caudally directed portion of the loop marks the inferior margin of the tonsil, which can be situated beneath the level of the foramen magnum either as a sign of herniation or as a normal anatomical variant (see also p. 108).

If both vertebral arteries are filled with contrast, it is possible to visualize their point of union into the basilar artery on the lateral projection only if the intracranial segments run at different levels and are not projected upon each other. The first portion of the basilar artery is superimposed on the temporal bone so that branches originating at this level, namely the *anterior inferior cerebellar artery* and the *internal auditory artery* (C-2), become visible only on subtraction views. The basilar artery is situated 2–3 mm from the clivus. As it approaches the dorsum sella, this distance is increased since the artery passes posteriorly to a point 1 cm

above the level of the dorsum where it divides into the two posterior cerebral arteries. Just before its bifurcation the basilar artery gives off the two *superior cerebellar arteries* (C-3), which, on the lateral view, are split into many irregular branches running in the direction of the internal occipital protuberance. The bifurcation of the basilar artery into the *posterior cerebral arteries* in the lateral projection has a variable shape resembling loops and knots. Both posterior cerebral arteries proceed above the level of projection of the upper edge of the pyramid in an occipital direction and are superimposed upon themselves. Just posterior to their origin, the posterior cerebral arteries give off several fine branches – the thalamic arteries – which are stretched out in a parietal direction. At the approximate transition of the posterior cerebral artery from its proximal to its middle third, the medial and lateral posterior choroidal arteries branch off. Then the posterior cerebral arteries divide into an occipital (P-4) branch and a temporal (P-3) branch. The *posterior choroidal arteries* run first in an occipital direction, curve around the pineal, and then bend sharply under the splenium of the corpus callosum in an anterior direction. Here they branch into many fine twigs which run in the tela choroidea of the lateral and third ventricles until they are lost in this projection over the tip of the basilar artery.

The temporal branch of the posterior cerebral artery – the *lateral occipital artery* or *temporo-occipital artery* (P-3) – is seen on the lateral projection somewhat superior to the superior cerebellar arteries on which it is superimposed. The occipital branch – the *medial occipital artery* or the *internal occipital artery* (P-4) – runs superiorly to the temporal branch with which it makes an acute angle, opening posteriorly. After an initial course in the superior direction, which brings the vessel directly behind the pineal gland, it turns in a posterior direction and loses itself at approximately the level of the lambdoid suture. The course of these vessels can be explained by the fact that the temporal branches leave the ambient cisterns to supply the base and outer surfaces of the posterior temporal lobes, while the occipital branches run through the cisterns on the medial surface of the occipital lobes to supply the occipital poles. Approximately at the level where the posterior choroidal arteries bend anteriorly, the posterior cerebral artery gives off a small branch which lies on and outlines the *splenium of the corpus callosum* (SP).

Sometimes the *posterior communicating artery* (R) is demonstrated running from its origin at the posterior cerebral artery in the direction of the anterior clinoid process. Through this vessel portions of the carotid system are occasionally filled. Branches from the posterior communicating artery are usually well seen on the lateral vertebral study. They supply the chiasm, the tuber cinereum, the cerebral peduncle, the ventral nucleus of the thalamus, portions of the hypothalamus, and the tail of the caudate nucleus.

The Anteroposterior Projection

In order to portray the intracranial branches of the vertebrobasilar system distinctly and to free it from superimposition on the base of the skull, it is necessary to employ a *half-axial* projection in the anteroposterior view (see p. 80). In this projection (Figs 40, 43) the cervical segment of the vertebral artery in general appears as a taut band of contrast which runs in a straight line until it reaches the atlas (V-1). Short segments of this section may, however, form a semi circle and then return to the original course. Beneath the atlas the vessel takes a more or less lateral curve (V-2), rises through the foramen transversarium of the atlas to reach its superior surface (V-3), and turns again in a sharp curve medially (V-4). This is the section of the vertebral artery sulcus on the posterior rim of the atlas which in the lateral projection appears to run dorsally. The point at which the vertebral artery pierces the dura is not apparent on the half-axial view. It corresponds, however, to the point at which the vessel reaches the outer rim of the foramen magnum. In the lateral view the point of penetration is marked by a rostrally directed acute angular bend between V-4 and V-5. In the half-axial projection, the artery gradually approaches the midline (V-5).

If the vertebral artery from the opposite side is also visualized, the shape and the position of the point of junction can be determined. The end segments of both vertebral arteries show considerable asymmetry, as a result of which their point of junction may lie up to 1 cm off the midline. In such cases the basilar artery itself also continues in a paramedian position until it reaches its rostral third.

On either side the terminal segment of the vertebral artery gives off the *posterior inferior cerebellar arteries* (C-1). The *anterior inferior cerebellar arteries* arise from the proximal portion of the basilar artery and run laterally in an irregular curve. As a rule, they give off the auditory arteries. Most impressive on the half-axial projection, however, is the bifurcation of the basilar artery into the two posterior cerebral arteries (P-1). As an analogy to the carotid bifurcation, the basilar bifurcation is also designated the "basilar fork". Both *posterior cerebral arteries* surround the cerebral peduncles of the midbrain describing a medially concave curve in so doing, whereupon they again bend somewhat laterally dividing into their terminal branches. Here there are many individual variants, but in general one or more *temporal branches* run laterally (P-3) so that the continuation of the curve (P-2) in its peripheral portion no longer represents the main branch of the posterior cerebral artery, but rather its *occipital ramus*. Its terminal branches (P-4) run out as far as the lambdoid suture. The point at which both occipital rami of the posterior cerebral arteries come nearest to each other (the transition from P-2 to P-4) corresponds approximately to the posterior edge of the tentorial hiatus. If one follows the highest and most lateral edge of the temporal bone from this point laterally, one can outline the approximate posterior attachment of the tentorium.

Just before its division into the posterior cerebral arteries, the basilar artery gives off the *superior cerebellar arteries* to either side which are, however, occasionally doubled (C-3). These initially take a course similar to the posterior cerebral arteries, but they are usually finer branches and in their terminal ramifications are superimposed by the posterior cerebral arteries so that recognition of individual branches is very difficult.

The same goes as well for the posterior choroidal arteries and for the posterior communicating arteries. In the capillary and venous phases the choroid plexus of the lateral ventricles is visualized as a diffuse blush.

It cannot be stressed enough that all of these vessels – even the largest – are normally so variable in their twisting course, divide so asymmetrically, and are paired so unevenly that a diagnosis of vessel displacement secondary to a space-occupying process should be made only with the greatest of caution.

The Axial Projection

The axial projection, which is only occasionally employed, is used principally to clarify a complicated vertebrobasilar system (Fig. 44). However, in general only the vertebral arteries (V-1 to V-5), the basilar artery (B), and the initial segments of the posterior cerebral arteries (P-1) are sufficiently portrayed to be analyzed clearly. The visualization of the smaller vessels is complicated because of superimposition by the petrous bone and the cervical vertebrae.

Also on this projection the vertebral artery is first visualized within the canal formed by the costotransverse foramen of the cervical vertebra within which it takes a straight line to the atlas (V-1). Here it bends laterally (V-2) and rises to the transverse process of the atlas (V-3) after which it turns on the posterior rim of the atlas, again medially (V-4), making a dorsal loop and finally swinging gradually in a frontomedial direction (V-5) crossing the lateral edge of the foramen magnum in the process. On the clivus it joins the opposite vertebral artery (when both are visualized) to form the *basilar artery* (B). This proceeds more or less in a frontal direction. Again, individual twists may

take the basilar artery away from the midline for variable distances. The length of this segment will change, quite naturally, according to the direction of the beam. At its rostral end, the basilar artery divides at right angles into its posterior cerebral artery branches (P-1) which in this projection are superimposed over the nostrils. The *posterior cerebral arteries* then proceed dorsally in a frontal convex curve (P-2), finally to be lost in a confusion of smaller vessels. The *posterior inferior cerebellar arteries* and the *superior cerebellar arteries* can usually be recognized near their origin from the vertebral and basilar arteries respectively. Farther laterally, they can be recognized only with subtraction films because of superimposition on other structures. This is also true for the demonstration of the posterior choroidal arteries.

e) The Venous Phase of the Vertebral Angiogram

The venous phase of the vertebral angiogram has achieved a diagnostic importance comparable to the study of the veins of the carotid circulation. Anatomical investigations and angiographic studies of subtraction views have contributed to such an extent that order has been brought to this area which was not apparent earlier. The lack of recognizable patterns until now prevented accurate analysis (HUANG and WOLF, 1964–1970). In this regard a distinction must be made between the *supratentorial* and *infratentorial* venous channels (Figs. 40c, 41c).

Of the supratentorial veins, the *ascending occipital veins* should be mentioned. These drain into the posterior third of the superior sagittal sinus. Of the descending veins, the *dorsal occipital descending veins* empty into the transverse sinus. They drain the occipital pole as well as its laterodorsal and laterobasal surfaces. The *medial occipital descending veins* drain the medial surface of the occipital lobe and empty into the sinus rectus.

Of the deep cerebral veins which are apparent on the carotid study, the great vein of Galen and the basal vein of Rosenthal are also well seen on the vertebral study, as is the sinus rectus. On the other hand, the internal cerebral veins and the choroidal veins are not so sharply outlined.

Of the infratentorial veins the following have diagnostic significance and should be identified on the lateral projection (Fig. 45):

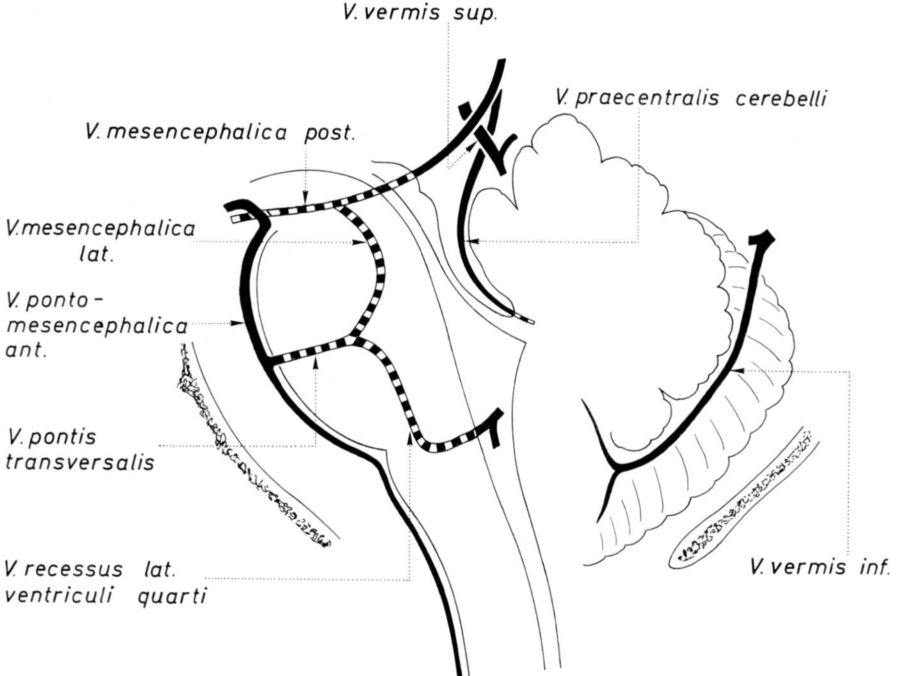

Fig. 45. a Schematic demonstration of the most important veins of the posterior cranial fossa, lateral view

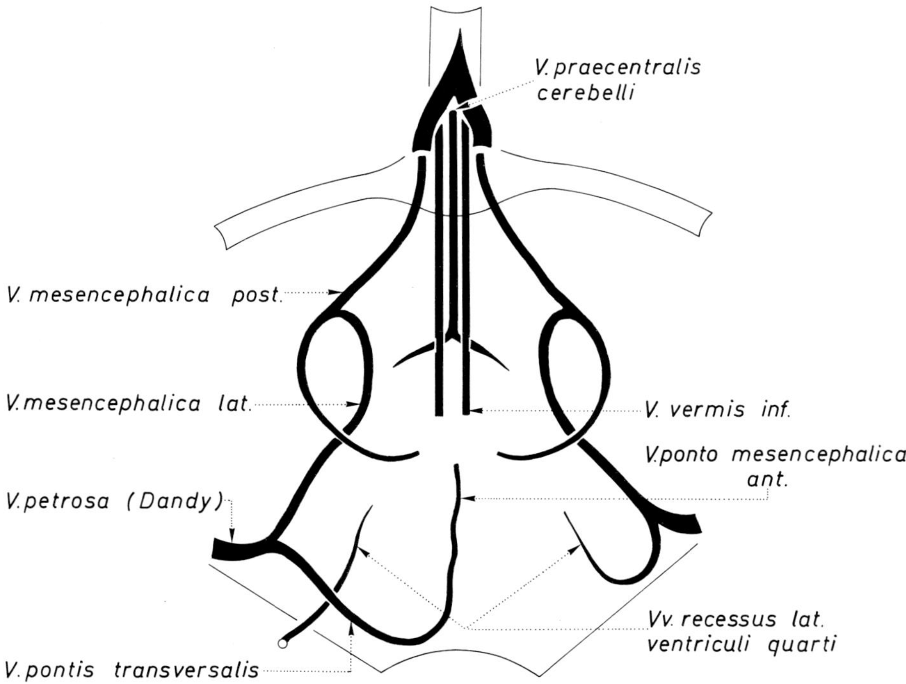

Fig. 45. b Schematic diagram of the most important veins of the posterior cranial fossa, sagittal view (half-axial)

The *anterior pontomesencephalic veins* and, continuing in a caudal direction, the *anterior medullary veins* and the *anterior spinal veins* which outline the anterior surface of the brain stem. These empty as a rule into the basal vein of Rosenthal, less commonly into the posterior pontomesencephalic veins.

The *precentral cerebellar vein* defines the posterior margin of the roof of the fourth ventricle, rising perpendicularly to a point below the quadrigeminal plate and emptying into the great vein of Galen.

The *inferior vermian vein* with its two tributaries, the *superior retrotonsillar* and *inferior retrotonsillar veins,* outline the posterior margin of the tonsil. They lie in the retrotonsillar fissure.

The *superior* and *inferior cerebellar veins* course on the dorsal and laterodorsal surfaces of the cerebellum and empty into the sigmoid sinus or into the petrosal and transverse sinuses.

In the anteroposterior projection the *precentral cerebellar veins* are shown running in a paramedian position similar to the *anterior pontomesencephalic veins,* which lie within the interpeduncular fossa. Of diagnostic significance are the *petrosal veins* which, on the half-axial projection, lie above the internal auditory canal. These are displaced with space-occupying processes of the cerebellopontine angle as well as of the cerebellar hemispheres (HUANG and WOLF, 1964–1970).

IV. The Pathological Intracranial Angiogram

The cerebral angiogram in general gives information about three types of pathological change within the intracranial space:
1. Displacements in the usual position of the normal cerebral vessels
2. Inherent changes in the vessels themselves, including:
   a) Dilation
   b) Constriction
   c) Occlusion with or without collateral circulation
3. Vessel malformations and new vessel formations

These pathological changes are of considerable diagnostic merit. They permit conclusions to be made on the one hand about vessel displacements, indirectly outlining space-occupying processes (such as tumors) and, on the other hand, they directly portray intravascular pathology. Frequently, these pathological processes exist simultaneously; the larger space-occupying processes displace adjacent normal vessels, but may also show pathological vessel formations within the lesion itself. There are also primary vessel diseases which can be associated with a mass effect. From this it is apparent that a sharp distinction between these overlapping processes cannot always be made from the angiogram alone. Each entity must therefore be carefully considered before it is discarded and appropriate ancillary studies (such as CT) performed. In the next section, practical application of the afore-mentioned pathological changes will be discussed – first, with respect to the space-occupying intracranial processes and second, with respect to the primary vessel diseases.

1. Intracranial Space-Occupying Lesions

a) Displacement of Normal Blood Vessels

The majority of the cerebral vessels show a relatively constant course in the normal state as they pass through the brain fissures. Changes within the adjacent brain substance are reflected by corresponding changes in the course of the affected vessels. The demonstration of a vessel on the arteriogram therefore gives indirect evidence about the condition of the adjacent brain. In other words, pathological distortions in the course of a vessel means pathological change in the adjacent brain. From a practical standpoint the most significant lesion in this regard is the space-occupying intracranial mass. The *presence of a mass effect* and the *precise location* of the lesion itself may often be surmised from the character of the vessel displacement, which is a most important consideration in the analysis of the cerebral angiogram.

Vessel dislocations are more apparent on the angiogram if *larger vessels* are involved (which are easily seen on the angiographic study) and also if the vessel is sufficiently *displaced;* however, such displacements are of diagnostic significance only if the vessels in question normally have a fairly *constant course.* These conditions are met with respect to the *internal carotid artery* itself as well as its *proximal branches.* The brain stem arteries, on the other hand, because of peculiarities in their course are more difficult to judge. The arteries of the cerebellum are only visible on the vertebral study and may require employment of the sagittal (anteroposterior) half-axial projection for clarification of apparent changes. This projection, above all, permits comparison with the contralateral side to be made. In the lateral projection these relationships are more complicated because of superimposition of the vessels of both sides.

Although the shape and course of the *cortical veins* are known to exhibit considerable variations, marked displacements of these veins are often clearly seen and diagnostically significant. A displacement of the deep cerebral veins brings to mind certain pathological states. The sinuses within the dura mater for the most part are so firmly fixed to bone that they cannot be displaced. Only in rare cases does this occur, as with displacement of the superior sagittal sinus from the inner table of the skull in an extradural space-occupying process.

From what has been said above, it is apparent from an angiographic standpoint that vessel displacements – especially those involving the *cerebral hemispheres* as well as those *near the base of the brain* – are better demonstrated with the arterial phase than with the venous phase.

The *angiographic study* begins with the *correct alignment* for each *projection* in order to minimize errors. One must carefully watch for *anatomical variants*. Then, one must try to recognize *larger mass displacements* in both projections of the arterial phase in order to give an overall perspective to the study. Next, one carefully observes the position and shape of individual vessel segments, *comparing both anteroposterior and lateral views*. Finally, there follows a study of the capillary and venous phases.

General Orientation

The sagittal (anteroposterior) projection. In the evaluation of the arterial phase on the anteroposterior projection it is first necessary to determine whether the *anterior cerebral artery* is in the *midline* or *displaced* (Fig. 46). This is of fundamental importance since a lateral displacement not only indicates that a space-occupying process is present, but also tells which side is involved. This sign is present with all but the smaller cerebral tumors. An exception to the rule is seen with unilateral cerebral atrophy, where the anterior cerebral artery is displaced to the side of the atrophy (Fig. 47). It is, however, essential that the alignment of the head be absolutely symmetrical in order to avoid the false suggestion of vessel displacement caused by rotation alone (see p. 63 and Fig. 179).

In addition to establishing which side is involved, the anteroposterior projection alone permits a more accurate localization in the medial to lateral direction. *Suprasellar* and *presellar* masses displace the normal horizontal course of the pars circularis of the anterior cerebral arteries superiorly (Fig. 46/2). The vertical segment of this vessel usually remains in the midline with such tumors. Masses sitting *above* or *in front* of the Sylvian fissure (especially frontal tumors) push the anterior cerebral artery and the middle cerebral artery inferiorly and apart (Fig. 46/3). *Temporal lobe masses,* by contrast, result in a "near" shift of the anterior cerebral artery and a characteristic displacement of the middle cerebral artery medially and superiorly (Fig. 46/4). Finally, the anteroposterior view permits the diagnosis of an extracerebral fluid collection to be made (usually a subdural or epidural hematoma) by demonstrating a pathological displacement of the peripheral cerebral vessels away from the inner table of the skull, which creates an angiographic "avascular" space (Fig. 46/5). In occipital tumors the

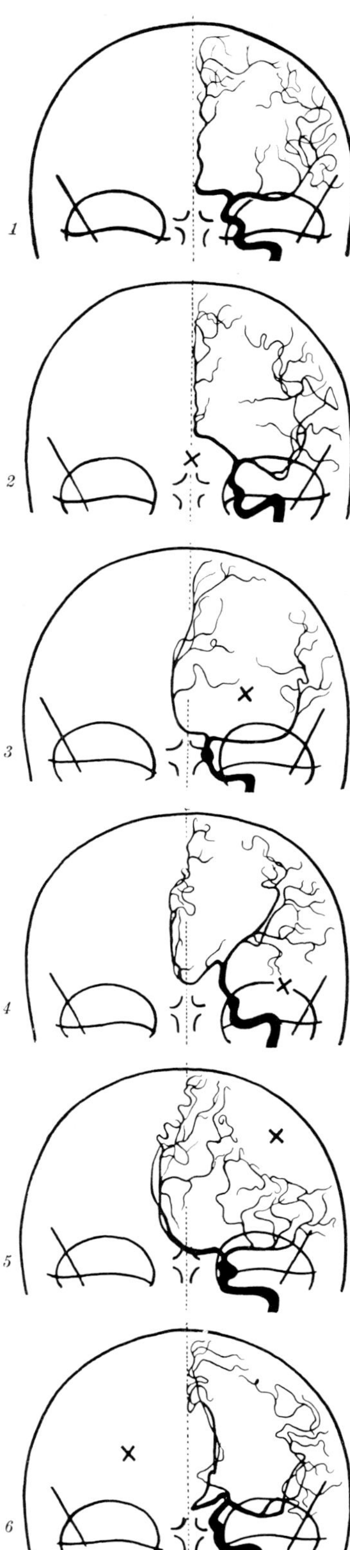

Fig. 46. Basic variations of the anteroposterior carotid arteriogram: *1*, normal; *2*, presellar midline tumor; *3*, frontal lobe tumor; *4*, temporal lobe tumor; *5*, subdural hematoma; *6*, tumor of the contralateral side. In each diagram the tumor is represented by "*X*"

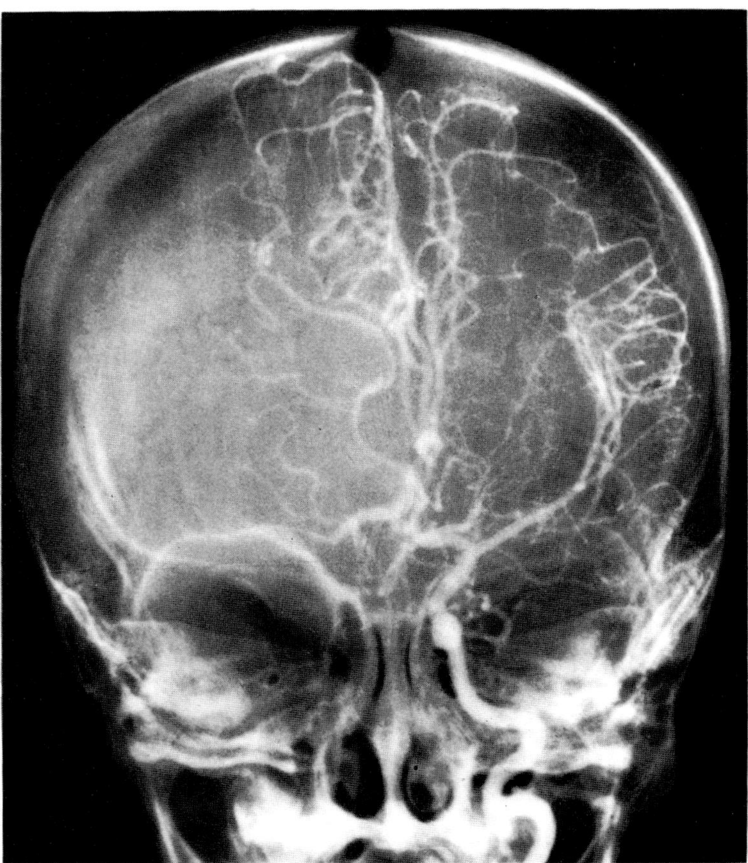

Fig. 47. Left-sided cerebral atrophy: displacement of the anterior cerebral artery to the affected side with hypoplasia of the left middle cerebral artery (see also Fig. 216)

displacement of the anterior cerebral and middle cerebral arteries in the anteroposterior view is often relatively small. A lateral displacement of the anterior cerebral artery to the side which is being studied implies that a space-occupying process exists on the contralateral side, i.e., on the side *which is not being studied* (Fig. 46/6). With bilateral space-occupying lesions – most commonly bilateral subdural hematomas or bilateral metastases – the course of the anterior cerebral artery remains undisturbed and follows its usual midline path.

The lateral projection. For the further localization of a space-occupying process in the anterior-posterior direction the lateral projection is necessary. Here the cerebral edema, which frequently accompanies mass lesions, becomes a factor in making the precise location of the tumor itself more difficult. It is recognized that the nearest vessels are most displaced and the farthest from the lesion least displaced. Those processes lying in the *parasagittal area* result in a definite displacement of the *anterior cerebral artery* (Fig. 48), while the more *laterally*

lying processes prevail in a similar fashion upon the *middle cerebral artery* (Fig. 49).

Tumors situated medially on the roof of the orbit push the pars circularis, the orbital segment, and the knee of the anterior cerebral artery (A-1, A-2, and A-3) posteriorly and superiorly (Fig. 48/1). Processes involving the frontal pole displace the knee of the artery (A-2 and A-3) posteriorly (Fig. 48/2). Parasagittal precentral processes push the horizontal callosal segment of the pericallosal artery inferiorly and posteriorly (Fig. 48/3). Turmors of the central parietal region displace this segment purely inferiorly (Fig. 48/4), while parieto-occipital lesions displace the terminal ramifications of the artery (A-5) inferiorly and eventually somewhat anteriorly (Fig. 48/5). Such displacements affect even the distally situated carotid siphon and middle cerebral artery, albeit to a much lesser degree (see Figs. 8 and 53).

The *middle cerebral artery* is a *sensitive indicator* of lesions lying in the frontoparietal region on the one hand, and in the temporo-occipital area on the other. Thus, on the lateral

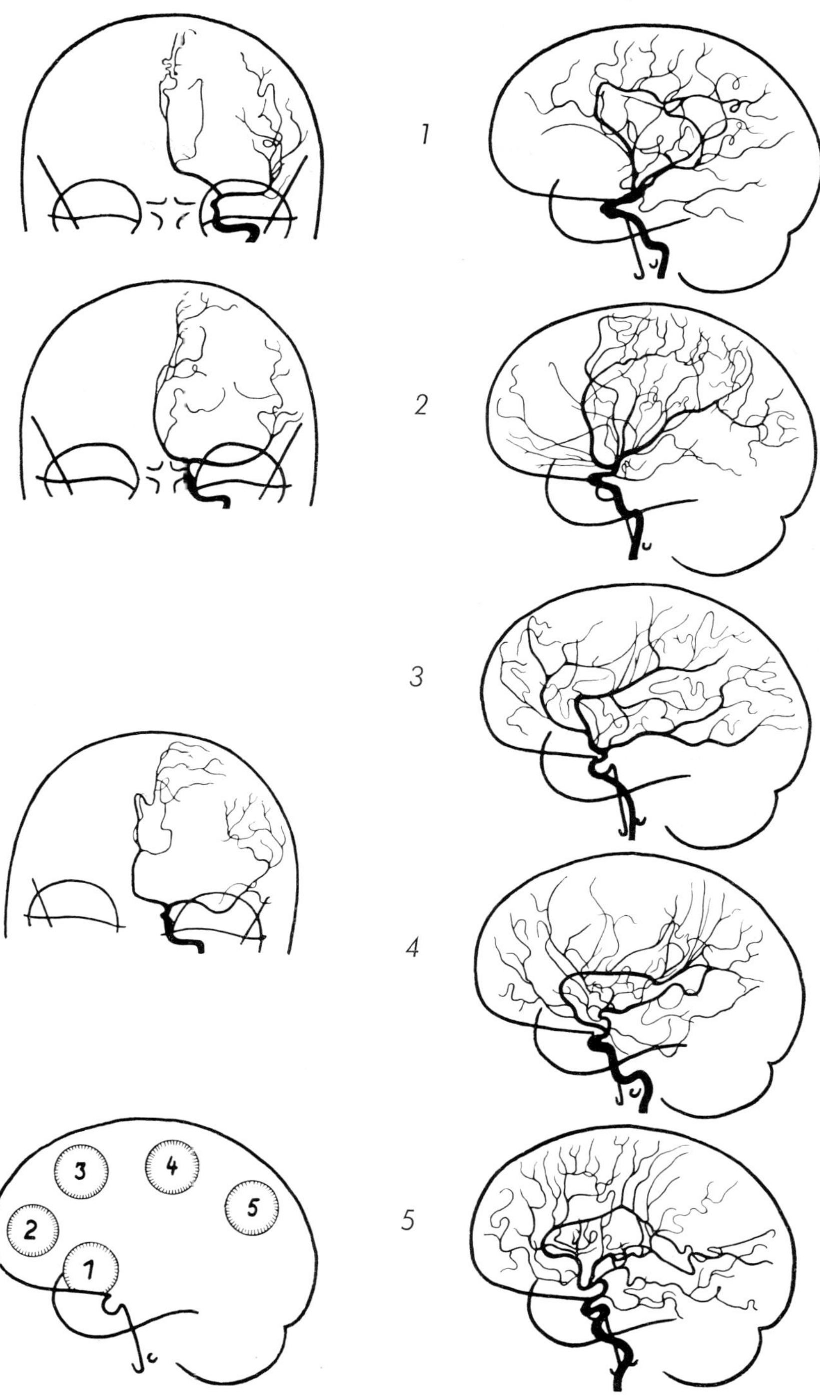

Fig. 48. Basic variations in arterial displacement caused by tumors in the territory of supply of the anterior cerebral artery

views the direction of the displacement of this artery will indicate which of these two areas of the brain harbors the tumor, just as the anterior cerebral artery in the anteroposterior view distinguishes between right and left hemispheric lesions. Space-occupying processes which are situated over or in front of the Sylvian fissure push the carotid siphon and the middle cerebral artery medially (Figs. 8, 49/1, 2). As a result it is recognized that frontal processes have more of an effect on the internal carotid artery and the proximal middle cerebral artery, while parietal

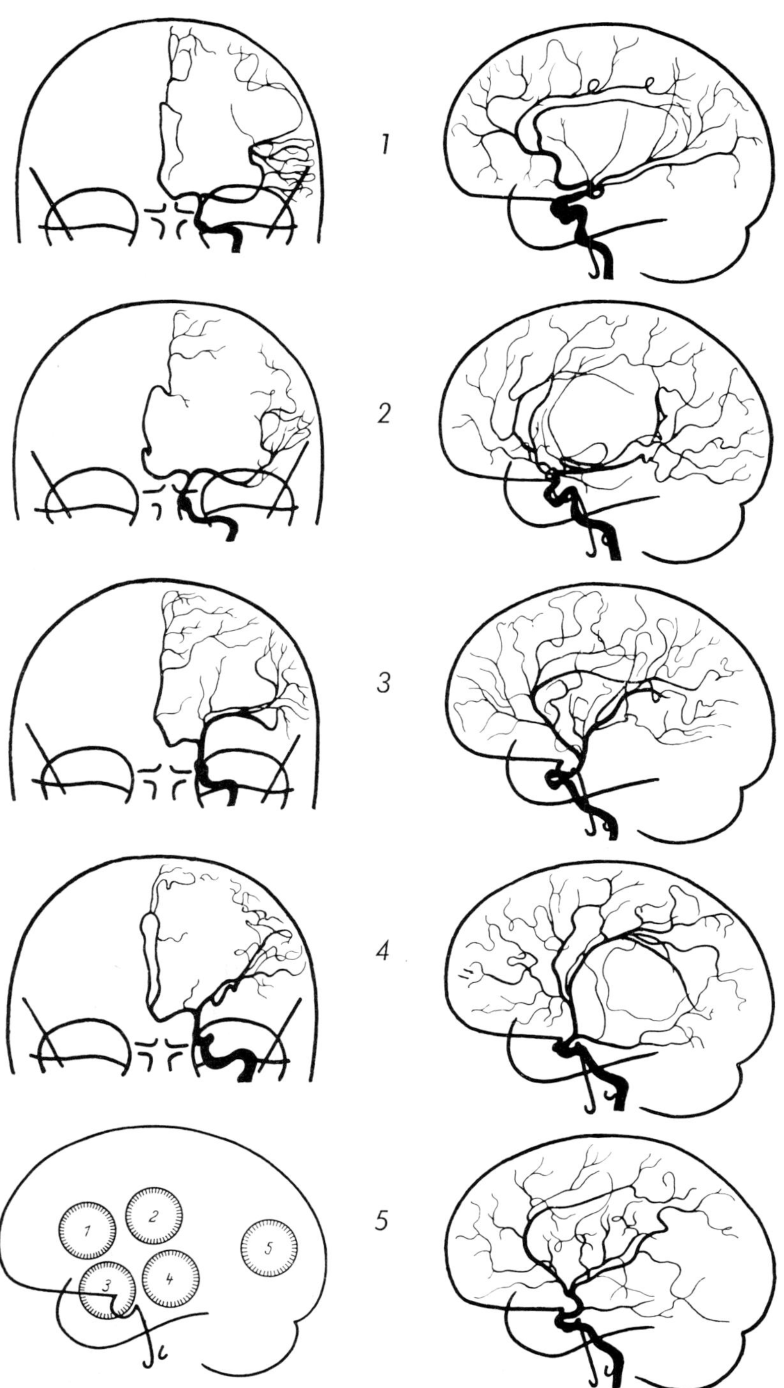

Fig. 49. Basic variations in arterial displacement caused by tumors in the territory of supply of the middle cerebral artery: *1*, frontolateral; *2*, central; *3*, frontotemporal; *4*, temporal; *5*, occipital. In *1* and *2*, the middle cerebral artery is displaced inferiorly; in *3*, posteriorly and superiorly (see p. 96); and in *4* and *5*, superiorly

tumors exert their influence more on the middle (M-2) or end segments (M-4 and M-5) of the middle cerebral artery. Temporal and occipital tumors which are situated under the Sylvian fissure affect corresponding segments of the middle cerebral artery (Fig. 49/3, 4, 5). The anterior cerebral artery with both of the last mentioned groups is less involved in the lateral projection. When it is involved, it is displaced upward and its curve exaggerated. In occipital tumors it is necessary to investigate changes in the course of the posterior cerebral artery and to interpret these according to the concepts just discussed. With such tumors it often seems as though the entire internal carotid artery tree in the lateral projection has been bent forward at the level of the terminal segment of the internal carotid artery trunk (C-3), as though it had been neatly "tipped" over.

Analysis of Individual Vessel Segments

An analysis of individual vessel segments in broad perspective follows.

The major portions of the internal carotid artery from an angiographic viewpoint are as follows:

Internal carotid artery: Displacements of the *cervical portion* of the internal carotid artery can be effected on the one hand by space-occupying processes in the region of the neck (glomus tumors, cysts, aneurysms, neurilemmomas, and malignant tumors); and on the other hand by space-occupying processes in the region of the floor of the posterior cranial fossa (meningiomas, glomus jugulare tumors, chordomas, etc.). With displacement of the *ganglion segment* (C-5) and the *intracavernous segment* (C-4) of the internal carotid artery, the carotid siphon is as a rule also displaced and correspondingly deformed. It is also true that with severe displacements the vessel lumen can be more or less *compromised*. Tumors which arise from the base of the skull, as well as extradural trigeminal neurilemmomas, can displace both the ganglion segment and the intracavernous segment superiorly together with the carotid siphon. In this case the ophthalmic artery may appear stretched (Fig. 50a). Parasellar tumors (chondromas, chordomas, epidermoids, teratomas, and also laterally extending pituitary tumors) can push the ganglion segment and the intracavernous segment of the internal carotid artery inferiorly and against the base of the skull, while displacing the upper limb of the siphon and usually the middle cerebral artery superiorly. The carotid siphon is thus "opened" and the intracranial segment of the internal carotid artery appears to have been unfolded (Fig. 50b). These segments of the internal carotid artery can also be displaced medially or even laterally – however only to a lesser degree – depending upon whether the disease process is extending laterally to one side or to the

other (as with a pituitary adenoma). It must be emphasized in this regard that all vessel displacements of the internal carotid artery must be considered very carefully since this vessel does not ordinarily vary in its course to any significant degree.

Of importance are the displacements which the *cisternal segment* of the carotid siphon (C-2) undergoes. They are best seen on the lateral view. These displacements can be brought about by adjacent tumors, i.e., in the region of the sella, or through more distant effects of frontal and temporal lobe processes. Presellar frontal and central tumors push the cisternal segment of the siphon posteriorly and inferiorly together with the knee (C-3). Parasellar, suprasellar, retrosellar, and above all temporal tumors elevate the upper limb of the siphon and "stretch" the siphon itself. In parasellar processes which elevate the internal carotid artery one can sometimes see a high position of origin of the ophthalmic artery whose normally stretched course would be angulated. Changes in the cisternal segment of the carotid siphon are so closely associated with those of the carotid bifurcation that they will be considered further in the following section (see p. 101 ff and Fig. 53).

Carotid bifurcation: The carotid bifurcation or carotid fork (C-1, A-1, M-1) is (especially for the beginner) easier to judge on the anteroposterior view (Fig. 51/1). It is obviously also necessary here to compare films obtained in both planes to gain an overall picture, an analysis of which can occasionally put considerable strain on the imaginative faculties. In the anteroposterior view the carotid bifurcation appears as a vertically rising trunk (C-1) with corresponding medial and lateral branches, the *pars circularis of the anterior cerebral artery* (A-1) and the *sphenoid wing segment of the middle cerebral artery* (M-1). All three parts of the carotid bifurcation take a more or less winding course, especially in the setting of arteriosclerosis and of cerebral atrophy. For tumor localization, dislocations of both branches are important, as has already been mentioned in the section on general observations (Fig. 46). Median parasellar processes elevate the chiasmal segment (pars circularis) of the anterior cerebral artery (Figs. 51/2, 52). Unilateral frontal pole processes push both branches of the fork inferiorly and laterally so that these appear stretched and more or less compressed (Fig. 51/3). The

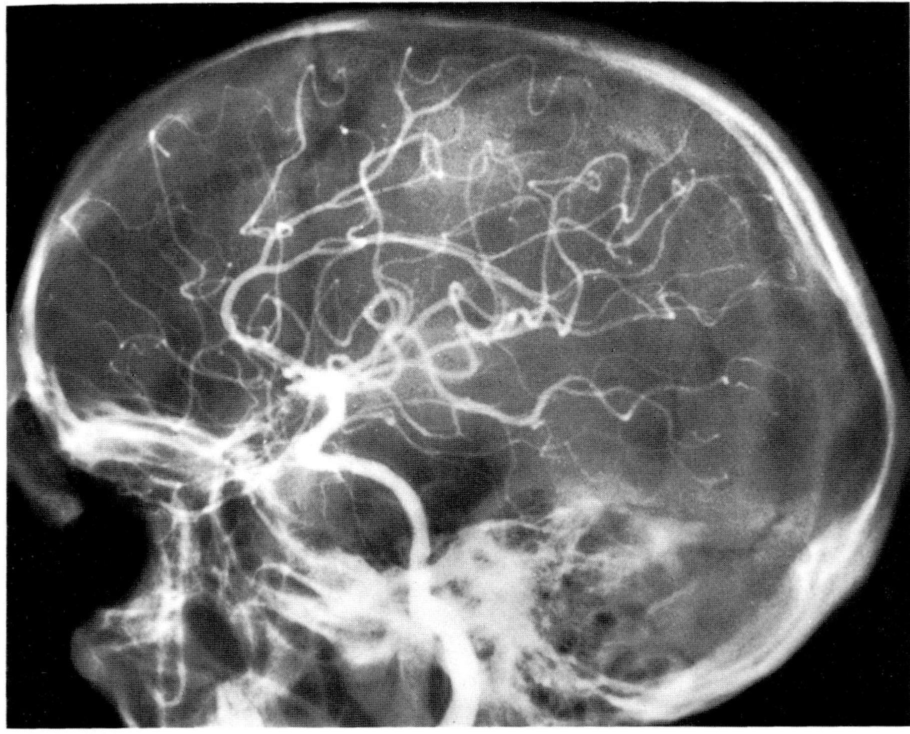

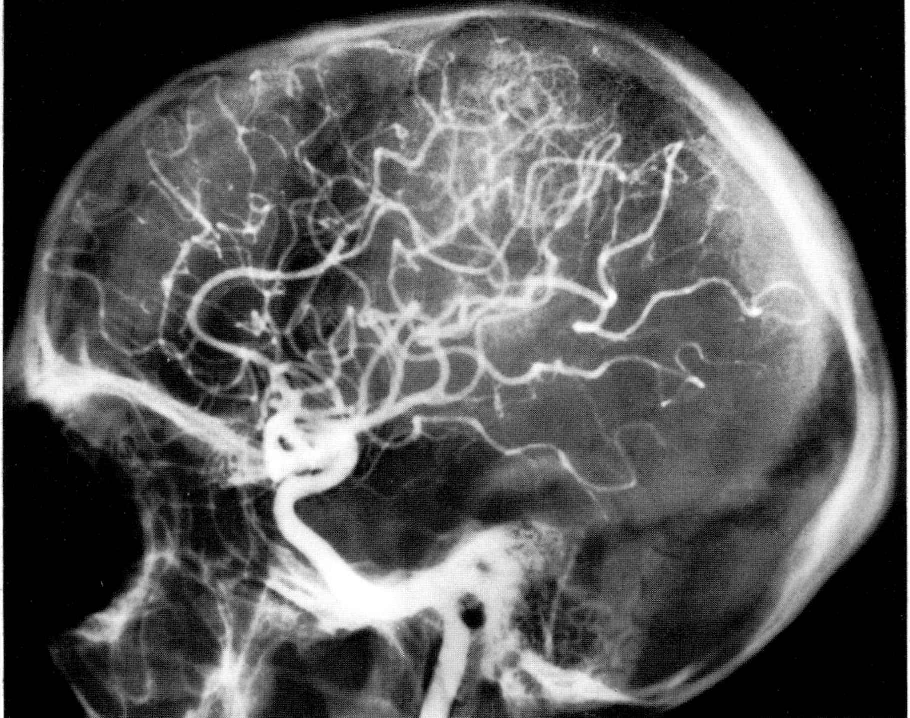

Fig. 50a, b. Displacement of the extradural segment of the internal carotid artery: **a** above, secondary to a trigeminal neurilemmoma; **b** below, secondary to a laterally growing pituitary adenoma

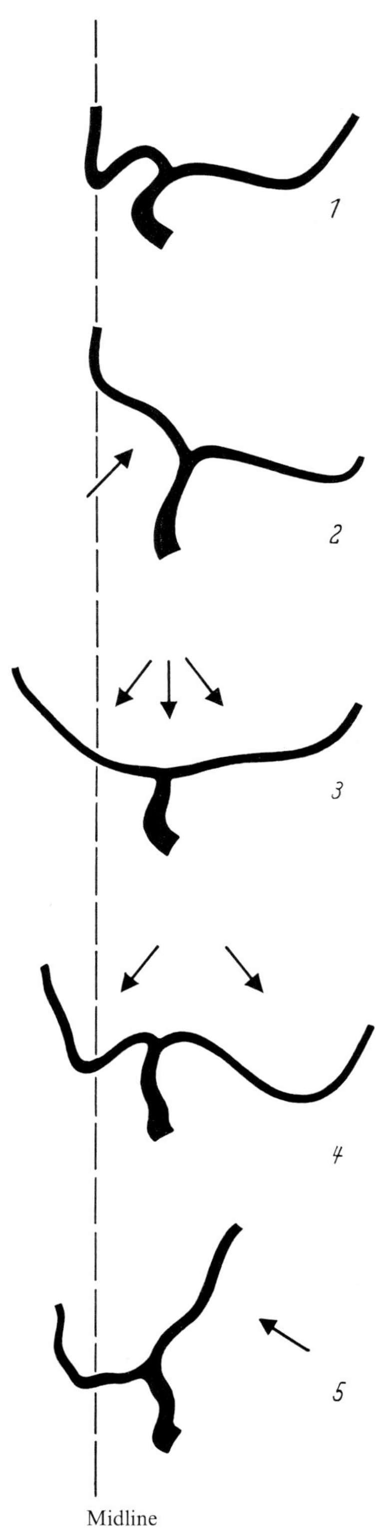

Fig. 51. Schematic demonstration of various changes in the carotid bifurcation, anteroposterior view: *1*, normal; *2*, elevation of A-1 with a presellar tumor; *3*, flattening of the carotid fork with a frontal lobe tumor; *4*, mushroom shape with a frontal tumor which has extended into the basal ganglia; *5*, temporal lobe tumor

picture of the carotid bifurcation in hydrocephalus is similar except that the anterior cerebral artery is not shifted from its midline course.

Farther posteriorly and deeper situated tumors (such as those of the basal ganglia) lead to the so-called mushroom deformity of the carotid fork (Fig. 51/4). This deformity, however, is occasionally also seen in occipital tumors or as an anatomical variant. Temporal tumors elevate the lateral branch of the fork, i.e., the proximal segment of the middle cerebral artery, in an exceptionally marked fashion (Figs. 51/5, 54).

In evaluating the carotid bifurcation on the *lateral projection* one must first consider the normal anatomy since superimposition of various vessel segments makes analysis difficult. The terminal segment of the internal carotid artery (C-1) is readily recognized in the lateral projection. However, the proximal segments of both the anterior cerebral artery (A-1) and the middle cerebral artery (M-1) are poorly seen in this view. The middle cerebral artery runs posterior to the lesser wing of the sphenoid in an anteriorly directed, mildly convex curve which, in addition, lies primarily in the horizontal plane (Fig. 37). Its outer and inner limbs tend, therefore, to be superimposed. In addition, it is also superimposed on the anterior cerebral artery (Fig. 53/1). FISCHER (1938, 1939) refers to this situation as a "covered" carotid bifurcation – however, with a slight alteration in the angle of projection, with a slight variation in the anatomical course, with hydrocephalus, and with all the various vascular displacements seen in the space-occupying processes, this "covering" is lifted and the individual vessels clearly distinguished ("opening" of the carotid bifurcation). In such situations both the pars circularis of the anterior cerebral artery and the proximal segment of the middle cerebral artery are likewise uncovered and can be better appreciated. This picture can be reproduced by means of two basic disease processes. *Frontal tumors* (especially with herniation into the cistern of the Sylvian fissure) can push the middle cerebral artery curve (M-1) posteriorly and inferiorly (Fig. 53/2). Then one looks at the carotid bifurcation from above. The branches of the fork (A-1 and M-1) form an obtuse angle with these tumors and the limbs of the carotid siphon (C-3) are pressed close together. In *temporal tumors* the bend of the

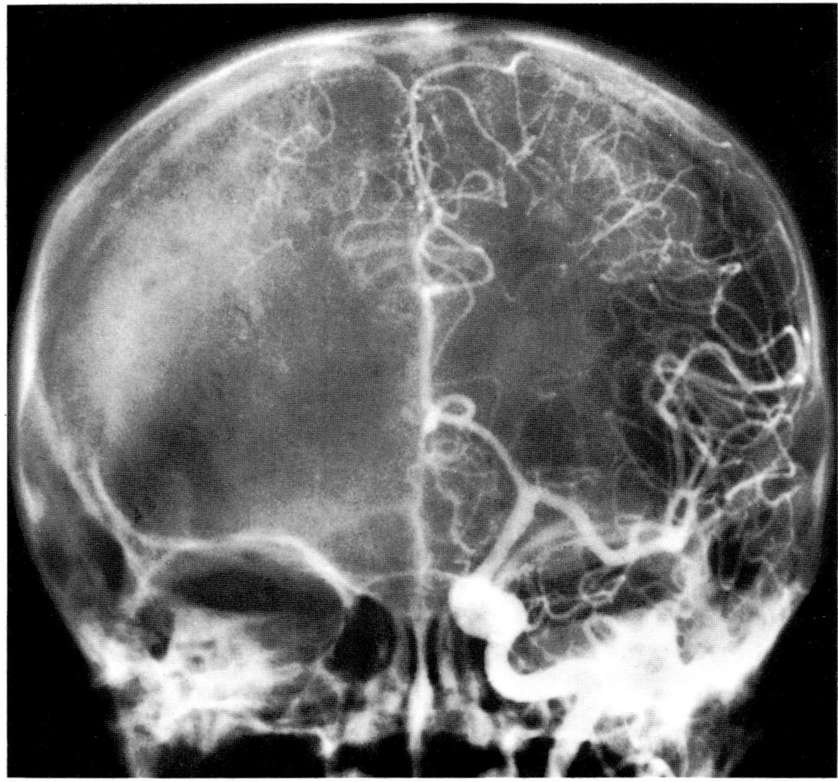

Fig. 52. Displacement of the pars circularis of the anterior cerebral artery with a meningioma of the tuberculum sella

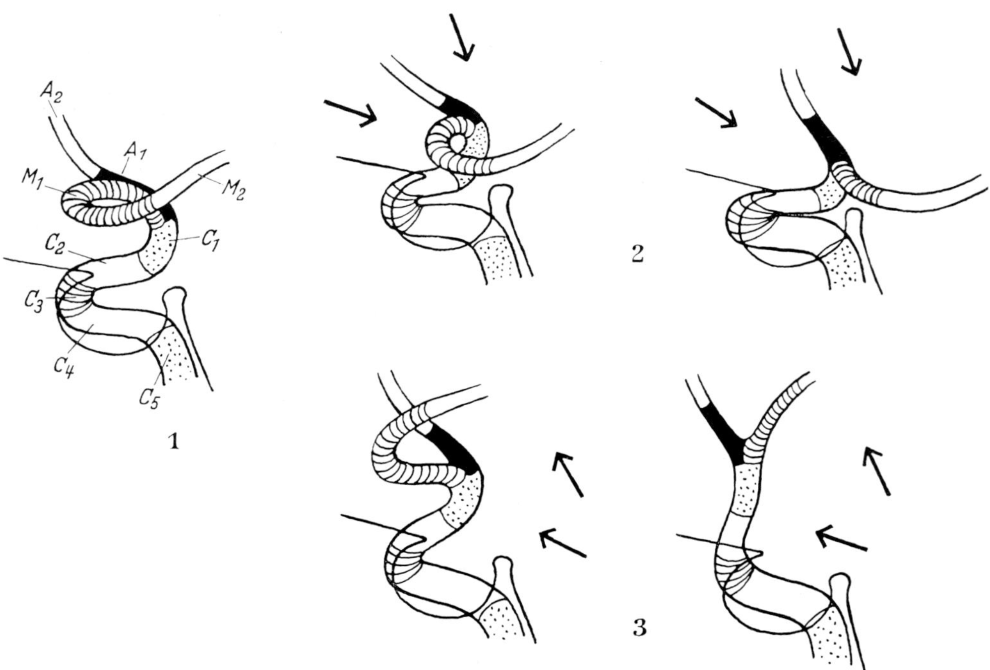

Fig. 53. Schematic demonstration of various changes in the carotid bifurcation, lateral view: *1*, normal; *2*, different degrees of opening of the carotid fork with frontal lesions; *3*, different degrees of opening of the fork with temporal lesions

Fig. 54a, b. Frontotemporal tumor (sphenoid wing meningioma)

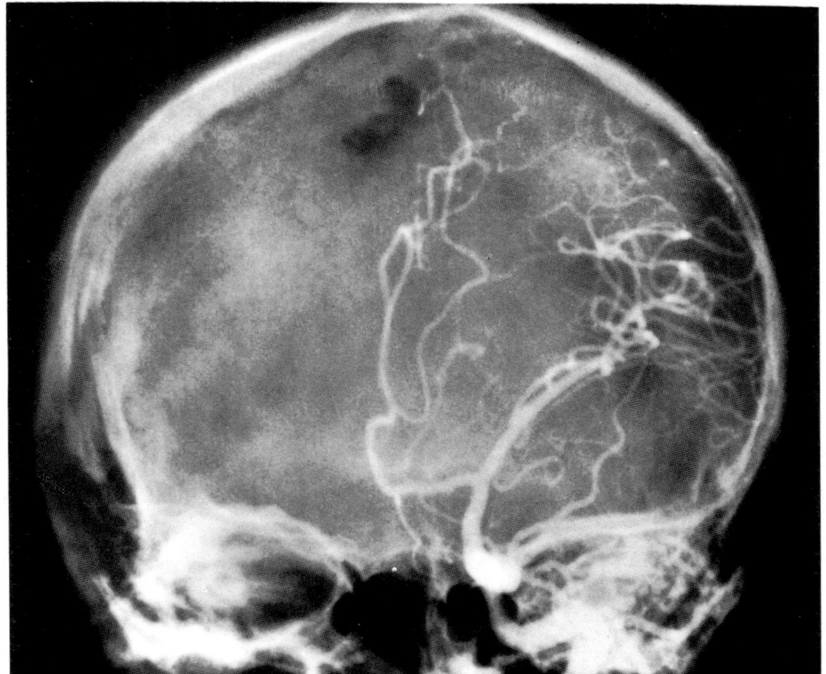

a

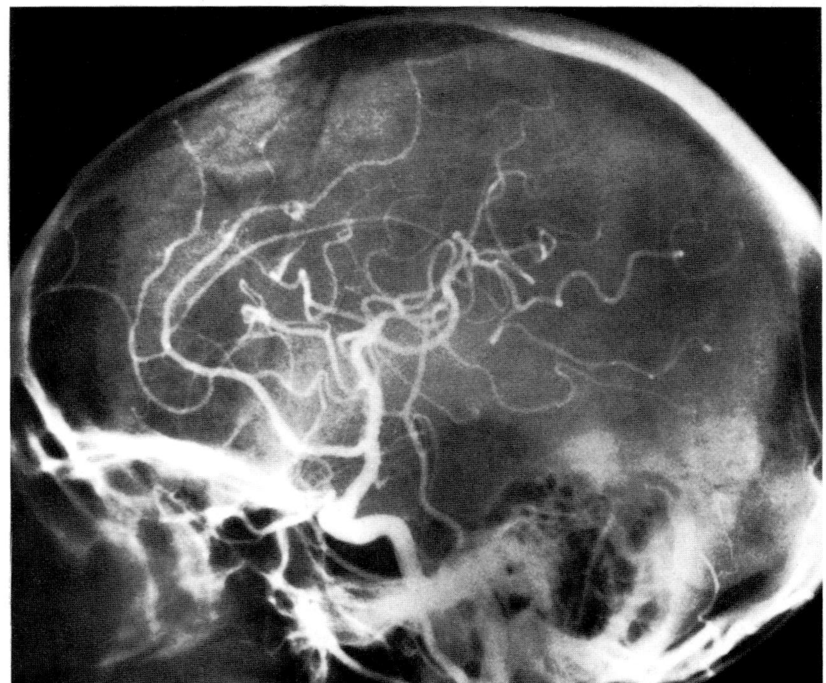

b

proximal middle cerebral artery and the upper limb of the carotid siphon are both displaced upward and the siphon opened. Here, one looks into the curve from below and outward. The angle between the proximal segment of the anterior cerebral artery (A-1) and the vertically displaced sphenoid wing segment of the middle cerebral artery (M-1) becomes acute (Fig. 53/3).

In extracerebral *frontotemporal tumors* the relationships are particularly difficult to interpret. Here a combination of the two displacements described earlier comes into play.

The following displacements are commonly seen in such tumors. The supraclinoid segment of the carotid siphon is pushed medially and inferiorly with a more marked frontal expansion of the tumor, but is elevated with a greater temporal involvement. The terminal segment of the internal carotid artery and the proximal segment of the middle cerebral artery are both drawn out around the medial and posterior surface of the tumor in an upward curve. In its further course the middle cerebral artery may be elevated by that part of the tumor which is growing within the middle cranial fossa from below. Normally, the proximal segment of the middle cerebral artery runs parallel to the lesser wing of the sphenoid. In tumors which arise from the lesser wing of the sphenoid the middle cerebral artery is displaced superomedially and posteriorly.

The anteroposterior projection on the arteriogram with such extracerebral frontotemporal tumors corresponds to that of intraaxial tumors of the temporal pole (Fig. 54a). The sphenoid wing segment of the middle cerebral artery is markedly elevated from its horizontal position so that it runs from its origin not laterally, but rather superiorly, and then gradually bends in a basal concave curve into the insular segment (M-2). On the lateral projection (Fig. 54b) the terminal segment of the internal carotid artery (C-1) and the proximal segment of the middle cerebral artery (M-1) are markedly elevated. In its further course the middle cerebral artery turns sharply to a horizontal position, but remains elevated. If the tumor is situated well within the middle cranial fossa, the supraclinoid segment of the carotid siphon together with the terminal segment of the internal carotid artery will be elevated so that the carotid siphon will have an "opened" appearance.

Middle cerebral artery: For all temporal space-occupying processes, the elevation of the middle cerebral artery is characteristic. In this situation, the anteroposterior view alone can show a definite localization within the temporal lobe. Tumors which are situated within the pole of the temporal lobe, especially those with a frontotemporal localization (the sphenoid wing meningiomas), push predominantly the sphenoid wing segment of the middle cerebral artery (M-1) superiorly, while the insular segment (M-2) is not involved at all or is less involved (Fig. 55/1). Tumors which arise in the middle temporal lobe displace the middle cerebral artery medially, anteriorly, and superiorly. Therefore, on the anteroposterior view the middle cerebral artery takes an oblique superolaterally directed course (Fig. 55/2). Tumors of the middle and posterior temporal lobe affect the sphe-

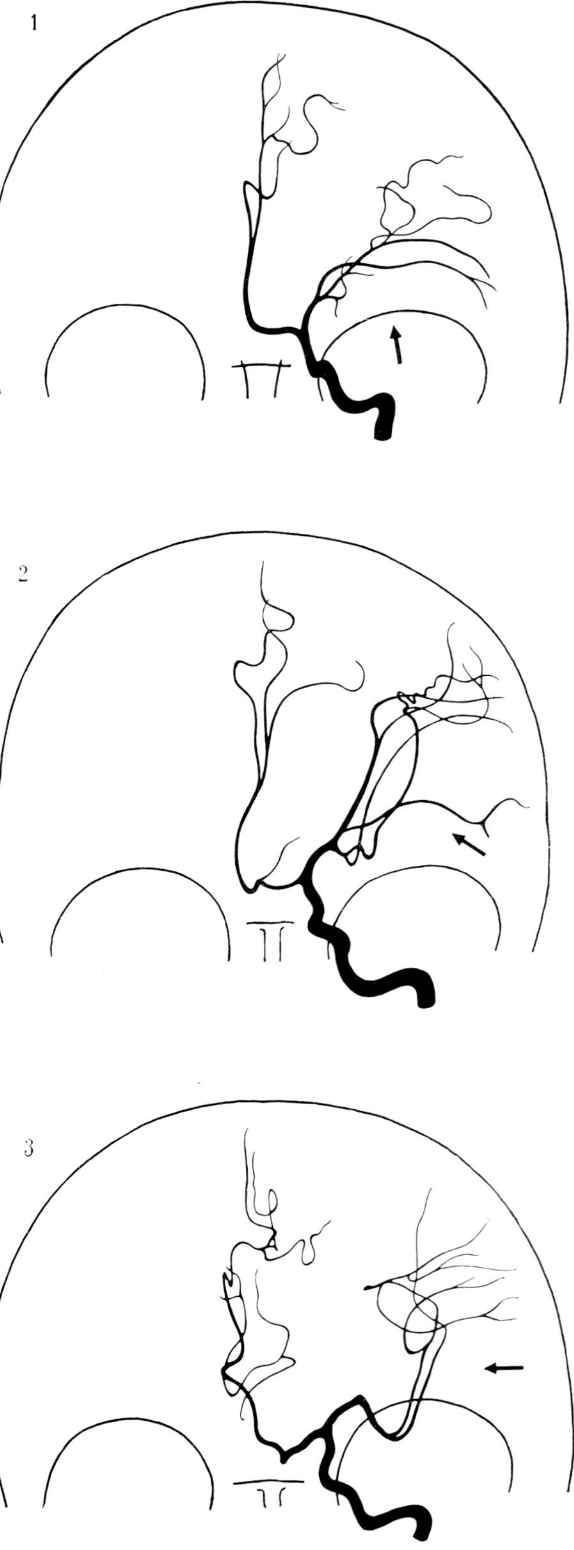

Fig. 55. Schematic representation of varying displacements of the middle cerebral artery, anteroposterior view: *1*, temporal pole tumor; *2*, tumor of the mid-temporal lobe; *3*, tumor of the posterior temporal lobe

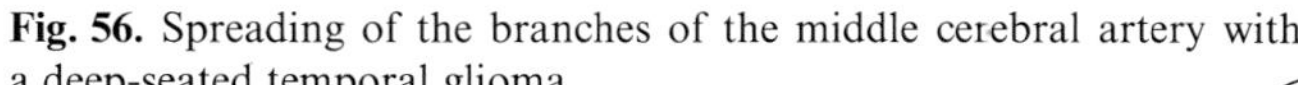

Fig. 56. Spreading of the branches of the middle cerebral artery with a deep-seated temporal glioma

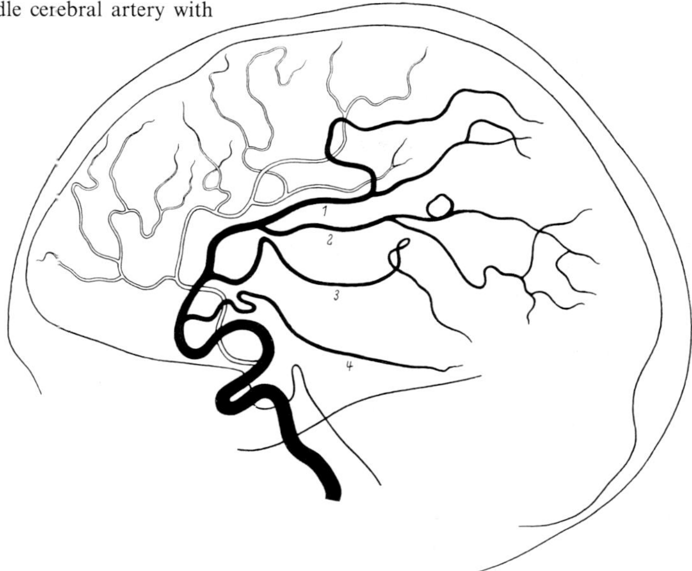

noid wing segment of the middle cerebral artery somewhat less but push the insular segment medially (Fig. 55/3).

A general description of the corresponding changes in the *lateral projection* have already been given (see p. 101). From the detailed individual analyses given above, one can generalize that *anterior* temporal lobe tumors *open* maximally the carotid siphon and the carotid bifurcation (right-hand diagram of Fig. 53/3).

In such cases the sphenoid wing segment of the middle cerebral artery will be strongly elevated, while the vessel segments lying more occipitally are less moved by this occurrence. *Posterior* temporal lobe tumors affect the carotid bifurcation, sphenoid wing segment, and insular segment of the middle cerebral artery to a *lesser degree* (left-hand diagram of Fig. 53/3), elevating instead the *terminal branches* of the middle cerebral artery. These tumors are easier to recognize in the lateral projection than in the anteroposterior view. It might be added that occasionally the branches of the middle cerebral artery are stretched out (Fig. 56). Such spreading is especially common in deep-seated gliomas lying between the involved branches. Occasionally meningiomas of the Sylvian fissure produce a similar picture. On the other hand, tumors of the convexity of the frontal lobe and of the anterior parietal lobe result in an inferior displacement of the insular branches (M-2) of the middle cerebral artery and cause stretching and unravelling of the normal vessel loops in this vessel group.

Deep-seated space-occupying processes of the central region produce a characteristic separating effect on the rising middle cerebral artery branches (M-3). Since they are all equally stretched they show an unusually parallel course. Tumors of the posterior parietal region push the posterior portion of the Sylvian group in a basal direction. As a consequence of this mass displacement the anterior temporal lobe is displaced forward and upward. Tumors in this region can thus be quite deceptive.

Tumors in the occipital region push the posterior branch of the middle cerebral artery and the anterior cerebral artery together in a superior and anterior direction. This tilts the entire carotid tree anteriorly with the siphon as the turning point.

Anterior cerebral artery: In the further analysis of individual vessel segments, the knee, the orbital segment, and the callosal segment of the anterior cerebral artery (A-2, A-3, and A-4) are of importance. Changes on the *lateral view* by tumors near the falx between the orbital roof and the occipital region have already been described (see p. 96). With meningiomas of the olfactory groove (Fig. 57) the pars circularis and orbital segments of the anterior cerebral artery are displaced backward and upward by the local pressure effect. Regarding the blood supply to these meningiomas, the ophthalmic artery is most important followed by the ethmoid branches. It should be noted that frontomedial and frontodorsal intracerebral tumors, especially when they involve the knee of the

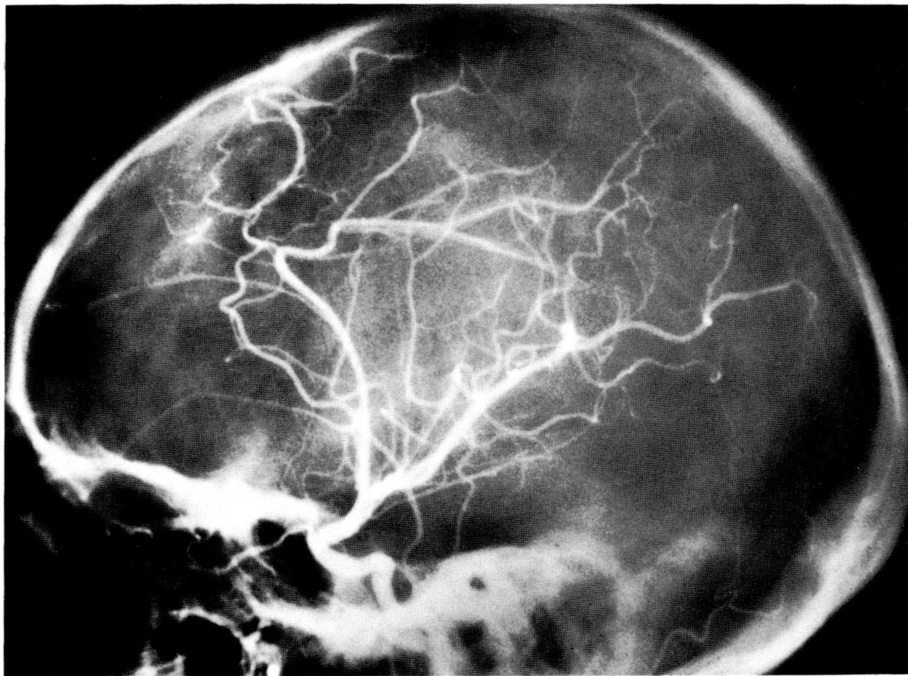

Fig. 57. Displacement of the anterior cerebral artery with an olfactory groove meningioma: posterior and superior displacement of the anterior cerebral artery (refer to Fig. 48/*1*)

corpus callosum, do not displace the anterior cerebral artery downward, but rather increase its frontodorsal curvature. Such intracerebral locations can often be appreciated by comparison of pneumoencephalography with the vascular picture. While the anterior horn is depressed in such cases the anterior cerebral artery is either stretched upward or is essentially uninvolved. In contrast, extracerebral tumors in this area, for example, parasagittal meningiomas, displace both artery and ventricle inferiorly.

The *lateral view* of the anterior cerebral artery is important for the recognition of advanced hydrocephalus. Mild degrees of hydrocephalus may not be recognized at all on the arteriogram. The changes consist of a widening of the anterior cerebral artery curve as well as that of the pericallosal artery. This vessel is – as are all other vessels in *hydrocephalus* – "stretched" (Fig. 58). A similar contour which can lead to confusion is seen in hypoplasia of the pericallosal artery, in which the callosomarginal artery seems to form the continuation of the anterior cerebral artery curve. The proximal middle cerebral artery with bilateral *occlusive hydrocephalus* can take a slight dorsally convex curve, which should not be misinterpreted as a temporal lobe tumor.

In aplasia of the corpus callosum, the anterior cerebral artery rises steeply so that it does not form an actual knee (A-3). The pericallosal artery is absent as well.

Of importance is the careful interpretation of the anterior cerebral artery on the anteroposterior view. Comment has already been made in the broad outline how important displacements of this artery are with respect to midline determinations. One should, however, not be confused by a filling of the contralateral anterior cerebral artery here. Also, one observes individual vessel twistings extending over the midline in strongly winding sclerotic vessels (Fig. 112). Unintentional angulation of the head to the opposite side during exposure gives the false impression of contralateral displacement of the anterior cerebral artery. One then looks into the anterior cerebral artery curve somewhat from the side.

Displacement of the anterior cerebral artery can be very slight or even lacking in tumors without cerebral edema and without general mass displacement, also with lesions in the *midline* or *occipital* areas, with *bilateral subdural hematomas,* with tumors in *both hemispheres,* and with *tumors in the elderly* (because of coexisting *atrophy*). A significant unilateral cerebral

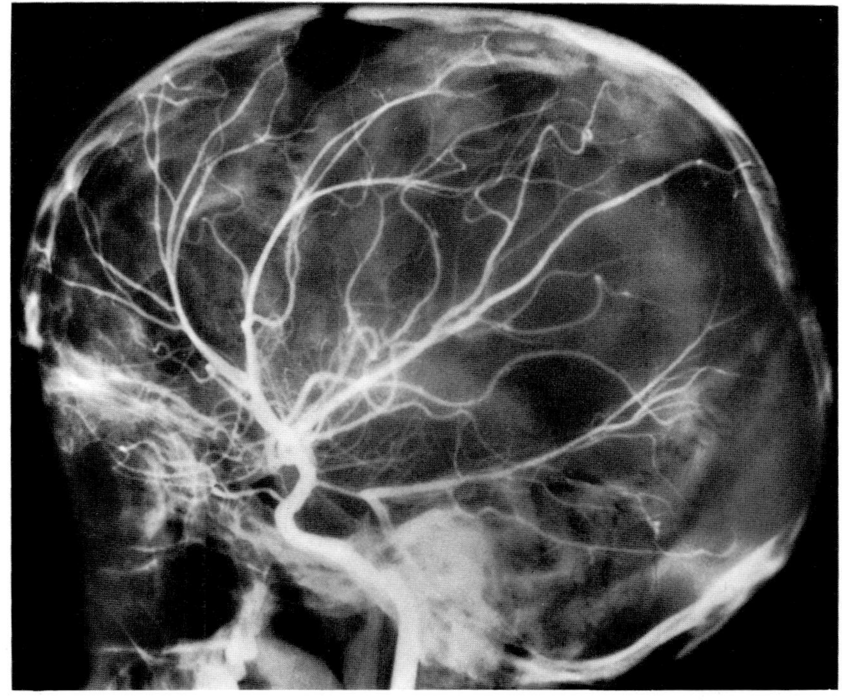

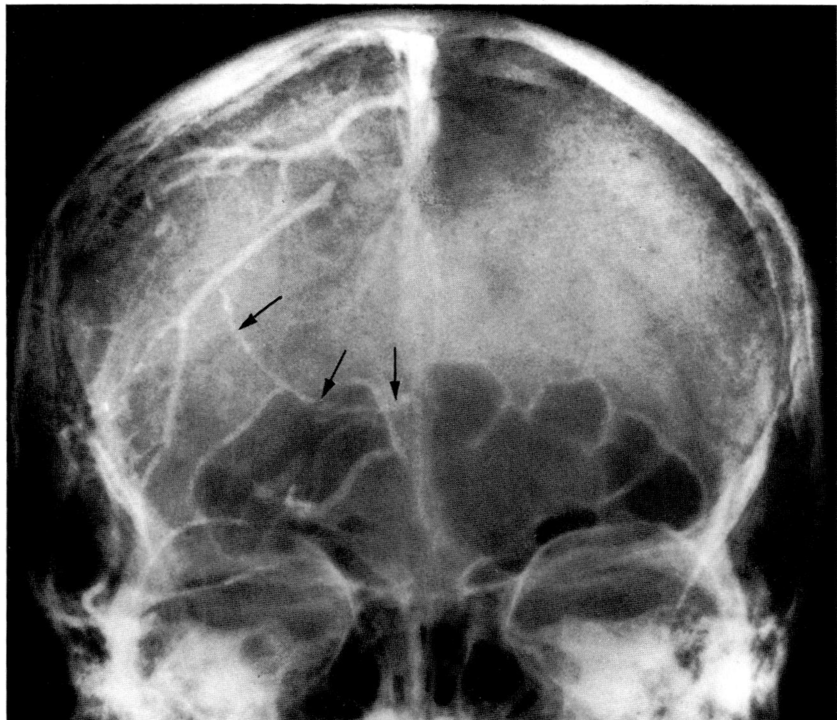

Fig. 58. a Arterial phase of an internal carotid arteriogram in a case with hydrocephalus: extreme widening of the bend in the anterior cerebral artery. The middle cerebral and posterior cerebral arteries are both stretched. **b** The thalamostriate vein as seen in the anteroposterior venous phase is forming a wide open curve

atrophy leads to displacement of the midline anterior cerebral artery in the direction of the atrophic hemisphere. Such a displacement can be mistaken for a space-occupying process on the opposite side (Fig. 47).

FISCHER-BRÜGGE (1950) has sought to localize more clearly the type of displacement of the anterior cerebral artery caused by space-occupying processes. He has proposed a variety of criteria for distinguishing the localization of a lesion either "near" or "distant" from the knee and callosal segment of the anterior cerebral artery, i.e., with the medial portion of the frontal lobe being considered the "nearest" position. As "distant" signs he has described a positive *falx sign,* a positive *frontopolar sign,* an increased *tortuosity* and *parallel* (vertical) *displacement* of the anterior cerebral artery and its branches, as well as *dissociation* of the pericallosal and callosomarginal vessels. As "near" signs he values the bowed displacement and stretched course of the anterior cerebral artery and its branches, the absent dissociation, the negative falx and frontopolar signs, and the absent tortuosity. More recent investigations have shown that of these signs only the opposing parallel and bowed displacement of the anterior cerebral artery are accurate criteria for localization in this regard (Fig. 59).

By *parallel displacement* is meant displacement of the anterior cerebral artery to the opposite side in a manner which keeps it parallel to the midline. This implies that the tumor lies "distant" from the knee and callosal segment of the anterior cerebral artery, and "distant" from the medial and dorsal portions of the frontal lobe. In an oblique placement of the falx the anterior cerebral artery and its branches are displaced together to the contralateral side in a typical *"bowed" fashion,* which is interpreted as a *"near" sign* and suggests localization of the pathological process in the medial or dorsal region of the frontal lobe (see p. 14, and Figs. 13, 59).

A short comment is still needed regarding the terminal ramifications of the anterior cerebral and middle cerebral arteries (A-5 and M-5). These are evaluated predominantly in the lateral views and are partly superimposed in the posterior parietal regions. This region therefore seems to be particularly "well-endowed with vessels" and can easily lead to errors in interpretation.

The posterior cerebral artery, usually a branch of the basilar artery, is filled by means of the posterior communicating artery in approximately 20%–30% of carotid arteriograms. The temporal pressure cone through the tentorial hiatus which accompanies temporal and parietal tumors can be diagnosed angiographically by characteristic distortions in the course of the posterior communicating and posterior cerebral arteries (Fig. 60).

The arterial phase of the vertebral angiogram. The vertebral artery is subject to displacement even during its course in the neck by space-occupying processes. Most frequently this results from a neurilemmoma which is partially intraspinal and partially extraspinal (the so-called dumbbell or hour-glass tumor) (Fig. 61).

The relatively small volume of the infratentorial space and the slight possibility of displacement of its contents results in only a limited displacement of vessels. Mass displacement is only possible through the tentorial hiatus upward and through the foramen magnum downward. However, occlusive hydrocephalus, common with tumors in this region, will resist upward herniation through the tentorial hiatus because of counterpressure from the dilated ventricular system.

Space-occupying processes on the *clivus* (meningioma, chordoma) displace the *basilar artery* posteriorly. If the process extends to the foramen magnum, the terminal segments of the vertebral arteries are not only displaced posteriorly as well, but are also separated from one another so that they simultaneously embrace the tumor (Fig. 62).

A high position of the basilar artery and a separating tendency of the terminal segments of the vertebral arteries can also be seen in a *basilar impression.* Deviations of the basilar artery from the midline must be interpreted with care, especially when these are the only changes present, since there can be a significant asymmetry in the position and shape of the terminal segment of the basilar artery as an expression of *anatomical variance* and particularly when arteriosclerotic change has occurred. On the other hand, the position of the basilar bifurcation is important since this is normally a midline structure.

A displacement of the basilar artery anteriorly and inferiorly so that it is pressed against the clivus and dorsum sella is seen in tumors of the cerebellum and brain stem. It is, however, not a dependable sign for a space-occupying process. An inferior displacement of the loop of the *posterior inferior cerebellar* artery beneath the rim of the foramen magnum is, as a rule, an expression of tonsillar herniation into the foramen magnum. A similar position can, however, occasionally also be seen as an anatomical variant or may result from arteriosclerotic change.

Space-occupying processes of the *cerebellopontine angle* displace the superior cerebellar artery and particularly the anterior inferior cerebellar artery, which in the sagittal half-axial

Fig. 59. "Far" and "near" signs with displacement of the ▷
anterior cerebral artery. *Above: Fa*, positive "falx sign";
Fp, positive "frontopolar sign"; *P*, parallel displacement
over the midline; *D*, dissociation. *Below: Fa*, negative
"falx sign"; *Fp*, negative "frontopolar sign"; *D*, no dissociation; *B*, bowed displacement across the midline

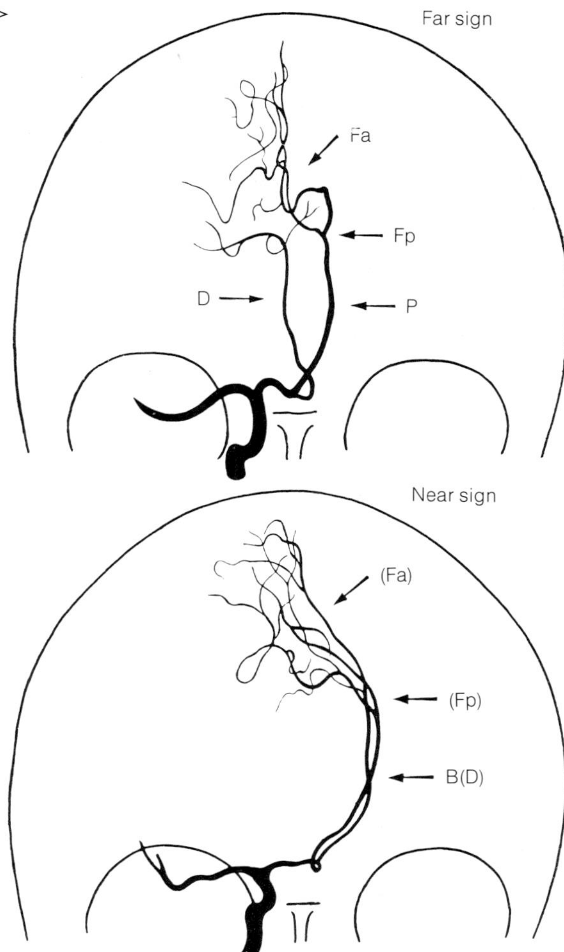

Fig. 60. Curved downward displacement of the posterior
communicating artery and the proximal portion of the
posterior cerebral artery as a sign of temporal lobe herniation

▽

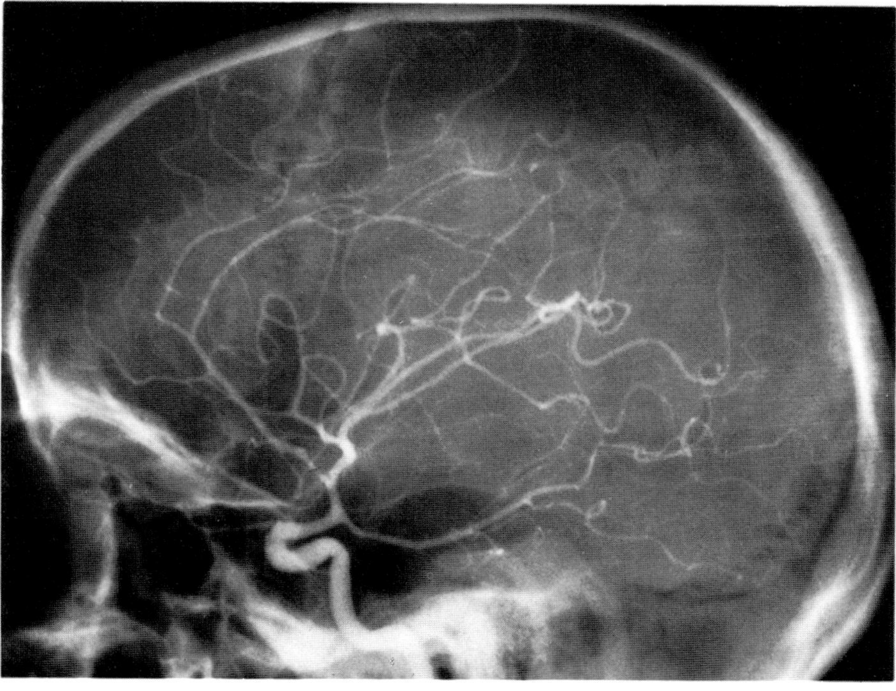

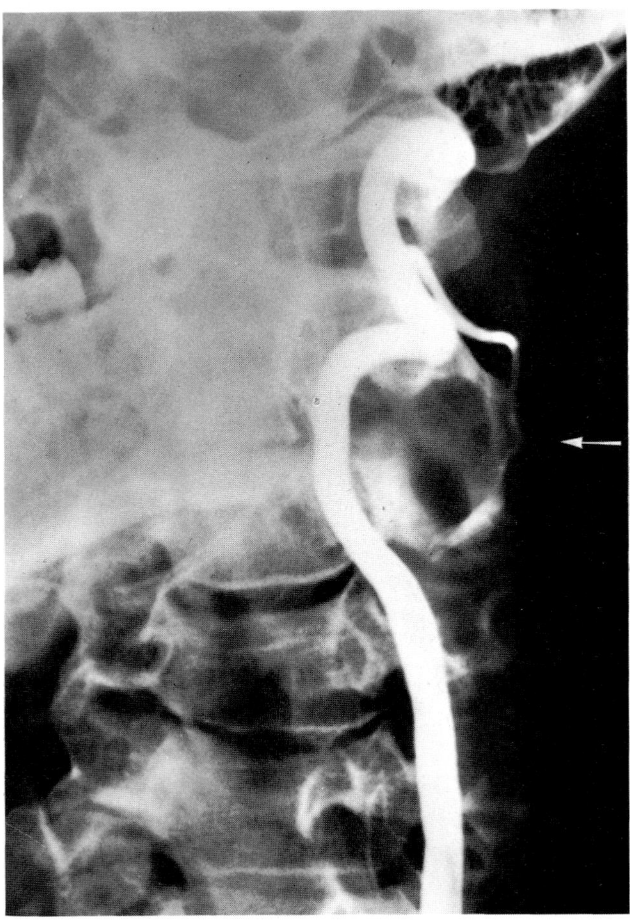

Fig. 61. Displacement of the left vertebral artery secondary to a large neurilemmoma of the third left cervical root

Fig. 62. Displacement of the basilar and vertebral arteries secondary to a meningioma of the clivus

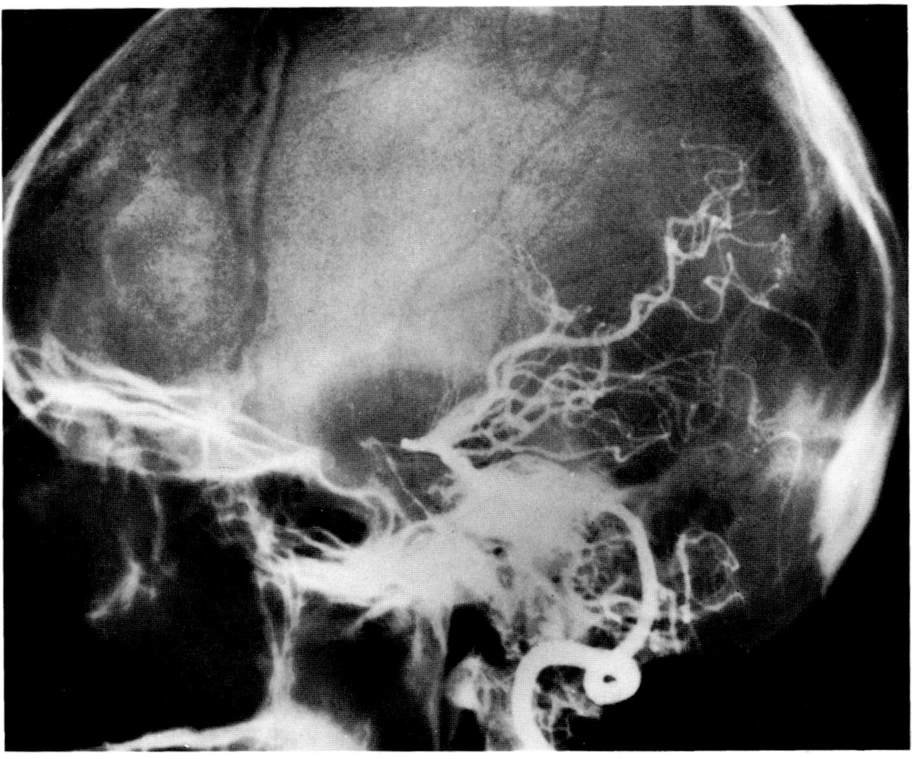

Fig. 63. Left-sided acoustic neurilemmoma (anteroposterior view with subtraction). Note the rounded shape (*arrows*) of the displaced anterior inferior cerebellar artery

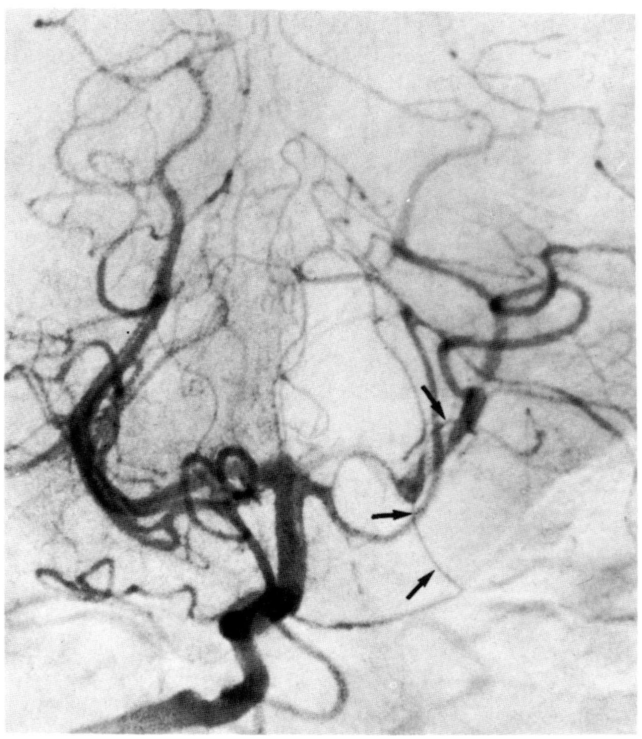

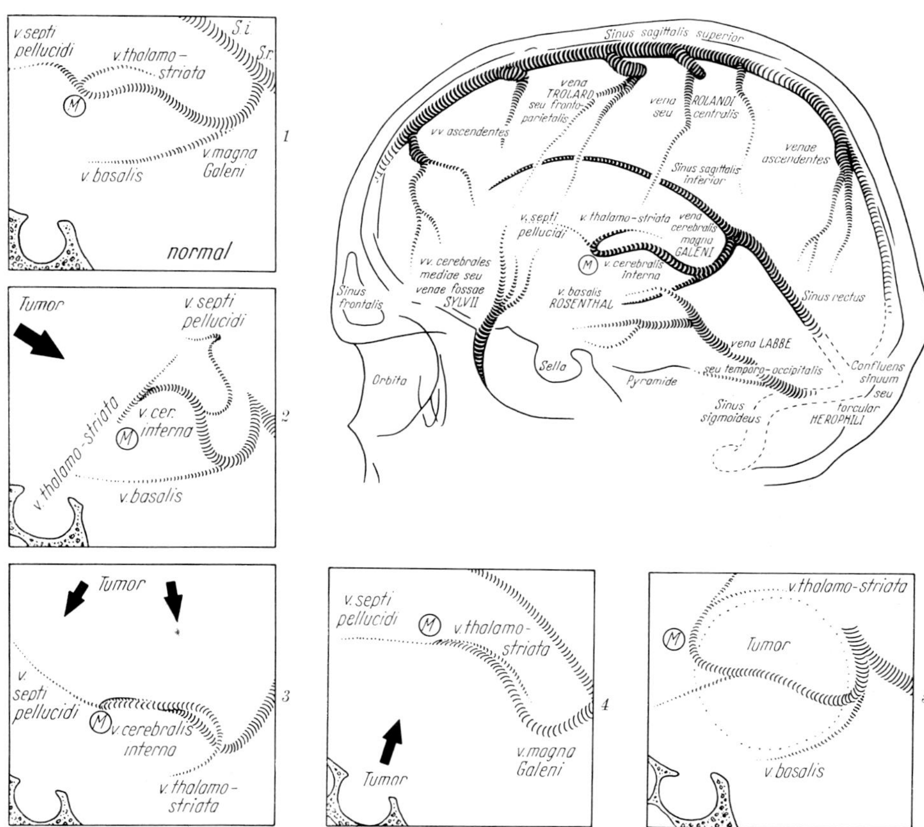

Fig. 64. Displacements of the deep venous system with various tumors. *Boxes: 1,* normal; *2,* frontal tumor; *3,* parietal tumor; *4,* suprasellar tumor; *5,* tumor of the basal ganglia.

Major diagram: normal venous anatomy from KRAYENBÜHL and RICHTER (1952)

projection is quite impressive when compared to the normal side (Fig. 63). In the lateral view the corresponding changes are less well appreciated.

The veins of the supratentorial and infratentorial spaces: In the diagnosis of space-occupying processes, displacements of the larger veins in both the carotid and vertebral angiograms can be as significant as that of the arterial displacements. Thus, displacements of the great *cortical* veins (Fig. 64/1) draining into the superior sagittal sinus point to the precise location of a corresponding space-occupying process.

The position of the great veins on the surface of the exposed brain during surgery provides better orientation as to the location of a tumor than the more deeply situated cortical arteries. Comparison of the venous phase of the angiogram with the exposed brain surface permits more ready identification of specific areas of the cortex with respect to the angiogram.

In the *anteroposterior view,* lateral displacement of the *internal cerebral vein* is a significant indication of the localization of adjacent space-occupying processes, which may affect the anterior cerebral artery very little or not at all. This is especially true for occipital tumors.

Enlargement of the curve of the thalamostriate vein in the anteroposterior view is indicative of enlargement of the lateral ventricle (Fig. 58 b).

In the *lateral view* a displacement of the venous angle in an occipital direction with compression of the internal cerebral vein suggests a frontal space-occupying process (Fig. 64/2). Parietal tumors displace the deep cerebral veins inferiorly (Fig. 64/3). In contrast to this, suprasellar space-occupying processes push the internal cerebral vein superiorly with the result that the venous angle usually becomes narrowed (Fig. 64/4). Thalamic and basal ganglia tumors open up the venous angle by displacement of the thalamostriate vein superiorly. The basal vein of Rosenthal is pushed inferiorly by such tumors (Fig. 64/5).

A widening of the curve between the posterior half of the internal cerebral vein and the vein of Galen is indicative of a growth in the splenium of the corpus callosum.

A high position of the internal cerebral vein with absence of the vein of the septum pellucidum is seen in agenesis of the corpus callosum.

In the angiographic evaluation of the posterior cranial fossa, the venous phase of the vertebral angiogram has particular significance.

These vessels are, however, difficult to evaluate and have only in recent years through the investigations of a couple of neuroradiologists (see HUANG and WOLF, 1964–1970) achieved diagnostic significance. The difficulty lies in the fact that the vessels are rather fine and the contrast filling not always optimal. Subtraction views are absolutely essential to eliminate superimposed bony structures (see also p. 91).

In the consideration of space-occupying processes of the posterior cranial fossa, distinction must be made on the one hand between tumors in the midline and lateral regions, and on the other hand between intracerebellar and extracerebellar growths. Indeed, localization of a tumor by displacement of an individual vein is not only more definitive, but also a much earlier indication of pathological change than arterial displacement. The veins of the posterior cranial fossa have already been mentioned in the description of the normal vertebral angiogram.

The pontomesencephalic veins outline precisely the contour of the pons and the anterior wall of the brain stem. They are readily recognizable on the lateral view. The demonstration of this venous system gives the same information as does an air study of the pontine cistern. Prepontine space-occupying processes displace the veins posteriorly, particularly the anterior pontomesencephalic veins and the precentral cerebellar vein. If the tumor is situated within the pons, veins which lie on the anterior surface of the pons are displaced anteriorly, while veins lying posterior to the pons are displaced posteriorly.

In intracerebellar space-occupying processes, displacement of the midline vessels is particularly apparent in the half-axial view. In this view the precentral cerebellar vein, which is a constant midline vessel, provides important diagnostic information. In the lateral view the distance between the precentral cerebellar vein and the clivus can be measured and is normally 36–43 mm. When the vein is situated nearer the clivus, this points to a space-occupying process in the dorsal and posterolateral regions of the posterior cranial fossa.

If the presence of a cerebellopontine angle tumor is suspected, evaluation of the petrosal vein of Dandy is particularly important. This vein lies constantly above the internal acoustic meatus and runs in the cerebellopontine angle region making it possible to evaluate this region (in the anteroposterior half-axial projection). If there is a tumor in this area, the vein is displaced superiorly. It is, however, also possible that the vein can be occluded as a result of pressure from the tumor and may not be seen on the angiogram.

Vessels in the vicinity of a tumor: We have seen that the displacement of large vessel trunks on the angiogram occurs in a similar fashion for all space-occupying processes albeit to different degrees. For *localization,* these changes are of decisive significance. Additional important information can be obtained through an evaluation of the *displacement of smaller vessels in the immediate vicinity of the tumor.* These vessels may seem to be *"stretched"* or *"bent",* since they lose their physiological tortuosity as a result of the displacement. In that their course is dependent to a certain extent on the pathological process present, information may be obtained not only regarding *localization,* but possibly also *tumor type.* In general, it can be said that pre-existing cerebral vessels tend to be pushed away from the area of a lesion with the result that this area appears poorer in vessels than the surrounding regions. That is only true, however, when the tumor itself is not rich in newly formed and clearly visible vessels. In well-circumscribed, superficial, noninfiltrating tumor growths there is displacement of the pre-existing cerebral vessels in a characteristic cup-shaped manner around the tumor bed (Fig. 65a). This is especially true in the case of meningiomas. In the deep-seated space-occupying processes, the individual vessels are so displaced from one another that the distance between them grows greater (Figs. 56, 65b). This is particularly seen in diffusely infiltrating tumor growths as a consequence of widening of the convolutions.

b) Pathological Vascularization in Space-Occupying Processes

The angiographic diagnosis of a tumor may also be made on the basis of *specific tumor vessels,* which can be distinguished from normal cerebral vessels by means of their shape and arrangement. Many tumor types may be recognized solely on the basis of their *characteristic vascularization.* If the pathological vessels are very fine, then the angiogram will not be able to distinguish between individual vessels, and there will be a diffuse enrichment of the contrast medium in the region of the pathological process, often referred to as a tumor "blush".

One must guard against mistaking calcifications within a tumor or the choroid plexus for such a tumor blush. Comparison of the plain X-rays with the angiogram will help prevent such errors.

The *precise timing of the X-ray exposure* will influence demonstration of the tumor. The *circulation time* in vessels in the region of pathological processes is often different than in normal vessels. Flow within the tumor may be slower than normal so that the tumor vessels are best demonstrated in the capillary or venous phases. On the other hand, there are tumor types in which the speed of flow is increased because of AV shunting and the tumor blush can already be seen in the arterial phase. There are techniques which permit the tumor vessels to be especially well-visualized (see p. 66).

The *pattern* of the tumor vessels can suggest the histology and malignant potential of the entire range of space-occupying processes. When the space-occupying process consists of a fluid collection, a *hematoma,* a *cyst,* or an *abscess,* there will be a complete absence of tumor vessels (Fig. 65b). Abscesses can, however, have a capsule which is rich in capillaries. Enlargement of the vessel-free zone is frequently indicative of surrounding cerebral edema.

It is also possible that an avascular space-occupying process may appear on the angiogram to have some vessels present as a result of projection into this area of vessels lying in front of or behind the tumor.

In solid tumor growths, dependent upon the tumor type present, the angiogram can show great variation in the number, type, and distribution of the tumor vessels present. An absence of tumor vessels is found not only in cystic processes, but is found as well in some solid tumors such as the intracranial *epidermoid* (cholesteatoma). These consist of a capsule which is filled with an avascular detritus. Also avascular are most of the *granulomatous processes,* for example, the tuberculoma and the gumma.

Of the gliomas, *the astrocytoma* is in general vessel-poor. The malignant anaplastic astrocytoma may reveal a specific vascular pattern in which pathological vessels appear as knots and blood lakes. These astrocytomas resemble the glioblastoma so closely that an angiographic differentiation between them is often not possible. The malignant degeneration which is pres-

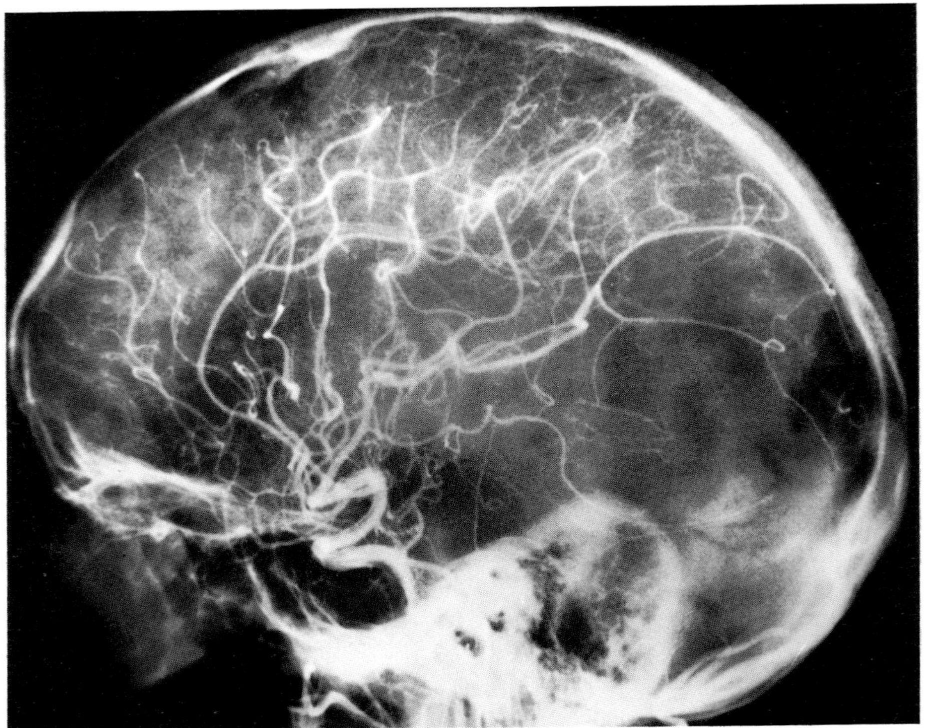

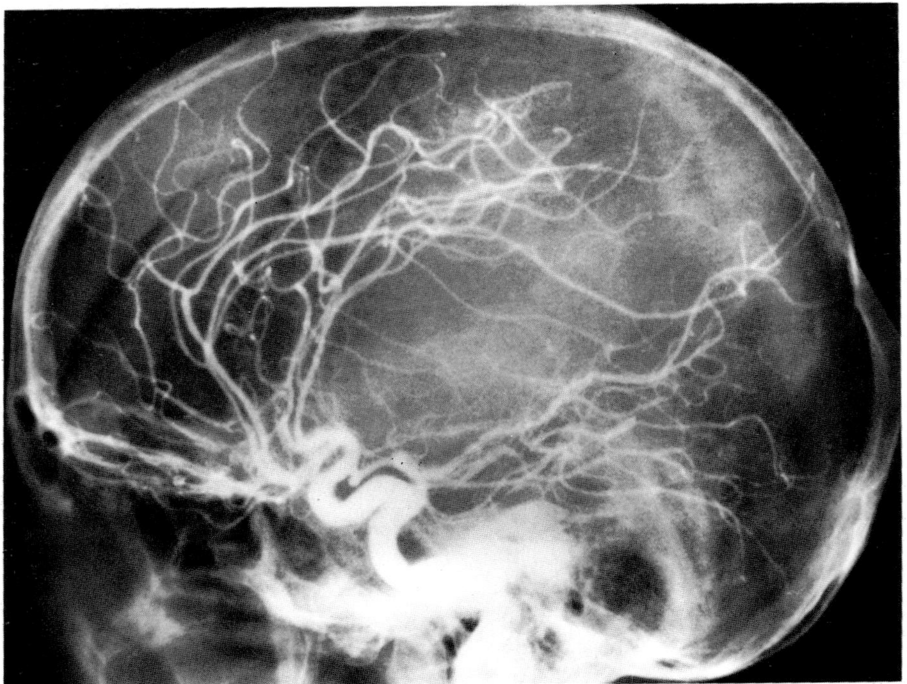

Fig. 65. a The temporal and occipital branches of the middle cerebral artery arch over an avascular occipital meningioma. **b** An intratemporal hematoma in the mid-temporal lobe elevates the middle cerebral artery and stretches its temporal branches

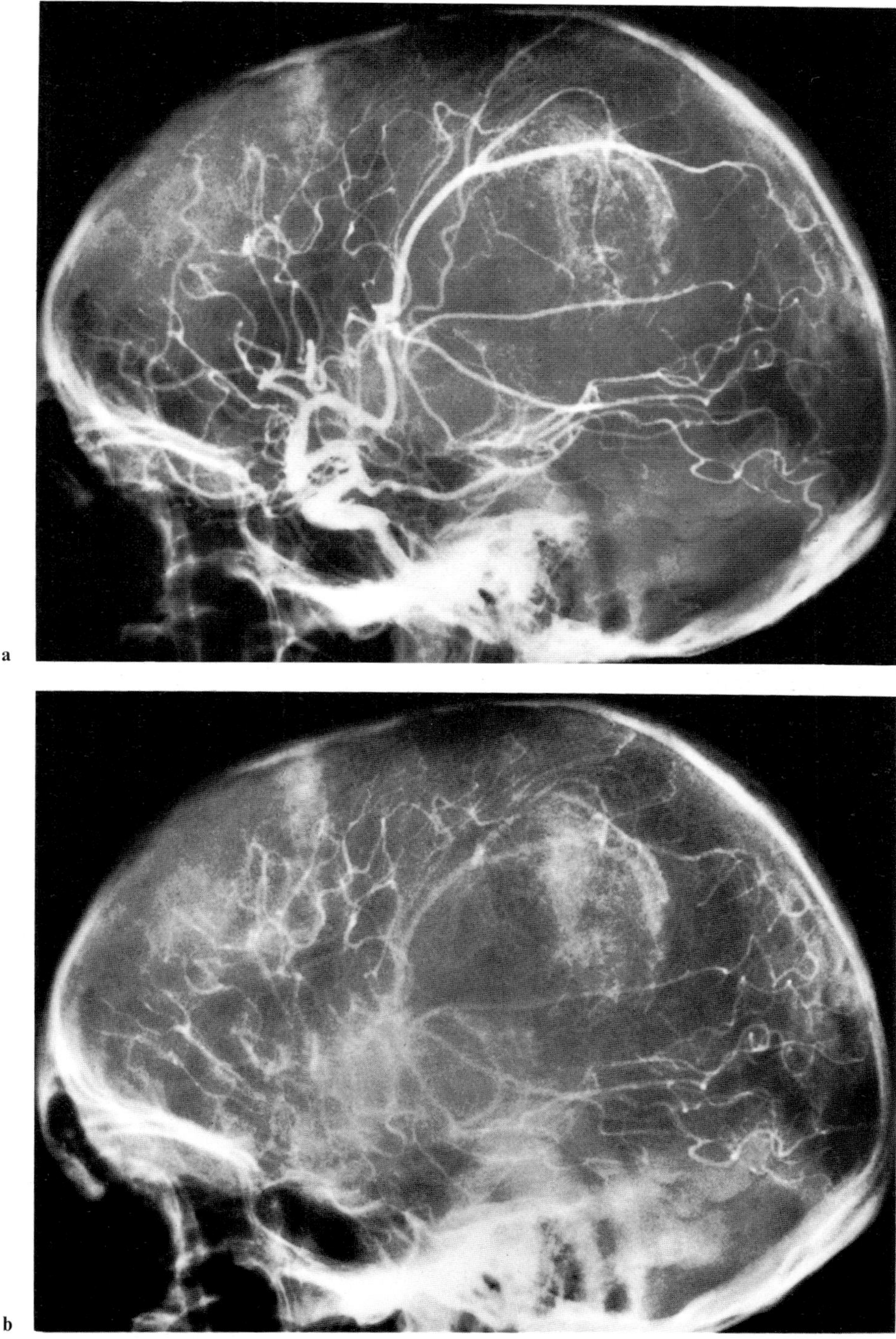

Fig. 66a, b. Parietal astrocytoma with malignant degeneration. There is marked separation of the branches of the middle cerebral artery and a definite partial tumor "blush"

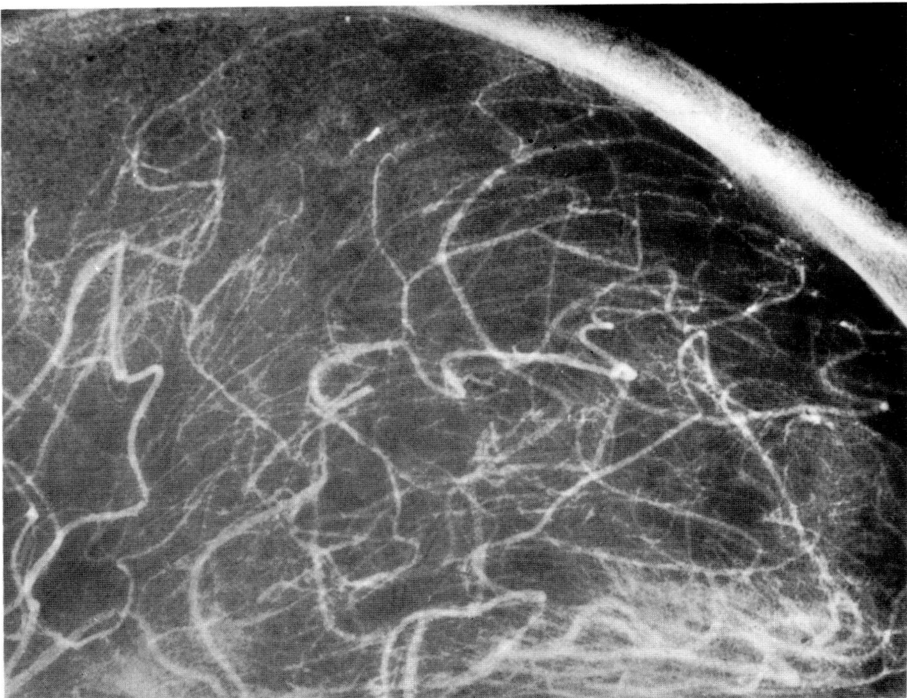

Fig. 67. "Brush stroke" tumor vessels in a glioblastoma (magnification technique, lateral view)

ent appears to be somewhat localized on the angiogram, which is confirmed by the pathological analysis (Fig. 66).

With respect *to oligodendrogliomas,* which are often calcified and apparent even on the plain films, there can be either vessel-poor types or vessel-rich types with a typical tumor blush. The angiographic findings are, however, not so characteristic as to be tumor-specific. Malignant anaplastic forms again may mimic the vessel picture of a glioblastoma.

Of particular significance is the vascular picture of the *glioblastoma multiforme.* Most of these tumors, whose preoperative recognition is so important, show characteristic vessel changes in a significant percentage of cases. Only a few – approximately 20% – are so poor in vessels that they do not permit themselves to be distinguished from other intracerebral or even extracerebral tumors. The vascular glioblastomas demonstrate a variety of angiographic pictures. The tumor blush can be in the form of a fine network with spotty enlargements at the intersections of the network. Occasionally, the pathological vessels run parallel to each other as a kind of brush stroke (Fig. 67). There are irregularly formed corkscrew vessels, as well as blood lakes and arteriovenous fistulas

(Fig. 68a and b). The blush can also consist of larger flecks of irregularly formed sinusoidal vessels, which can be so strongly developed that they resemble an arteriovenous malformation. In all cases, regular *variations in vessel caliber* are particularly characteristic. Occasionally, the pathological vessels are found predominantly at the periphery of the tumor, while the necrotic center has few vessels. Very frequently there is a differential time frame of blood flow through the tumor in comparison to the rest of the brain. The flow through the tumor can be speeded up by means of arteriovenous fistulae so that draining veins already appear in the arterial phase ("early vein"), and even visualization of venous sinuses can take place (Fig. 68b). In cases with a slower circulation time, differentiation between arteries and veins can be difficult because contrast medium remains well into the later venous phases, at a time when the normal brain is no longer visible.

The tumor vessels of the *meningioma* are usually readily differentiated from those of the glioma. This fact is explained by virtue of the structural differences between the two tumor groups, which is of practical importance in considering the operative approach to each type. While the glioma is usually supplied only by

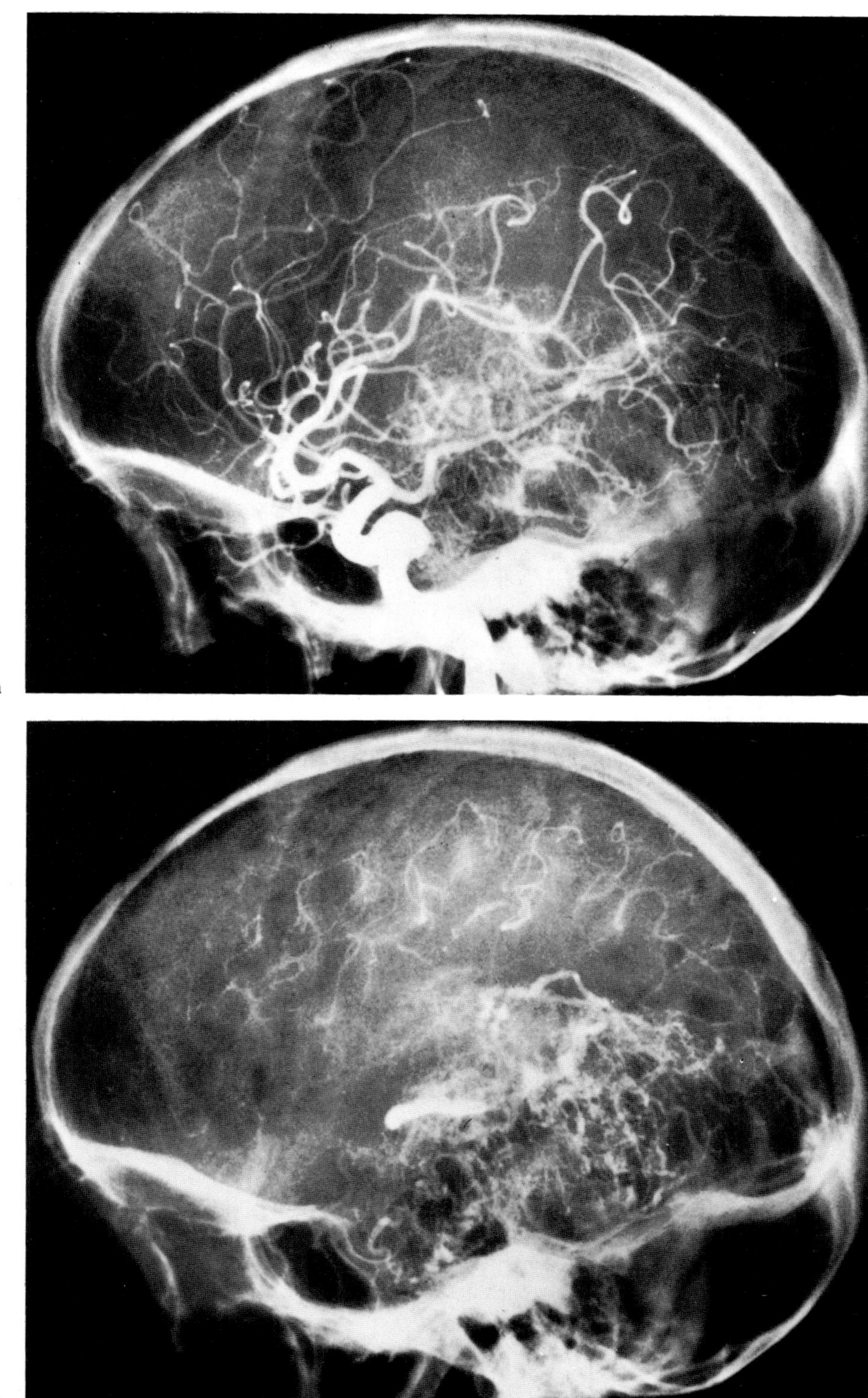

Fig. 68a, b. Glioblastoma: **a** Note the irregular course and variable size of the pathological tumor vessels with "blood lakes" in the center. **b** Early filling of the venous structures and the transverse sinus (small arteries are still apparent in the frontal and parietal regions)

branches of the internal carotid or vertebral arteries, the meningiomas of the cerebral hemispheres are frequently fed in addition by branches of the *external carotid artery*. As a result of this, there follows an enlargement and greater tortuosity of the branches of the middle meningeal artery which is feeding the meningioma. Often a typical dural "star" results (Fig. 69). The intensity of the tumor blush depends on which vessel was injected with the contrast medium (common carotid, internal carotid, external carotid, vertebral). In cases where a meningioma is suspected, it is particularly important to perform a selective catheterization of the external carotid artery (Fig. 70). As noted above, the vessel-rich meningioma results in a relatively rapid appearance of a blush involving the entire tumor, which is usually well-circumscribed. The architecture of the tumor can appear to be spotty, reticulated, or even radiating. In the late capillary phase the blush is often diffuse. It usually outlines the actual extent of the tumor (Fig. 71). In addition, "capsule veins" may be apparent. Occasionally, a nonmalignant meningioma may show some "pathological" vessel changes or an "early" vein.

A strong, diffuse, well-circumscribed blush is seen with *hemangioblastomas*. These are found almost exclusively in the cerebellar region and are fed by the cerebellar arteries. It is characteristic of these tumor types that there are well-defined, round, contrast-free compartments within them which can be readily recognized within the almost homogenous tumor blush (Fig. 72). In rare cases the vessel picture of a hemangioblastoma and an arteriovenous malformation can be similar.

A pronounced proliferation of tumor vessels is also seen in the *glomus jugulare tumors*. The demonstration of small tumors of the glomus tympanicum which are situated at the base of the skull, i.e., in the region of the petrous bone, is made difficult by superimposition of bony structures. It is especially recommended in these cases that subtraction views be used (Fig. 73).

The angiographic picture of the *sarcoma* is variable. The well-circumscribed monstrocellular sarcoma, which arises from the cerebral vessels themselves, can show characteristics of the glioblastoma though this is not common. The primary *fibrosarcoma* of the dura, as well as the malignant meningioma, has some character-istics of the meningioma tumor group but is a mixture of both tumor types.

Cerebral *metastases* of malignant tumors can show a variable angiographic picture. In some cases they cause only displacements of the pre-existing normal cerebral vessels as a result of the intense, accompanying cerebral edema. In other cases they are characterized by a marked proliferation of tumor vessels as well. Frequently, the angiographic picture of a metastasis is similar to that of a glioblastoma. "Early veins" are also characteristic of these tumors. A spherical tumor blush suggests the presence of a metastasis, while a wedge-shaped blush indicates a glioblastoma. When metastasis is suspected, the angiogram should be carefully checked for the presence of additional tumors (Fig. 74).

With reference to the demonstration of pathological vessels, the same rules apply to the angiogram of the vertebral artery as have been laid down for the carotid system. Tumors of the cerebellum (medulloblastoma, pilocytic astrocytoma, ependymoma) have no typical vascular picture on the angiogram. A distinct tumor blush is seen with hemangioblastomas as well as with meningiomas and metastases. On the outer surface of the acoustic neurilemmoma, a network of vessels is usually found within the capsule. It is significant that tumors of the pineal region as well as of the thalamus and basal ganglia are often better demonstrated on the vertebral angiogram than on the carotid study.

2. The Angiogram in Head Injuries

In the *acute* and *subacute* phases of a head injury, the angiogram primarily gives information pertaining to hemorrhages, space-occupying cerebral contusions with vessel displacements and their accompanying edema, vascular lesions, and acute traumatic cerebral abscesses. From a diagnostic standpoint, therefore, the angiogram gives much practical information.

Extracerebral hematomas, as a rule, show an avascular zone in the anteroposterior view which is displacing the superficial cortical vessels away from the inner table of the skull. Hematomas which are localized in the frontal or occipital regions may often be seen only on oblique views. In such cases the head should

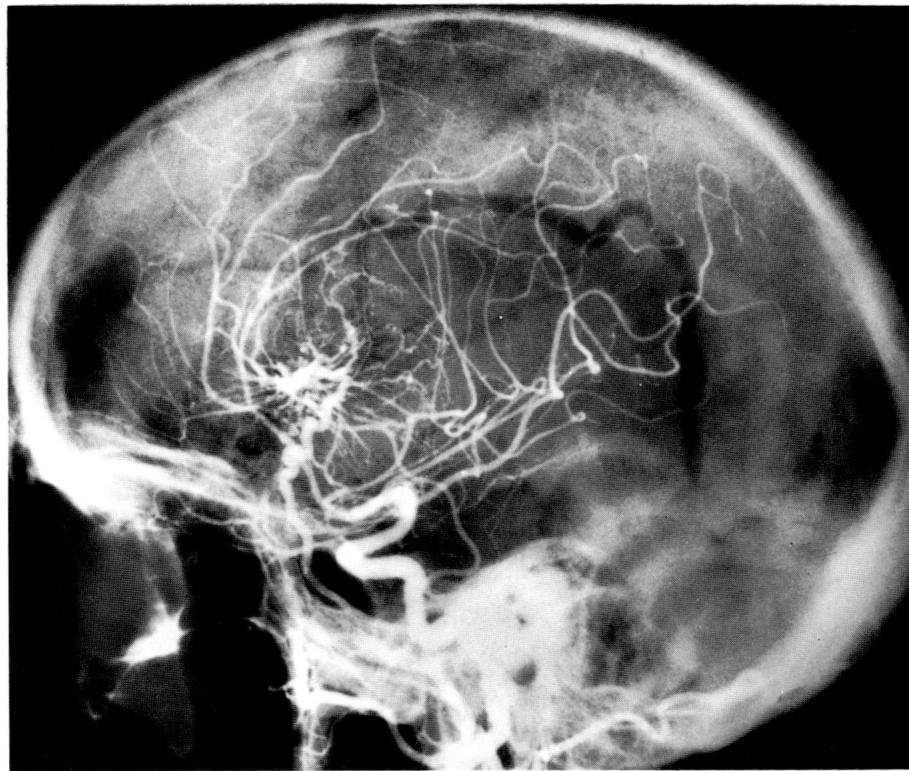

Fig. 69. Frontolateral convexity meningioma. Note the pathological star-shaped pattern of the tumor vessels, which are supplied by hypertrophic branches of the middle meningeal artery

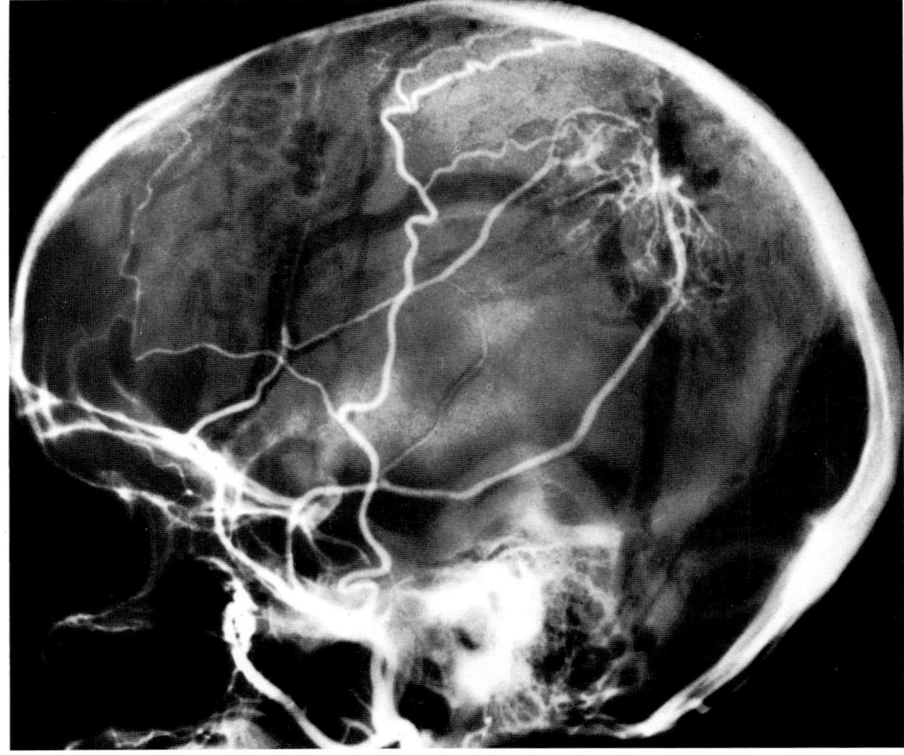

Fig. 70. Selective contrast filling of the external carotid artery showing a convexity meningioma (note the widened diploic venous channels)

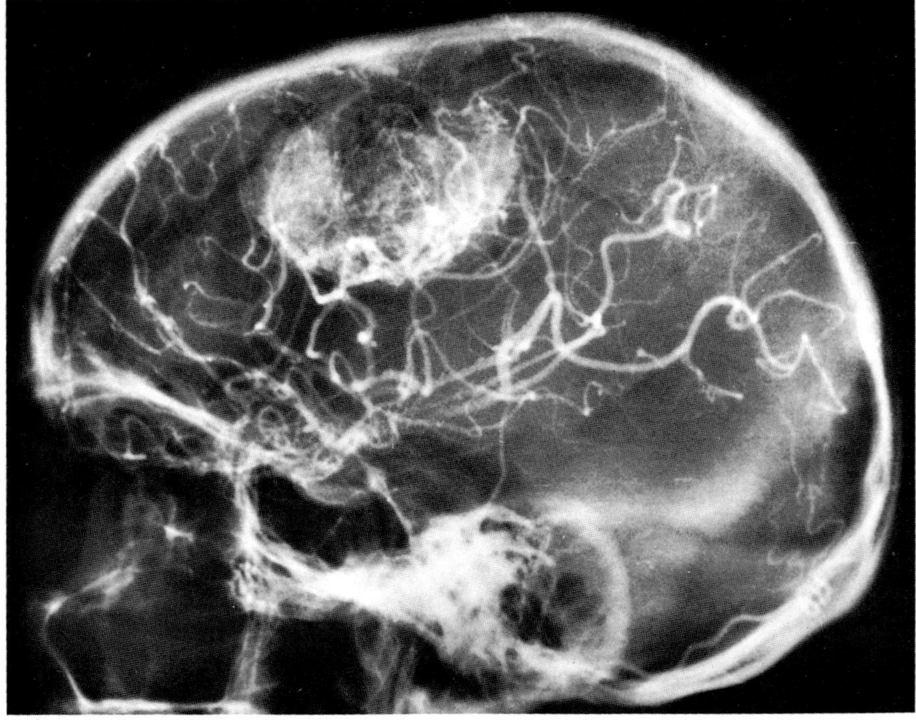

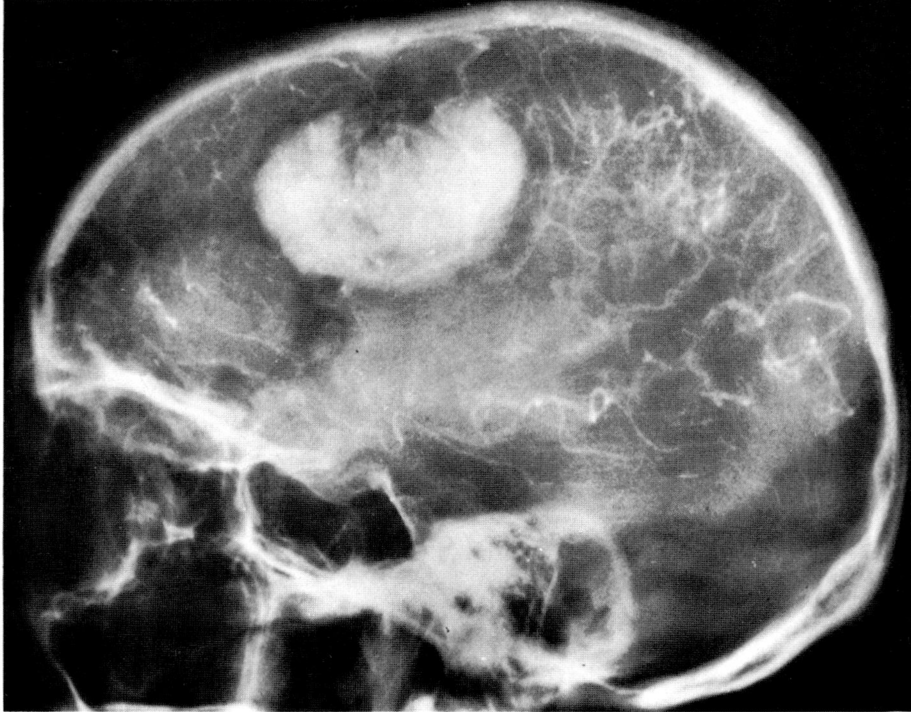

Fig. 71a, b. Arterial and venous phases of an angiogram with a convexity meningioma

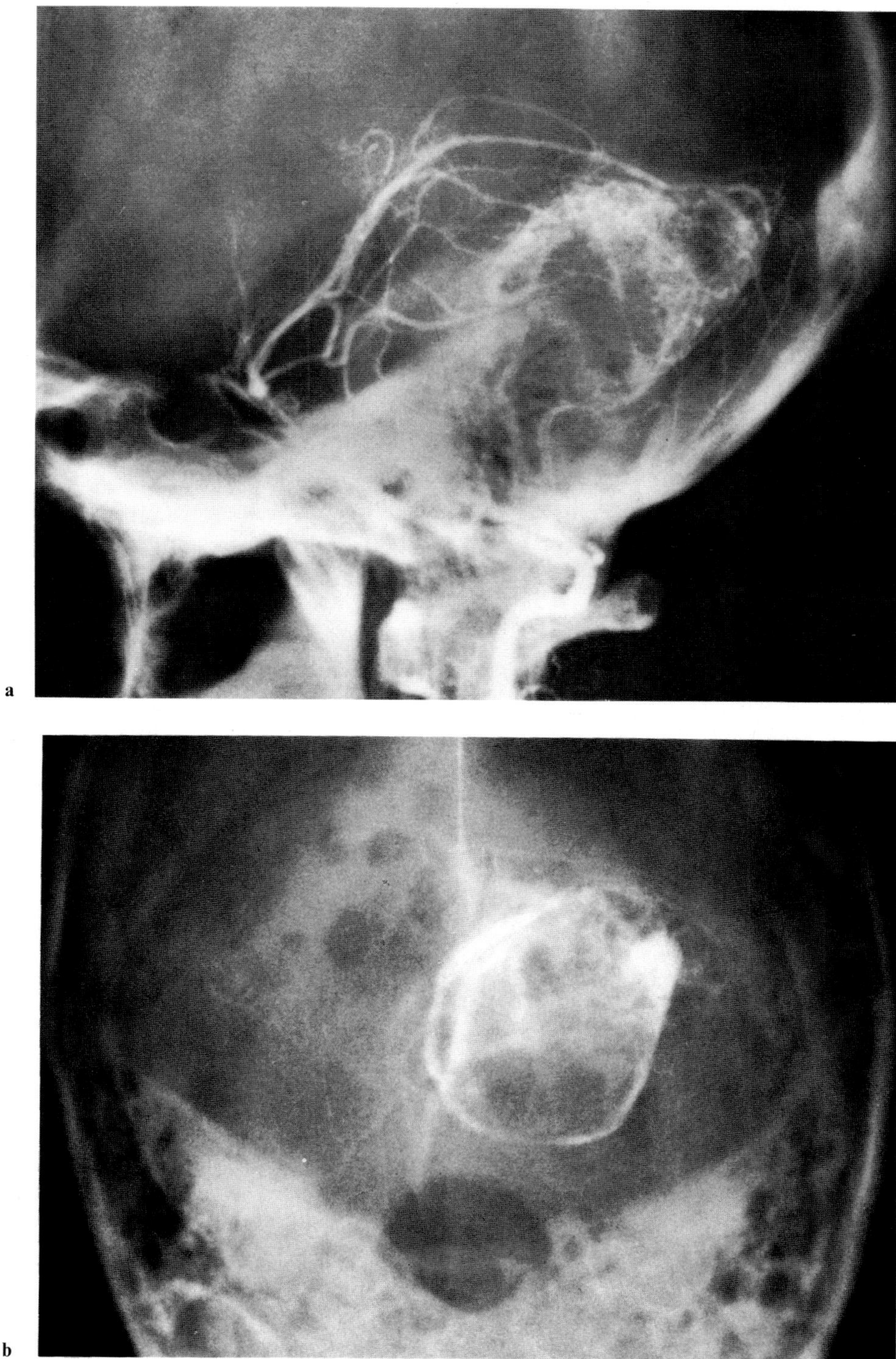

Fig. 72a, b. Cerebellar hemangioblastoma: **a** lateral view, arterial phase; **b** half-axial view, venous phase

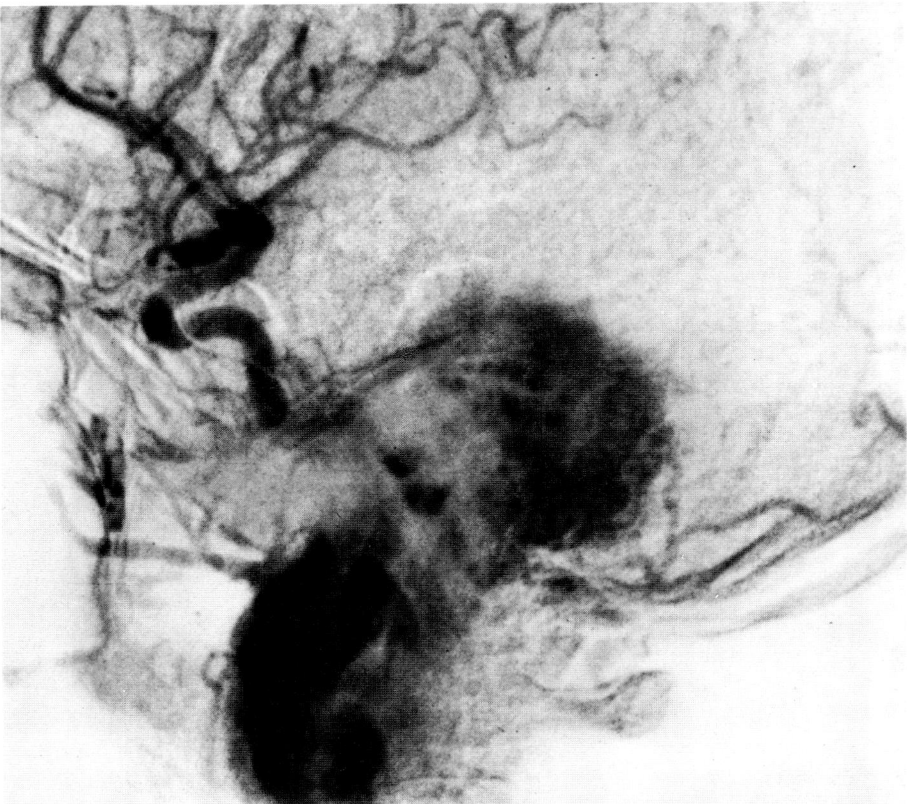

Fig. 73. An enormous intracranial/extracranial glomus jugulare tumor

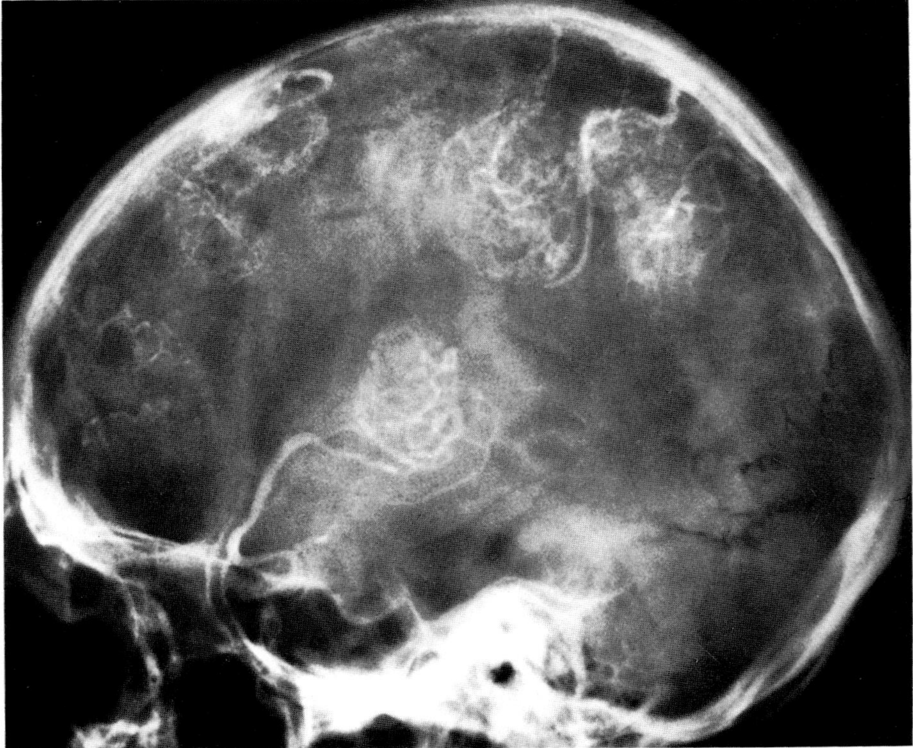

Fig. 74. Multiple metastases with intense contrast filling of the draining veins

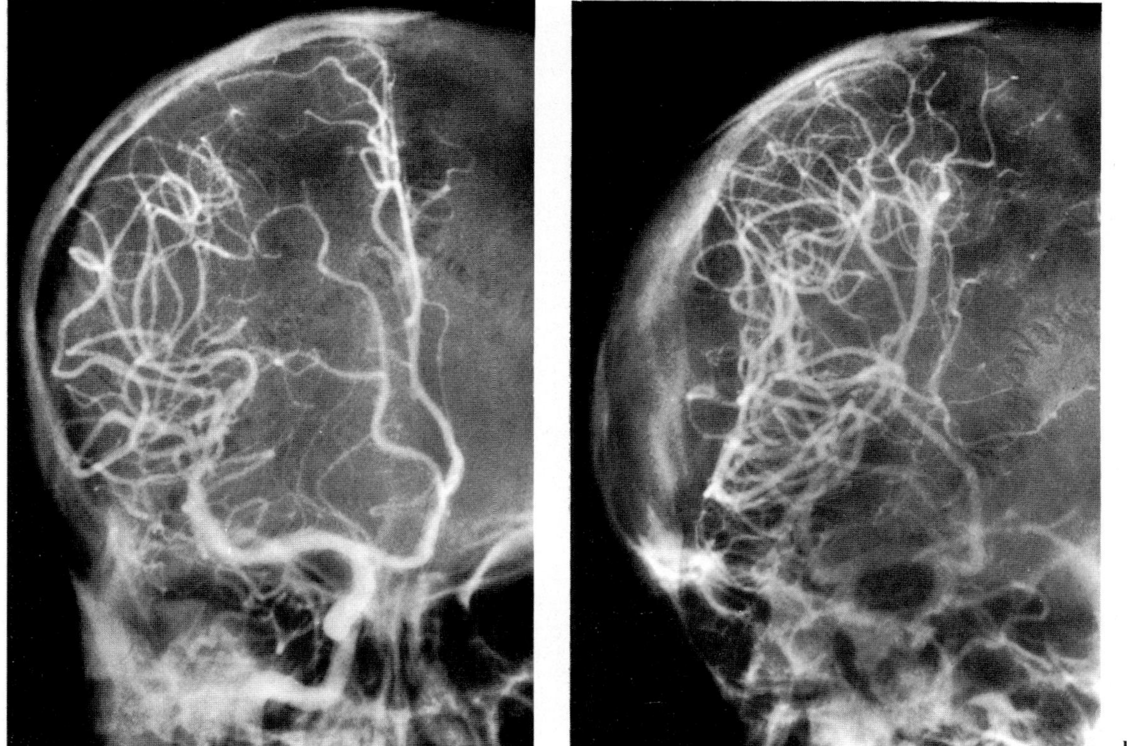

Fig. 75a, b. Frontal epidural hematoma: **a** barely visible in the anteroposterior view; **b** well demonstrated in the oblique view as a large peripheral avascular zone

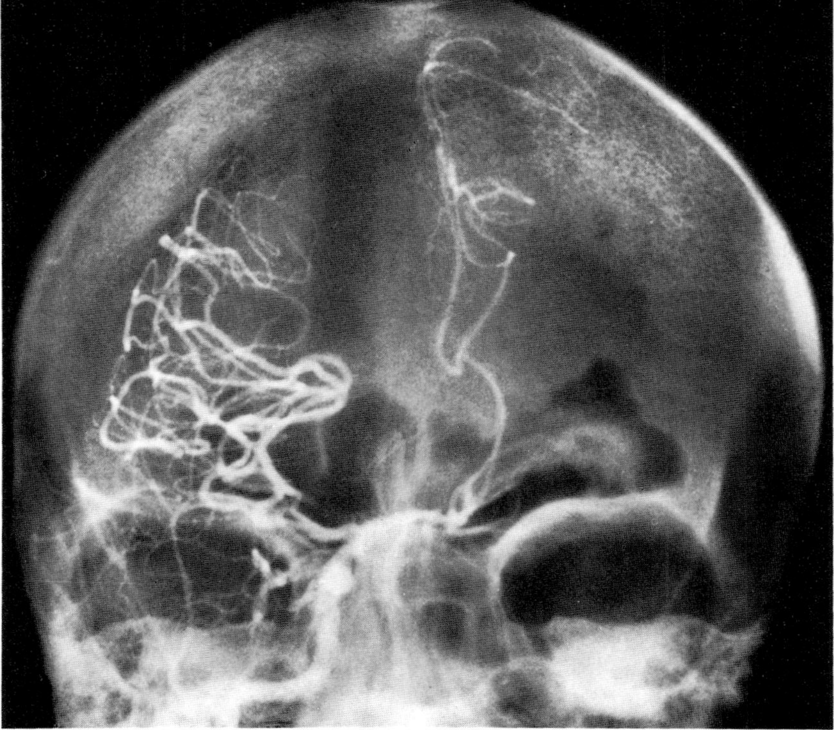

Fig. 76. Avascular halfmoon-like peripheral zone with an acute temporoparietal subdural hematoma

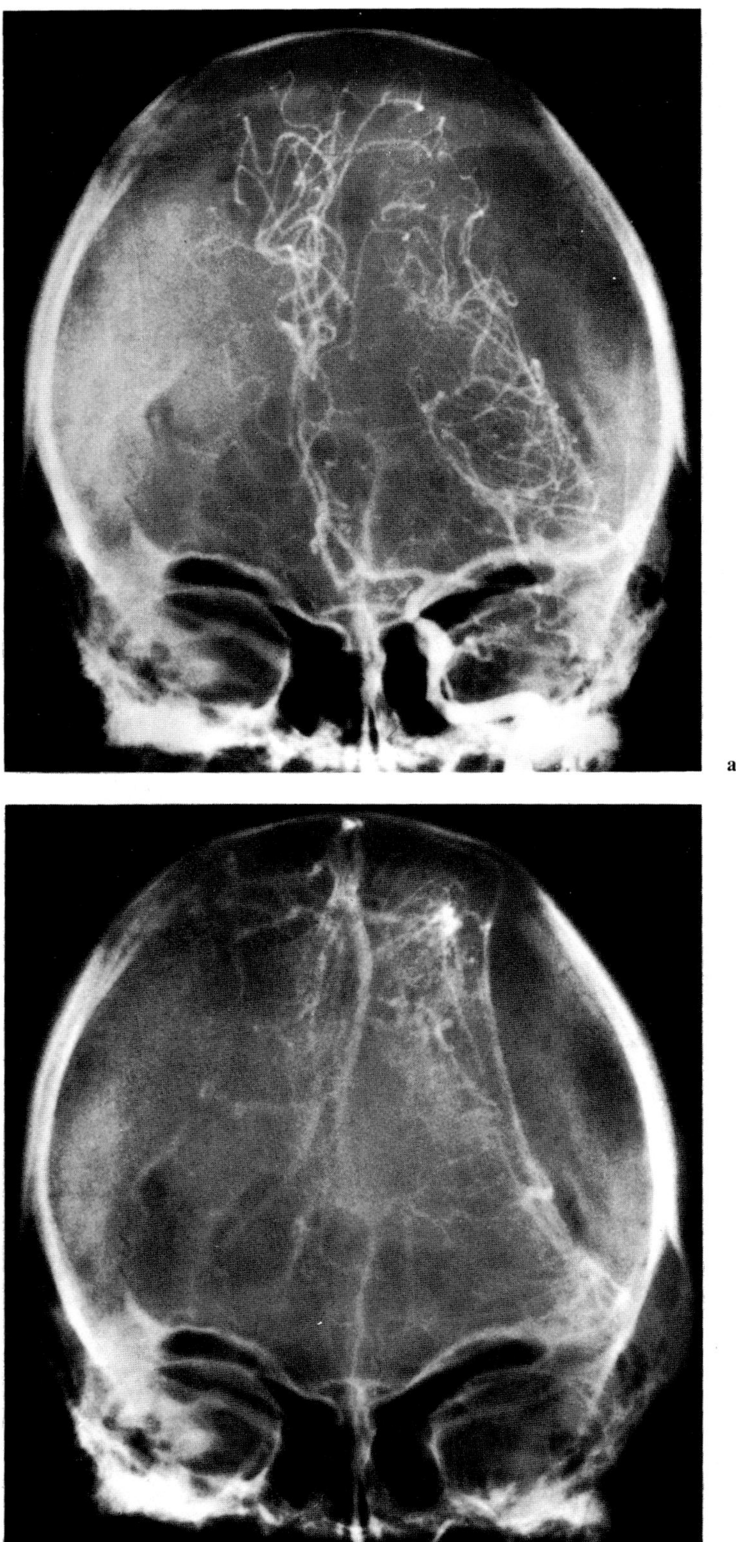

Fig. 77 a, b. Arterial and venous phases of a chronic subdural hematoma. Note the lenticular shape

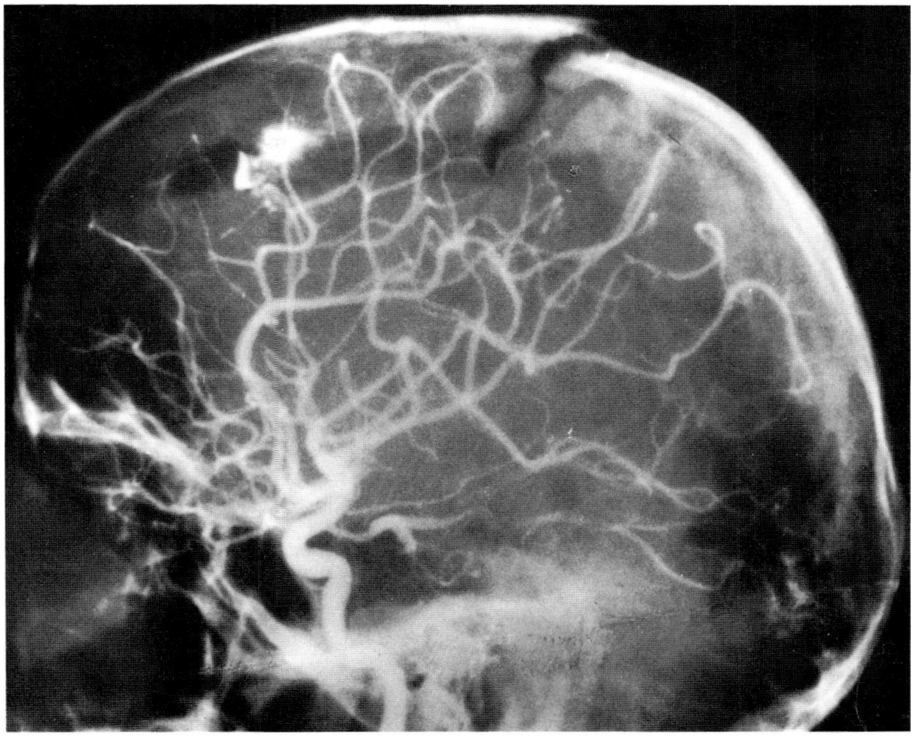

Fig. 78. Contrast leakage into a blood pocket: intracerebral hematoma in association with a skull fracture

be turned to the side being angiogrammed for frontal hematomas, and for occipital hematomas to the opposite side (Fig. 75).

Acute subdural hematomas usually follow a cerebral contusion with laceration and tearing of vessels, particularly ruptures of the bridging veins. They extend over the convexity of the brain fairly uniformly and thus form a sickle-shaped zone of avascularity (Fig. 76). The anterior cerebral artery and the internal cerebral vein are shifted to the opposite side to varying degrees, depending on the size of the mass effect. The acute subdural hematoma cannot always be distinguished from an epidural hematoma on the angiogram. An *epidural* localization, however, is assured if the superior sagittal sinus or branches of the middle meningeal artery are displaced away from the inner table of the skull.

In *chronic subdural hematomas* the avascular zone assumes a lenticular form (Fig. 77), so that the cortical surface of the frontotemporo-occipital region seems to be indented.

The *intracerebral hematoma* has the same appearance as an avascular space-occupying process on the angiogram. It is often difficult to differentiate this lesion from a well-localized

cerebral contusion or from a localized area of edema. The diagnosis of an intracerebral hematoma is assured, however, if the contrast medium runs out into the avascular space (Fig. 78). In large hematomas or with extensive cerebral edema there may be a slowing of the circulation time as a result of the accompanying increase in intracranial pressure. In patients who are receiving anticoagulant therapy, intracerebral hematomas may follow unimportant injuries or may occur spontaneously.

Two special types of injury to the internal carotid artery must still be mentioned. First is the traumatic injury of the intracavernous segment with formation of either an *aneurysm* or a *fistula to the cavernous sinus* (for details, see the chapter on carotid-cavernous sinus fistulae, p. 133, Fig. 79). A second relatively rare and therefore less well-known vessel injury comes from blunt trauma to the cervical vertebrae and the internal carotid artery in the upper third of the neck, approximately at the site where the vessel enters the transverse process of atlas. Through tearing and bruising of the artery at this location an *intimal tear* can arise, which can then form a dissecting aneurysm or a berry-type aneurysm. At the point of injury a throm-

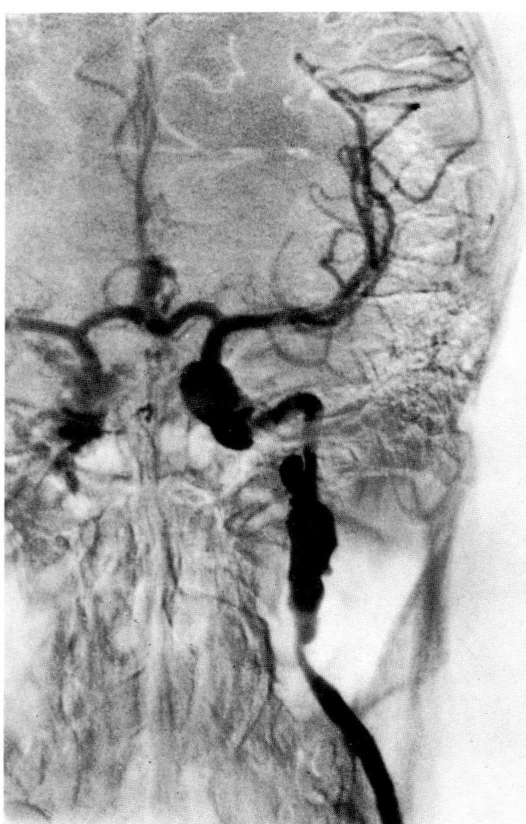

Fig. 79. Damage to the left internal carotid artery at the level of the transverse process of the atlas after blunt trauma. Note the retrograde filling of the right internal carotid artery as far as the cavernous sinus, where a carotid/cavernous fistula has formed

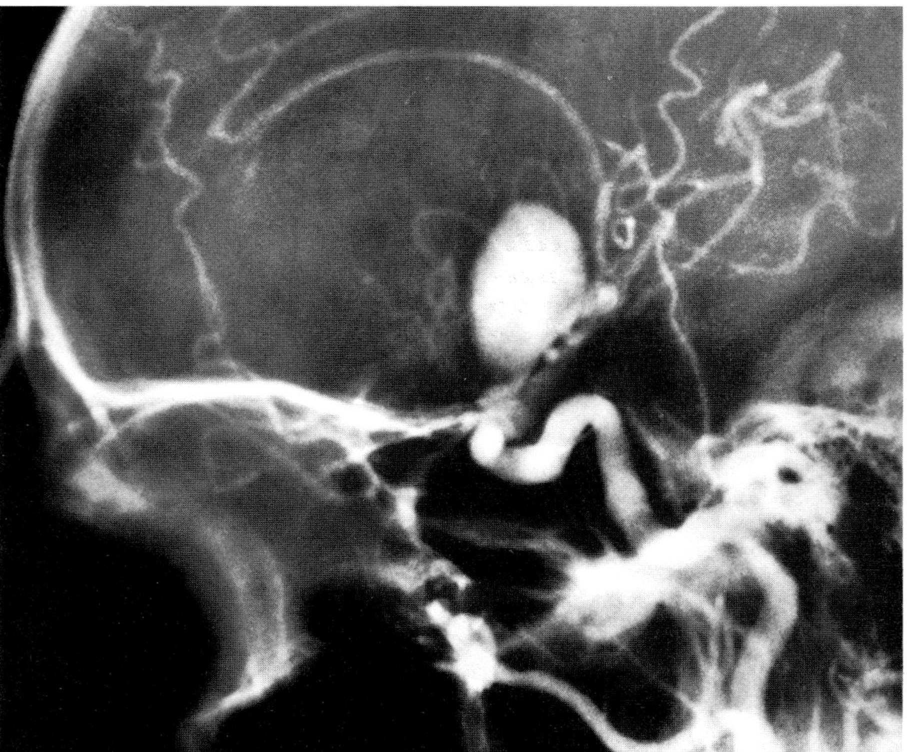

Fig. 80. Partially thrombosed, giant aneurysm arising from the anterior cerebral artery. The extent of the lesion is indicated by the arched displacement of the anterior cerebral artery

bus may also form, which can either lead to an *occlusion of the internal carotid artery* in the neck or to *embolic phenomena* in the carotid distribution. Such emboli are primarily disseminated to the middle cerebral artery territory.

3. The Diagnosis of Primary Intracranial Vascular Disease

a) Arterial Aneurysms

Berry aneurysms develop for the most part as a result of inherent localized defects in particular layers of the vessel wall. Rarer than the congenital aneurysms are those which follow trauma, inflammatory processes, or arteriosclerotic lesions of the arterial wall.

Angiography gives one the ability to demonstrate the origin, shape, and size of aneurysms. The berry aneurysm can have a diameter of a few millimeters or may reach many centimeters. In evaluating these aneurysms, it is necessary to keep in mind that the contrast-filled portion is sometimes only a part of the whole aneurysm, since its outer portions can be thrombosed. One can get a true indication of such partially thrombosed aneurysms from the angiogram if calcifications within the wall exist or if adjacent vessels are displaced more than they should be (Fig. 80). Significant stretching of neighboring vessels can, however, arise as a result of aneurysmal bleeding alone.

Superimposition of other structures in many cases obscures the origin of berry aneurysms in both the anteroposterior and lateral views. Such superimpositions also occasionally prevent determination of the shape of an individual aneurysm, particularly the size and location of the neck. Under such circumstances it is necessary to employ oblique projections as recommended by LOEFSTEDT (1950), axial exposures, or angiotomography for clarification (Figs. 81, 82).

Aneurysms can also be *multiple in location,* so that it is advisable to carry out bilateral carotid angiography. This will also ensure visualization of the anterior communicating artery. In some situations it is necessary that compression of the opposite carotid artery be carried out to facilitate demonstration of this vessel. If after bilateral carotid angiography the source of a subarachnoid hemorrhage is not apparent, a

vertebrobasilar study should certainly be undertaken.

In spite of a great degree of variability there are sites of predilection for arterial aneurysms. Most frequently these are found on the intracranial carotid branches of the circle of Willis and the middle cerebral artery. Proportionally more rare are aneurysms in the vertebrobasilar distribution. Very rare are aneurysms of the small branches of the carotid or basilar system. Within the areas of predilection mentioned on the internal carotid artery and circle of Willis, there are again especially preferred sites. One of these is on the internal carotid artery at the origin of the posterior communicating artery; this aneurysm is in the immediate vicinity of the third nerve as it enters the dura, a fact which explains its frequent paralysis in such lesions (Fig. 83). In this region it is necessary to be on guard against calling a funnel-shaped widening of the posterior communicating artery at its origin from the internal carotid artery (infundibular dilatation) an aneurysm, which it is not. Less frequent are the *infraclinoid* carotid aneurysms, which lie within the cavernous sinus and often reach considerable proportions. The most frequent intracranial site for an aneurysm is on the *anterior communicating artery.* These aneurysms can be fed by one or both anterior cerebral vessels (see also Fig. 87).

Aneurysms of the *middle cerebral artery* are frequently found at points of division of the artery, either at a bifurcation or a trifurcation (Fig. 84). Here, it is particularly important to guard against mistaking a vessel loop for an aneurysm. Aneurysms in the intracranial segments of the vertebral arteries are rare. They can arise on either vertebral artery and therefore both arteries should be studied if such a lesion is suspected. Berry aneurysms of the *basilar artery* are most frequently found at the bifurcation (Fig. 85). Aneurysms of the branches of the basilar artery are quite rare.

Individual variations in flow characteristics are not uncommon in large aneurysms, especially when the neck of the aneurysm is small (Fig. 86). Under these circumstances the periphery of the aneurysm may be the first part to fill with the contrast-containing blood and the first part to empty. In other cases the aneurysm remains visualized well into the venous phase, possibly as a result of laminar-flow.

Relatively rare are the *fusiform aneurysms* which are more or less uniform enlargements

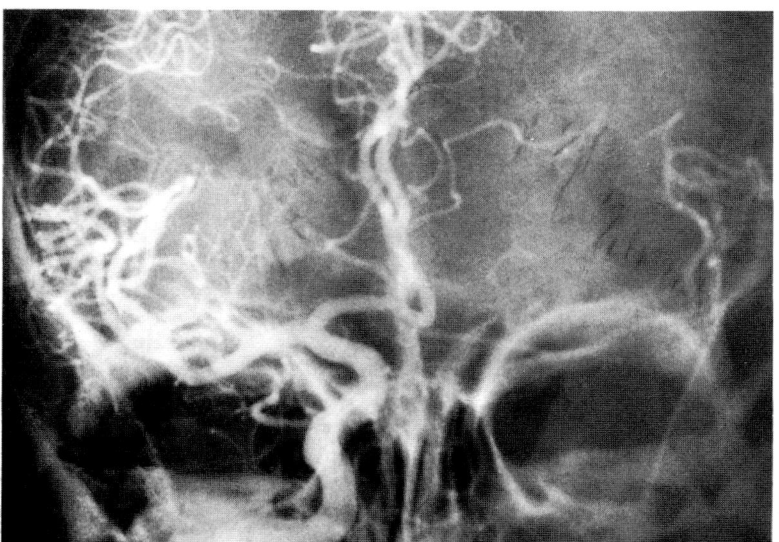

a

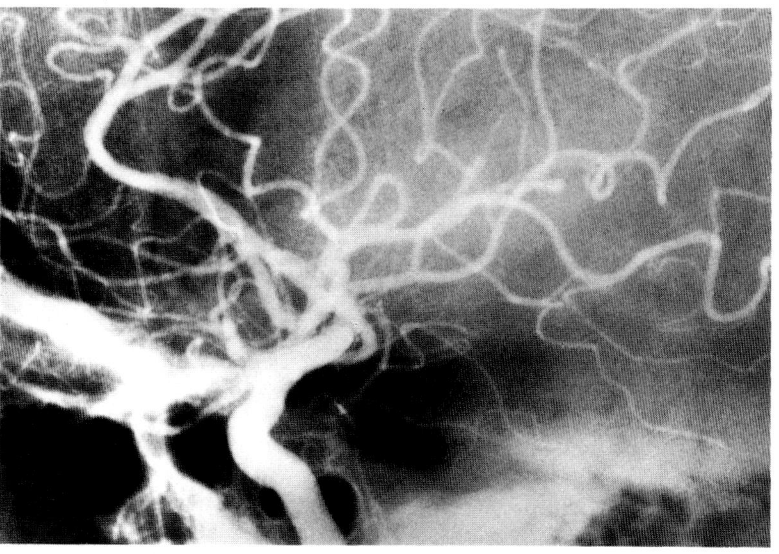

b

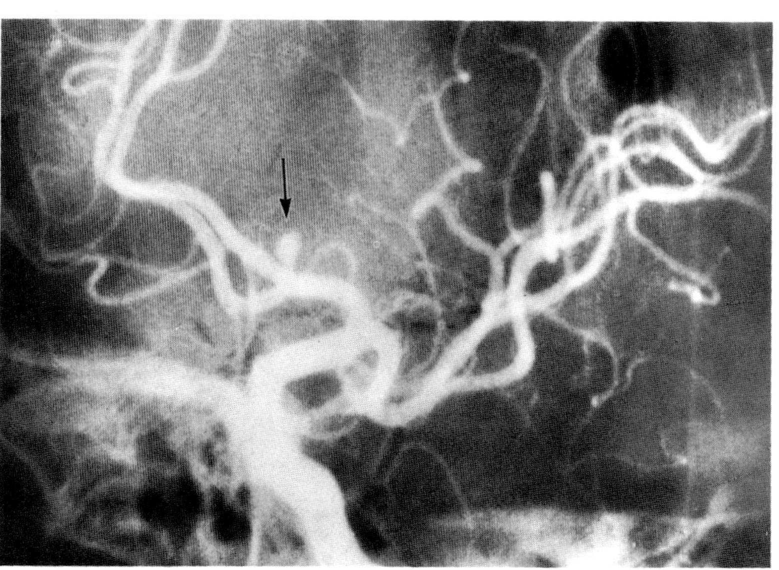

c

Fig. 81 a–c. Small aneuryms of the anterior cerebral artery, which can only be seen in the oblique view (Loefstedt)

of a long segment of vessel. This is especially true for the basilar artery.

Bleeding from a ruptured aneurysm can lead to alternating spasm of adjacent vessels, which may last 1–4 weeks (Fig. 87). This can cause hemodynamic sequelae by slowing down the circulation time or by decreasing blood flow in the territory of supply of the affected vessel. When hemorrhage from a ruptured aneurysm collects in the brain substance, the angiographic

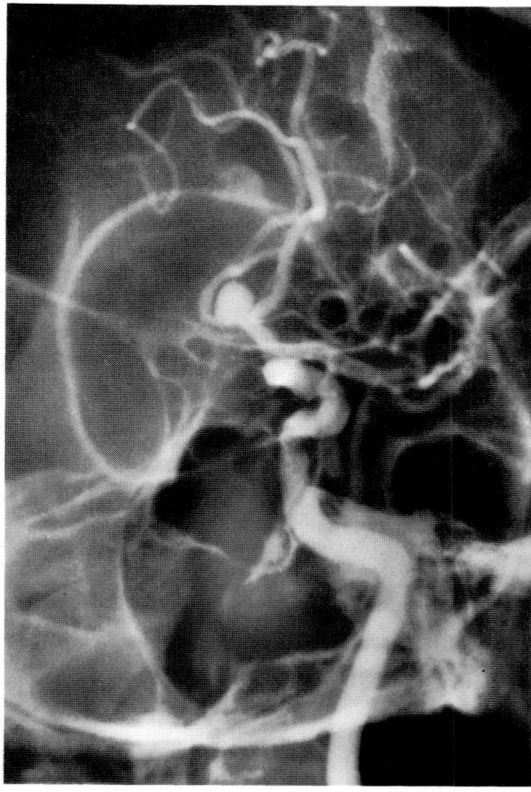

Fig. 82. Aneurysm of the anterior communicating artery projecting into the orbit in this oblique view (reverse Loefstedt position, see p. 64)

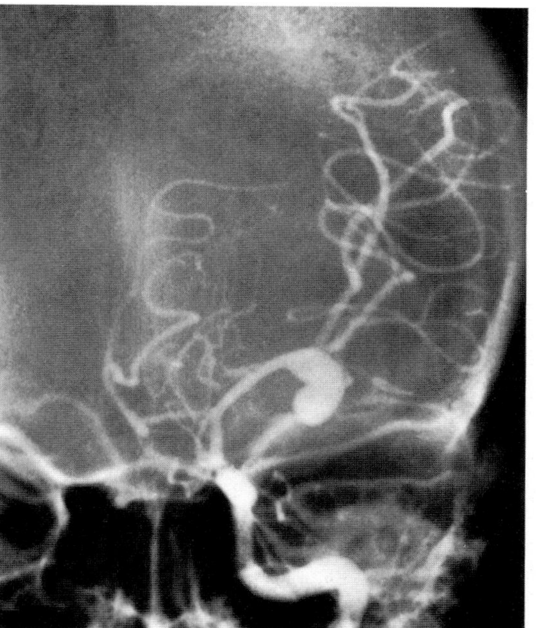

Fig. 84. Aneurysm at the bifurcation on the middle cerebral artery. The displacement of the adjacent vessels suggests an associated intratemporal hemorrhage

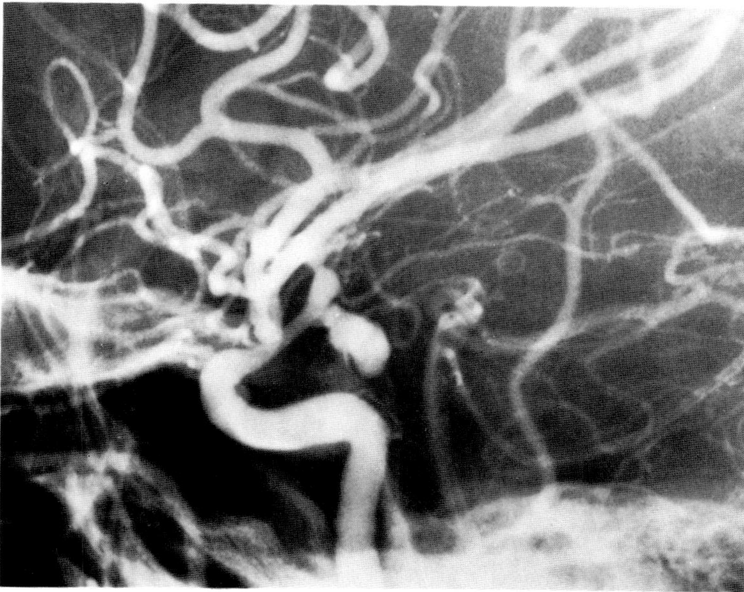

Fig. 83. Aneurysm of the internal carotid artery at the origin of the posterior communicating artery. (Note the spasm of the terminal segment of the internal carotid artery)

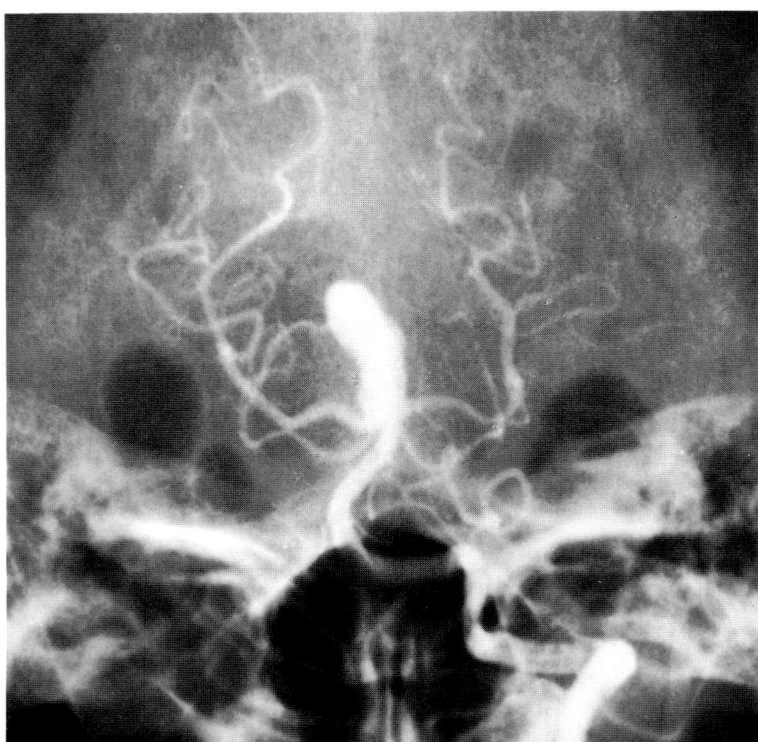

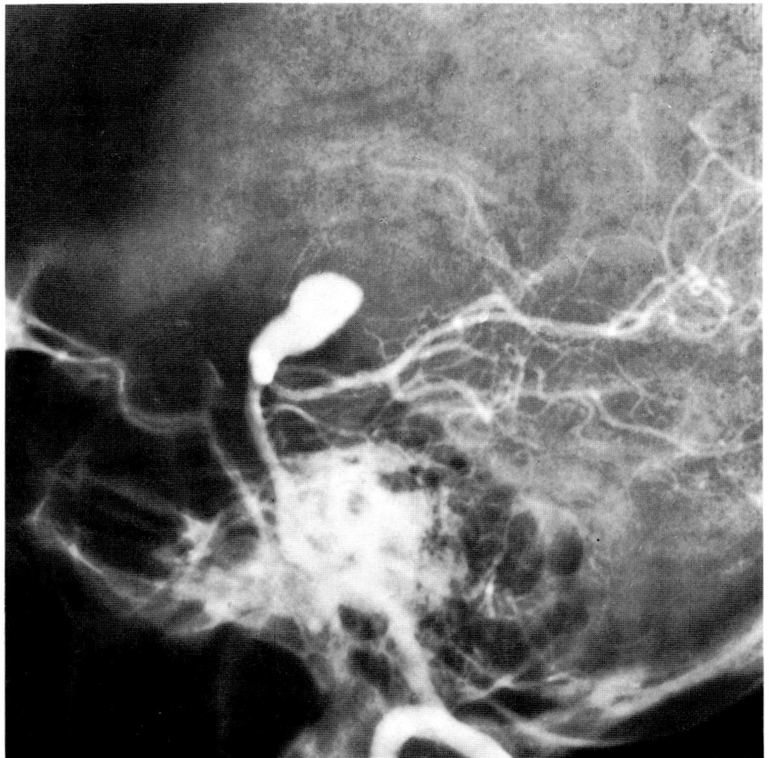

Fig. 85a, b. Aneurysm of the basilar bifurcation

Fig. 86a–c. Turbulence in a large aneurysm
of the internal carotid artery

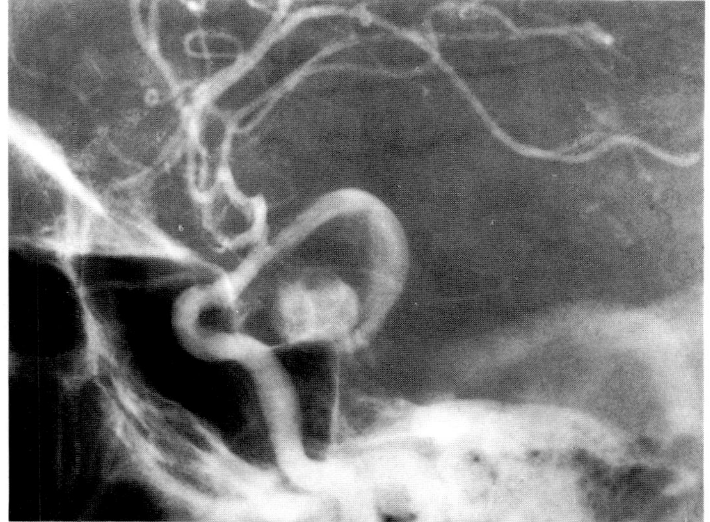

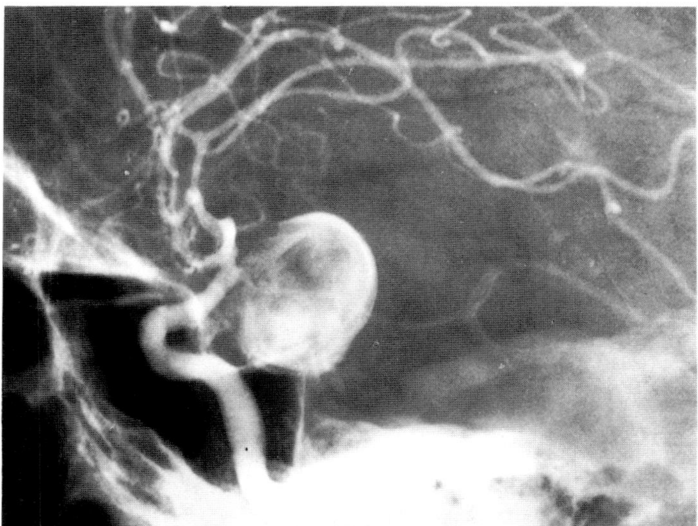

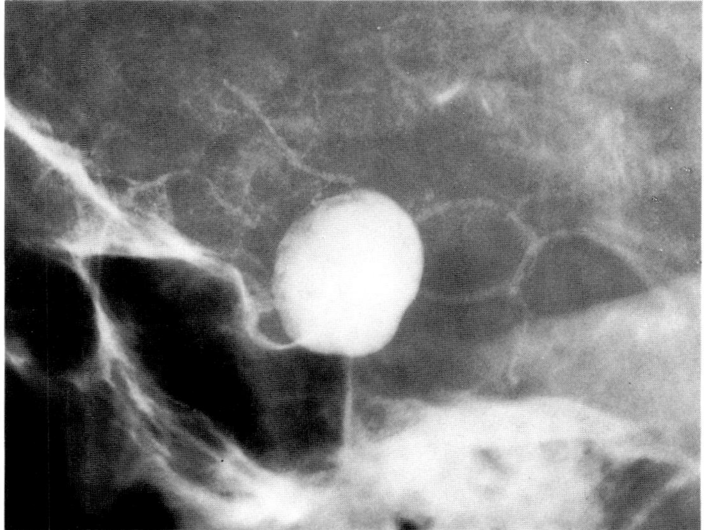

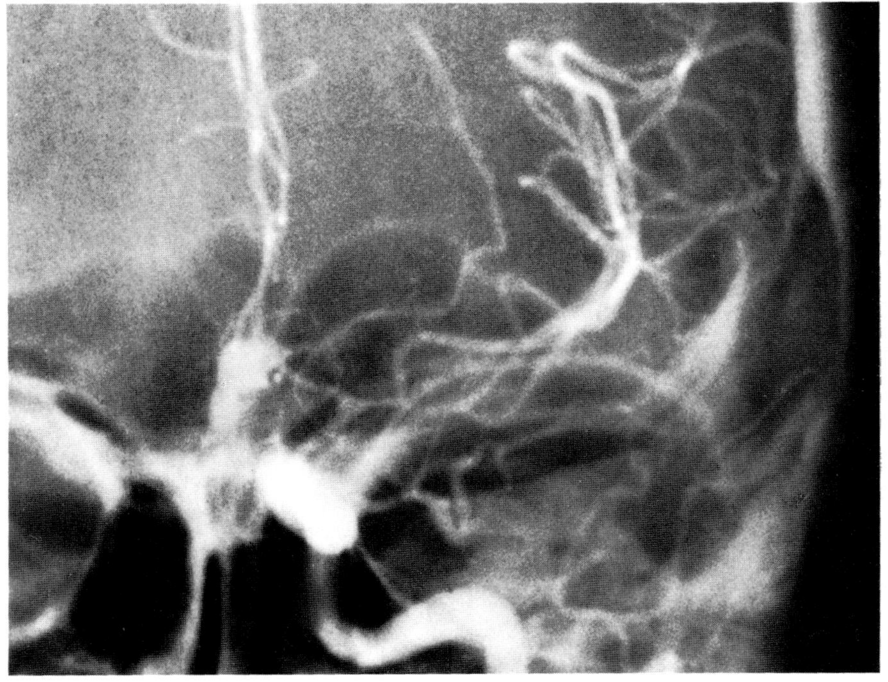

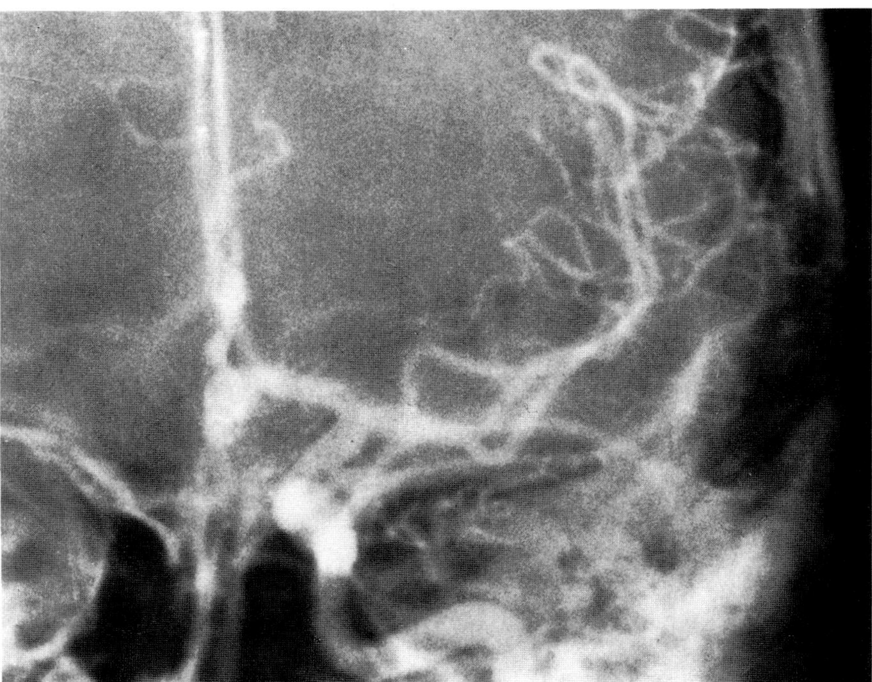

Fig. 87a, b. Anterior communicating artery aneurysm with **a** marked spasm of the carotid bifurcation; **b** repeat angiography 4 weeks later, showing resolution of the spasm

picture resembles a space-occupying process. *Venous aneurysms* (phlebectasia) appear most commonly in the region of the great vein of Galen where they can reach enormous size and may present as a space-occupying process obstructing the CSF pathways.

b) Arteriovenous Malformations

The precise angiographic demonstration of an arteriovenous malformation (AVM), earlier known as the arteriovenous aneurysm or arteriovenous angioma, is particularly important with respect to its operative excision. Because of this not only are the identification, the position, and the extent of the AVM itself of interest, but especially also the position of the vessels which supply them with blood. These lesions arise from a congenital vessel maldevelopment resulting in persistence of embryonic conditions in which countless fistulous connections exist between arteries and veins. Because of this, the histological differentiation of arteries and veins in the AVM is accomplished only with great difficulty. The inherent weakness of these primitive vessel walls explains the tendency to hemorrhage into brain substance, the subarachnoid space, or the ventricle.

The angiographic picture usually consists of one or more pencil-thick branches which merge into an entangled network of large and small vessels, out of which many dilated veins exit. In the operative exposure of such angiomas, bright red blood is seen within the veins.

The *shape* and *size* of an AVM may vary considerably. A supratentorial localization is more common than an infratentorial. They may be supplied by only one of the large cerebral vessels (anterior cerebral artery, middle cerebral artery, posterior cerebral artery) or by many; the external carotid artery may also contribute blood to the lesion. The extent of the actual involvement of individual large vessels in supplying an AVM can only be determined through selective contrast study of the internal and external carotid arteries and of the vertebrobasilar system (Fig. 88). As a result of local blood pressure decreases resulting from fistulae, AVMs (such as one supplied primarily by the anterior cerebral artery) will also draw blood from the opposite internal carotid artery circulation. During surgery on a supratentorial AVM it is recommended that intraoperative angiography be carried out, both in the interest of safety and in order to insure that complete removal has been accomplished. In such situations, the contrast medium is injected by means of an indwelling catheter within the internal carotid artery. Although most AVMs appear on the cerebral surfaces, they do receive considerable blood supply from the depths, such as from branches of the choroidal arteries. As a result, blood drains also by way of the deep cerebral veins and the picture of the lesion on the anteroposterior view may appear wedge-shaped. The remaining cerebral vessels, which do not take part in supplying the lesion, are often poorly filled with contrast or not seen at all. This apparent decrease in flow results because the effect of the low pressure AV shunts is to steal blood from the surrounding brain. These same AV shunts create a significant burden on the entire circulation with corresponding changes in the heart.

On the other hand, there are AVMs that are so small that they are nearly invisible on the angiogram. These "microangiomas" can be recognized by the early appearance of their draining veins (Fig. 89). These small AVMs can result in massive intracerebral hemorrhages, an etiology which is frequently recognized only from operative specimens or from autopsy material. It may also happen that such a hematoma does not clot off, but rather remains encapsulated and persists as an aneurysmal sac in free communication with the AVM.

Occasionally, the differential diagnosis between glioblastoma, metastasis, hemangioblastoma, and arteriovenous malformation is quite difficult. The angiogram can be quite helpful also for surgical follow-up of these lesions. After extirpation of an AVM, it is advisable to perform postoperative studies to insure that a radical removal has in fact been accomplished. In such studies it is interesting to see that the enormous dilated vessels supplying and draining the lesion can in time shrink. Similarly, the removal of the AVM is followed by disappearance of the fistulous channels which were present in the adjacent healthy brain substance with resumption of normal circulatory conditions.

c) The Carotid-Cavernous Fistula

A *rupture* of the internal carotid artery at the level of the intracavernous segment results in arterial blood entering the cavernous sinus, which will lead to a corresponding increase in local pressure. In the overwhelming majority of cases the rupture is traumatic, although it may rarely originate from arteriosclerotic vascular change. The pulse beat of the internal carotid artery is then carried into the cavernous sinus and is further transmitted to the orbital vein so that a "pulsating exophthalmus" results. In the angiogram one sees in the early arterial phase an irregular deposition of contrast medium in the region of the cavernous sinus. As a rule, contrasted blood flows from

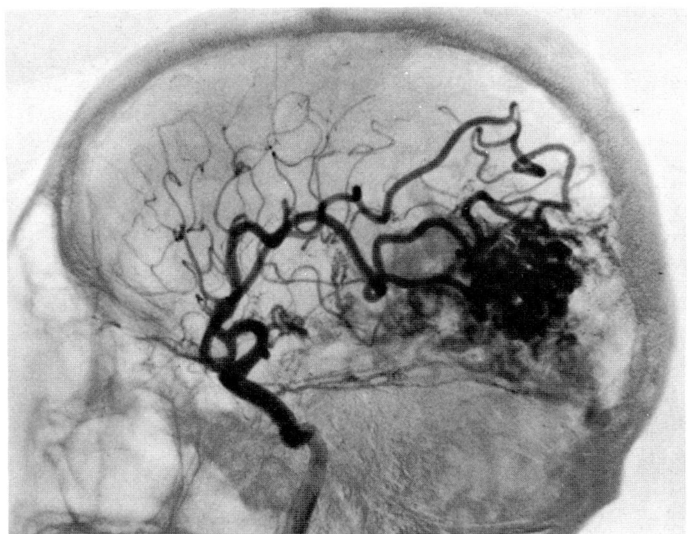

a

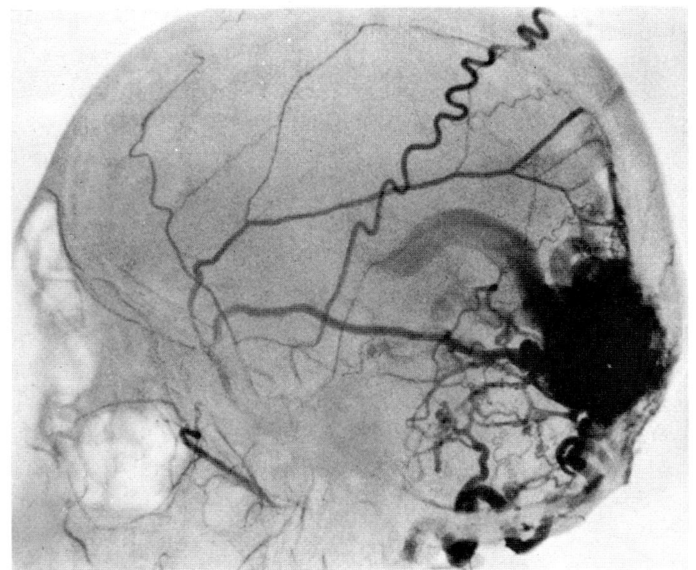

b

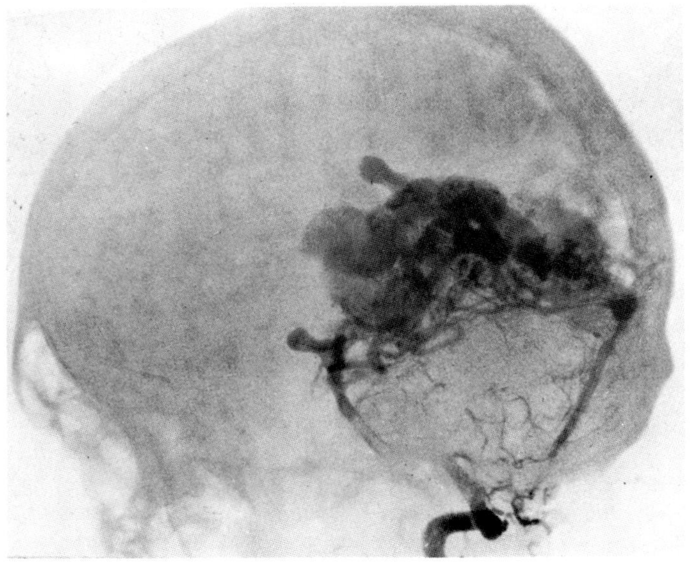

c

Fig. 88a–c. Prominent arteriovenous malformation of the occipital region: **a** being fed by the internal carotid artery; **b** by the external carotid artery; and **c** by the vertebral artery

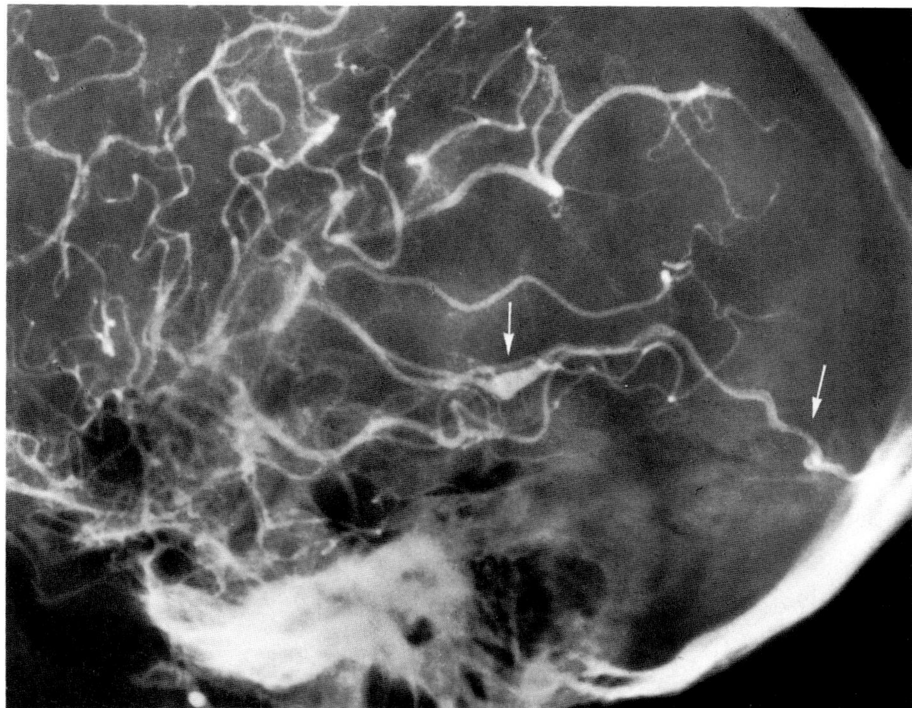

Fig. 89. Microangioma in the temporal lobe being supplied by branches of the middle cerebral artery. Note the "early vein" running to the transverse sinus indicative of an arteriovenous fistula. Spreading of the middle cerebral branches suggests an associated intracerebral hematoma (*arrows* point to the AVM and its draining vein)

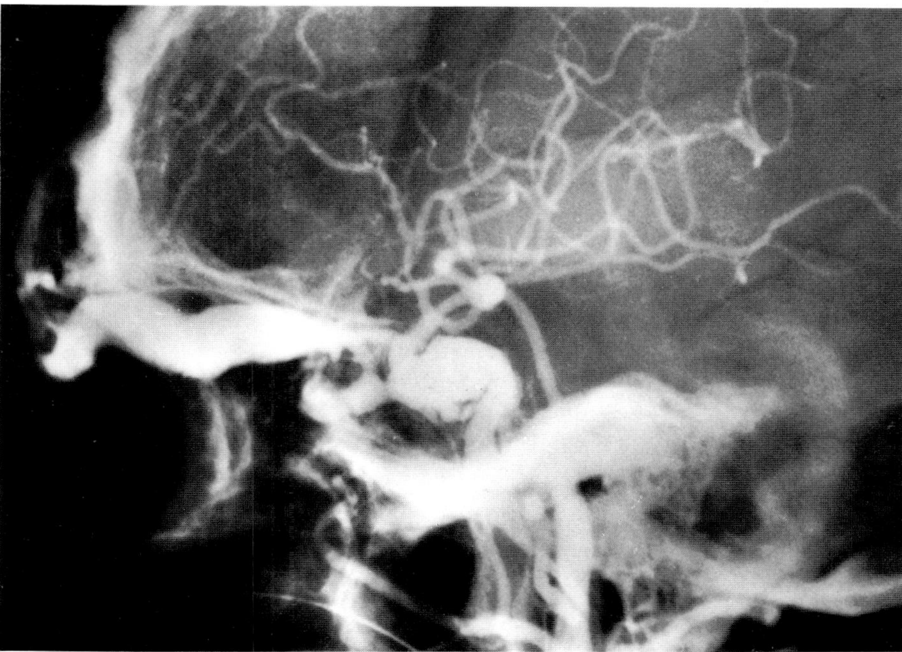

Fig. 90. Carotid/cavernous fistula: note the contrast medium from the carotid siphon filling the cavernous sinus and the dilated superior ophthalmic vein in retrograde fashion

here into the dilated ophthalmic veins (Fig. 90). Other veins may also fill with contrast and empty into the superior petrosal sinus, as well as the superior sagittal sinus and sigmoid sinus. As a result of the arteriovenous fistula and the corresponding decrease in pressure within the internal carotid artery, the territory supplied by this vessel is poorly demonstrated with contrast.

d) Vascular Stenoses and Vascular Occlusions

Special Dangers and Complications of Angiography in Patients with Disorders of Cerebral Blood Flow

The complication rate for angiography in patients with disturbances of the cerebral circulation is in general higher than that for healthy patients. It is therefore necessary to consider carefully the positive indications for the invasive neuroradiological procedure on the one hand, and the negative risk of complications on the other. In the case of an operable, life-threatening lesion (such as an epidural or subdural hematoma), angiography remains the method of choice in the absence of CT despite advancing age, since it is the only certain means of establishing the diagnosis. Only in dire emergencies when time is of the essence should such lesions be *surgically explored without* the benefit of angiographic confirmation or CT.

Another absolute indication for angiography exists in distinguishing subacute vascular processes in the elderly from cerebral tumors. Such an angiogram will not only localize the site of the lesion but also give insight as to the pathological diagnosis. For the demonstration of an operable arterial lesion, e.g., a stenosis, an aneurysm, or an AVM, only angiography is of value. Yet one must decide beforehand whether such an operative procedure is still feasible and whether the patient is willing to permit.

The remaining indication for angiography – evaluation of disturbances in cerebral blood flow – should be considered in the light of the commonly associated complications presented below.

Local Complications

These are usually seen in association with puncture of a carotid or vertebral artery in the elderly, but may as well occur in the younger age groups. A careless puncture in the presence of advanced arteriosclerosis can certainly result in a dissecting aneurysm or a deposition of contrast medium between an arteriosclerotic plaque and the arterial wall (Fig. 99). Such occurrences are not uncommon in the case of the carotid artery and can lead to a transient occlusion of the vessel lumen. The catheter technique is also associated with an increased risk of complications in elderly patients: ulcerated plaques can be dislodged or thrombi formed and disseminated with resultant infarcts. In the case of *selective catheterization of a given artery,* the catheter itself can transiently interfere with local blood flow and can lead to ischemic symptoms. Such disturbances are not tolerated as well in the older age groups as in the younger and are of considerable significance in the selective catheterization of spinal arteries.

Generalized Complications

Even in healthy tissues the passage of contrast-filled blood can lead to *tissue damage,* usually through changes in the *blood brain barrier.* These are primarily dependent upon the type and concentration, the amount, and the speed of flow of the contrast medium. These influences, together with a simultaneous ischemia resulting from decrease in the oxygen content of the contrast-filled blood, can be magnified by any pre-existing tissue injury. The investigation of cases with genuine neurological complications following correctly performed angiography leads one to conclude that tissues which have already suffered hypoxic damage or are edematous tend to tolerate poorly the additional insult of the angiographic procedure. Although these possibilities must be considered when angiography is deemed necessary, the overwhelming majority of cases are in fact free of complications. Occasionally, the *poor risk vascular patient* can even experience an improvement in his clinical picture following the angiogram.

Anesthetic Complications

If general anesthesia is employed, it is *necessary to insure that the blood pressure is kept stable throughout the procedure.* Any fall in blood pressure should be immediately corrected since acute hypotension may lead to cerebrovascular insufficiency and secondary neurological abnormalities. This is especially true for patients with labile hypertension and coronary vascular disease. Following the procedure, careful monitoring should continue for a period of observation, particularly in patients with significant stenotic lesions (Intensive Care Unit, see p. 157).

Injuries Secondary to Vascular Lesions

Statistics in the world literature lead to the conclusion that cerebral angiography in comatose "stroke" patients – especially when multiple vessels at one sitting are studied – results in an especially high risk of complications (MCDOWELL, 1966). It must further be pointed out that the patient experiencing a *migraine attack* will also tolerate angiography less well than the normal patient (see PATTERSON et al., 1964).

Hypotensive Crises

It cannot be emphasized enough that patients with disturbances in cerebral blood flow and especially "older" patients with pre-existing vessel disease should be carefully monitored throughout the procedure. Hypotensive crises, i.e., drops in blood pressure, should be carefully avoided. Should the angiogram show a significant stenosis in a large vessel or an occlusion with collateral circulation, such monitoring of vital signs should be continued over the next 24 h under carefully controlled conditions, such as in an intensive care unit. This is even more important if the angiogram was associated with any fall in blood pressure during the procedure itself.

Complications with Cerebral Angiography

In a table published by KAZNER et al. (1969) complication rates were broken down according to the different lesions studied as follows: in 42,395 patients with neurological or neurosurgical disease the mortality was 0.11%. Those suffering transient or permanent deficits constituted another 1.28%. However, in 3073 patients with vascular disease alone, the mortality was higher at 1.9%, with a corresponding elevation in morbidity to 4.5%.

In the literature, neurological complication rates following angiography in patients with cerebrovascular insufficiency vary from 3% to 5% (BAUER et al., 1962). A detailed presentation of this subject has been made by SCHIEFER (1972).

The Goal of Neuroradiological Investigation in Cerebrovascular Insufficiency
(see also p. 49)

The size, shape, and course of the cerebral arteries and veins, as well as any inherent vascular abnormalities, are readily demonstrated on the cerebral angiogram. This permits conclusions to be drawn regarding the cerebral circulation itself. In this way, much valuable information is obtained with respect to the pathogenesis and therapy of disturbances in cerebral blood flow. The angiogram is indispensible when one is contemplating surgery for any reason on any of the "four major cerebral vessels".

There are two goals in the angiographic evaluation of disturbances in cerebral blood flow, namely: (1) to demonstrate the normal and pathological morphology of the vascular network itself; and (2) to explain functional disturbances of blood flow through the brain. Thus, neuroradiology allows both anatomical and physiological diagnostic analyses to be made.

These analyses can be enhanced even further by use of the brain scan, CT, and "regional" cerebral blood flow measurements. These methods will not be given detailed consideration here.

Indications and *goals* of the angiographic investigation are determined on *clinical* grounds in order to provide information about the *pathogenesis* of disturbances in cerebral blood flow. Three generalizations must be made with respect to any discussion of pathogenesis:

1. A disturbance in cerebral blood flow can arise on a predominantly hemodynamic basis through the combined effects of a local vessel abnormality – usually a stenosis – and a generalized circulatory disturbance (for example, a critical drop in blood pressure). The local vascular lesion is usually arteriosclerotic, but may be thromboembolic, or may result from a more distal primary or secondary arterial thrombosis. The goal of the study is to demonstrate radiographically these morphological changes and their consequences. General circulatory disturbances, on the other hand, arise for cardiovascular reasons and are mainly diagnosed on clinical grounds. Hemodynamic disturbances can be transient in nature (transient ischemic attack, TIA) or more permanent, although many of these will eventually resolve (reversible ischemic neurological deficit, RIND).

2. Cerebrovascular ischemia can be caused by a generalized or localized spasm of the smaller intracranial arteries and arterioles, in the sense of an angiospastic "insult" with an associated disturbance in the blood-brain barrier. One cause of this is an acute hypertensive crisis, which is surely a rare event. In such cases neuroradiology may be misleading because this type of spasm – in contrast to the visible segmental spasm of the larger vessels after aneurysmal bleeding (see p. 169 and Fig. 87) – is only temporary and affects smaller vessels. Thus, by the time the angiogram is performed any abnormality may already have resolved for the most part; however, if the study is performed early enough, there is a demonstrable slowing of the flow of the contrast medium. A similar situation is seen immediately after a convulsion or when blood viscosity is increased.

3. Cerebrovascular ischemia can also be caused by a dissemination of microemboli. These, however, elude all attempts at angiographic demonstration. In any event, one can postulate thrombi from ulcerated arteriosclerotic plaques, e.g., at the carotid bifurcation in the neck, as a possible source for microemboli (see Fig. 111). A decrease in regional cerebral blood flow is rarely recognized.

The following abnormalities may also be demonstrated by cerebral angiography:

1. Direct visualization of a stenosis or an occlusion of an artery as well as a "saddle" embolus. Here, one attempts to ascertain whether the occlusion was caused by thrombosis or an embolus. Occasionally, only the *"absence"* of a *single branch vessel* is found.

The previous remarks are especially applicable to the demonstration of *all extracranial arterial stenoses, occlusions, or ectasias* which constitute the common vascular anomalies amenable to surgical therapy (endarterectomy, vessel reconstitution, bypass procedures, and segmental resections; Fig. 91).

2. Demonstration of disturbances of flow in terms of the rapidity and degree of regional filling of the vascular tree, prolongation of the arterial filling time, or the "early" visualization of normal veins, or regional hyperemia (blush).

3. Demonstration of retrograde filling of an artery, or more extensive flow patterns such as effective anastomoses and collateral circulation.

4. Evidence of localized absence of veins or of a sinus segment with prolongation of the venous phase of the angiogram, or an abnormal pattern of venous emptying.

5. Global prolongation of the circulation time.

To fulfill these goals it is necessary to perform a complete study of both *the extracranial and intracranial* (four-vessel) circulation, em-

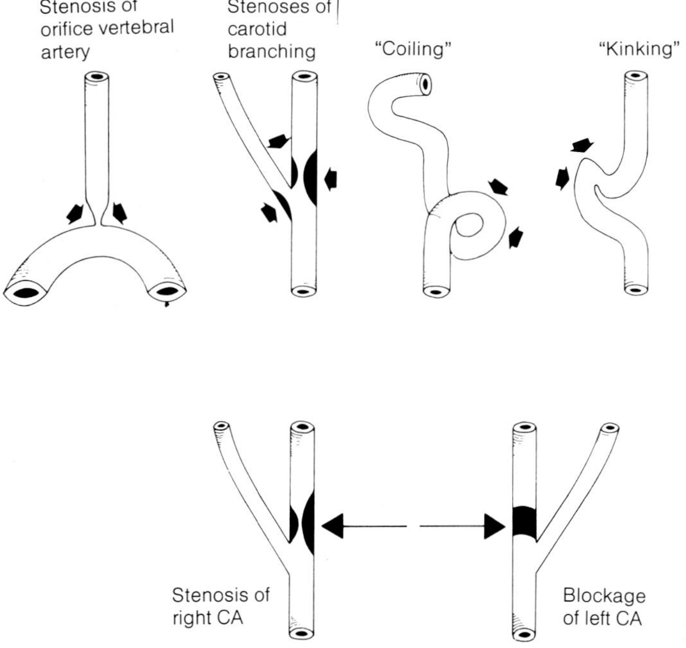

Fig. 91. Diagram depicting operable lesions of the four major cerebral arteries

ploying magnification and subtraction techniques as needed (for example see Fig. 124).

Indication, Timing, and the Technique of the Neuroradiological Examination

For catheterization of the aortic arch, see p. 59; for brachial or subclavian catheterization studies, or for retrograde pressure injections, see p. 60; for direct carotid and vertebral punctures, see pp. 58, 59.

Diagnostic Functions: The General Determination of Circulation Time

One of the most accurate methods of determining the cerebral circulation time is that described by GREITZ (1956). Here, one measures on the serial films the time elapsed between the maximal filling of the siphon with contrast medium (at the level of its passage through the dura) and the maximal filling of the first bridging veins in the anterior parietal region. In this manner it is possible not only to demonstrate delay in the circulation time (as well as any existing collateral circulation), but also to define clearly any delays in venous outflow. These delays can either be regional, as with an occluded vein, or global, as with loss of a major sinus (see p. 172, sinus thrombosis; see below, circulation time), with increases in intracranial pressure, or with increased viscosity of the blood.

Determination of Regional Circulation Time

In serial studies employing retrograde brachial angiography with filling of both the right carotid and vertebral systems, it is generally accepted that under normal conditions the carotid system is usually filled approximately 1 s *prior* to the vertebral system. With a significant carotid stenosis of the right side, a reversal of this sequence is seen in the retrograde angiographic study; on the other hand, should the delay exist in the vertebrobasilar system, there is a prolongation of the normal interval between the filling of the carotid and vertebral systems. This differential, however, is only a useful point of reference and should not be considered inflexible, since it also depends on the position of the neck.

More important are the *regional* disturbances of flow in individual arteries and their branches by a tight stenosis of more than 80% (see pp. 49, 157). Thus, it is possible that the

filling of vessels in the territory of the anterior cerebral artery might only be beginning at a time when the Sylvian vessel group is already completely filled. On the other hand, the filling of the entire middle cerebral artery and/or its peripheral branches can be greatly prolonged, especially in the anterior and posterior parietal arteries and the artery of the angular gyrus. In such cases, the peripheral branches of both arterial trees will still be visible well into the venous phase.

This prolongation of regional circulation time in individual branches of the middle cerebral artery is particularly significant when there is close correlation with neurological symptoms, such as in aphasia, Gerstmann's syndrome, or the parietal lobe syndrome.

It is also accepted that the last arterial branches to be visualized on the normal carotid arteriogram are found in the *parietal region* in the border area between the parietal, occipital, and temporal lobes. This corresponds to the common watershed area of the anterior cerebral, posterior cerebral, and middle cerebral arterial territories. From a hemodynamic standpoint, this watershed zone is particularly liable to injury from generalized circulatory disturbances affecting the brain. Here, one also finds transient disturbances of cerebral blood flow and occasionally an actual infarct.

The *venous* outflow can also show regional differences. It is reasonable from a physiological standpoint that first the frontal veins fill, then the parietal, and finally the occipital. This can be seen from the progress of flow through the territory of supply of the anterior cerebral artery, which drains into the sagittal sinus. GREITZ (1956) has, however, shown that with occlusion of an artery and its subsequent retrograde filling via collateral flow, transient differences can also occur in the topography of the venous drainage. These observations permit conclusions to be made regarding the topographical basis for clinical symptoms.

Morphological Diagnosis: Anatomical Variations in Arteries and Veins

Before a decision is made about changes in vessel morphology or even the absence of a vessel, it is first necessary to determine that the anomalies are not due to anatomical variants. Recognition of such variants is thus quite important. It is also necessary to keep these variants in mind when evaluating differences in blood flow patterns of the major brain arteries and sinuses, and to look for them when the indications warrant it.

In the carotid system there are variations in the diameter of the lumen of the neck arteries. Farther on, there are variations in the curvature of the siphon which are quite important in that they may mimic the changes seen in mass displacements. In 20%–30% of the cases, the *posterior cerebral artery* is predominantly filled from the carotid artery, the "embryonal" origin of the posterior cerebral artery. In another variation, a thin stream of blood enters the posterior cerebral artery by way of the posterior communicating artery, but the major contribution comes from the vertebrobasilar system (Fig. 92). Most frequently, however, the posterior cerebral artery is supplied almost exclusively by the vertebrobasilar system. Occasionally, the posterior communicating artery alone is visualized on both the carotid and vertebrobasilar injections (Fig. 93).

A quite frequent variation in the *anterior cerebral artery* occurs when both arteries are filled from *one side*. This anomaly is usually associated with aplasia or hypoplasia of the opposite A-1 segment (see p. 77).

In such cases the dominant carotid will almost never fill the posterior cerebral artery at the same time, so that both anterior cerebral arteries and the posterior cerebral artery are rarely seen from a single injection. These morphological variations with respect to channels of flow through the circle of Willis can be demonstrated more clearly if, during the injection, the opposite carotid artery is compressed.

A rarer occurrence is the presence of a third anterior cerebral artery which is for the most part quite delicate and is situated in the midline (middle anterior cerebral artery; KRAYENBUEHL and YASARGIL, 1965; KRAYENBUEHL et al., 1979).

Extremely rare are other variations such as an *oblique supracallosal anastomosis* between both anterior cerebral arteries. In this situation, both parietal regions are filled from the same anterior cerebral artery. Although the opposite anterior cerebral artery exists, it does not supply its own parasagittal parietal territory. This anastomosis takes place on the corpus callosum and may be of significance in the pathogenesis of infarcts in the anterior cerebral territory.

In analyzing the middle cerebral artery, it is necessary to identify its various ascending branches accurately. It is often quite difficult to diagnose the absence of a branch on the angiogram. For this reason, it is important to keep in mind certain rules of thumb as outlined by FOIX and LEVY (1927), RING and WADDINGTON (1967), and SALAMON (1971). Variations are commonly found in the three frontal branches, which occasionally exit as a single large branch or may consist of several branches from the main middle cerebral trunk. The most common variation in the parietal and temporal branches is the omission of one of the branches, which can be mistaken for an occluded trunk. In fact, the normal population of vessels in this region may at times seem sparse.

Variations in the origin of the *posterior cerebral artery* from either the *carotid* or *vertebrobasilar systems* have been discussed. The frequent appearance of the "embryonal type", i.e., a carotid origin for the posterior cerebral artery, can be of particular significance when the vertebral study is being attempted by means of a left retrograde brachial injection. If the posterior cerebral artery of one side fails to fill in such a study, the physiological variant of a carotid origin must be suspected and verified by means of a carotid injection. Only when the posterior cerebral artery fails to fill during the carotid study can one assume that it is occluded (for genuine occlusion of the posterior cerebral artery, see p. 152).

The variations of the *circle of Willis* are particularly important and will be described below (see p. 161). The potential for anastomosis between both carotid arteries and the vertebrobasilar system is extremely important in the event of a major vessel occlusion (see Fig. 93, and collateral circulation, p. 159). Also important is the situation in which one vertebral artery, usually the right, is hypoplastic, and the other enlarged. The complete absence of one or the other vertebral artery is, on the other hand, seldom seen.

Variations are also frequently seen involving the cerebellar arteries. The superior cerebellar arteries are often doubled, while the anterior inferior cerebellar artery is often absent or so thin that it cannot be identified on the angiogram. On the other hand, the posterior inferior cerebellar arteries should be readily demonstrated on both sides. They usually arise from the vertebral arteries, but can originate from the lower basilar artery segment. The posterior inferior cerebellar artery can also divide early or may even originate as a double vessel. In such cases each branch supplies its own portion of the medulla oblongata and cerebellum.

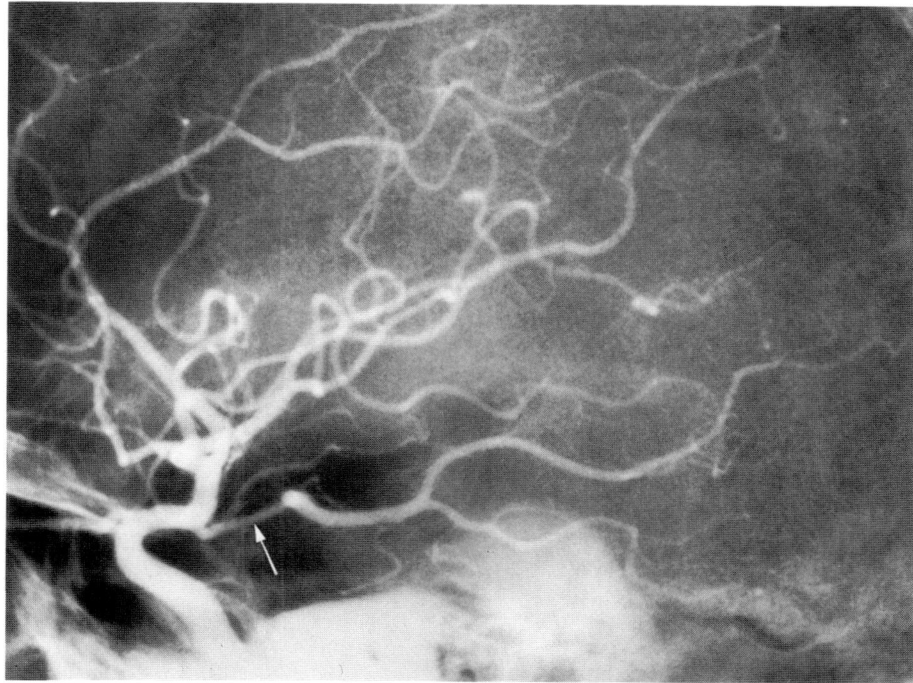

Fig. 92. The posterior cerebral artery originates from the basilar artery in 80% of cases. In the remaining cases it may be supplied fully by the internal carotid artery – as in this example – or by both systems, with varying contributions

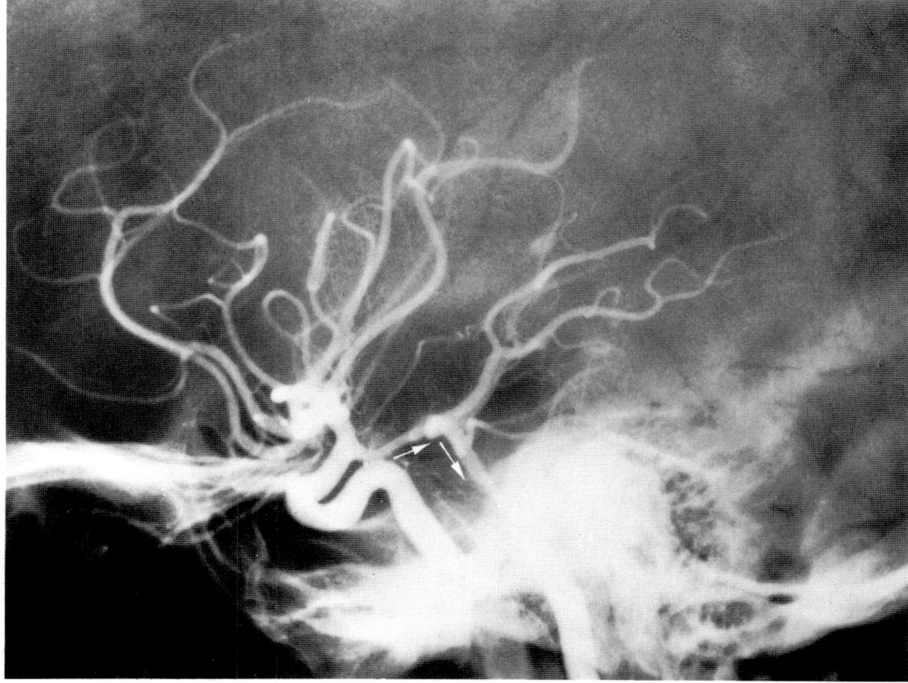

Fig. 93. Carotid arteriogram demonstrating relative stenosis of the basilar artery. There is retrograde filling of the distal basilar artery and its branches from the carotid system over the posterior communicating artery

The apparent absence of one of the posterior inferior cerebellar arteries (artery of Wallenberg) does not always indicate an occlusion, since this artery can be represented by two or three fine vessels originating partly from the basilar and partly from the vertebral arteries. These may not be visualized on the normal arteriogram.

Such fine discriminations of detail are not always possible on the routine angiographic study. In such cases use of the magnification view with subtraction or angio-tomography will frequently demonstrate the missing vessels.

Pathological Vessel Changes in Arteriosclerosis

The major effect in such cases is on the arterial wall in which arteriosclerotic plaques form, resulting in stenosis of the vessel lumen. This stenosis can lead to total occlusion either through arteriosclerotic changes alone or through thrombus formation in a narrowed lumen. Because of this fact, occlusions and stenoses of vessels have the same sites of predilection. Finally, macroemboli may "hang up" at areas of stenosis and may also be responsible for an occasional occlusion.

It is important also to recognize the factors contributing to the local predilection for stenosis formation. This abnormality is found wherever "turbulence" exists, namely: (1) a change in the direction of flow; (2) where changes in the vessel wall have taken place; and (3) through loss of vessel elasticity. One therefore finds arteriosclerotic changes particularly at vessel curvatures, bifurcations, at the origin of branches, where two vessels join and flow streams are mixed, and at points of constriction such as the opening in the dura for passage of an artery, a bony canal, or a point of impingement by another structure (i.e., a cranial nerve). Such turbulence can be demonstrated especially well on the cine-angiogram. At such points the contrast medium often remains longer than usual.

Extracranial Arteriosclerotic and Thrombotic Vessel Changes:

The Stenosis. The most proximal stenosis (less frequently occlusion) is found at the origin of the vertebral artery from the subclavian artery (Fig. 94). This is seen more often than a similar stenosis at the origin of the common carotid. At the termination of the stenotic seg-

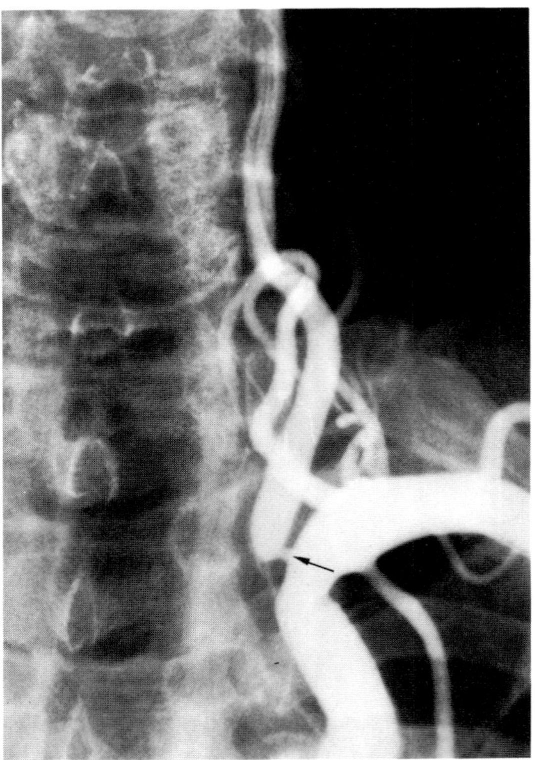

Fig. 94. Stenosis (see *arrow*) at the origin of the left vertebral artery from the subclavian with poststenotic dilatation

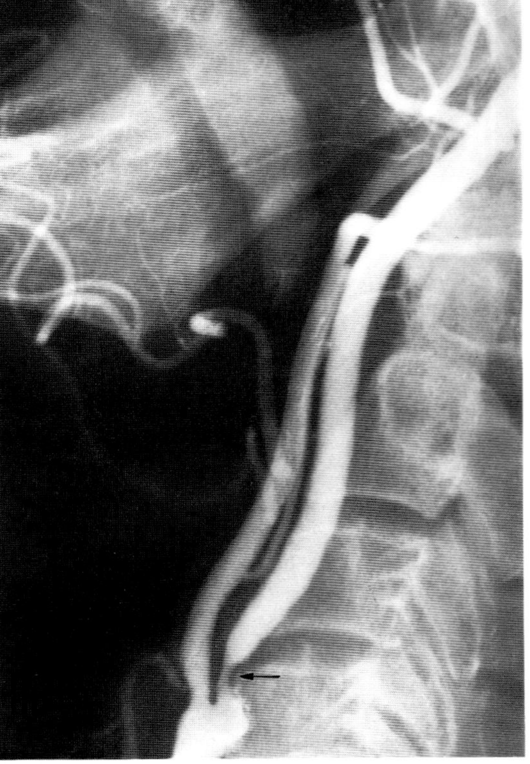

Fig. 95. High-grade (80%) stenosis of the internal carotid artery near its origin. Note also the constriction (25%) of the external carotid artery at its origin

Fig. 96. Occlusion of the internal carotid artery in the neck (*arrow*)

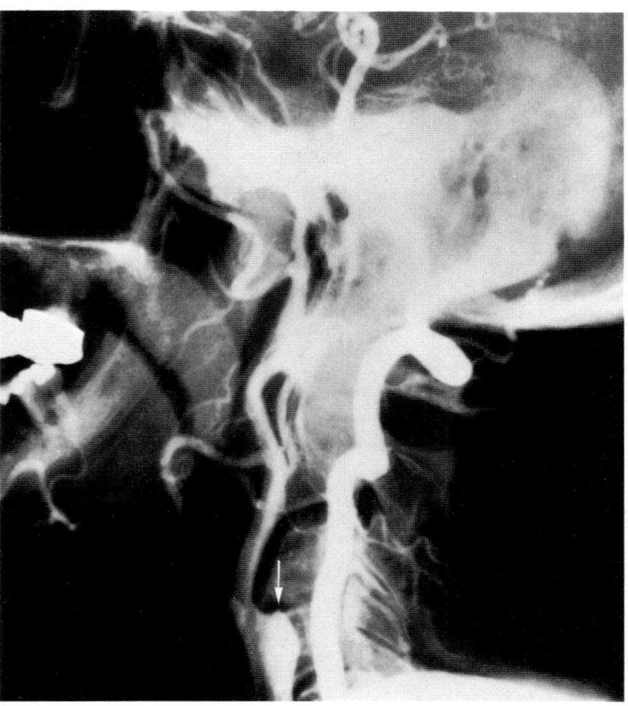

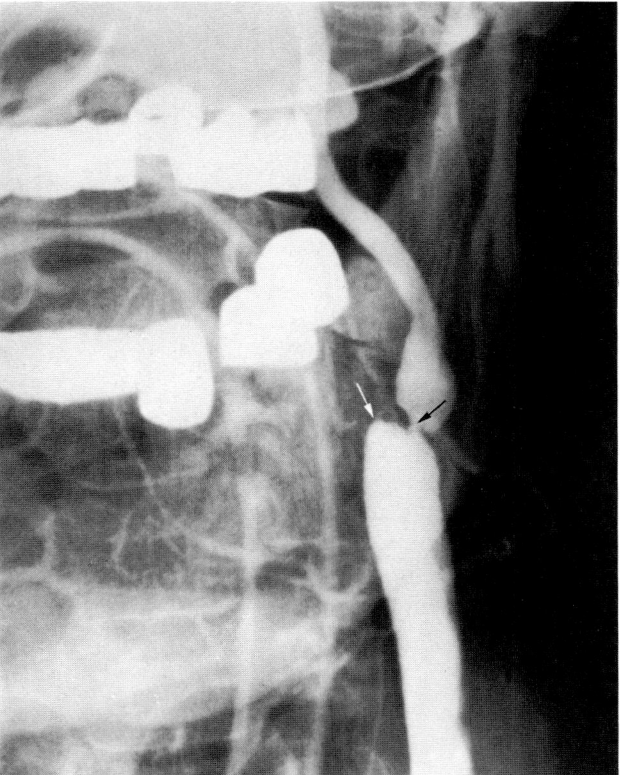

Fig. 97. Occlusion of the external carotid artery just distal to the bifurcation of the common carotid with a large common carotid artery. High-grade stenosis (70%) of the internal carotid artery at its origin (*arrow*) with poststenotic dilatation

ment on the vertebral artery, a poststenotic dilatation is often found, or later a lengthening of the artery with loop formation.

A lesion which occurs at a more distal location in the neck is seen at the bifurcation of the common carotid into the internal carotid and external carotid vessels (Fig. 95). Here the *stenotic plaque* lies for the most part on the medial "carina" of the internal carotid artery, less commonly in a similar location on the ex-

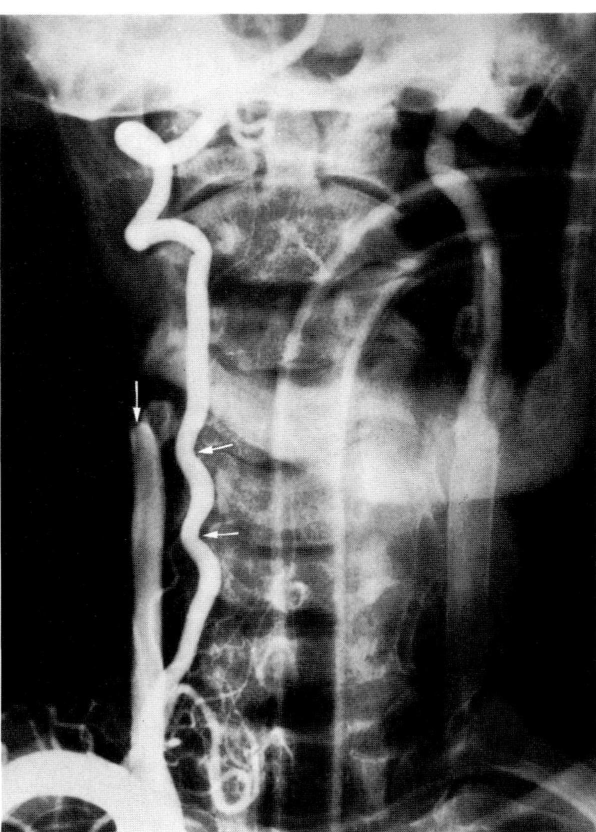

Fig. 98. Right retrograde brachial arteriogram depicting occlusion of the right common carotid artery. Moderate filling of the left carotid artery. The right vertebral artery shows two indentations (*arrows*) secondary to osteophytic spurring of the cervical vertebra (C-4/5 and C-5/6)

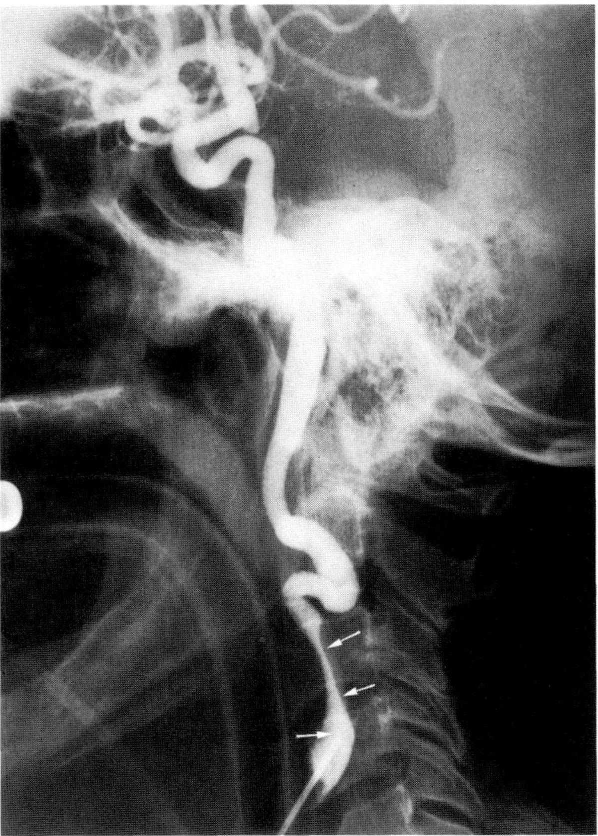

Fig. 99. Intramural hemorrhage (*arrows*) with iatrogenic stenosis of the internal carotid artery in the neck secondary to needle puncture (*arrow*). This vessel in addition shows coiling with moderate kinking

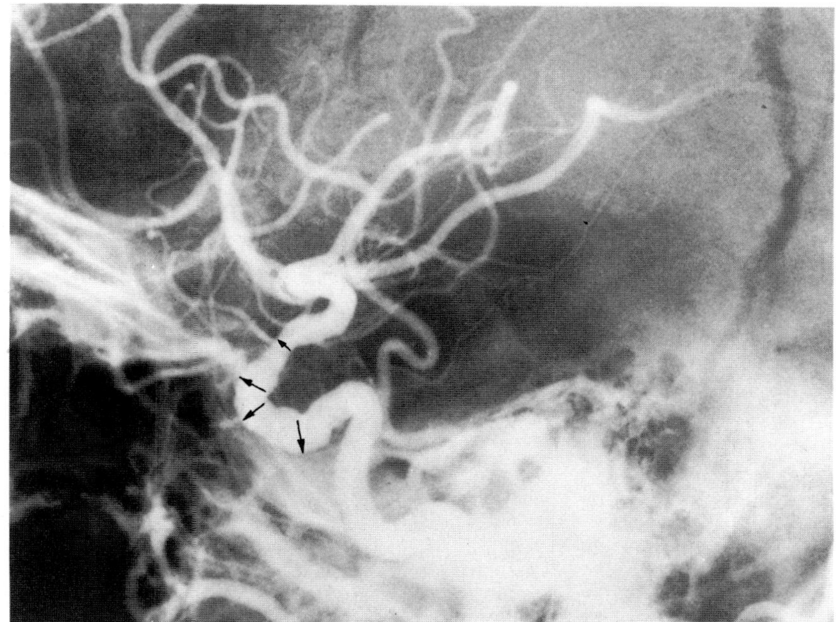

Fig. 100. Irregular narrowing of the entire internal carotid artery siphon

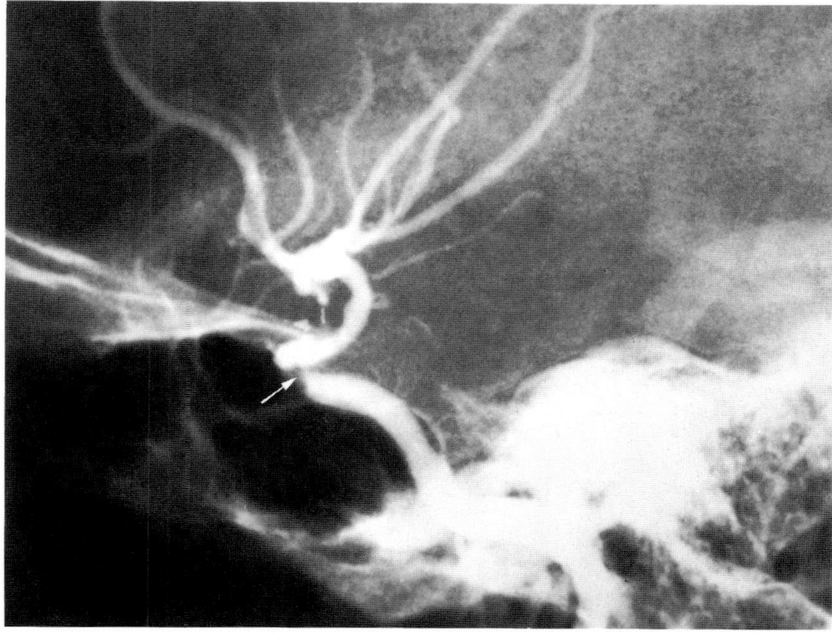

Fig. 101. Stenosis of the siphon (*arrow*) proximal to the knee (intravenous segment)

ternal carotid artery. Corresponding to these plaques, occlusions are also found predominantly in the internal carotid artery which usually remains only as a short stump (Fig. 96). This infrequently occurs in the external carotid (Fig. 97) or in the common carotid just proximal to the bifurcation (Fig. 98). An arteriosclerotic plaque can be simulated by an intramural injection of contrast medium or through a dissecting hematoma (Fig. 99).

An occlusion of the vertebral artery is occasionally seen at the level of the 6th cervical vertebra as the artery enters the costotransverse foramen.

After entering the skull, a stenosis of the internal carotid artery at the level of the siphon

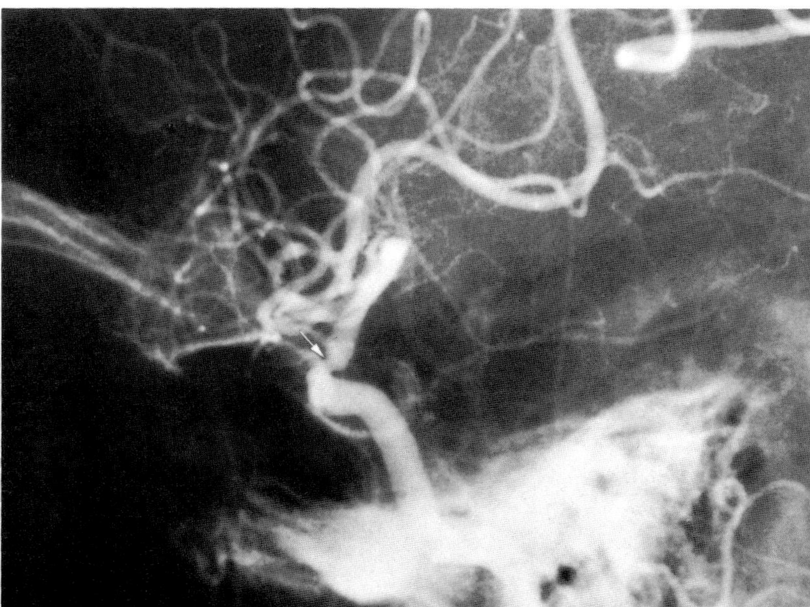

Fig. 102. Stenosis of the internal carotid artery in the region of the siphon (*arrow*) at the point where the artery perforates the dura

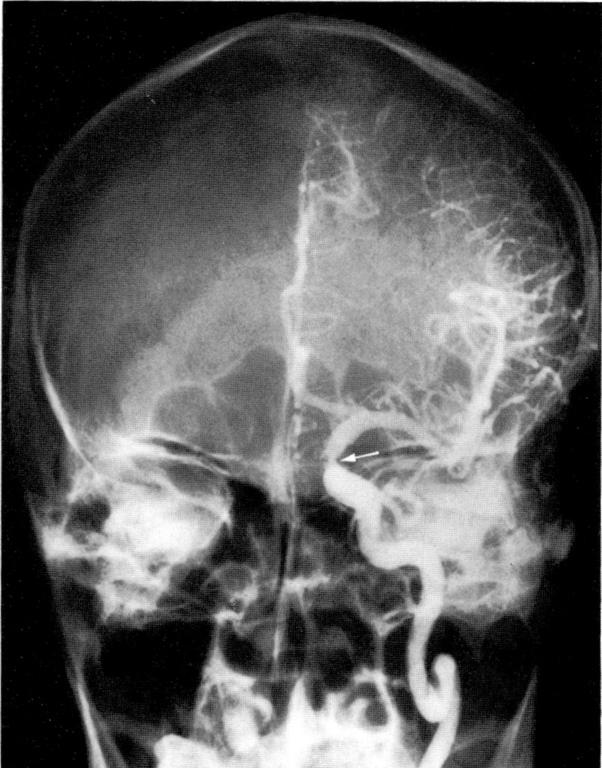

Fig. 103. Stenosis of the internal carotid artery at the siphon as it pierces the dura (*arrow*). Note the coiling of this vessel which is apparent in the cervical area

Fig. 104. Stenosis of the internal carotid siphon in its cisternal segment

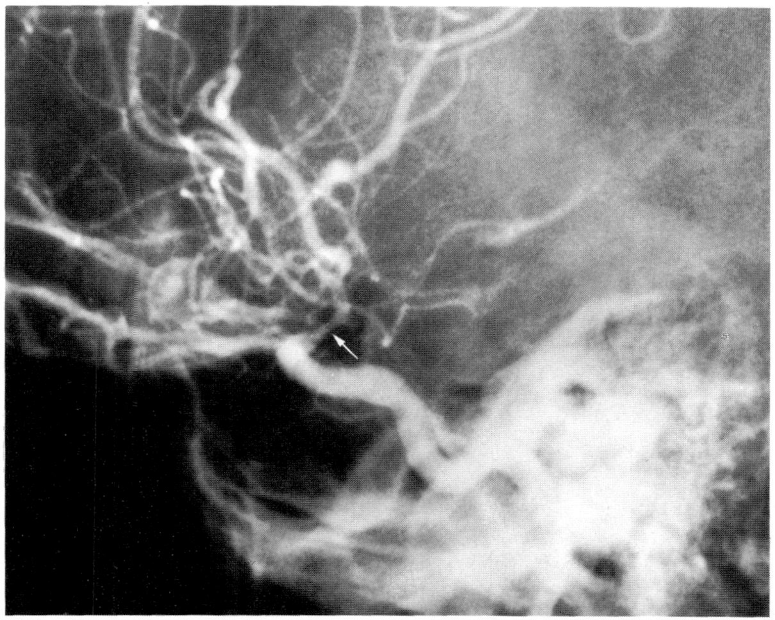

Fig. 105. Occlusion of the internal carotid artery from an embolus at the level of the most distal siphon segment

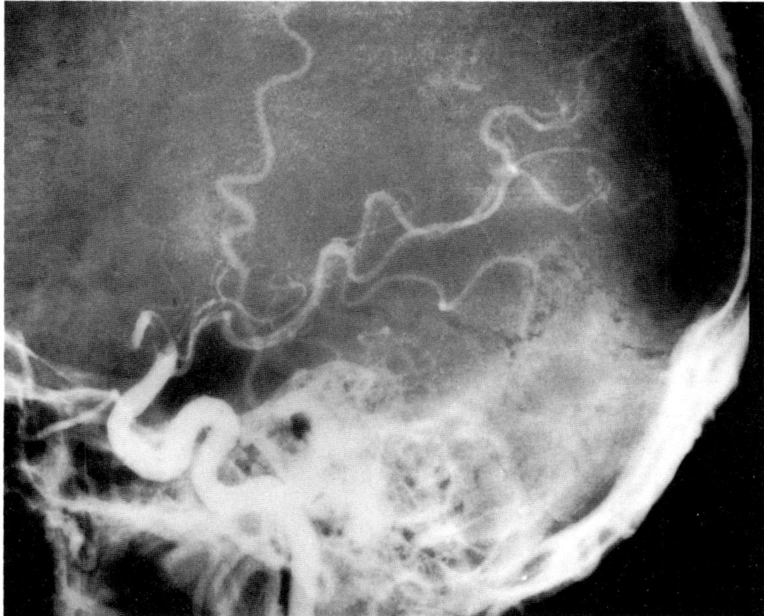

is quite common and involves either the entire loop (Fig. 100) or, more frequently, is localized to one of the three segments forming the siphon (ganglion-cavernous-knee, Figs. 101, 102, 103; cisternal segment, Fig. 104; most frequently the cisternal segment after penetration of the dura, Fig. 105 and also 116).

It should be stressed that two kinds of arteriosclerosis involve the "cerebral arteries" – the *stenotic type* and the predominantly *ectatic type*. The latter runs the gamut from a lengthening of the vessel – so often the case with the superficial temporal artery overlying the temporalis muscle – to a winding tortuosity (Fig. 106), a coiling (Figs. 103, 107), or even a kinking of the vessel (Fig. 91). Coiling to the point of loop formation is seen frequently involving the internal carotid artery just distal

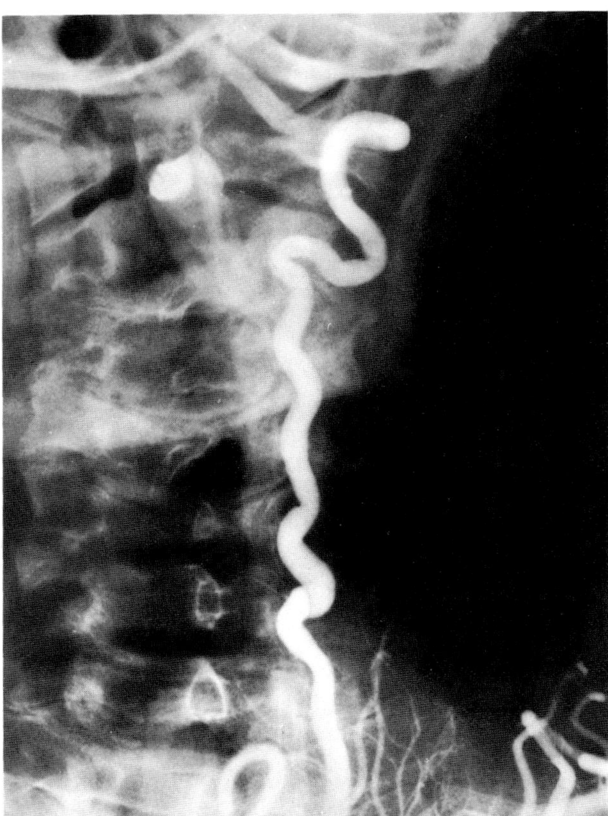

Fig. 106. Ectatic arteriosclerotic change with tortuosity in this left vertebral artery study (left retrograde brachial angiogram)

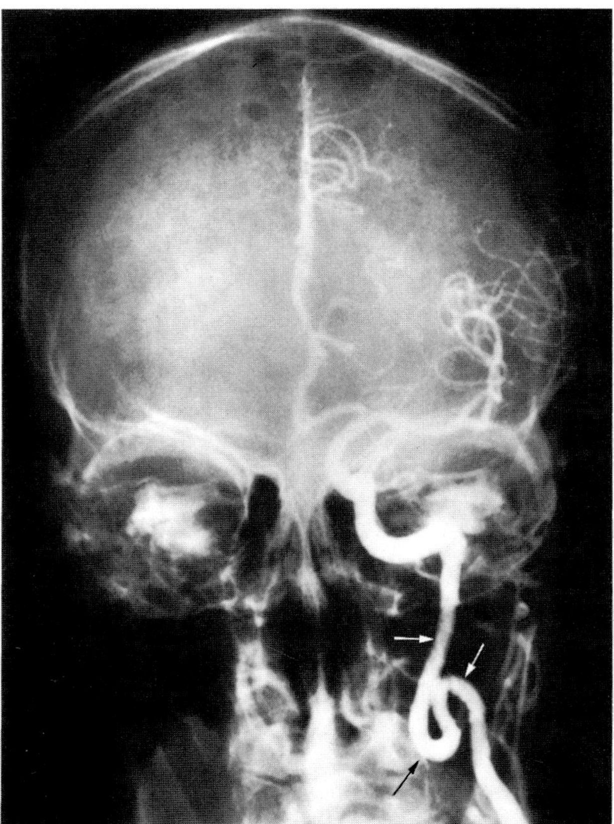

Fig. 107. Considerable arteriosclerotic change with stenosis and coiling in the mid-portion of the cervical segment of the internal carotid artery (*arrows*)

Fig. 108. Marked stenosis (90%) of the internal carotid artery siphon (*arrow*) caused by an embolus (on birth control pills). The lenticulostriate vessels are completely patent. Note the 6-cm long "stenosis" (*arrows*) of the internal carotid artery in the neck well above the puncture site

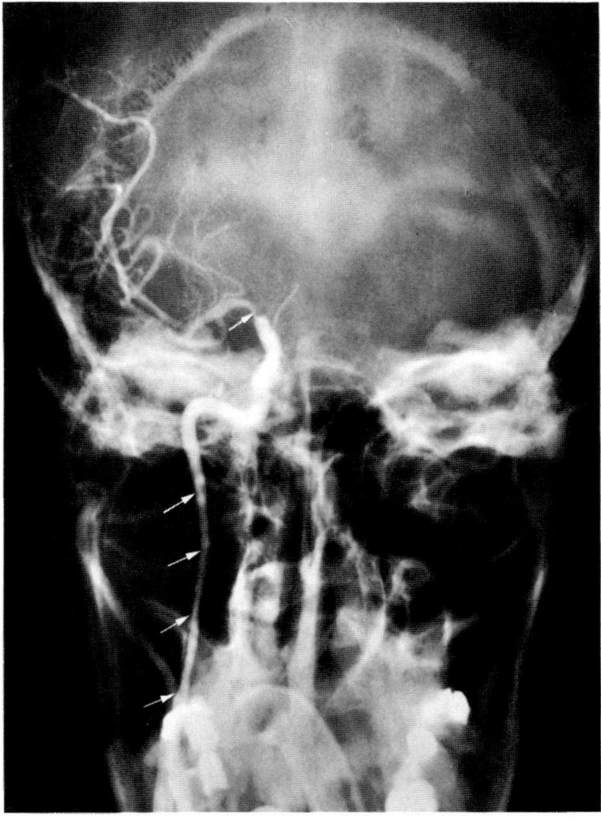

to its origin in the neck, as well as on the vertebral artery between the foramen magnum and the atlas. Such coils could certainly result in genuine disturbances of cerebral blood flow, depending upon the position of the head.

A tortuosity involving the entire vessel may be seen in both the carotid and vertebral arteries (Fig. 106).

Many authors consider tortuosity or even coiling to be congenital. In any case a heightening of this abnormality is seen with old age or arteriosclerosis.

Finally, there is in the frame of these ectatic types of arteriosclerosis a true kinking of the vessel which is occasionally an indication for surgical resection. Coiling, on the other hand, is less commonly an indication for surgery because it is less frequently associated with clinical symptoms. Such anomalies are found as often on the internal carotid artery as on the vertebral artery (usually the distal third of its extracranial course). Both sides are involved with equal frequency.

The "Narrow Carotid Artery". Vessel narrowing or "stenosis" over a rather long stretch is especially common in the internal carotid artery in the neck. It is difficult to determine from the angiogram alone in a given case whether the abnormality is secondary to fibromuscular dysplasia or is simply an extensive recanalized thrombosis (Fig. 108). A functional transient narrowing involving several centimeters of vessel may also occur above the needle puncture site in the internal carotid (Figs. 109, 110; see also angiospasm, p. 169). Moreover, it is important to ascertain in cases of internal carotid artery hypoplasia whether a simultaneous hypoplasia of the opposite site is present as well. Most of the remaining arteries show changes only in individual segments.

Thrombosis and Embolism:

Thromboses of the carotid artery preferentially involve the bifurcation in the neck at the site of a pre-existing arteriosclerotic plaque. These plaques can ulcerate and can serve as a source for microemboli (see p. 138 and Fig. 111).

Next in frequency and involving the same sites are thrombotic occlusions of "youthful" vessels which appear not to be involved with arteriosclerosis. This type of thrombosis is pre-

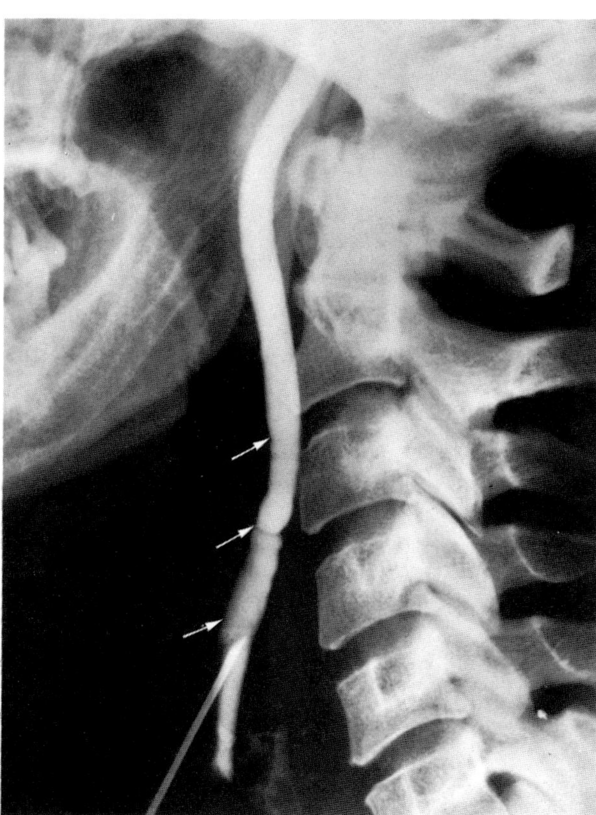

Fig. 109. Typical "string of pearls" deformity of the internal carotid artery above the puncture site. This is thought possibly to be a spastic phenomenon

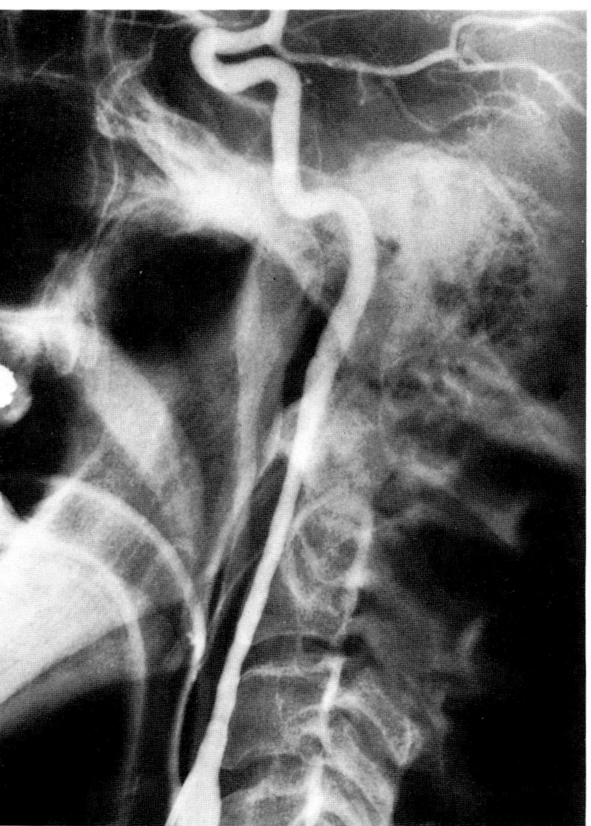

Fig. 110. Stenosis of an elongated segment of the internal carotid artery in the neck, possibly a spastic phenomenon related to the puncture site

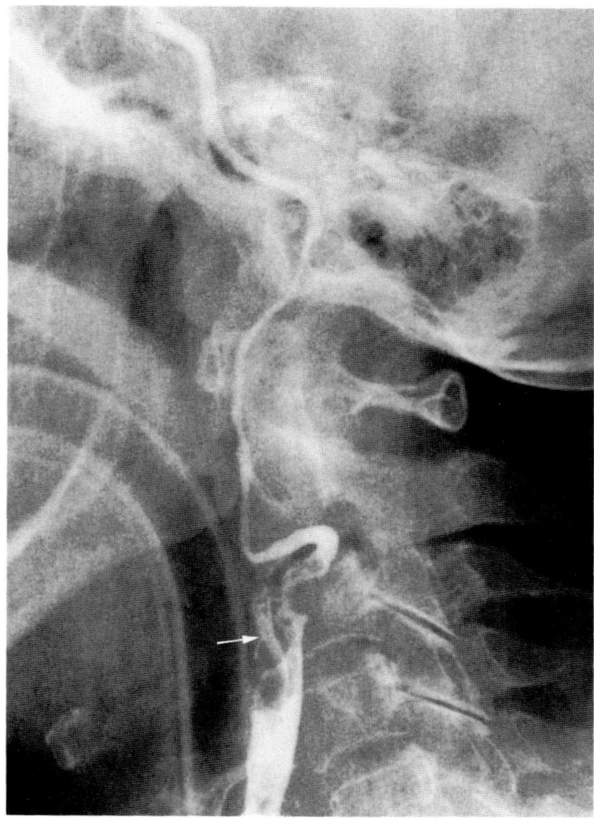

Fig. 111. Irregular stenotic lesion involving the internal carotid artery distal to the bifurcation with occlusion of the external carotid artery. This picture is typical of that seen with secondary thrombosis of an arteriosclerotic plaque (the needle lies in the common carotid artery far below the lesion)

valent among young people and is frequently of uncertain etiology.

Acute *emboli* occasionally lodge at the bifurcation of the common carotid artery (see Fig. 105), but rarely lead to internal carotid artery occlusion. They primarily involve the distal segment of the siphon (Fig. 105), the middle cerebral artery (see p. 158) or its branches, and are less commonly seen in other arteries. Embolism is found frequently in association with incompetent or artificial heart valves, arrhythmias, and not uncommonly in women taking birth control pills.

Only occasionally can a thrombosis ("cone-like") be distinguished with some certainty from an embolus ("pointed"). An embolus is definitely present when it is found "riding saddle" at a vessel fork (see Fig. 124). An iatrogenic embolus may be disseminated during angiography if it arises at the site of a needle puncture.

Intracranial vessel changes:

The predilection for intracranial stenoses is well known (see also siphon of the carotid artery, Fig. 100–104). The most frequent site on the middle cerebral artery for stenotic occlusion to occur is 1–2 cm beyond its origin from the internal carotid artery (Fig. 112). Since thrombotic occlusions usually involve areas of pre-existing stenosis, it is possible to predict from the presence of stenoses four distinct localizations for *occlusion* of the middle cerebral artery:

1) Proximally at its origin, in which case the branches of the basal ganglia and thalamus are also involved (Fig. 113/I).
2) More distally at the exit of the lateral lenticulostriate branches, the medial lenticulostriate branches remain open (Figs. 113/II and 114)
3) Still more distal at the trifurcation of the middle cerebral artery, with the deep nuclei branches uninvolved (Figs. 112 and 113/III)
4) Furthermore, branch occlusions may involve any of the vessels of the Sylvian group (see Fig. 115).

As a result of highly effective "meningeal anastomoses", some 20% of middle cerebral artery occlusions – both proximal and distal – occur without associated neurological symptoms.

Stenoses involving the *anterior cerebral artery* are particularly prevalent in the bend of

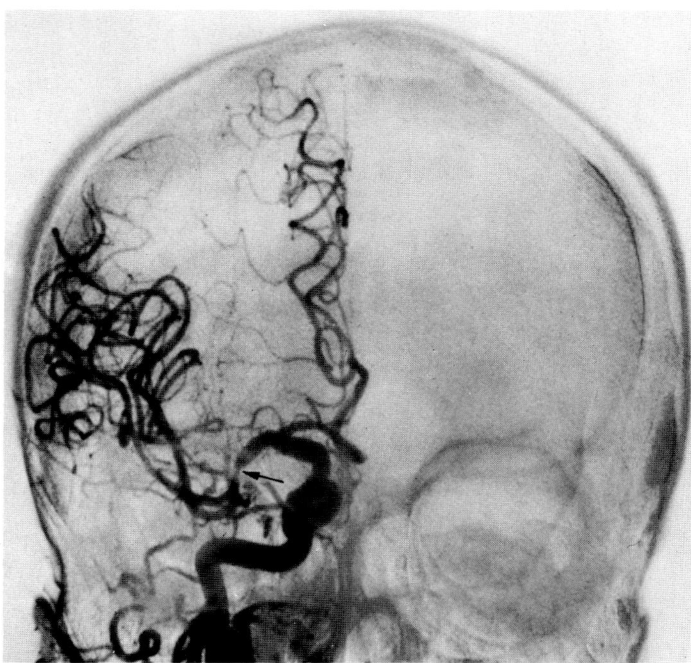

Fig. 112. Subtraction technique showing a stenotic lesion (60%) of the middle cerebral artery (location corresponds to Fig. 113/*III*)

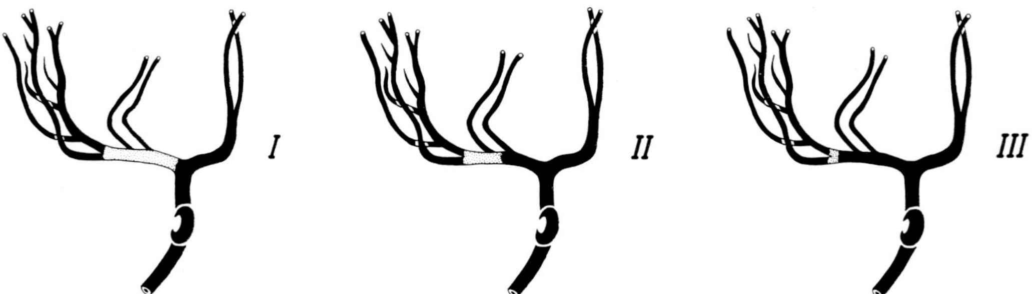

Fig. 113. The major types of middle cerebral artery occlusion. Rarely seen is the occlusion at the origin in which all lenticulostriate vessels are patent (see text)

the artery at the rostrum of the corpus callosum, either just beneath or just above this structure (Figs. 116, 124). Total occlusion in this area is uncommon.

The *vertebral artery,* on the other hand, is most frequently involved with a stenotic lesion just as it penetrates the dura (Fig. 117). Not infrequently there follows a post-stenotic dilatation which can be so large as to mimic a fusiform aneurysm. Also, the *basilar artery* is frequently the site of a major stenosis, usually in its middle or distal segment (Fig. 118).

The *posterior cerebral artery* is likewise involved with stenoses and occlusions just as it curves around the peduncle. Occlusions are particularly prevalent on the posterior cerebral artery at the following three sites (Fig. 119):

1) *Proximal* at its origin from the basilar artery as it begins to course around the peduncle (Figs. 119/I, 120, 121)

2) Just *distal* to this point at the site of the attachment of the posterior communicating artery, which is also occluded (Fig. 119/II)

3) Slightly more distal at the *apex* of the curve around the peduncle, in which case the posterior communicating artery is uninvolved (Fig. 119 III).

4) Again "*distal branch occlusions*" are known to occur (Fig. 119/IV).

Both posterior cerebral arteries can be stenosed or occluded at the same time, usually at different sites.

Ectatic changes with arteriosclerosis: Ectasia as a result of arteriosclerosis with regard to the

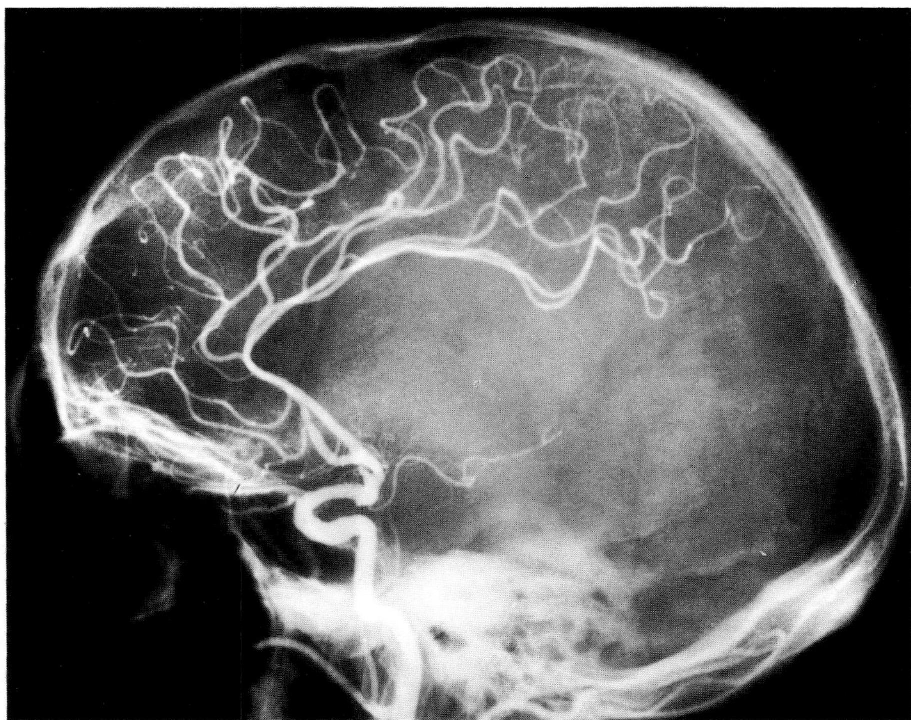

Fig. 114. Occlusion of the main trunk of the middle cerebral artery (Fig. 113/*II*), with sparing of some medial lenticulostriate branches

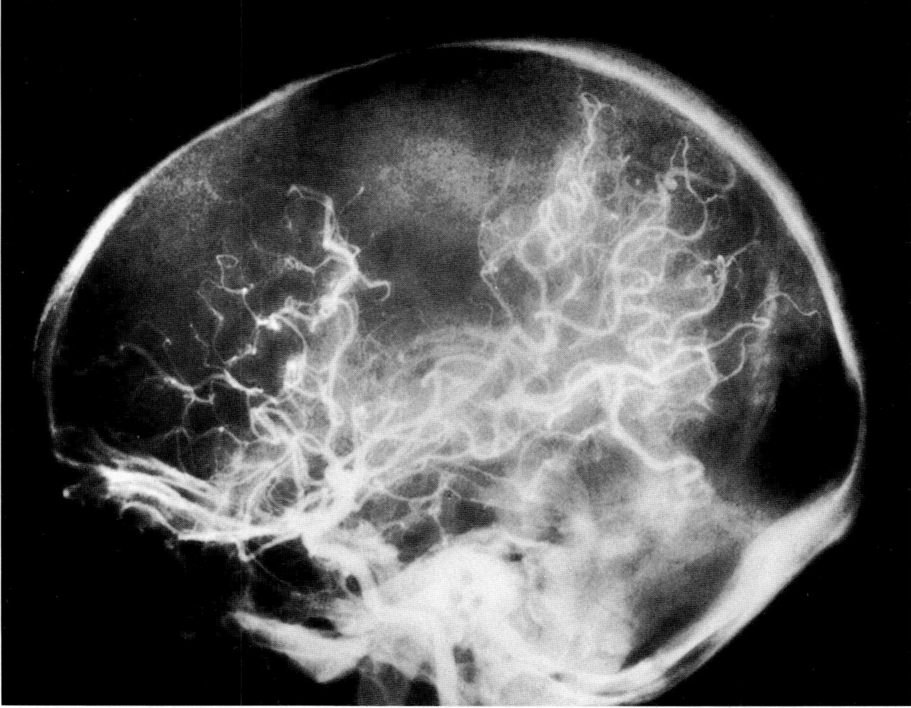

Fig. 115. Branch occlusion (Rolandic and pre-Rolandic arteries) in the middle cerebral artery territory. Note that the anterior cerebral artery is absent in this study

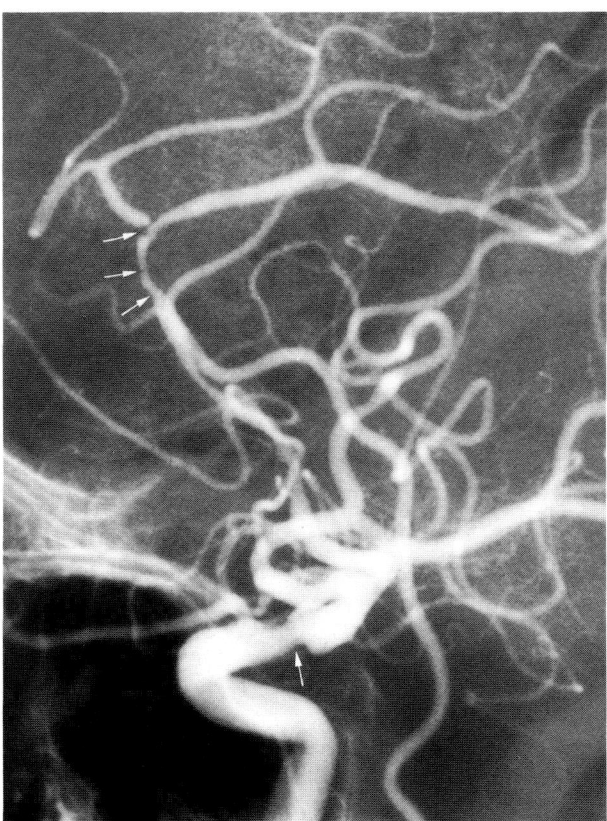

Fig. 116. Stenosis involving the siphon of the internal carotid artery as it pierces the dura. Narrowing also occurs at several points along the anterior cerebral artery as it curves over the rostrum of the corpus callosum, particularly at the origin of the callosomarginal artery (*arrows*). These stenotic lesions are caused by arteriosclerotic plaques

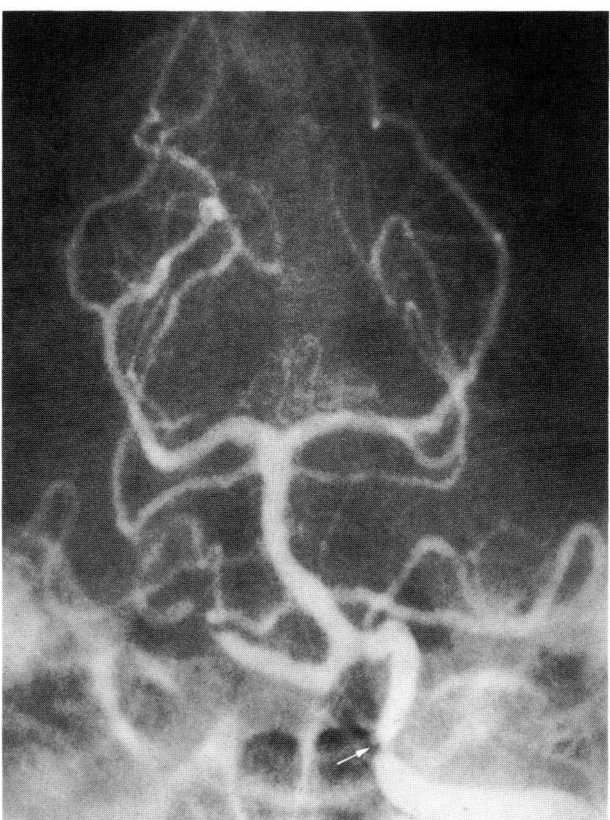

Fig. 117. Distal stenosis of the left vertebral artery as it pierces the dura (*arrow*). Note the retrograde filling of the opposite vertebral artery

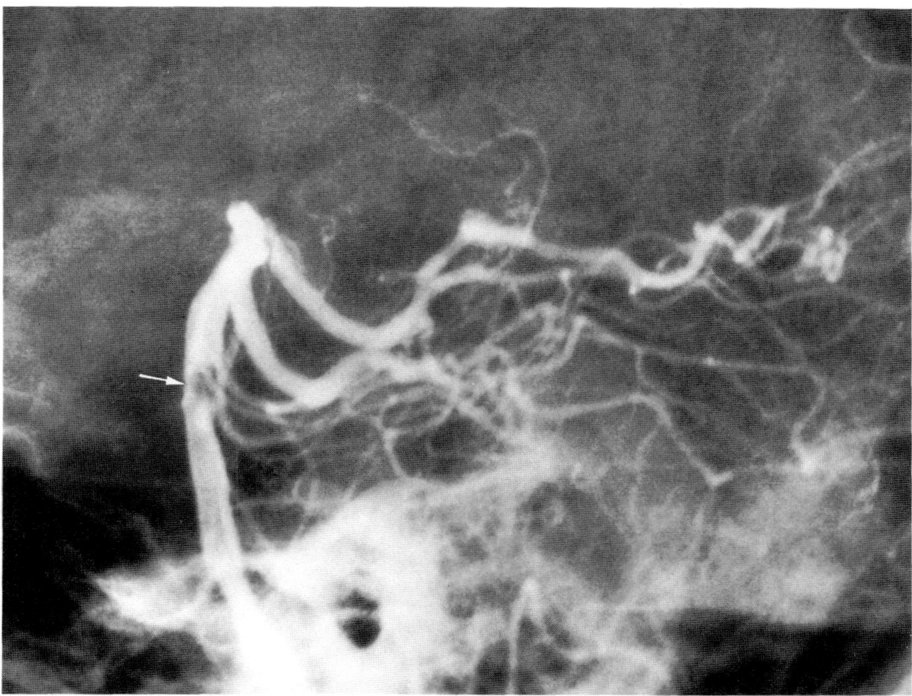

Fig. 118. Large stenotic plaque in the middle segment of the basilar artery (this patient was rendered quadriplegic by this lesion)

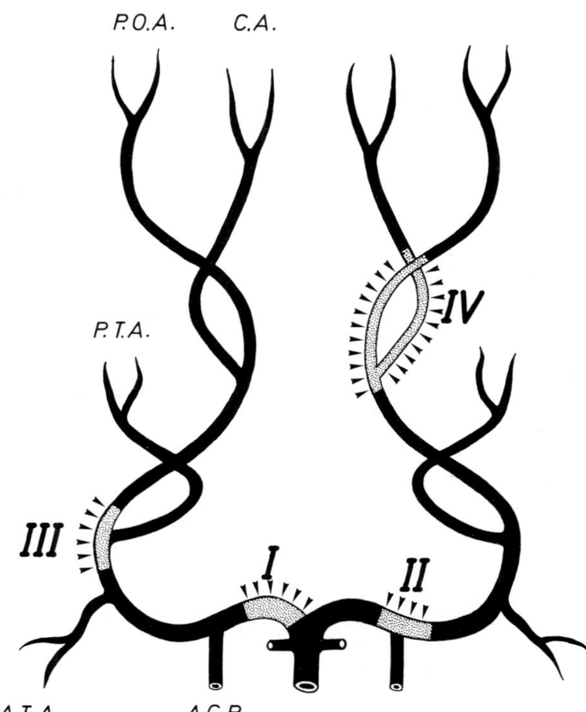

Fig. 119. The four major sites for stenosis and occlusion of the posterior cerebral arteries: *I*, proximal to the posterior communicating artery, which remains patent; *II*, at the origin of the posterior communicating artery; *III*, at the apex of the curve around the peduncle; *IV*, distal branch occlusions

extracranial vessels has been described above. *Intracranially* such changes are especially evident on the vertebral arteries just beyond their penetration through the dura where they often form large fusiform aneurysms. These ectatic changes also involve the basilar artery to a significant degree. As a result this vessel assumes a tortuous course which can appear to be quite marked on the anteroposterior views (Fig. 106). In such cases the basilar artery will frequently

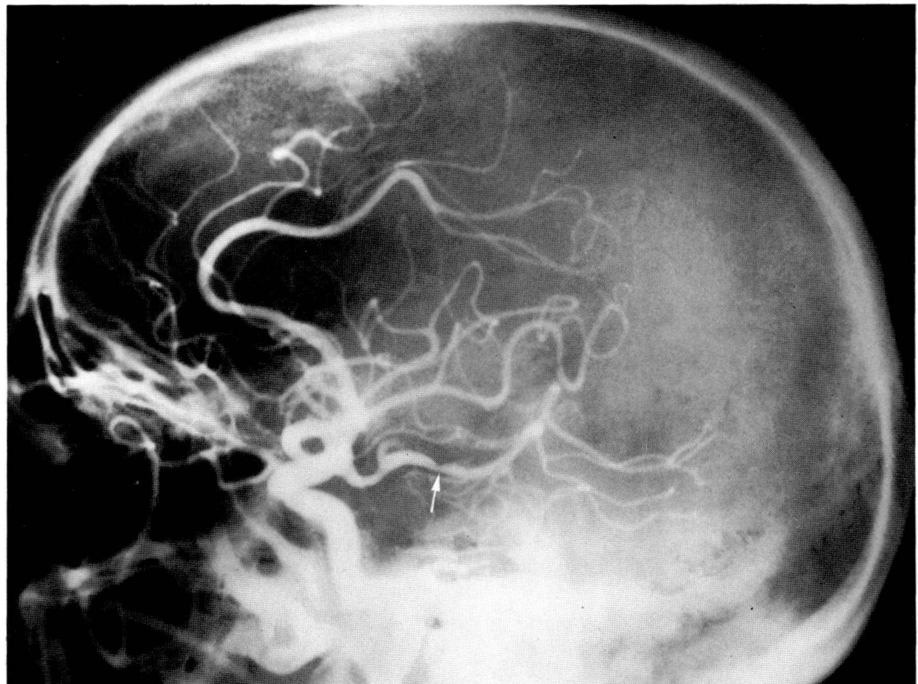

Fig. 120. Stenosis of the posterior cerebral artery ("embryonal type") corresponding to Fig. 119/*III* (*arrow*)

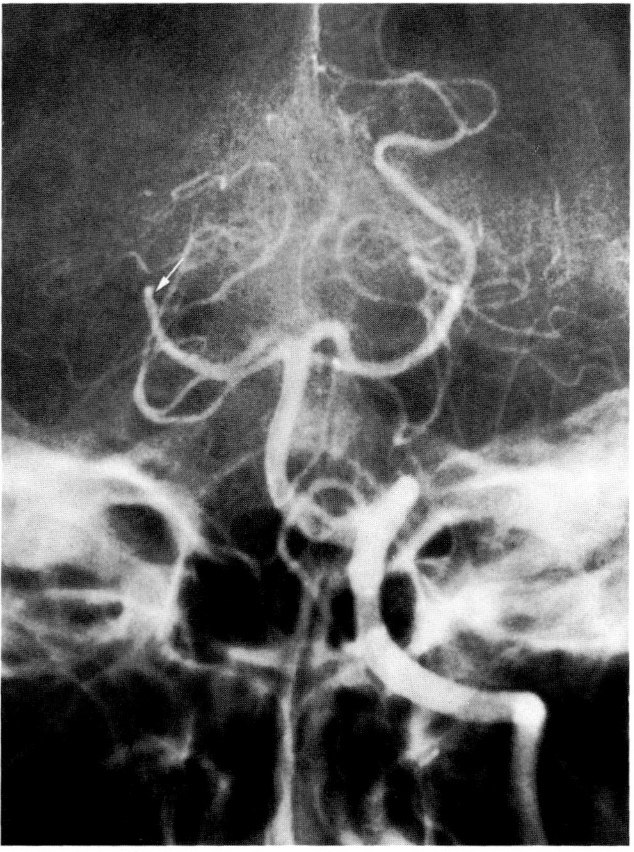

Fig. 121. Occlusion (*arrow*) of the posterior cerebral artery (Fig. 119/*III*)

Fig. 122. Marked tortuosity of the left ectatic vertebral artery, with shifting of the basilar artery far across the midline and then back to its original side. Stenotic lesions are apparent throughout the length of this vessel. This is an example of "megadolichobasilaris"

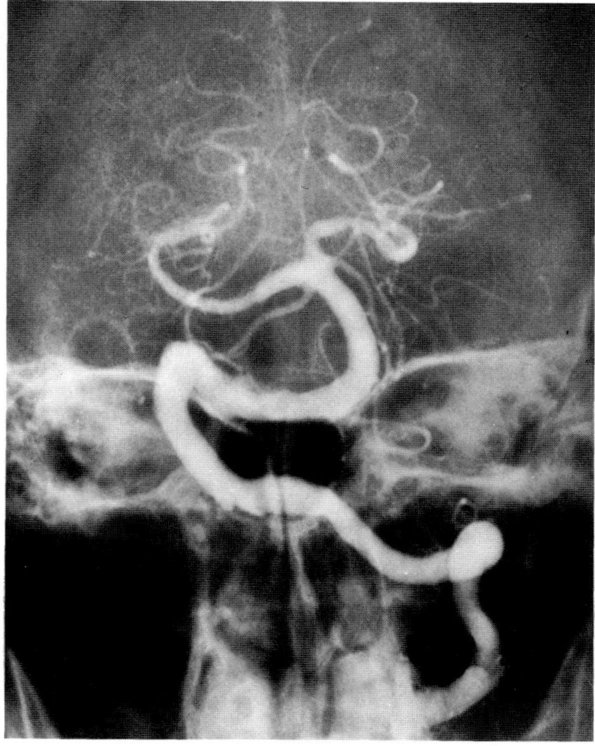

assume an S-shaped curve (Fig. 122) with the middle third of the vessel often displaced 1–3 cm from its usual midline course. The displacement is generally to the side of the smaller vertebral artery, mostly to the right since the left vertebral is statistically the dominant vessel. In this situation, the basilar artery appears to be merely a continuation of the larger vertebral artery traversing the pons in circuitous fashion and returning to the midline just at the point of bifurcation into the posterior cerebral arteries. Despite its marked tendency to tortuosity, true coiling of the basilar artery is not seen. However, giant fusiform aneurysms of the basilar artery are occasionally encountered.

Only rarely are the ectatic changes described above found in association with significant vessel wall changes and stenoses. In rare cases, the elongation of the basilar artery is so marked that the vessel is not only tortuous in its lower portion (Fig. 122), but is also distorted in its distal segments (Fig. 123). In the lateral views the basilar bifurcation may be situated well above the dorsum sella, occasionally at the level of the foramen of Monro. Generally, the bifurcation is no more than $1^1/_2$–2 cm above the dorsum. Italian authors have described this phenomenon as "megadolichobasilaris". With pneumoencephalography followed by angiog-

raphy it is possible to demonstrate in such cases that the artery indents and elevates the floor of the third ventricle. Similar ectatic changes can also be found involving the carotid siphon (megadolichocarotis).

The degree of stenosis: It is important to determine the approximate percentage of stenosis present, not only to estimate its effect on the circulation, but also ultimately to determine whether surgical intervention is required. Such evaluations are always made on the basis of changes seen in two planes on the angiogram. It is generally accepted that a 50% narrowing will lower the blood pressure distal to the stenosis, but that a narrowing of 70%–80% is required to diminish regional cerebral blood flow. However, it is not known whether this rule of thumb also applies with hemodynamic changes, such as "hypotensive crises". In our experience acute drops in blood pressure will frequently lead to flow changes with minor degrees of stenosis. It is especially important to be on the lookout for such changes during angiography of the elderly under anesthesia. A hypotensive episode under such conditions can be extremely dangerous.

For similar reasons, any patient with an 80% stenosis of a major vessel should be carefully observed in an intensive care unit for 24 h after the angiography.

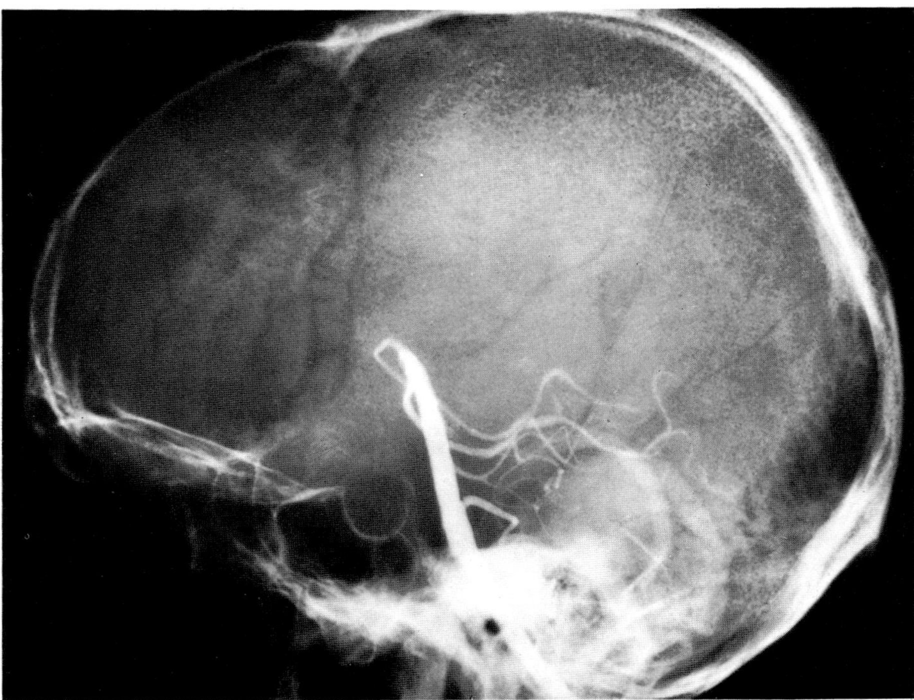

Fig. 123. High-grade ectasia of the basilar artery with so-called "megadolichobasilaris." The basilar bifurcation is elevated far above the posterior clinoid processes at the level of the foramen of Monro

Difficulties can arise in estimating the degree of stenosis, since it is frequently difficult to determine the caliber of the lumen from the angiogram. Even in normal situations the information received from two plane angiograms is frequently relative, depending on the degree of "laminar" flow present. There are cases – as we have seen with both right and left vertebral injections – when only a wedge-shaped quarter of the basilar artery lumen is outlined with contrast medium. In such cases the false conclusion might be reached that a high degree stenosis of the basilar artery was present. This error can be avoided by simultaneously injecting the other side, although an occasional case remains "unclear" despite this maneuver (Einsiedel – Lechtape et al., 1977). Laminar flow is especially marked just at the vertebrobasilar junction, as contrasted blood from one vertebral artery mixes with the noncontrasted blood from the other. There are even cases where a right-sided vertebral injection filled only the right posterior cerebral artery and vice versa. Only in exceptional cases is the reverse seen, i.e., a right vertebral injection fills only the left posterior cerebral artery, and vice versa.

Distal arterial stenosis and magnification angiography: In the "distal" portions of arteries, that is, the smaller branches, one occasionally sees spotty stenotic patches, mainly at vessel forks or curves. They are more apparent in the lateral exposure and are better demonstrated with magnification techniques (Fig. 124). Careful attention should be paid to determining whether the lumen is excentrically or concentrically narrowed, in both planes. The recognition of this type of "distal" *intra*cranial stenosis is particularly important when one is considering surgical intervention to correct a proximal *extra*cranial stenosis on one of the major vessels in the neck.

Vessel occlusions (thrombosis and embolism) – The question of dissolution of the thrombus and thromboembolus: As we have noted, the most frequent factor associated with arterial occlusion is thrombosis, either primary in the relatively narrowed vessels of youth, or as the final phase of a stenotic lesion on the arterial wall. The final occlusion in such situations can also be caused by an embolus. In intracranial occlusions, repeat angiography a few days later has demonstrated that the thrombotic occlusion may undergo rapid dissolution. Certainly emboli may be expected to break up rapidly (Figs. 105, 124) and be disseminated to smaller branches where they are either dissolved or are

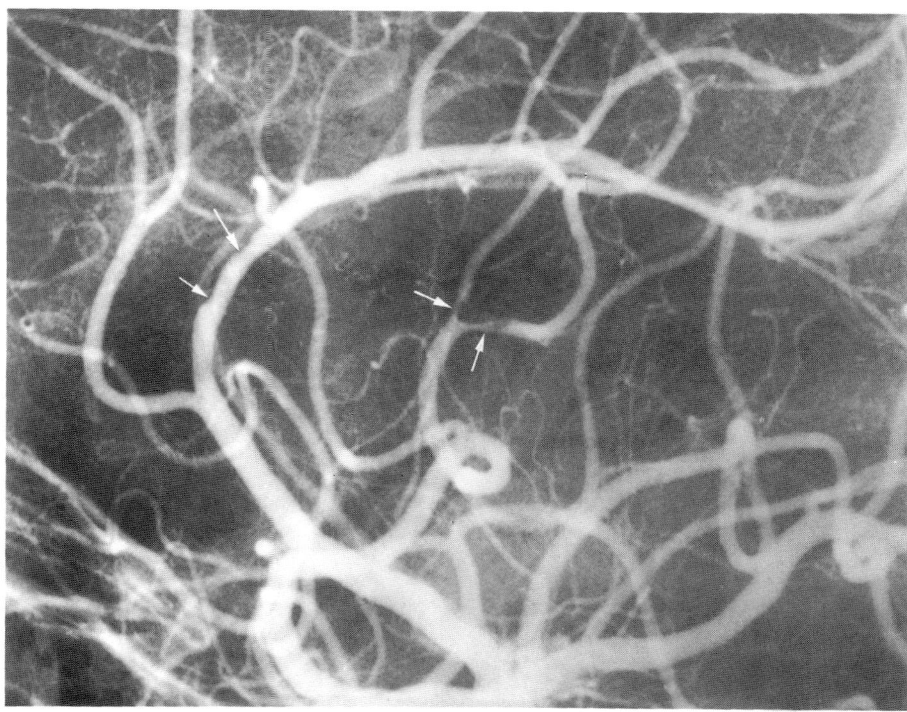

Fig. 124. Stenotic change in the anterior portion of the pericallosal artery (*arrows*). In addition there is a saddle embolus involving the anterior parietal artery (*arrows*). Magnification technique

no longer apparent on the angiogram. Occasionally one recognizes a saddle embolus at a point of bifurcation (Fig. 124). We have, however, also seen delayed " secondary arterial thromboses follow infarcts which had resulted from hemodynamic disturbances alone (see p. 158).

Anastomoses and collateral circulation (including the Moya-Moya syndrome): The four extracranial and the intracranial cerebral arteries communicate in a netlike web at various levels distal to the aortic arch. Not all these anastomoses are functionally patent initially because of the small size of their lumen; when needed, they must first undergo a process of enlargement.

Extracranial anastomoses: Channels of communication between both external carotid arteries and the intracranial circulation become functional in the presence of a stenosis, and particularly an occlusion of the common carotid artery.

With respect to anastomoses between the carotid and vertebral systems, the vertebral artery gives off numerous muscular branches during its course in the neck which can serve as anastomotic channels with other major cerebral vessels or with the external carotid artery. Thus, a vertebral occlusion at the level of the anterior

tuberculum of C-6 where the artery enters the costotransverse foramina can be compensated for distally by such anastomoses.

A direct anastomosis between the occipital artery and the vertebral artery can work in either direction depending on whether the vertebral artery or the common carotid artery is closed (Fig. 125). Occasionally, a thyrocervical-vertebral artery anastomosis develops with a proximal occlusion of the vertebral artery.

A communication can also form from the external carotid artery over the ophthalmic artery to the internal carotid artery, the so-called ophthalmic anastomosis (Fig. 126). In such cases three main channels from the external carotid artery to the ophthalmic artery may be employed, namely the ethmoidal arteries, the A. dorsalis nasi and the superficial temporal arteries, and to a lesser extent the middle meningeal. Through these anastomoses the stump of the siphon can be filled (Fig. 127) with its branches of supply to the hypophysis, to the trigeminal ganglion, to the tympanic membrane, and to the tentorium. Distally, the ophthalmic artery will often fill in a retrograde fashion a large portion of the territories supplied by the middle cerebral and anterior cerebral arteries (Fig. 127).

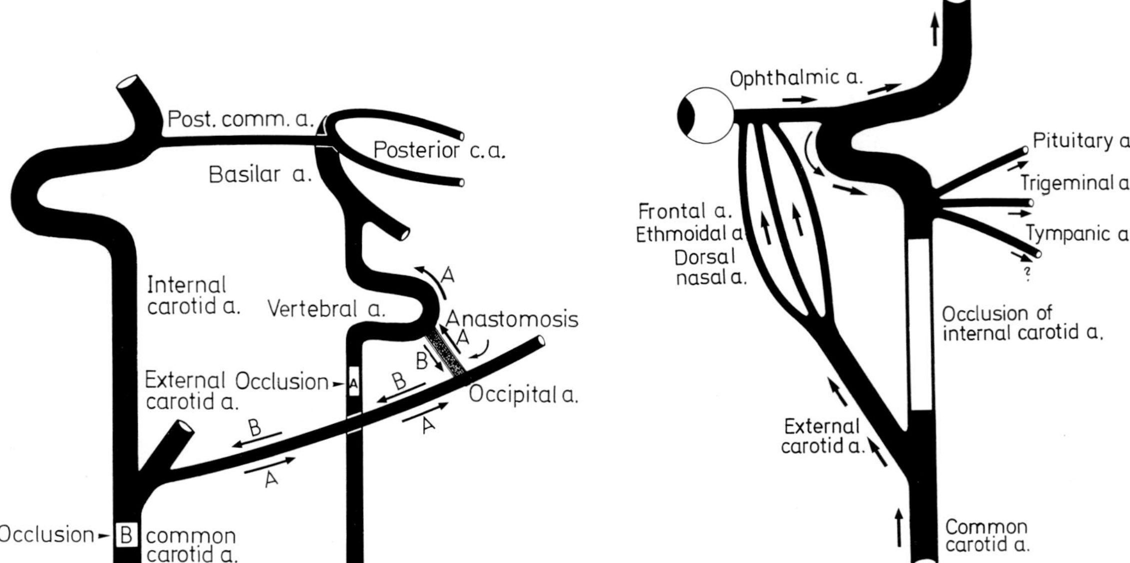

Fig. 125. Schematic representation of possible occipitovertebral anastomoses: *A*, with occlusion of the vertebral artery; and *B*, with occlusion of the common carotid artery (see Fig. 133 a)

Fig. 126. Schematic representation of possible anastomoses between the external carotid and internal carotid arteries via the ophthalmic artery

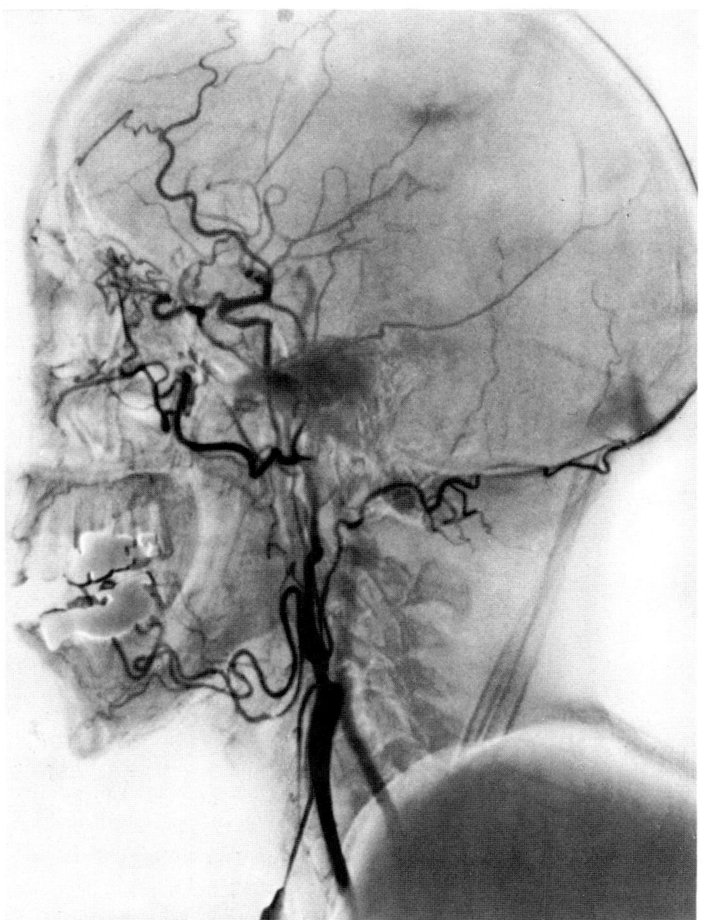

Fig. 127. Occlusion of the internal carotid artery. Note the excellent anastomotic network via the ophthalmic artery. The internal carotid artery with its three "intracanalicular" arteries (see Fig. 126) is filled in retrograde fashion. The anterior and middle cerebral arteries are both already demonstrated and are better opacified later in the study

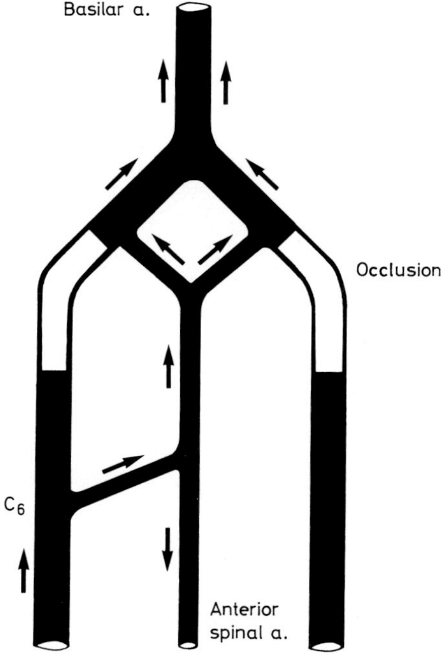

Fig. 128. Schematic representation of potential anastomoses over the anterior spinal artery in occlusions of both vertebral arteries

With occlusion of both vertebral arteries in their extracranial course, an anastomotic channel by way of the spinal arteries can open up to permit filling of the intracranial vertebral system (see Fig. 128).

Intracranial anastomoses: According to the textbooks of anatomy the *circle of Willis* is a complete circle joining the three major arteries of the brain – both carotid arteries and the basilar artery – to one another. In point of fact, however, a "complete" circle is present in only 25% of the cases. The other 75% consist of numerous variants in which an incomplete circle is found, any one of which can be disadvantageous to the individual. Because such anatomical variants will restrict the number of potential anastomotic channels available in the event of a stenotic arteriosclerotic lesion (especially prevalent on the posterior communicating artery), the anatomical makeup of the circle of Willis is of considerable importance (Figs. 129 and 130).

The meningeal anastomoses: The meningeal anastomoses, first described by HEUBNER (1872, 1874), are between the terminal branches of the large intracranial arteries, resulting in numerous weblike 1–2 mm interconnections over the cerebrum and cerebellum. In the case of a mid-

dle cerebral artery occlusion, there is extensive retrograde filling of the compromised region over this anastomotic network predominantly from the anterior cerebral artery (Fig. 131), or from the posterior cerebral artery (Fig. 132), or from both (Fig. 133). On the other hand, with occlusion of the anterior cerebral artery or posterior cerebral artery a retrograde filling from the middle cerebral artery takes place.

Angiographic demonstration of a meningeal anastomosis was reported for the first time by FISCHER-BRÜGGE (1949), who described a communication from the posterior cerebral artery over the corpus callosum to the anterior cerebral artery territory (Fig. 134).

"Meningeal anastomoses", especially if still visible in the venous phases, are indicative of an impediment in flow to neighboring arteries. "Meningeal anastomoses" from the posterior cerebral artery to the middle cerebral artery territory point to an occlusion of the middle cerebral artery, or internal carotid artery, or one of their larger branches. It is therefore indicative of a regional disturbance in cerebral blood flow, but must be correlated with the neurological deficit present. The demonstration of Fischer's callosal anastomosis on the vertebral angiogram must be interpreted as sign of disturbed flow to the anterior cerebral artery, or to the entire carotid system on that side (Fig. 134).

Similarly there are other numerous, very complicated anastomoses possible which may become functional collateral channels when the need exists. For example, a communication develops by way of the posterior inferior cerebellar arteries to the superior cerebellar artery in cases of occlusion of the basilar artery in its middle segment (Fig. 135a, b; see the complete description by WEIBEL and FIELDS, 1969).

The "arachnoidal ring anastomoses": The smallest anastomotic network joining the cerebral arteries exists within the outer layers of cortex and is called the arachnoidal ring anastomoses (SCHMIDT, 1955). This system joins the smaller arterial branches on the cortical surface directly with one another through connecting channels in the millimeter range.

To what extent this smallest network of arterial connections is functional under normal conditions is not known. Under pathological conditions (see below p. 164) it plays a definite role.

In hyperemic states, many of these small channels become visible on the angiogram as a diffuse blush. In thromboangiitis obliterans,

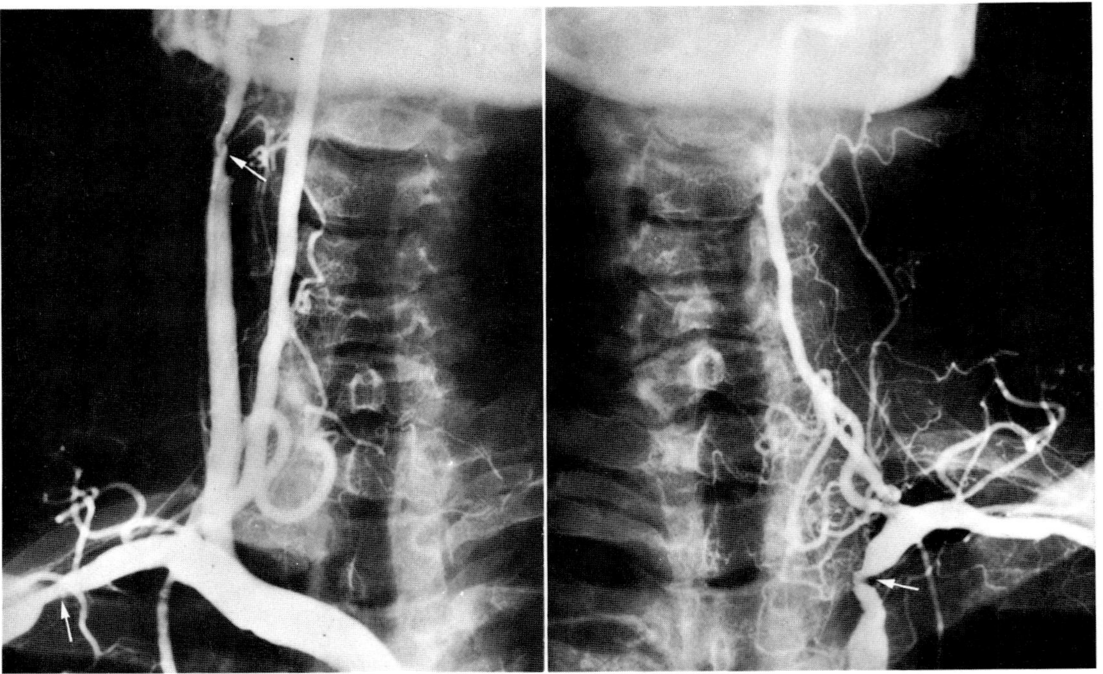

Fig. 129a, b. Retrograde brachial arteriogram: **a** Occlusion of the right internal carotid artery with high-grade stenosis (*arrows*) of the external carotid and subclavian arteries. **b** High-grade stenosis of the left subclavian artery (see also Fig. 130)

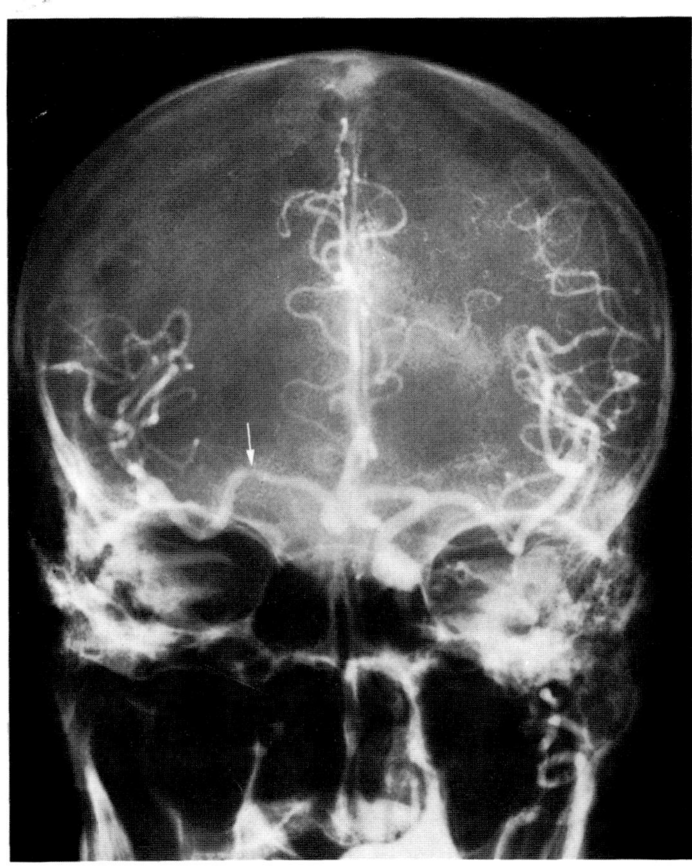

Fig. 130. Same case as Fig. 129. The left carotid angiogram fills both carotid systems, the right via the anterior communicating artery. Note the stenosis of the right middle cerebral artery (*arrow*). This patient suffered from *left* hemisphere insufficiency

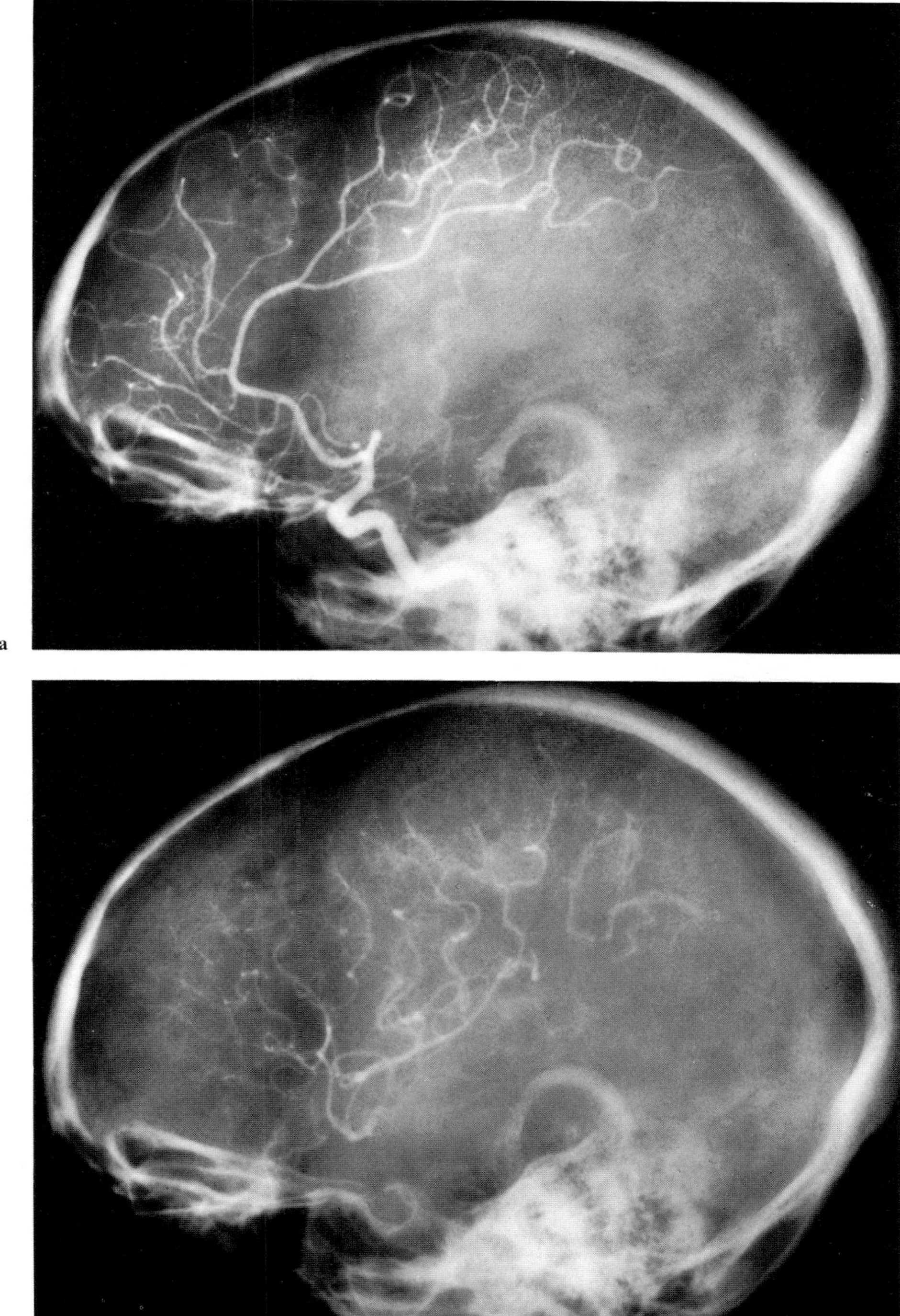

Fig. 131 a, b. Occlusion of the middle cerebral artery: **a** with sparing of the medial lenticulostriate arteries. **b** In a later phase there is almost complete filling of the proximal two-thirds of the middle cerebral artery territory via meningeal anastomoses from the anterior cerebral artery

such a hyperemic state is found in the capillary phase in the border zone between the middle cerebral artery territory on the one hand, and the anterior cerebral artery and posterior cerebral artery territories on the other (see page 161).

Intracerebral anastomoses: The Moya-Moya syndrome of the basal ganglia: After the

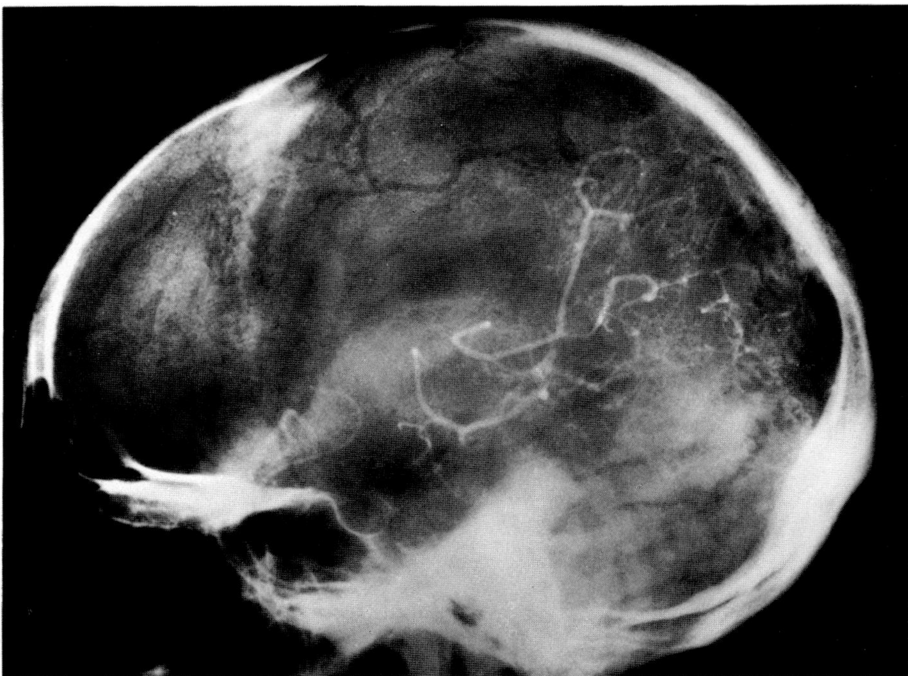

Fig. 132. Occlusion of the middle cerebral artery similar to Fig. 131. There is filling of the posterior one-third of the middle cerebral artery territory via meningeal anastomoses from the posterior cerebral artery

branches to the basal ganglia penetrate the brain substance, the possibility of developing significant anastomotic communications between these vessels and other similar vessels is generally lost with the exception of capillary anastomoses. Therefore, the entire system of perforating median and paramedian arteries along the central axis of the brain is a system of *true end arteries.*

An exception to this rule is found in a very rare vessel disease in which a proliferative arteritis is associated with a stenosis of major arterial trunks (Moya-Moya). Usually involved by the stenosis or occlusion are the carotid siphon as well as the proximal stumps of both the middle cerebral and anterior cerebral arteries. In this situation an extensive network of collateral vessels is formed from the median and paramedian basal ganglion and thalamic branches. These branches dilate and make fistulous connections in the "fashion of an angioma" (AVM) and eventually may join cortical arteries of the convexity through their deep penetrating smaller arterial branches to the centrum semiovale. Thus, a collateral circulation may develop between the cortex and the deep perforating branches to these nuclei, consisting of 1–2 mm diameter arteries radiating from the depths of

the hemisphere to its surface. The presence and location of this collateral system, the so-called Moya-Moya syndrome, depend directly upon the existence and location of a high-grade stenosis or occlusion of a major cerebral artery (Figs. 136, 137).

One must assume that the frequency of this type of case in Japan and China reflects the frequency of closely associated disease entities – "allergic" arteritis – of which the common Takayashu disease is another prime example. In spite of this, individual cases of the Moya-Moya syndrome (although still rare) have been found in many countries.

We have demonstrated by means of repeat angiography that the Moya-Moya type of collateral circulation can also develop in the white race in middle age, even as a "secondary" phenomenon 23 months later.

In this case a 52-year-old woman suffered an occlusion of the middle cerebral artery with sparing of the branches to the basal ganglia and thalamus. Repeat angiography 23 months later showed that the branches to these nuclei had been converted to Moya-Moya vessels which were unequivocally supplying the temporoparietal cortex. There was also retrograde filling of the posterior cerebral artery from this region.

Zones of "hyperemia and of rapid circulation (blush, early veins): Regional blood flow determinations in an area of impaired circulation

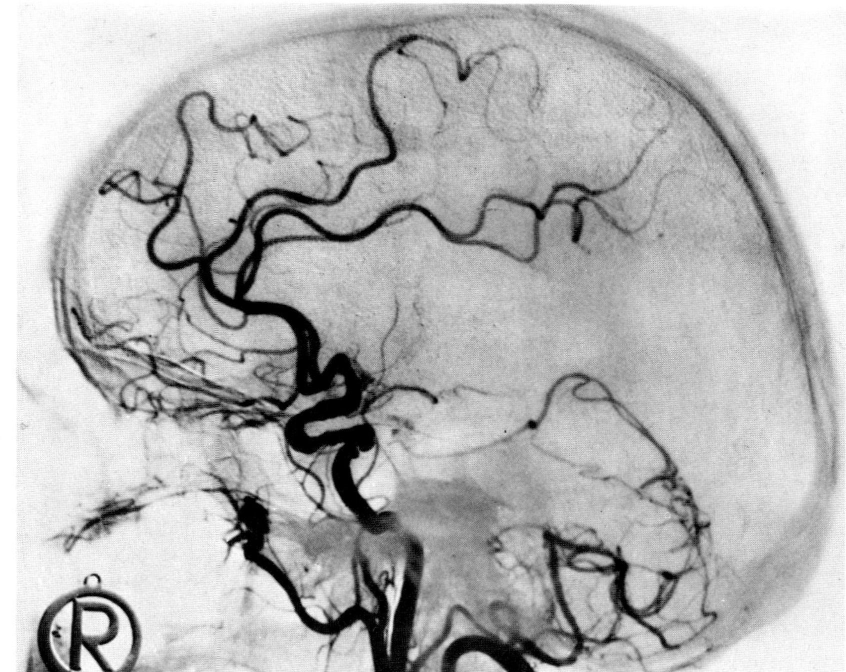

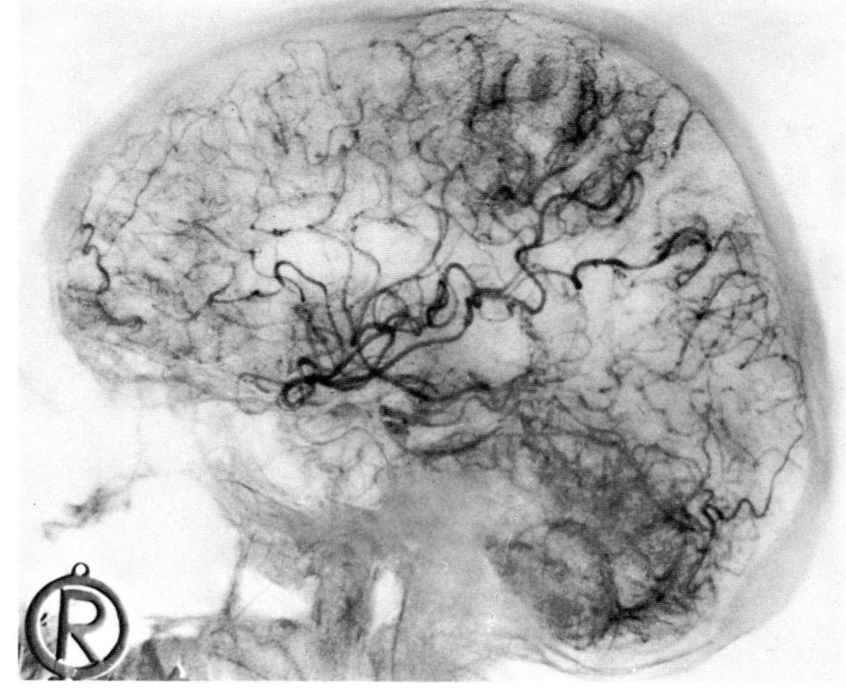

Fig. 133a, b. Right retrograde brachial angiogram with occlusion of the middle cerebral artery and with retrograde filling of its territories via anastomoses from the anterior cerebral arteries. There is also occlusion of the vertebral artery with an effective occipitovertebral anastomosis filling the posterior inferior cerebellar artery, the superior cerebellar artery, and the posterior cerebral arteries in that sequence (see Fig. 125)

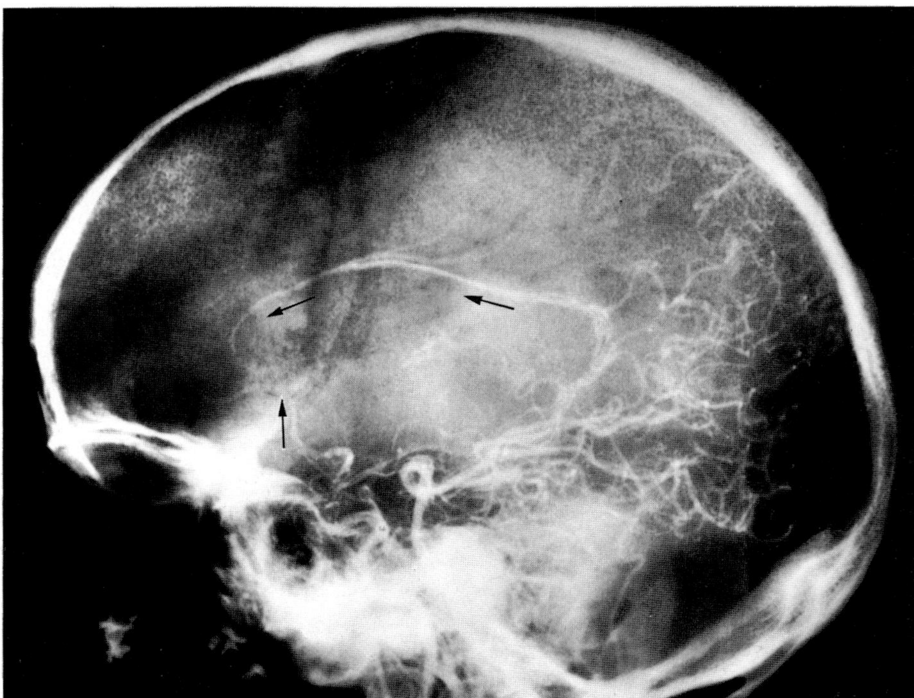

Fig. 134. Occlusion of the internal carotid artery at the siphon. There is retrograde filling of its territory of supply via an anastomosis between the posterior cerebral artery and the pericallosal artery (the so-called Fischer's callosal anastomosis). At the same time, the proximal portion of the anterior cerebral artery (*arrow*) is filled by way of the posterior communicating artery

later reveal a "hyperemic zone", the so-called "luxury perfusion". This develops as a result of a "reactive hyperemia" which has been described with respect to the extremities by BIER (1897/1898). Radiologically this zone is recognized as a diffuse "blush" (see p. 113 ff.), which is most apparent in the subtraction films. Here the arterioles, capillaries, and venules are dilated, the flow time is especially rapid, and the filling of the veins seems not only "too early" on the angiogram, but also "too red" on the surgically exposed surface ("red", "early" veins). The "early veins" of the cerebral circulatory disorders (Fig. 138) represent the same phenomenon as that found in the arteriovenous fistulas, in AVMs, and in malignant tumors (glioblastomas and metastases) (see p. 113 ff.).

Thromboangiitis obliterans: Cerebral thromboangiitis obliterans is a rare disease. Early radiological descriptions do not correspond to the actual morphological changes. The thromboses occur in vessels which are otherwise normal and have a definite topographical predilection, in that they are found in the watershed areas of the larger arteries. In the cerebral hemispheres they prefer a zone with fixed boundaries. They originate from thrombotic occlusions of the distal branches of the middle cerebral artery, as well as the anterior cerebral, posterior cerebral, and cerebellar arteries. In the watershed zone they establish a collateral circulation consisting of circular anastomoses (see p. 161). This gives the picture of a hyperemic zone, i.e., a blush.

"Steal" syndromes: The preceding discussion has dealt with the various collateral circulatory systems which can be developed from existing anastomotic channels in a short time (extracranial anastomoses, circle of Willis, Heubner's meningeal anastomoses, etc.). In the course of the development of these systems with their later, sometimes unnaturally dilated and circuitous channels, a most remarkable hemodynamic phenomenon is occasionally seen, the "steal" syndrome, in which blood is drawn away from another vessel system to the detriment of the donor vessel.

Best known is the "subclavian steal" syndrome. With occlusion of one (usually the *left*) subclavian artery, a collateral flow develops from the right vertebral to the basilar to the left vertebral and back to the left subclavian artery (Figs. 139, 140, 141). When flow into the

Fig. 135. a Schematic representation of potential anastomoses over the inferior and superior cerebellar arteries with occlusion of the basilar artery. **b** Right retrograde brachial angiogram with occlusion of the internal carotid and vertebral arteries in the neck, as well as basilar occlusion. Anastomoses have developed from the external carotid artery (*1*) to the internal carotid artery by way of the ophthalmic; and (*2*) to the vertebral artery by way of the occipital artery. Note also (*3*) the collaterals from the posterior inferior cerebellar artery to the superior cerebellar artery and then to the distal basilar stump

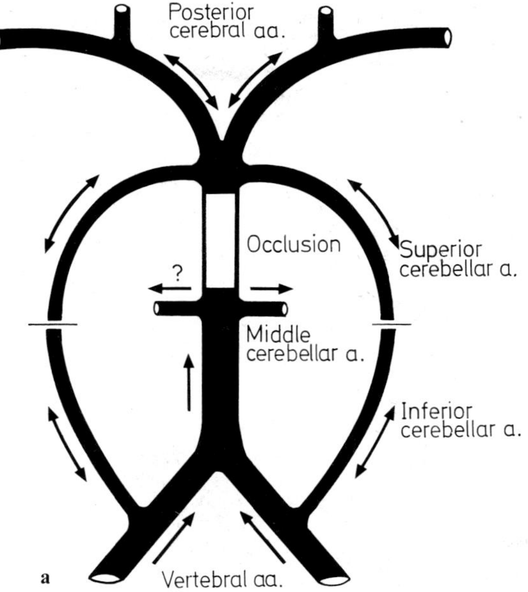

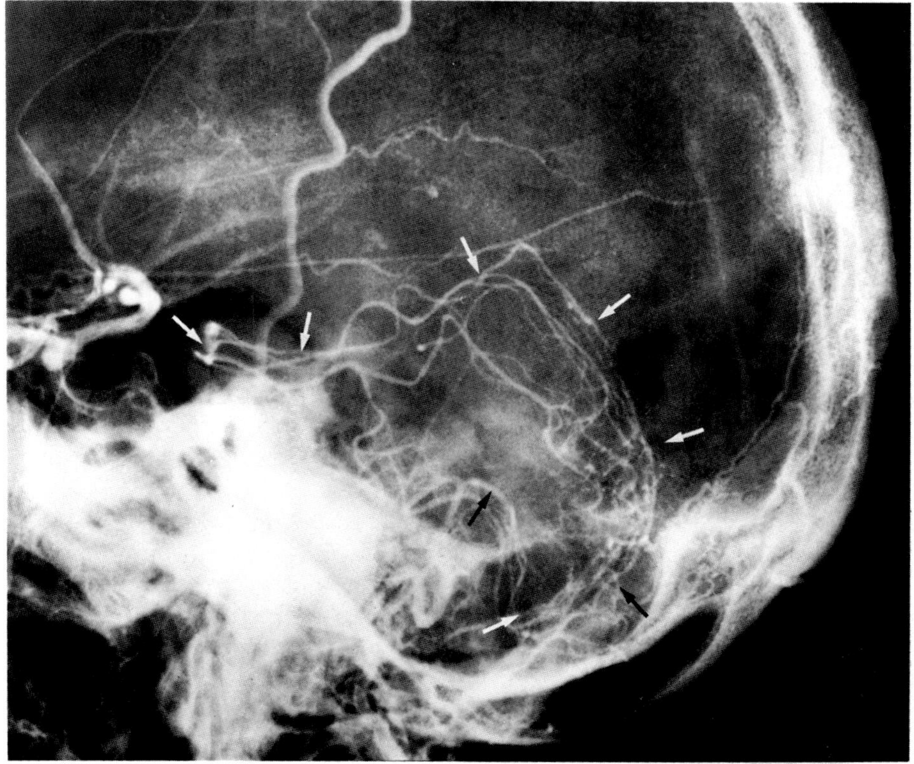

territory of supply of the left subclavian artery is increased through muscle activity, a steal phenomenon develops in approximately half the cases from the basilar circulation with corresponding clinical symptoms.

A recently recognized steal syndrome is seen in occlusion of the internal carotid artery from a predominantly hemodynamic effect. Through the anterior communicating artery and through interarterial anastomoses between both anterior cerebral arteries over the corpus callosum, blood is distributed from the contralateral carotid system to the occluded carotid system (Fig. 98). The development of this collateral circulation is quite understandable; however, this may lead to a very unusual clinical situation

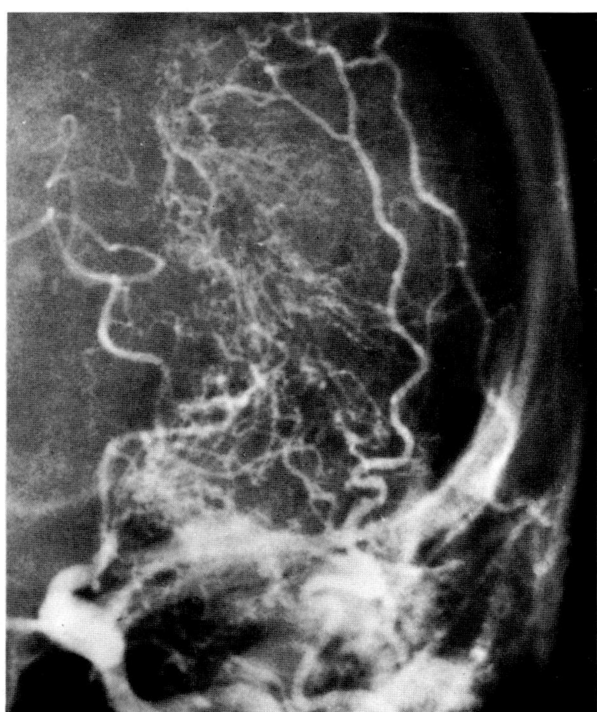

Fig. 136. Angiographic demonstration of a system of anastomoses developed in a 52-year-old woman over a 23-month period. This has the morphological appearance typical of Moya-Moya disease (anteroposterior view, photographic enlargement)

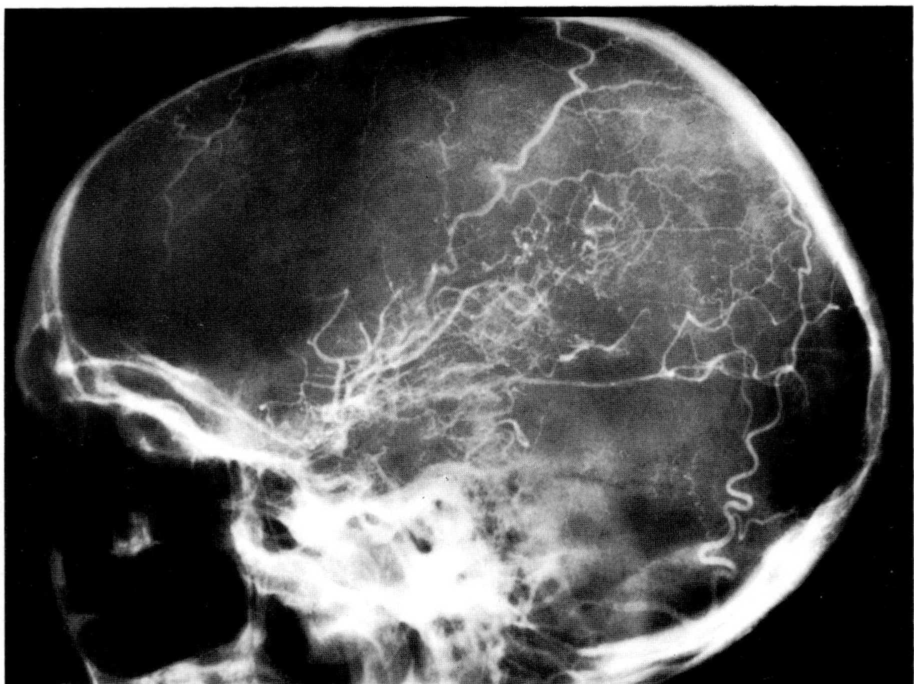

Fig. 137. Lateral view of Fig. 136

in which the neurological symptoms do not correspond to the hemisphere with the occluded internal carotid, but rather to the contralateral side because of blood loss via the anterior communicating and anterior cerebral arteries to the occluded side. This is called an interhemispheric steal syndrome.

A similar steal syndrome between the two hemispheres has been described with AVMs. In this situation the EEG confirmed the presence

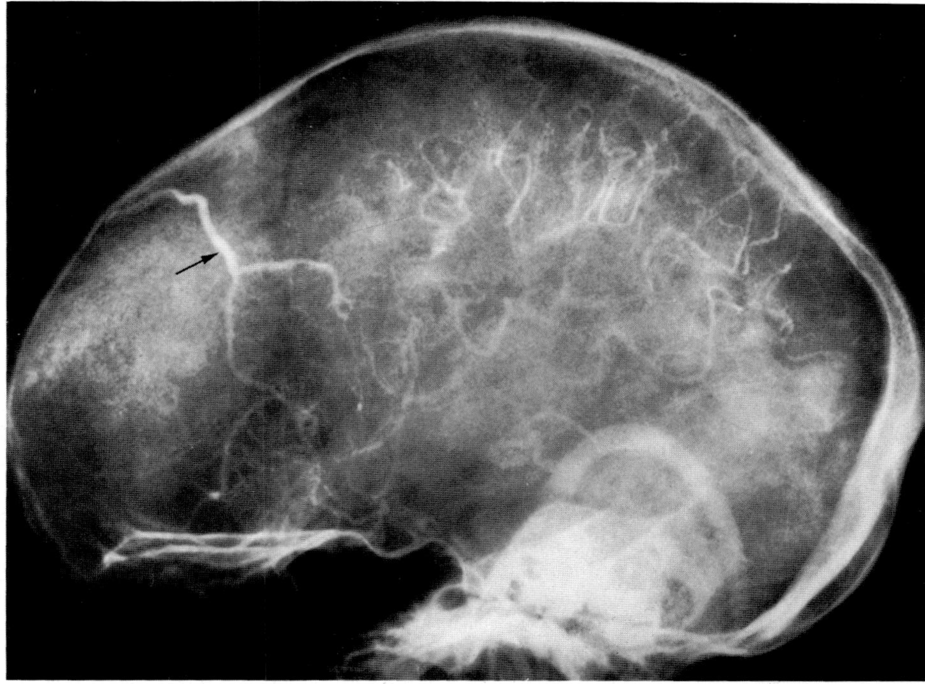

Fig. 138. "Early vein" in an infarct without apparent arterial occlusion

of impaired circulation to the opposite hemisphere, while the hemisphere containing the AVM showed no signs of a functional disturbance.

Functional changes in the lumen through arterial spasm: It has been confirmed by observations at the time of surgery, in experimental studies, and also by angiography that specific segments of the cerebral vessels may undergo angiospasm. The phenomenon has a varied etiology.

The cerebral vessels seem to have a peripheral type of innervation being outfitted with alpha and beta receptors which respond to their corresponding transmitter substances, as well as to local metabolic products, and finally also to metabolites in the blood. There are also mechanical stimulants, i.e., surgical manipulation or changes in the vessel wall by experimental emboli of glass splinters, which result in truly recognizable narrowings. Also known is the spastic narrowing of a large vessel in the vicinity of a needle puncture, as with carotid and brachial artery punctures. Such spastic segments can occupy several centimeters of vessel or more (see also Fig. 110). Occasionally one finds a vessel so involved that it resembles a "pearl necklace" (Fig. 109). A controlled vasoconstriction and dilation is part of the physiological mechanism regulating cerebral blood flow, known as "autoregulation". The autoregulatory effect is to maintain a relatively constant cerebral blood flow under a variety of conditions. Ordinary constituents of the blood and chemical metabolites from the tissues (CO_2, O_2, lactic acidosis), as well as internal arterial pressure variations, i.e., blood pressure changes, control autoregulation even in the "vessels of the elderly". Since the vessels of older individuals are often heavily encrusted with arteriosclerotic plaques in their proximal portions and are thus relatively "rigid", one must postulate that the autoregulatory mechanism works through vessels with smaller lumens (1–3 mm diameter?). There is even reason to postulate that a rapid rise in blood pressure with resultant vessel stretching might result in a pathologically excessive narrowing of the vessel lumen, i.e., spasm, within the framework of a "physiological autoregulatory" response followed by segmental dilatation and "breakthrough" of the blood brain barrier.

Such autoregulatory vasospasm in a hypertensive crisis would explain the occasional appearance of local areas of poor perfusion; such a situation has also been confirmed by regional cerebral blood flow measurements.

In neuroradiology the spastic narrowing of a large vessel at the needle puncture site is especially significant (for example, the carotid artery or brachial artery), as is hemorrhage into the vessel sheath at such a site. Here, the spastic segment can extend over several centimeters. Also well-known is the often marked and extensive vasospasm which can follow subarachnoid hemorrhage and can persist for long periods (in terms of weeks). Such vascular narrowings can be definitely confirmed as vasospasm only if they subsequently disappear on repeat angiography.

Mechanical compression of vessels from without (secondary stenosis): In many individuals

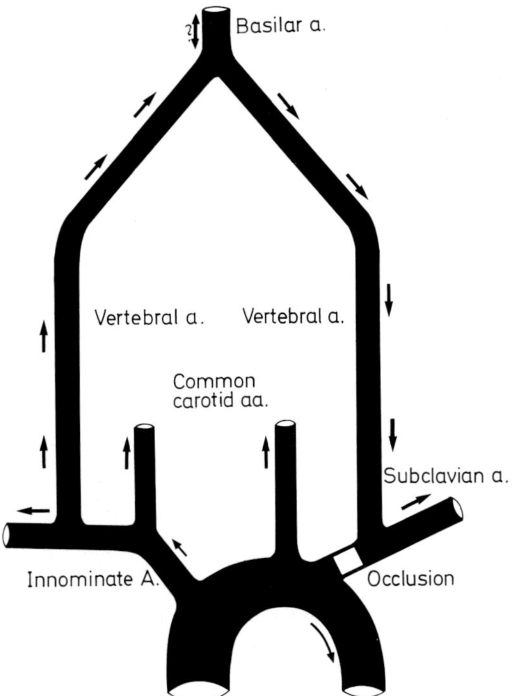

Fig. 139. Schematic demonstration of the anastomoses in effect in the "subclavian steal" syndrome (see Fig. 140)

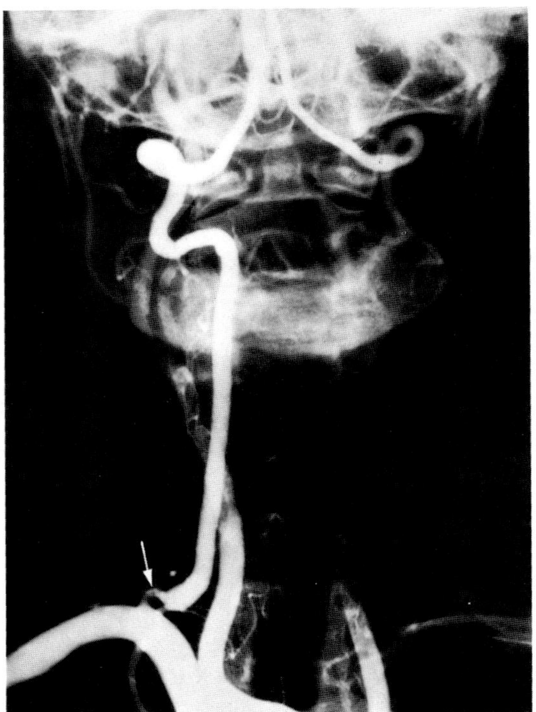

Fig. 140. Angiographic demonstration of a subclavian steal syndrome resulting from occlusion of the left subclavian at its origin (right subclavian to right vertebral to left vertebral to left subclavian anastomosis) in an early arterial phase. Note the marked stenosis of the proximal right vertebral artery

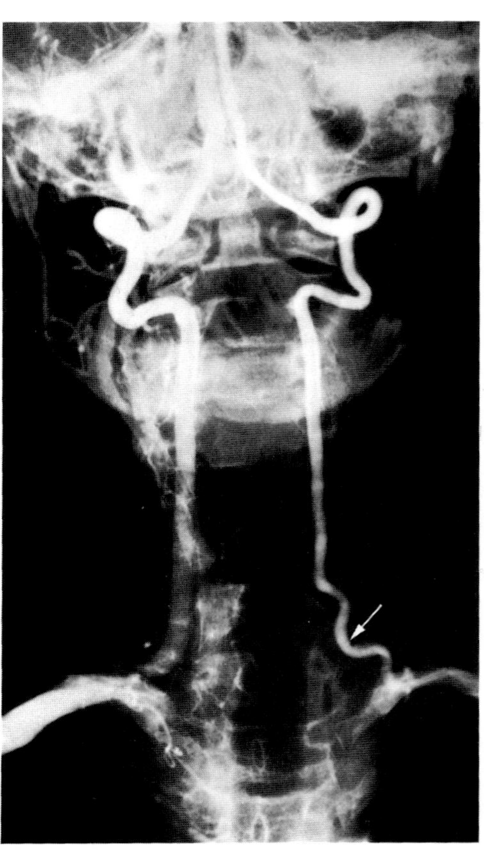

Fig. 141. Later phase of the same angiogram shown in Fig. 140. The left vertebral artery shows considerable tortuosity

a "temporary compression" to the point of complete occlusion can affect the major cerebral arteries under certain physiological conditions. Such a condition exists with respect to the vertebral arteries in certain extreme positions of the head and neck.

Similarly, hyperostotic spur formation on the lateral margins of the vertebral bodies can indent and narrow the vertebral artery at certain segments (C-4/5, C-5/6, C-6/7) as it passes by. A sharper spur may even impinge upon the costotransverse foramen through which the artery passes (Figs. 26b, 98).

During angiography it is possible to demonstrate through appropriate turning or positioning of the head that the lumen of the vertebral artery can be not only slightly compromised by these mechanical maneuvers, but also completely obstructed in extreme positions, especially in the presence of associated arteriosclerotic change. The clinical history of such patients corresponds well with the angiographically demonstrable mechanical obstructions.

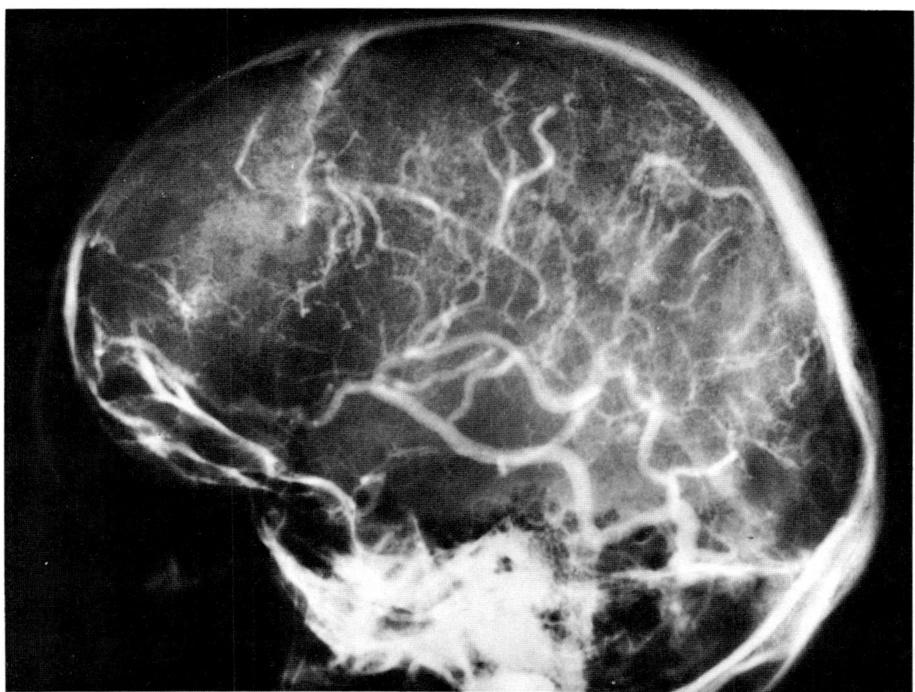

Fig. 142. Development of an abnormal corkscrew-shaped venous drainage with occlusion of the proximal third of the sagittal sinus (as a complication of pregnancy)

When the neck is extended, the carotid arteries are extremely taut. However, it appears – as the angiogram confirms – that their lumens are not so significantly narrowed as the vertebral arteries were in the preceding discussion. The clinical disturbances, which suggest impaired flow to the cerebral hemispheres and accompany hyperextension of the neck, may well be caused instead by an unusually hypersensitive carotid sinus reflex.

e) Intracerebral Hemorrhage

The diagnostic confirmation of an intracerebral hemorrhage is occasionally of clinical importance. If such a hemorrhage is "atypical" in location, lying outside the putamen-claustrum region (as is common in younger patients without hypertension), it is usually possible to identify it with certainty only as a "space-occupying process" (rather than "hemorrhage") unless a source of bleeding, e.g., a microangioma, is also demonstrated. Such hemorrhages can involve the frontal, parietal, or temporal regions. Occasionally, contrast medium will be seen to "leak" into the hemorrhage, which serves to confirm the pathology.

When hemorrhages occur in elderly patients with hypertension, the site of predilection in over 80% is the "striatum". In this setting the diagnosis of a space-occupying process in the proper location with displacement of the lenticulostriate arteries anteriorly and medially confirms the diagnosis. It is also possible to demonstrate "leakage" of the contrast medium into the hemorrhage when the procedure is performed "early" enough. Such a demonstration is essential if neurosurgical removal of the clot is being contemplated, or if the differential diagnosis includes other possibilities. Less frequently, hypertensive hemorrhages are also found in the thalamus, in the white matter of the cerebellum, or in the pons.

Setting the stage for such "striatal hemorrhages" one is occasionally able to demonstrate a microaneurysm (Fig. 27).

f) Disturbances in Venous Outflow

With serial angiography it is also possible to analyze the late venous phase intracranially, while retrograde jugular and sinus studies permit evaluation of the larger, more proximal venous pathways (see p. 63). Venous thrombo-

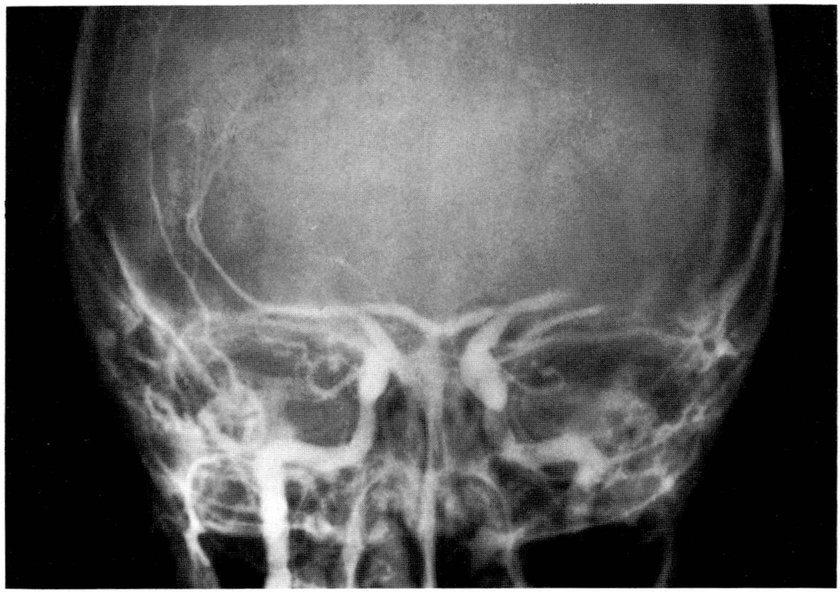

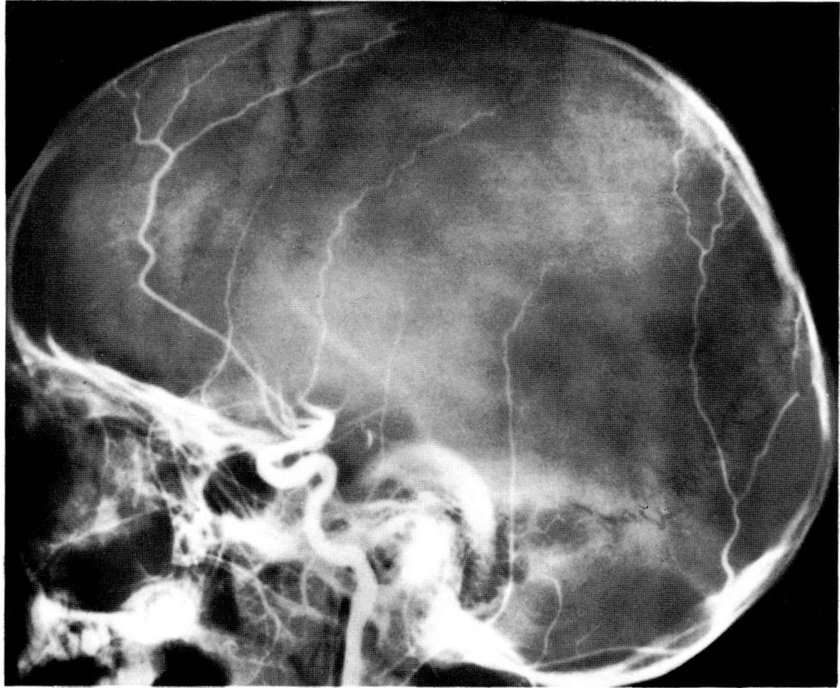

Fig. 143a, b. Cerebral circulatory standstill: **a** anteroposterior view: both carotid arteries and the proximal portion of both middle cerebral arteries are opacified, but no further intracranial filling occurs. **b** Lateral view: note the normal filling of the external carotid artery

sis and sinus occlusion can significantly alter the venous outflow on the angiogram. This is especially true for acute occlusions of the sinus through which the majority of blood passes. The torcular Herophili, as described on p. 83 permits free communication between the superior sagittal sinus, the straight sinus, and the transverse sinuses in only 10% of cases. In two-thirds of the cases, the major venous outflow from the cerebral hemispheres traverses only the right transverse sinus. Its occlusion, therefore, will lead to massive cerebral edema secondary to the damming effect.

This effect is also, as has been shown, undoubtedly responsible for the abducens nerve palsy seen in the so-called Gradenigo's syndrome. In a similar manner, the brachiofacial syndrome seen in "otitic hydrocephalus" is most certainly caused instead by cortical venous stasis in the face and arm region.

Serial angiograms in patients with sinus occlusions will show prolongation of venous emptying, sometimes as long as 20 s or more. If, on the other hand, the sinus occlusion is incomplete or only a part of the sinus is involved as, for example, in occlusions of the initial third of the sagittal sinus, collateral channels will form over the adjacent convexity which should be easily recognized by virtue of their tortuosity and their obvious function as an alternative drainage system (Fig. 142). Occasionally, it is possible to demonstrate the thrombotic occlusion of an individual vein in the late venous phase as, for example, a bridging vein in the parasagittal area.

For literature, see: ALAJOUANINE et al. (1961), BAUER et al. (1962), DECKER (1955, 1958), DENNY-BROWN (1951, 1953), EINSIEDEL-LECHTAPE et al. (1977), FIELDS et al. (1965), FISHER (1954), FOIX and LEVY (1927), GREITZ (1956), HEUBNER (1872, 1874), KAZNER and SCHIEFER (1966), KRAYENBÜHL and YASARGIL (1957, 1965), KRAYENBÜHL et al. (1979), KUBIK and ADAMS (1946), LECHTAPE-GRÜTER and ZÜLCH (1971), LOEB and FAVALE (1962), McDOWELL (1966), METZINGER and ZÜLCH (1971), PATTERSON et al. (1964), PFEIFER (1931), RIGGS and RUPP (1963), RING (1962), SALAMON (1971), SCHÜRMANN (1954), VAN DER EECKEN (1959), VAN DER EECKEN and ADAMS (1953), WEIBEL and FIELDS (1969), YATES and HUTCHINSON (1961), ZÜLCH (1950, 1971), ZÜLCH et al. (1974). For details of cerebrovascular pathology and pathophysiology see ZÜLCH (1981).

4. Cerebral Circulatory Standstill and Brain Death

The total cessation of cerebral blood flow is a consequence of excessive increased intracranial pressure, which can have a varied etiology. It can follow an intracranial hemorrhage, massive cerebral edema, or, with unilateral involvement, a brain tumor. Cerebral circulatory standstill can also be caused by a severe primary ischemic episode (such as a cardiac arrest) with onset of high-grade cerebral edema and marked increase in intracranial pressure following cardiac resuscitation. The cerebral circulation will eventually be altered by rising intracranial pressure with impairment of flow first in the capillaries and then in larger vessels, until finally all flow ceases. This situation leads directly to cerebral anoxia which is poorly tolerated by the brain. If the anoxic state persists more than a few minutes, permanent brain damage ensues. After as little as 10 min, the damage is irreversible and brain death occurs even if resuscitation of the cardiac and respiratory and other organ systems is successful.

The angiographic picture of cerebral circulatory standstill is characterized by failure of the contrast medium to pass beyond the circle of Willis in both the carotid and vertebrobasilar systems (Fig. 143). This is confirmed by serial exposures over a suitable length of time. Since the diagnosis of "brain death" has serious clinical consequences, it is important to analyze carefully the pictures in order to avoid any possibility of error.

For example, a similar picture can follow a partially intramural injection of contrast medium. The intramural deposit causes gradual obstruction of arterial flow so that the contrast medium tapers off at the level of the internal carotid artery, as in cerebral circulatory standstill, or flows slowly as far as the origin of the ophthalmic artery. To avoid this source of error it is necessary to ascertain specifically the patency of the vessel at the puncture site.

Another potential source of error follows catheter injections in which the diameter approximates the lumen of the carotid or vertebral artery being injected. In this situation the contrast medium is injected under relatively high pressure such that filling of the circle of Willis and its distal branches (anterior cerebral artery, middle cerebral artery, and posterior cerebral artery) can follow despite circulatory standstill. However, the contrast medium remains stagnated within these vessels after the injection.

For literature, see: BÜCHELER et al. (1970), NEWTON and POTTS (1974), PENIN and KÄUFER (1969).

V. Special Angiographic Procedures

1. Angiography of the Ophthalmic Artery

MONIZ described the angiographic picture of the ophthalmic artery as early as 1934. In the following years, CURTIS (1949), SCHURR (1951), BREGÉAT et al. (1952), DECKER (1955), YASARGIL (1957), DICHIRO (1961), KRAYENBÜHL (1962), and VIGNAUD et al. (1975) reported on the anatomy, angiographic techniques, and pathological findings in the distribution of the ophthalmic artery.

Prior to the advent of CT, demonstration of the ophthalmic artery had significant diagnostic value in orbital lesions. Following the injection of contrast medium into the internal carotid artery, the whole of the ophthalmic artery can be visualized in the majority of cases (see p. 71 for angiographic anatomy of the ophthalmic artery). The demonstration of the choroid layer of the eye is also possible in approximately 30% of cases.

Until recently, ophthalmic artery studies were required whenever a retro-orbital or intraorbital tumor was suspected, and particularly if demonstration of collateral flow was desired (see p. 159). It should be pointed out that the ophthalmic artery lies on the medial wall of the orbit and that tumors which originate here are very rare. Furthermore, only a few orbital tumors show a tumor blush. The distinction usually has to be made between an angioma or a meningioma (Fig. 144) and in such cases hypertrophy of the ophthalmic artery will be apparent. It should further be emphasized that every case of ophthalmic artery angiography requires subtraction studies. An external carotid study is also necessary in every angiographic investigation of ophthalmic tumors, since many orbital tumors are supplied exclusively by branches from the external carotid artery. In recent years CT has largely supplanted the need for orbital angiography.

For literature, see: BRISMAR (1974), DICHIRO (1961), DILENGE et al. (1965), LASJAUNIAS et al. (1975), LOMBARDI (1967), NEWTON and POTTS (1974), SCHOBER and BENDER (1968).

2. Orbital Venography

For the diagnosis of intraorbital and retro-orbital processes in the absence of CT, orbital venography is the method of choice since tumors in the region of the orbit frequently cause displacement of the superior ophthalmic vein. In contrast, the inferior ophthalmic vein lying directly on the orbital floor is of no diagnostic significance.

DEJEAN and BOUDET (1951) opacified these veins by puncturing the angular vein. In subsequent years, the technique has been modified and perfected.

Investigative Technique

The radiological demonstration of the superior ophthalmic vein is easily accomplished through percutaneous puncture of the angular vein. It is also possible to opacify the inferior petrosal sinus by way of a catheter in the internal jugular vein. Contrast medium injected by this route results in visualization of the orbital veins. Another relatively simple method is to insert a catheter into the frontalis vein and to pass it from there to the angular vein. In the hands of experts each of these techniques can yield excellent results.

Puncture of the Angular Vein

The angular vein is punctured with a thin-walled needle similar to those used for infant venipuncture. A spontaneous flow of blood into the physiological salt solution filling the catheter confirms the position of the needle within the vessel lumen. After injection of approximately 3 ml of a 60% concentration of contrast medium, serial exposures are made in the anteroposterior and lateral directions. The anteroposterior exposure should be made with the head lightly reclined so that the upper margins of the petrous pyramids are projected beneath the orbits. Additional axial views can be of value as well.

During injection of the contrast medium, manual compression of the frontal, frontolateral, and facial veins is desirable. With obstruction of the draining veins, bilateral visualization of the superior ophthalmic veins may be expected. The anteroposterior view will thus provide the opportunity for comparing both sides.

Puncture of the Frontalis Vein

If angular vein puncture is unsuccessful, the frontalis vein on the forehead at the level of the hairline should be tried. In these cases, a catheter is inserted far enough for the tip to be palpable in the region of the glabella.

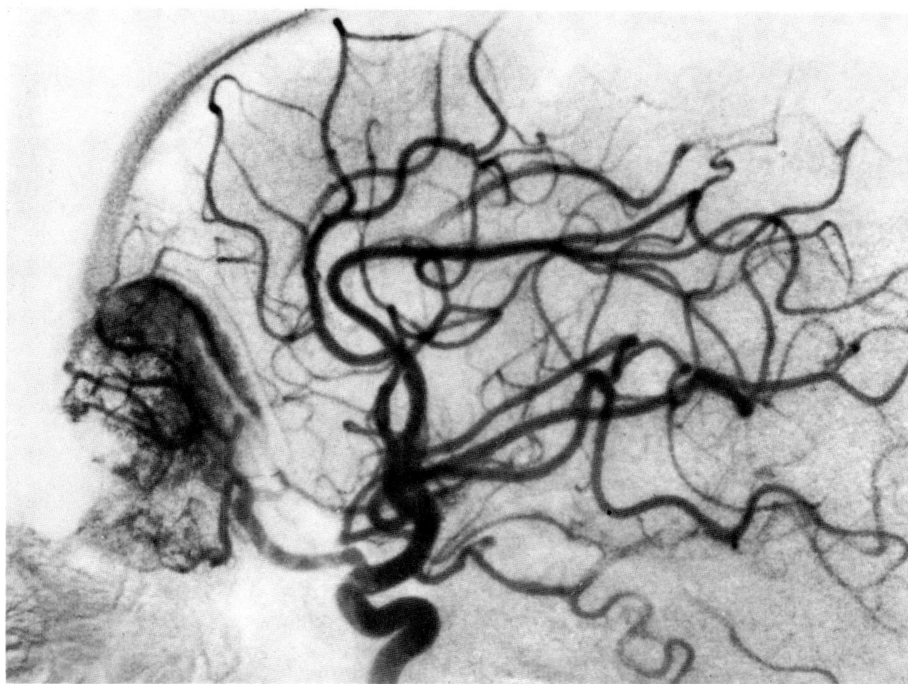

Fig. 144. Orbital hemangioma. Arterial phase with demonstration of the dilated ophthalmic artery (subtraction technique)

Radiologic Anatomy

The superior ophthalmic vein initially runs in a caudal direction near the medial wall of the orbit (prebulbar portion = first segment) and then directly beneath the superior rectus muscle belly laterally (superior rectus loop = second segment). Then it turns in a sharp posteromedial angle (postbulbar portion = third segment) and ends in the cavernous sinus after leaving the orbit through the superior orbital fissure. Normally the superior ophthalmic veins take the shape of a butterfly in the anteroposterior exposures (Fig. 145). This figure is characteristically distorted in space-occupying processes.

Indications for orbital venography include unexplained cases of exophthalmus and papilledema. The technique is not dangerous and serious *complications* have not been reported.

The *pathological venogram* is of great significance. The changes which accompany space-occupying intraorbital processes consist of changes in the position of the veins, changes in vein caliber, and also the addition of pathological vessels (Fig. 146). Displacement of the first segment medially is compatible with a lateral process as, for example, a tumor of the tear gland. Displacement of the second segment laterally is seen in medially situated tumors, while compression and stenosis with dilation of the third segment is common in tumors of the posterior orbit.

While the *localization* of a space-occupying intraorbital process is possible with orbital venography, the determination of tumor type is more difficult. It is not always easy to distinguish between an inflammatory process and a tumor. An increase in venous filling, a less characteristic displacement picture, and an open communication between the superior ophthalmic vein and the cavernous sinus is more suggestive of chronic inflammation. In intraorbital neoplastic processes, obstructions with distinct venous dilation and definite displacements are the rule. In addition, pathological vessels are often apparent.

3. Direct Sinography

The first description of a contrast demonstration of the sinus was that of FRENCKNER in 1934. Regarding improvements in the investigative technique, see FISCHGOLD et al. (1953).

Direct sinography is indicated if the venous phase of the carotid arteriogram does not clearly differentiate individual segments of the

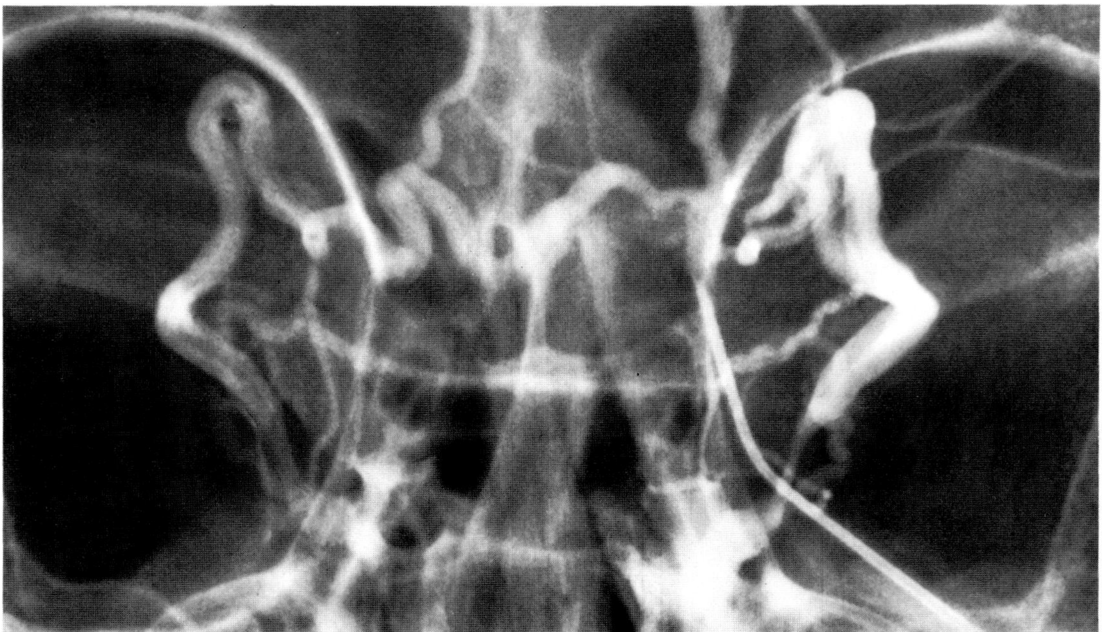

Fig. 145. Normal ophthalmic venogram

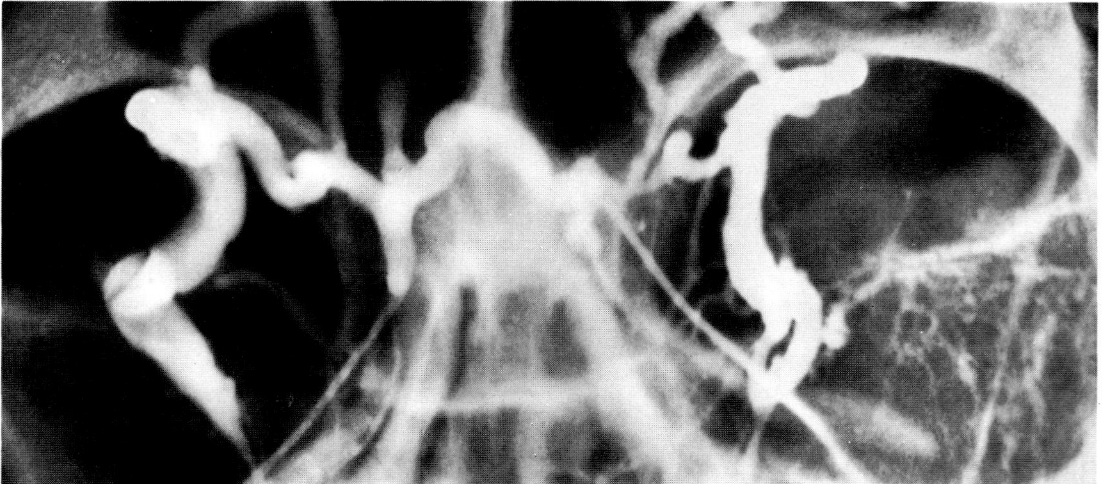

Fig. 146. Tumor in the lateral portion of the left orbit. Note the displacement of the second segment of the superior ophthalmic vein as well as the pathological vessels within the tumor

superior sagittal sinus, the transverse sinus, or the sigmoid sinus. The most important indication is encroachment on the aforementioned sinuses by meningiomas, other primary tumors, or metastases to the vertex of the skull.

Investigative Technique

Under local anesthesia, a burr hole is made in the midline of the forehead at the hairline. Through a small punctate incision, a thin cathe-ter is introduced into the superior sagittal sinus. Then the wound is closed and the patient brought to the X-ray room. It is recommended that the catheter be flushed with a heparin solution at short intervals. The same contrast medium used for cerebral angiography is injected in 5–6 ml boluses. Serial angiography is then performed in both planes. When the contrast medium is being injected directly into the superior sagittal sinus and when the flow within the sinus is relatively strong, it is recommended that

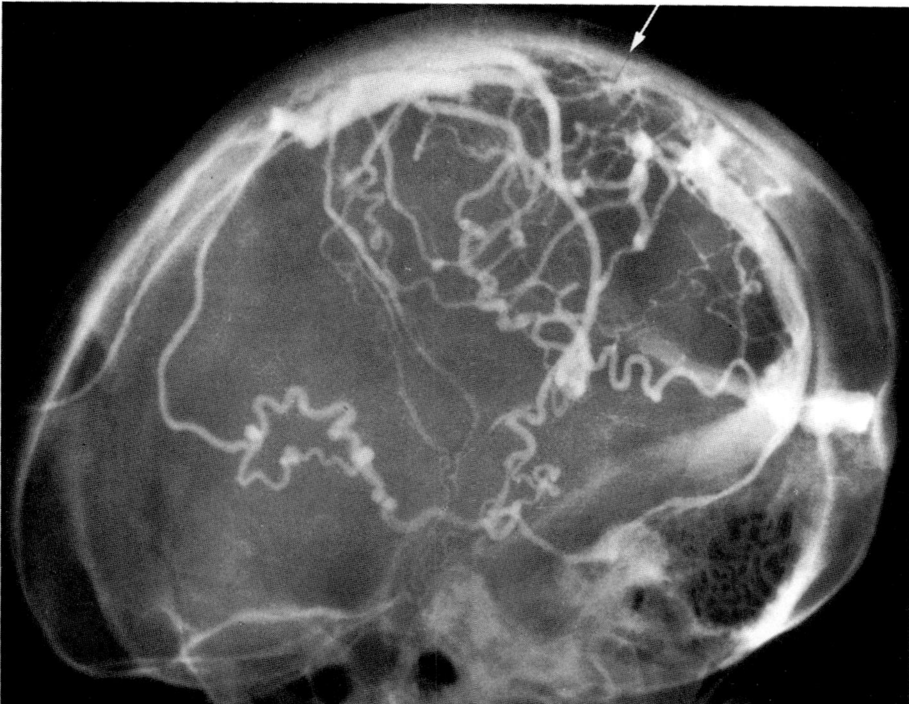

Fig. 147. Direct sinography, demonstrating occlusion of the middle third of the superior sagittal sinus because of invasion by a meningioma. Note the collateral venous channels connecting the anterior and posterior thirds of the sinus (the posterior sinus segment stands out clearly because of the oblique projection used)

exposures begin at the moment of injection so that the path of the contrast medium may be followed throughout. The position of the patient depends on the site of the expected lesion, which is already suspected from plain films or antecedent carotid angiography. If one wishes to visualize the upper wall of the sinus clearly on the lateral exposure, i.e., to avoid superimposition of other structures, it is recommended that the head of the patient be inclined slightly to the right or left. Similarly, the superimposition of the anterior and posterior portions of the superior sagittal sinus with the usual anteroposterior positioning is undesirable. Consequently, it is also necessary here to incline the head of the patient slightly to the right or left.

Changes in the lumen of the superior sagittal sinus can occur as a result of a stenosis or a complete occlusion. Of great value for a subsequent surgical procedure is precise information of position and direction of flow in collateral channels following sinus occlusions – as for example, with meningiomas involving the middle third of the sinus (Fig. 147).

If the anterior third of the superior sagittal sinus is not fixed or is very short, its puncture and/or introduction of the catheter may prove to be unsuccessful. Information about variations in the anterior sinus segment must be obtained beforehand through the carotid study. In aplasia of the anterior third of the sinus or with encroachment on this area by a frontally situated tumor, it is necessary to place the burr hole posterior to the occluded segment.

Primary or secondary tumors of the skull first displace the sinus, and then infiltrate it in later phases.

Complications

With the exception of a light warm feeling, the investigation is carried out without complaint. TALAIRACH et al. (1951) have reported an extravascular injection of the contrast medium into the subdural space, in which the contrast medium spreads out along the falx and on to the tentorium. Such complications can be avoided if one injects the contrast medium through a catheter and if one is convinced by aspiration of blood that the catheter is in an intravascular position.

For literature, see: FISCHGOLD et al. (1953), TÄNZER (1971).

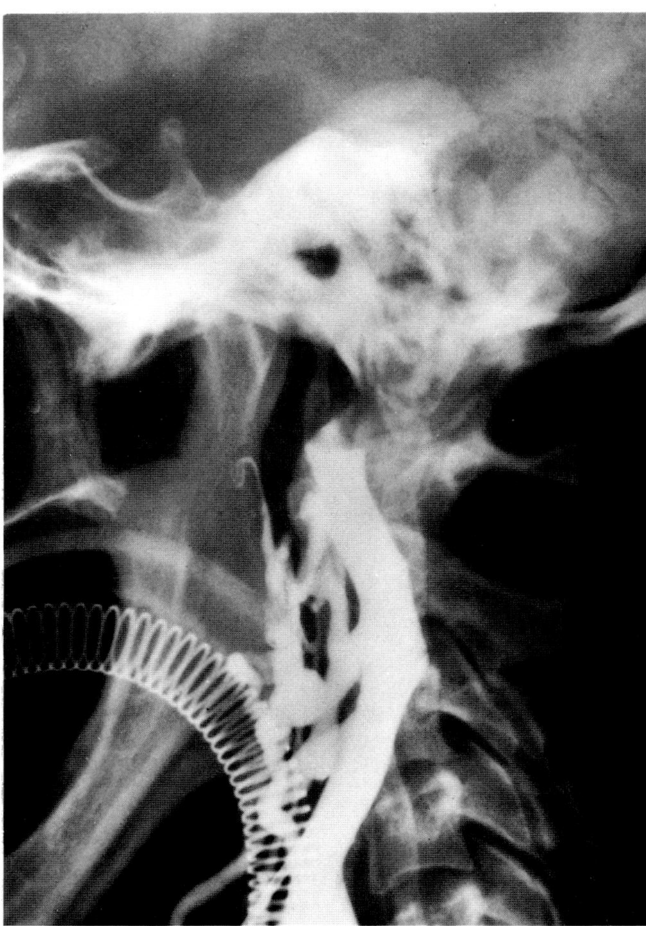

Fig. 148. Note the smooth cut-off in this occlusion of the internal jugular vein due to a glomus tumor (jugular venogram)

4. Angiography of the Jugular Vein

GEJROT and LINDBLOM (1960) have for years recommended retrograde jugular venography as the procedure of choice for demonstration of a glomus tumor. To accomplish this, a catheter is introduced into the jugular vein in a cranial direction, and then contrast medium is injected under pressure against the direction of flow.

Indications

With this technique, the extracranial venous segments are especially well portrayed. If one encounters a complete, rounded occlusion or indentation of the internal jugular vein, the presence of a glomus tumor is considered certain (Fig. 148). Since the intracranial sinuses also fill with contrast medium (Figs. 149, 150), this procedure can be used as well for the diagnosis of sinus occlusion or sinus stenosis (for example, by a tentorial meningioma). In addition, jugular venography is of value in the diagnosis of tumors at the base of the skull. With a growth in the region of the sella, definite changes are found including indentations and flattening of the cavernous sinus from an anterosuperior direction. These changes are most striking with parasellar extensions. The greatest value of the anteroposterior view is to demonstrate the lateral extension of a pituitary tumor by unilateral obstruction or indentation of an affected sinus. Nonfilling of the cavernous sinus does not necessarily imply occlusion, since technical difficulties may be solely responsible.

Technique

The internal jugular vein is usually punctured at the level of the upper rim of the thyroid cartilage, medial to the sternocleidomastoid muscle and laterodorsal to the common carotid artery.

Fig. 149. Normal jugular venogram (lateral view)

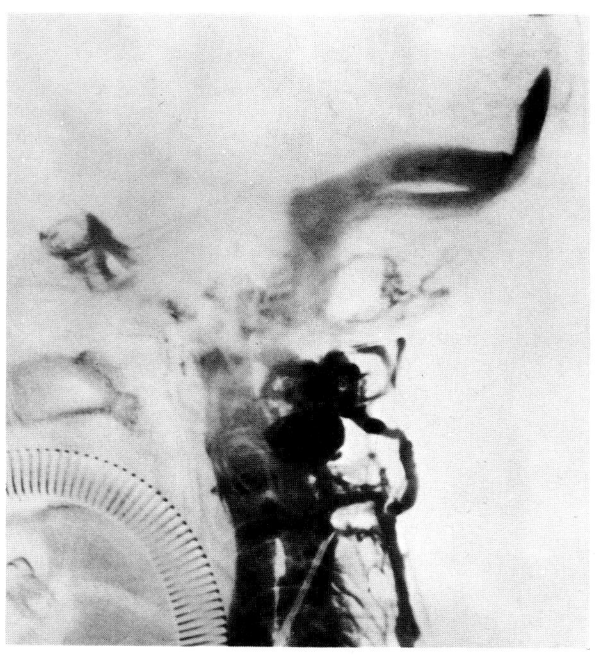

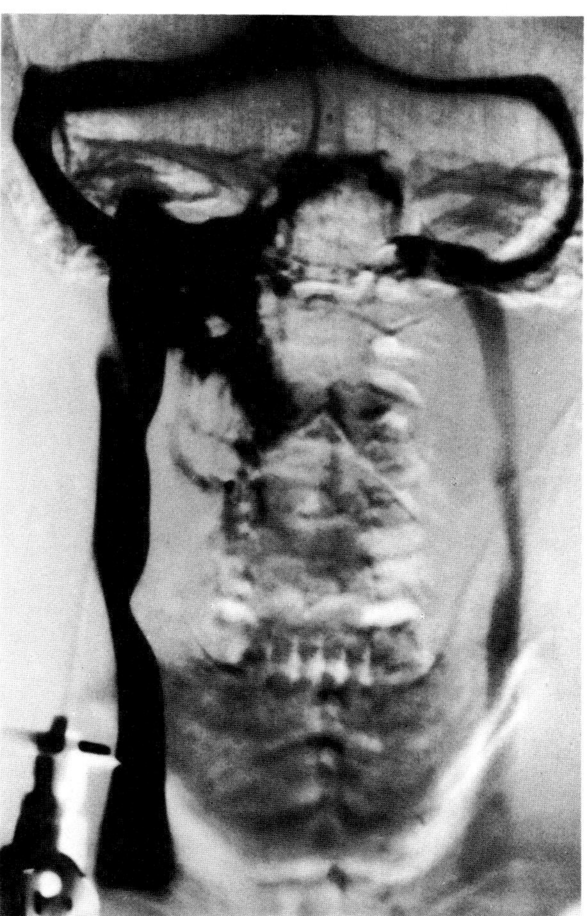

Fig. 150. Normal jugular venogram (anteroposter or view)

First, the carotid artery is pushed medially with the finger. The puncturing needle should have a lumen of 1.5 mm so that the manually injected contrast medium may flow into the vessel quickly with sufficient pressure. After the puncture, a syringe filled with a sterile saline solution is attached to the needle, which is then advanced 1–2 cm in a cranial direction while gently aspirating blood. A good intravascular position of the needle is confirmed by the fact that aspiration continues to yield large quantities of blood. The puncture and also the injection of contrast medium (10–15 ml of 60% contrast medium) is simplified by having the patient hold his breath and blow against a closed glottis (Valsalva maneuver). This results in a decrease in flow from the jugular vein and facilitates the introduction of the contrast agent into the intracranial space (Fig. 150). Obviously, the injection of contrast medium can also be accomplished by insertion of a catheter into the jugular vein.

For literature, see: GEJROT and LAUREN (1964a, b).

D. Pneumoencephalography

I. History

Luckett appears to have been the first person (1913) to visualize air in the ventricles of a living person. The demonstration of air in the ventricles of a corpse is without question attributed to Chiari (1891). In June 1918, Dandy reported on the introduction of air into the ventricle through puncture of a fontanelle or through burr holes ("ventriculography","pneumoventriculography", later also "cerebral pneumography"). In 1919 he demonstrated for the first time the possibility of introducing air into the cerebrospinal fluid (CSF) pathways by means of a lumbar puncture.

Encouraged by Dandy's results, Wideröe (1921) attempted to demonstrate spinal cord tumors by introduction of air into the spinal canal. Simultaneously he noted visualization of air within both ventricles and the cisterns. Independent of Dandy and Wideröe, Bingel reported in 1921 on a "new technique for the radiological demonstration of the brain" and described filling of the ventricle with air by the lumbar route, which he called "encephalography" or "pneumoencephalography". He elevated the lumbar introduction of air to a useful diagnostic procedure by his systematic technique. Under the designation of "pneumoencephalography", this bloodless demonstration of the CSF pathways by air has achieved prominence. On the other hand, when the air is introduced by means of a brain puncture directly into the ventricle, the term "ventriculography" is employed.

A "cisternal technique" with respect to air studies was popularized by Schaltenbrand et al. (1932). A particularly safe method proposed by him was the "limited" pneumoencephalogram, which enhanced the diagnostic capabilities of this technique. He stressed spontaneous sucking of air instead of forced filling of the cisterns.

With these techniques, air or some other gas was employed as a "negative" contrast agent. Under certain circumstances nitrous oxide (after antecedent ventricular drainage) was employed. In addition to the "negative" contrast agents (i.e., exchanging CSF for air), "positive" contrast agents which absorb the X-rays have also been injected into the CSF pathways. Most are iodine compounds, like the water-soluble Metrizamide or the water-insoluble oil Pantopaque.

The introduction of "fractional" pneumoencephalography, in which a small amount of air is positioned at will within the ventricular system or subarachnoid pathways, was an important advance (Robertson 1941; Lindgren 1948–1954).

Our knowledge of the normal and pathological encephalogram has come from the work of Dandy (1918, 1919), Bingel (1921/1922), Foerster (1925), Dyes (1934–1937), Lysholm et al. (1935), Schlesinger (1937), Tönnis (1939), Robertson (1941–1957), Davidoff et al. (1946–1950), E. Lindgren (1948–1954) and Liliequist (1959a, b). Lysholm and his school have made great contributions to this field as a result of their systematic analysis of ventriculography in space-occupying processes.

II. Injection Technique

At present, *"fractional"* lumbar positive pressure pneumoencephalography is most widely used. However, in earlier years the majority of studies were carried out through suboccipital puncture, since this method at that time was considered to be safer. With the methods now in use it is possible to direct the flow of air into the ventricular or subarachnoid spaces at will. The process of advancing air can be monitored through X-ray exposures or through fluoroscopy, so that the greatest possible diagnostic information is obtained from the smallest amount of air.

Pneumoencephalography is in every instance an invasive procedure, that is, it should not be performed on an outpatient basis. The same is true for *ventriculography,* which requires surgical trepanation and direct puncture of a ventricle.

1. The Lumbar Pneumoencephalogram

In carrying out lumbar pneumoencephalography, the following four points are of significance:

a) The air injection is accomplished by the positive pressure method without preliminary reduction in the quantity of CSF. From the beginning, air is injected under moderate pressure. By so doing, collapse of the subarachnoid spaces is prevented. Any pre-existing pressure cone can hardly be increased and ventricular filling is facilitated.

b) The air is injected slowly. The time span of the injection is extremely important. In a given time unit, only a certain amount of air can enter the foramen of Magendie from the cistern: with an excessive injection the surplus spills over out of the cisterna magna into the adjacent subarachnoid spaces.

c) During air injection, changes in the position of the head are possible. ROBERTSON (1941) was the first to show that the admission of air into the CSF compartments is dependent upon head position. With mild forward flexion of the head, the air predominantly enters the ventricular system. With more acute flexion of the neck, the air is directed over the dorsal surface of the cerebellum, while extension of the neck and head results in passage of the air ventrally into the basal cisterns. Then it separates, with some air passing into the midline spaces and some over the convexities.

d) The progress of the air filling is radiographically controlled.

The determination of how well the cisterns and ventricles are filling is made by routine X-ray exposure after each injection of 10 ml air. The entire procedure is considerably simplified if fluoroscopy is available. The rising air is then seen to enter the CSF spaces very clearly. The fluoroscope also permits the pulsations of the larger vessels to be seen as well as pulsations of the CSF. Because of the presence of the basilar and carotid arteries, CSF pulsations are stronger in the basal cisterns.

Keeping these rules in mind, the following procedure for *fractional lumbar pneumoencephalography* is recommended:

On the evening before the study, a sleeping pill is administered. The patient is thus calm in the morning. An hour before the beginning of the procedure a strong sedative is given, for example, Nembutal. In addition, Atropine or Scopolamine are given to counteract autonomic disturbances caused by the presence of the air. During the examination, the patient sits in front of the X-ray apparatus on an ordinary chair or, preferably, a special chair devised for this procedure. The X-ray tube is horizontal with a cassette placed to the side of the head. The lumbar puncture is carried out in a routine fashion, but only 1 ml of CSF is drained. From this, a cell count is obtained since the presence of air will incite leukocytosis and later quantities of CSF will thus be useless. In addition, a protein analysis is obtained. A special injection syringe facilitates this part of the study. Throughout the remaining procedure as little CSF as possible is withdrawn to permit additional necessary analyses to be performed.

Prior to injection of the first air, the head of the patient is lightly flexed so that the orbito-meatal line is approximately 15° below the horizontal (Fig. 151 b). For the lateral views, it is important to position the head until the orbital roofs are superimposed. Then, 8–10 ml of air is slowly injected. The air is injected slowly since only then will it all enter the ventricle and since rapid pressure injections tend to cause headaches. Each time air is injected, there is a corresponding brief increase in CSF pressure, which remains only for a few minutes and then quickly disappears. Following this, a lateral exposure

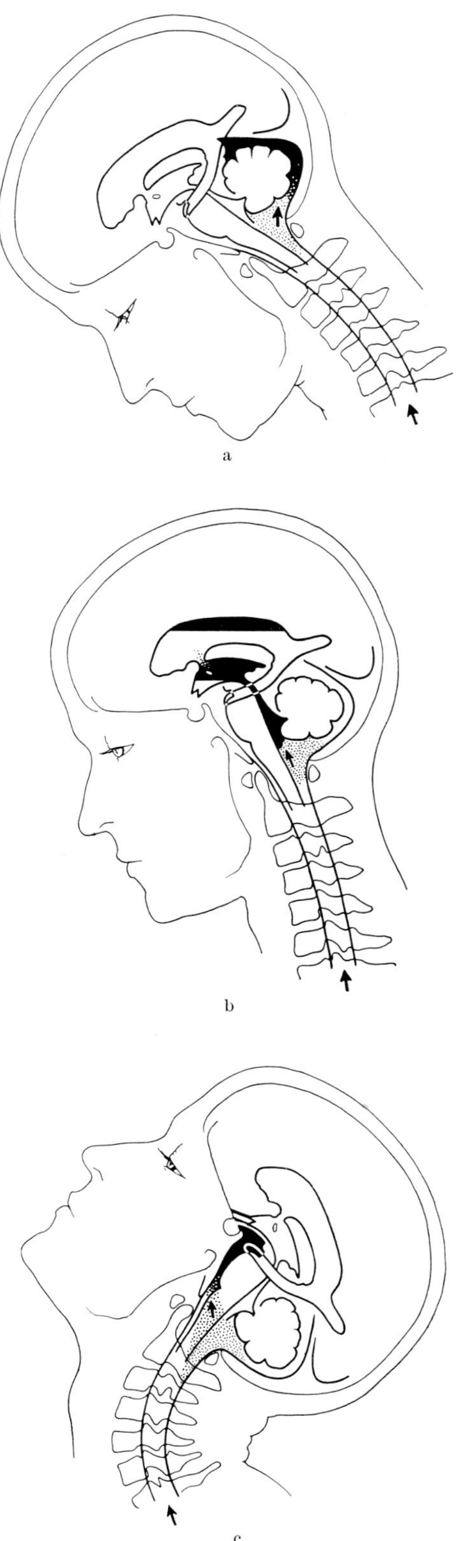

Fig. 151 a–c. The route taken by air after lumbar injection is dependent on the position of the head: **a** with maximal flexion of the neck – to the surface of the cerebellum (position A); **b** in the neutral or slightly flexed position – into the ventricular system (position B); **c** with extension of the neck – into the basal cisterns (position C)

is made to ascertain the position of the air. It is usually found within the posterior cranial fossa in the cisterna magna, from which it passes directly into the fourth ventricle, rising to the aqueduct and posterior portion of the third ventricle.

At this point, tomography or autotomography of the fourth ventricle should be carried out (see p. 192), especially if the mastoid air cells are large and interfere with visualization of the ventricle.

Occasionally, air will already be visible in the lateral ventricle. In this case, more air is injected. Afterward, additional X-ray exposures are made not only in the lateral position, but also in the half-axial anteroposterior view.

On the other hand, if no air is found within the ventricular system, the position of the head must be corrected. If air lies in the cisterns above the cerebellum, this is because the head is flexed too strongly (see Fig. 151 a) and correction is made by slowly extending the neck until the head rests in the position in Fig. 151 c. In this manner, the head will at some point automatically achieve position B with the result that the existing air will enter the fourth ventricle without having to inject additional air. The other possibility, however, is that the position of the head at the time of the air injection corresponded to C and the air went directly into the basal cisterns. This means that the head was extended too far at the time of the initial injection. Correction is made by a greater degree of flexion and repeating the air injection.

If the test exposure shows that only one ventricle is filled, the head is inclined to the filled side and several more injections of air are carried out until both sides are adequately filled. In position B, air in 10 ml quantities continues to be injected until sufficient ventricular filling is obtained.

If one wishes to fill the subarachnoid spaces instead, injection is carried out with the head further extended. In this position, the clivus should be vertical. In such a position, injected air quickly reaches the subarachnoid spaces of the anterior spinal and basal cisterns and outlines the anatomic structures in this region. Here, the injection of air may be carried out more quickly than when ventricular filling is desired. Of special value in this study is the demonstration of the chiasmatic cistern.

If visualization of the cerebellum is needed, i.e., the cistern above the vermis and the spaces between the folia, it is necessary to carry out the air injection and take the exposures with the head more flexed (Fig. 151a).

The needle is now removed and the patient positioned on a X-ray table for the remaining exposures.

With this technique for a routine air injection, it is obvious that only a portion of the entire ventricular system is visualized at any one time. The next step is to position the head of the patient so that the injected air will move into and outline all parts of the ventricle. In this fashion a picture of the entire ventricle is obtained from its individual parts, like the pieces of a puzzle. This part of the procedure is simplified by using a special apparatus which permits easy positioning of the patient for the various views and has an adjustment for tomography.

2. Suboccipital (Cisternal) Pneumoencephalography

The patient is prepared as for lumbar pneumoencephalography (see p. 184). The nape of the neck is shaved as far as the occipital protuberance. The patient sits facing away from the doctor on a chair in a comfortable upright position with the back arched slightly forward and with the neck initially erect. This chair should be fitted with fixed arm rests, if possible, which the patient can hold. The site of needle insertion is found as follows: the index finger of the left hand is placed on the spine of the axis and this part is marked or the index finger is left in place. Directly over this point is the puncture site. The chin of the patient is now tucked in sharply so that most of the ligamentum nuchae stands out posteriorly as a long ridge. For this position, the head is held by an assistant, who stands between the patient's legs and places the palms of his hands over the patient's temples with the fingers on the back of the head, helping to hold the chin in its proper position. Next, the skin of the neck is cleansed with disinfectant and a skin wheal made by local anesthetic (1%–2% Novocaine). A thin, sharply pointed cannula is then inserted in the direction of the line joining both mastoid prominences. The hand of the physician is supported by bracing the wrist against the patient's neck. The needle is then advanced deeper into the soft tissues,

which yield with a familiar resistance as they are penetrated. Upon reaching the dura there is usually a springlike resistance. As the dura is slowly penetrated, a grinding noise is occasionally heard in elderly patients. After penetration, the needle will be so firmly held by the dura that a funnel will form around it when pressure against the needle and adjacent skin is relaxed simultaneously. Also, upon lightly pushing or pulling the needle, it will return to the same position relative to the skin surface. This contrasts with the situation which exists before the dura is penetrated when such maneuvers would result in an advance or withdrawal of the needle, and confirms that the dura has in fact been punctured. Then, the needle is slowly advanced through the dura a further 2–3 mm. Removal of the stylette at this point will usually be followed by a flow of CSF.

One should attempt this "direct" puncture of the cistern only after much experience and only if the technique has been mastered. For the beginner, or if difficulties are encountered with the direct method, it is recommended that the "indirect" method of AYER and ESKUCHEN (1930) be employed. In this method the needle is directed diagonally upward after skin puncture and is advanced until the bone of the posterior fossa is encountered. Then, the needle is "walked" down the bone until the rim of the foramen magnum is reached, after which the bony resistance gives way to an elastic resistance. With further advancement of the needle, the fused dura and atlanto-occipital membrane are pierced simultaneously.

If no CSF is obtained, the needle should be turned. The patient is instructed to strain or cough, or the jugular veins are compressed. Gentle aspiration with a syringe may also be attempted. If these maneuvers fail to yield CSF, then the procedure should be repeated. The second procedure should follow the "indirect" method and the position of the head should be carefully controlled. The needle, however, does not need to be withdrawn from the outer skin layers.

After successful cisternal puncture, the head of the patient may be brought to a more comfortable position with the orbitomeatal line inclined forward at an angle of 15° to the horizontal.

To aspirate the CSF, a 5–10 ml syringe is employed. After removing approximately 5 ml, it is not necessary with this procedure to inject air; rather the syringe is removed and air is spontaneously sucked into the open needle, occasionally in large amounts. The spontaneous sucking effect can be augmented by having the patient breathe deeply at regular intervals. From time to time 5 ml CSF is again withdrawn and the process repeated. Aspirations are carried out when the air sucking ceases and CSF begins to drip from the open needle.

Usually 20–40 ml CSF is withdrawn during suboccipital pneumoencephalography, although in massive hydrocephalus additional air may be necessary. The injection of air is not recommended with cisternal punctures, except in cases where the spontaneous sucking effect is insufficient. If bloody CSF is aspirated initially, usually a small dural vein or the rim sinus has been torn, either of which should clear spontaneously after a short period. If not, it is recommended that the needle be advanced an additional 1–2 mm. If the bleeding still continues, the procedure must be terminated. The patient is allowed to recline and is observed. If his clinical condition deteriorates – which is rare – then a lumbar puncture is performed to see whether the bleeding is continuing. A deterioration in the conscious state with associated nuchal rigidity may, under certain circumstances, require immediate neurosurgical intervention to expose and control the hemorrhage, which may be coming from an injured artery.

A "dry" cistern with a correct needle puncture is a danger signal (the position of the needle should be verified and other sources of error eliminated). It may reflect a filling of the cisterna magna with the cerebellar tonsils, which occurs in tonsillar herniation (see p. 10). In such a situation, continued attempts to puncture the cistern can easily lead to brain damage or further herniation of the tonsils with a resultant herniation syndrome (see p. 10). Tonsillar herniation is a condition where only ventriculography is permitted.

If acute deterioration of the patient or a seizure occurs during the course of the procedure, it should be terminated immediately and appropriate therapy instituted.

3. Ventriculography

Ventriculography is accomplished by direct puncture of the ventricle and direct injection of the contrast agent. It is used only when injection via the lumbar route is not possible or is considered too risky. There are a variety of methods available which differ as to the type of contrast medium employed and its route of introduction into the ventricular chambers. Analogous to myelography, there are both positive and negative contrast agents. To the first group belong the water-soluble or oily iodine-containing contrast agents, while the second group consists of gases like oxygen, nitrogen, nitrous oxide, helium, and air. Nowadays, most neurosurgeons prefer atmospheric air as a negative agent since it is the least irritating and most comfortable of the gases to use. As positive contrast agents, Metrizamide is currently popular.

Originally, both ventricular trigones were punctured by way of occipital burr holes and air was introduced by this route. Rarely were frontal trephines used for this purpose, the choice of a puncture site depending upon the diagnostic goal. In the course of the years, this goal has changed with the increasing significance of angiography, isotope brain scans, and recently CT. In the overwhelming majority of cases today, ventriculography is no longer employed for the diagnosis of space-occupying cerebral hemispheric lesions, but has contributed greatly to the diagnosis and localization of tumors of the brain stem and cerebellum, as indicated by their effect on the third ventricle, aqueduct, and fourth ventricle. For this reason, the classical method of ventriculography has been modified to permit more ready visualization of these structures.

The method involves two steps:

1) Introduction of a rubber catheter into the third ventricle in the operating room

2) Fractional introduction of air or positive contrast medium in the X-ray department.

The fasting patient is placed in a supine position and, under local anesthesia, a 3 cm incision is made behind the hairline (a finger breadth in front of the coronal suture and 2 cm lateral to the midline). The incision is made through the skin, galea, and periosteum and a burr hole made in the skull.

It is not important which side is chosen. We generally prefer the left side in order to leave the right side free for a possible ventricular drainage procedure. The dura is coagulated by diathermy and is punctured with an ordinary scalpel. The dural incision is then enlarged so that a catheter may be easily inserted. Beneath the dural incision, the exposed cortex appears

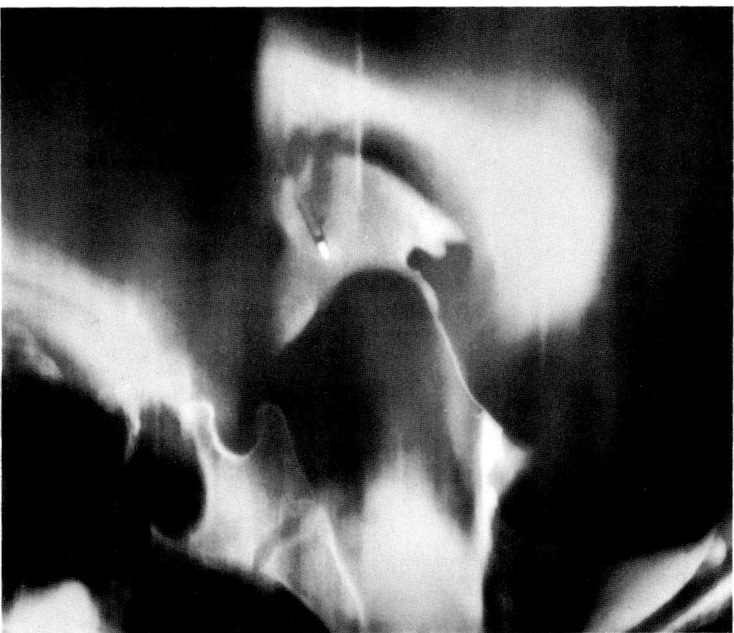

Fig. 152. Positive contrast demonstration of the third ventricle, particularly the middle and posterior portions. The contrast medium also opacifies the fourth ventricle via the aqueduct

with its arachnoid membrane and pial veins. The latter should be carefully avoided when the cortical incision is made, which is accomplished by inserting a pointed blade and coagulating the exposed cortical surface. Occasionally, when the intracranial pressure is elevated, a little brain tissue will issue forth. The described puncture of the leptomeninges is necessary so that the blunt ventricular catheter may be inserted with ease. For this purpose one may employ the blunt metal cannula favored by Cushing. It is closed at its tip, has many openings on the side, and a stylette. When all bleeding has been controlled, the cannula is inserted in the direction of the outer ear or the middle of the zygoma with a slight medial angulation. Just before entering the ventricle, a light resistance is encountered from the subependymal glia. After this has been overcome, CSF will frequently appear in spite of the presence of the stylette, or after its removal, indicating a successful ventricular puncture. Since these cases are almost always associated with ventricular enlargement, the puncture is usually not difficult and is further facilitated by the comfortable supine (brow-up) position of the patient in contrast to other methods.

At the first appearance of the CSF, the cannula is rapidly withdrawn and a rubber catheter inserted to a depth of 9 cm (previously marked by tying a thread on the catheter) through the same channel with minimal loss of CSF. Only after the catheter has been positioned and the flow of CSF resumes should any CSF be taken for analysis. If the CSF does not flow spontaneously, the possibility of inadequate ventricular pressure exists. To verify this, the catheter is filled with a sterile physiological saline solution, alternately raising and lowering its distal end. With a correct intraventricular location, the solution will run into the ventricle when the catheter is raised and will re-appear when it is lowered. One can also look for pulsations of the fluid and for pressure changes associated with breathing.

As a rule, this method of insertion will cause the tip of the catheter to rest within the third ventricle. To accomplish this, it is important that the catheter be directed anteromedially rather than posterolaterally, so that it may slide into the funnel-shaped foramen of Monro rather than the cella media of the lateral ventricle. At this point the catheter is closed off. It is recommended that the catheter contains only a single side hole, since any additional openings will interfere with later ventricular filling. The skin incision should then be closed in two layers and the catheter fixed to the skin. The thread can be either passed through the wall of the catheter, avoiding the lumen, or wrapped

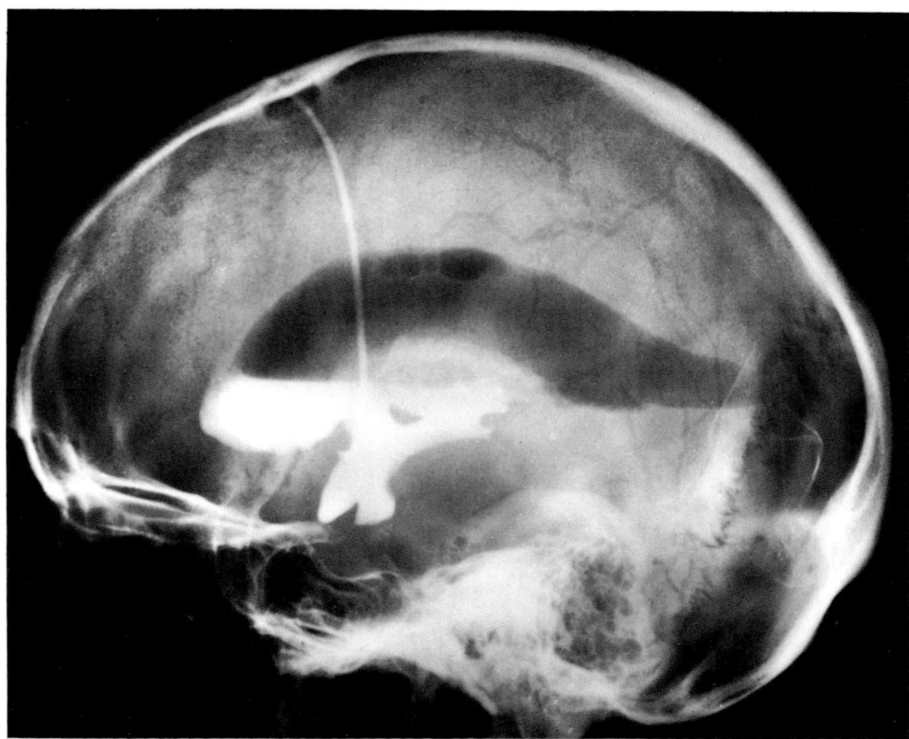

Fig. 153. Positive contrast demonstration of the third ventricle using a water-soluble contrast medium. The middle portion (with the massa intermedia) and the frontobasal portions of the third ventricle are well seen. The positive contrast agent fills the frontal horns of the lateral ventricles as well. Air is also present in both lateral ventricles

around the catheter. The wound is then covered with a sterile dressing and the exposed catheter wrapped in sterile gauze. The patient is then taken to the X-ray department.

The occipital route is used only in frontal processes, which prevent insertion of a catheter into the frontal horns.

The first step is to verify the position of the catheter by obtaining X-ray exposures in two planes. If one has a portable X-ray unit with an image intensifier in the operating theater, this verification can naturally be accomplished at the time of the catheter insertion (Figs. 152, 153). In the X-ray room, air or Metrizamide is injected with minimal pressure into the ventricle under fluoroscopic control. For this injection, the Metrizamide concentration for adults should be 170 mg/ml. A maximum of 5 ml of this concentration is then injected. In order to avoid complications, it is essential that no Metrizamide be injected before the position of the catheter within the ventricular chambers is unconditionally verified! Such verification can be simply carried out by injecting 2–3 ml air into the ventricular catheter under fluoroscopic control.

III. Radiologic Technique

It is important that a definite "standard" positioning technique be part of the procedure routine. Only by mental comparison of similar abnormal and normal views can one hope to recognize the pathological study and distinguish it from "normal" variants, such as the senile atrophies. The following standard technique comprises one such routine. It must be emphasized, however, that the concept of a "routine technique" in no way implies that the procedure may be left in the hands of ancillary personnel. Each case should be dealt with individually and should be personally directed by the responsible physician himself, who reviews the exposures and varies the technique as needed to obtain the necessary information.

a) Recommended Standard Technique

1) A fixed focus film distance of 80–100 cm.
2) A head holder, as with the Lysholm table
3) A film size of 18 × 24 cm or 24 × 30 cm
4) A similar exposure technique corresponding to the physical capabilities of the X-ray machine

b) Positioning the Patient and Setting of the Apparatus for the Films

After taking the initial films in the anteroposterior and lateral views following air injection in the sitting position, the following exposures should be carried out for all patients on the X-ray table (Fig. 154).

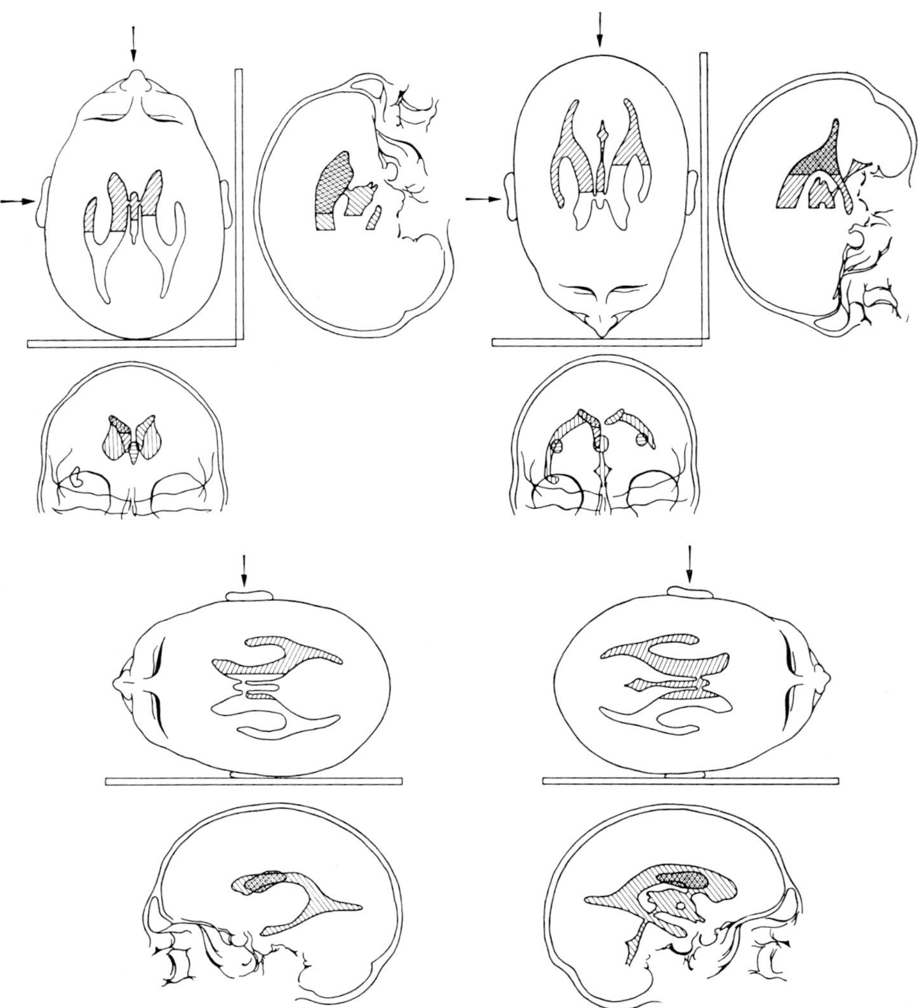

Fig. 154. Comprehensive diagram showing the major brow-up, brow-down, and lateral positions for demonstration of the ventricular system. The *arrows* show the direction of the X-ray beam while the *parallel lines* indicate the placement of the film in each case

1. X-Ray Exposures in the Supine (Brow-Up or Back) Position

a) Anterior-posterior position = "anteroposterior view". The back of the head rests against the cassette. The orbitomeatal line[1] is vertical, as is the X-ray beam. The central beam is directed at the nasion (Fig. 155).

b) Lateral position = "Lateral frontal horn view". The position of the patient is similar (head position must not be changed between the two exposures!). The cassette lies to the side of the head. The X-ray beam is horizontal, centered on the upper margin of the ear. On occasion a "hanging head" view is necessary to visualize adequately the anterior-inferior portion of the third ventricle (see p. 235).

c) Sometimes an exposure in the "anteroposterior half axial (Towne's) view" is also required. The position of the patient is the same as for the normal anteroposterior view, but the tube is tilted 30° in the caudal direction so that the central beam is directed toward the feet. It enters approximately at the hairline on the forehead and exists in the vicinity of the foramen magnum (Fig. 155).

2. X-Ray Views in the Prone (Brow-Down or Abdominal) Position

a) Posterior-anterior position = "posteroanterior view". The patient lies with forehead and nose on the cassette and chin tucked in. The orbitomeatal line is vertical, as is the tube. The central beam is directed at the external occipital protuberance (Fig. 155).

b) Lateral position = "Lateral occipital horn view". The position for the patient is the same (again head position must not be changed between exposures!). The tube is horizontal, the cassette lies to the side of the patient, and the central beam is horizontal and directed at the upper margin of the ear.

c) Again, an exposure in the "posteroanterior half-axial (reverse Town's) view" may be obtained. The position of the patient is the same as for the normal posteroanterior view, but the tube is tilted 30° in a cranial direction so that the central beam is directed toward the head.

---

1 The orbitomeatal line (auriculo-orbital line) joins the lateral corner of the eye with the external auditory canal. This line corresponds nearly to the "German horizontal" and runs parallel to the "Frankfurt horizontal", which have been established as standard radiologic reference points.

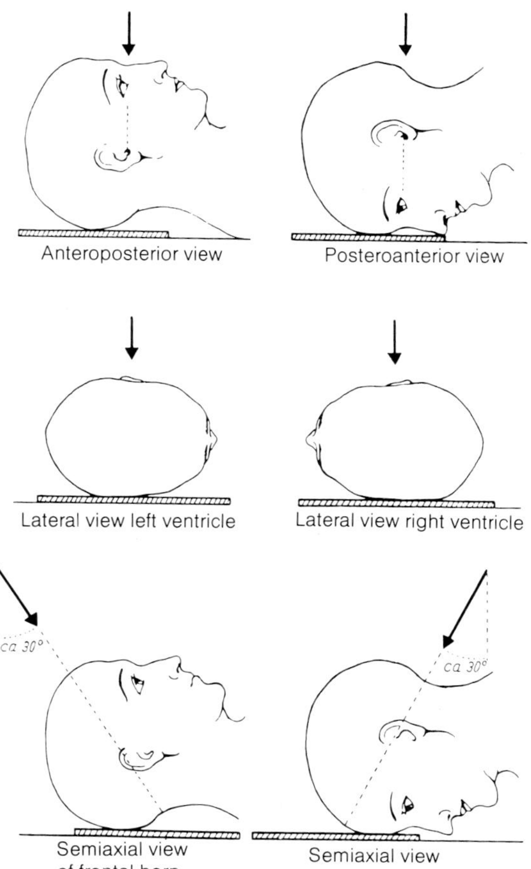

Fig. 155. Position of the head and direction of the incident X-ray beam for the various views

It is pointed at the foramen magnum and exits at the hairline of the forehead (Fig. 155).

3. X-Ray Views for the Temporal Horns

Earlier it was the custom following the routine methods to obtain two exposures with the head turned to either side in order to visualize the temporal horns better ("right" and "left" lateral views). A more dependable method is to perform a frontal "somersault", following which both temporal horns will be filled simultaneously. This method is commonly used in young children and is tolerated by them. With both temporal horns filled by air, superimposition on the lateral view is prevented by tilting the head of the supine patient slightly toward the right or left shoulder. In doing this, the temporal horns are projected one above the other, rather than superimposed. This permits comparisons of shape to be made, but prevents comparison of their position relative to one another. For the anteroposterior position, the head is placed as with the plain anteroposterior skull films. The chin is, however, raised until the petrous pyramids lie beneath the orbits and the air-filled temporal horns are projected within each orbit. The X-ray field should be narrowed and the central beam directed 1 cm below the nasion.

In the technique described by E. LINDGREN (1948), the examination is begun with the patient on his back with the head positioned beyond the edge of the table so that it is unsupported and hangs free. Then the patient is turned to the side, resting on one shoulder, depending on which temporal horn is to be filled. In this manner, the head hangs down over the shoulder placing the temporal horn being studied at the highest point in the ventricular system. After that, the patient again rolls onto his back taking care that the head is never raised above the horizontal. In a similar fashion the opposite temporal horn is filled with air. Then exposures in anteroposterior and lateral positions are obtained.

4. Tomography

The tomogram represents a valuable diagnostic tool. With the patient in either the sitting or the recumbent position, tomography permits precise definition of individual segments of the ventricular system and cisterns in the antero-posterior and lateral views. It effectively eliminates superimposed bony structures, which would otherwise impede the study of these areas. Tomography requires special apparatus, but is performed without difficulty.

It is also possible in the lateral view to demonstrate the midline structures by a variation of this technique called "autotomography". Here, the head is rotated 10° to each side on the long axis of the body (similar to shaking the head to signify "no"). The exposure time is usually 3–4 s depending upon the machine. Varying the position of the patient (sitting, recumbent, brow-up and brow-down) permits sharp visualization of various midline ventricular segments without interference of overlying structures. During this procedure, a headband greatly simplifies the turning of the head from side to side.

5. Transverse Pneumoencephalography

By means of a special tomography apparatus, tomograms can be obtained in a transverse di-

rection. This enhances the recognition of indentations of the ventricular system from either side and is especially valuable in recognizing space-occupying processes in the region of the medulla oblongata.

6. How Much Air Should be Injected?

The more air that is injected, the more detailed and more complete will be the contrast demonstration. Too much air will cause confusion by superimposition of the various ventricular segments or by superimposition of the subarachnoid spaces on the ventricular pathways. In addition, immediate and delayed autonomic reactions are proportionately related to the quantity of air present. As a general rule, the answer to the question is *"as much air as necessary, as little as possible"!* In the majority of cases 30–40 ml air is considered sufficient to study a ventricular system which is not markedly dilated.

c) The Causes of Nonfilling of the Ventricular System

Failures of filling of the ventricular system are primarily dependent upon technical difficulties inherent in the methods employed, particularly the position of the head during the air injection. In a small percentage (up to 5%) of patients without space-occupying processes, air fails to enter the ventricular system in spite of a flawless technique. In these cases an abnormal position of the foramen of Magendie is occasionally responsible.

If repeated vomiting occurs during the procedure, it is an indication that the air is primarily entering the subarachnoid spaces and that ventricular filling is impaired. If the ventricular spaces are narrowed by increased intracranial pressure secondary to cerebral edema, incomplete filling of the ventricular system may follow unless a dehydrating agent has been given beforehand.

In the event that ventricular filling does not take place, it is important to visualize the various cisterns since these will sometimes reveal the location of a space-occupying lesion (see above, Mass Displacements and Space-Occupying Lesions, p. 6, and pp. 208ff., 213). It is recommended that these cisterns be sharply defined, their positions verified, and any displacement ascertained (as by tomography, see above).

d) Unilateral Filling

If only one lateral ventricle is filled, which is in its normal position and not enlarged, it may be assumed that nonfilling of the other side is caused by some technical difficulty and is not necessarily pathological. Further attempts should then be made by varying the head position and reinjecting air to fill the side in question. Only when repeated attempts also fail to accomplish the desired filling should this be considered a pathological finding. In such cases, a narrowing or scarring will rarely be found at the foramen of Monro, since a true occlusion or even a relative narrowing would be expected to impede the flow of CSF and result in a unilateral mass-producing hydrocephalus.

e) The 24-h Pneumoencephalogram

When the routine pneumoencephalogram fills only the subarachnoid spaces and no ventricular filling occurs, additional exposures should be made 24 h later. Occasionally, air will then be found in the ventricular system. Also, these delayed views will tend to fill out unsuspected arachnoid "cysts" which would not otherwise be found.

With the 24 h pneumoencephalogram, deviations of the septum and dilations and constrictions of the ventricular system will all become apparent. In addition to the cerebral atrophies, which are responsible for the majority of nonobstructive ventricular dilations, other cases have been described in the literature where technical error has been the sole responsible factor. It should be noted that a slight asymmetry in size of the lateral ventricles – with the left usually larger – may be seen as a variant of normal (p. 216 ff.).

IV. Gas Resorption

The resorption of injected gas depends upon both the resorption coefficient of the gas and other conditions peculiar to the individual patient. The time element may vary from several hours to several weeks. Individual patients can frequently discern a clicking sound on movement of the head when ventricular air is present. Usually, the subarachnoid air is first to disappear. After 24 h, approximately half of the residual air has been resorbed. Although the primary site for gas resorption is undoubtedly the subarachnoid space, ventriculography done in the presence of occlusive hydrocephalus proves that gas resorption can also take place through the ventricular walls.

V. Autonomic Reactions

Autonomic reactions secondary to pneumoencephalography can be divided into early and late reactions. The early effects are undoubtedly due to changes in the intracranial pressure and to irritation of the autonomic centers by the injected gas. Irritation of the meninges is also possible. When the air exclusively enters the ventricular system, the systemic reactions are much reduced. The severity of these early reactions is directly related to the quantity of injected air, as well as to the quantity of CSF removed and the speed of injection of the gas.

During the lumbar injection there is at times a brief rise in intraventricular pressure which can be quite impressive. This is, however, rapidly compensated for and is therefore not associated with any clinical change or, if present, such change is of brief duration.

With aspiration of a large amount of fluid (for example, 10–20 ml), there is a significant fall in the CSF pressure which lasts about 30 min or longer and cannot be compensated for by injecting additional air. Disturbances of this type are considerably reduced with the fractional positive pressure lumbar technique (p. 184).

The speed of injection of the gas is an additional factor of importance. This is shown by the fact that fractional lumbar pneumoencephalography with its *slower* air injection is accompanied by a *marked reduction* in the number of systemic reactions; however, the severity and the type of the early reactions seen are also dependent to a large extent on the clinical condition of the patient.

Finally, the emotional make-up of the patient and his psychological reaction to the procedure are also of significance. It is therefore important to calm the patient before beginning the procedure and to divert the patient's attention through conversation or some other means during the actual air injection. Deep breathing during the injection of air alleviates not only problems associated with the introduction of air into the CSF spaces (by enhancing venous drainage), but also stabilizes a labile autonomic response.

The Early Reactions

Entry of air into the CSF pathways is accompanied by: headaches, nausea and vomiting, pallor and coolness of the skin, excessive sweating, shivering, slowing of the pulse followed shortly by tachycardia, and occasionally even circulatory collapse with loss of consciousness. During injection, significant variations in blood pressure are seen (up and down). It is important to keep in mind that the lumbar puncture alone can lead to marked circulatory changes. The initial autonomic disturbance recognized is usually skin pallor. The disturbances mentioned above usually resolve in 1–2 h.

The *headaches* are most likely secondary to irritation of the arachnoid and sensitive nerves traversing the subarachnoid space by the injected air. They are experienced by the patient in certain well-defined areas, dependent upon the position of the irritating air. *Suboccipital* headaches point to overfilling of the cisterna magna, and *temporal* headaches to a filling of the basal cisterns including the Sylvian fissures. *Retro-orbital* headaches accompany the presence of air over the frontal convolutions, while *parietal* headaches are occasionally seen with ventricular filling. A syncopal episode requires cessation of the injection, but is not an emergency. The patient is laid flat or is given a pressor agent. Recovery is usually rapid.

The Late Reactions

Even after the air injection has stopped, autonomic reactions can persist or begin anew. Apparently these are related to the length of time the gases remain in the CSF spaces – the shorter the stay (as with O_2, a rapidly resorbed gas), the less severe are the associated problems.

Also of importance is the *speed of resorption*. The reactions noted in this second phase – like the first – consist of disturbances in regulatory mechanisms (such as temperature rises),

to redness and increased warmth of the skin, to a rise in the basal metabolic state. The pulse may be rapid, but remains full. Within 5–6 h of injection, the patient's temperature can reach 38.5° C, but is rarely higher and generally returns to normal on the same day. A similar temperature rise rarely occurs on day 2, or even days 3 or 4. With O_2 injections, the initial temperature elevation is usually missing. Occasionally, neck and shoulder pains are felt.

Headaches may also be experienced on day 1 despite a recumbent position, but are controlled by medication. To the autonomic disturbances of the second phase belong a series of central autonomic reactions which are best represented by changes in the hematological picture. Between 1 and 5 h after injection there is a neutrophilic leukocytosis with a shift to the left, which tapers off between hours 7 and 10. Occasionally one sees hyperglycemia, rarely glucosuria.

CSF Changes

Whenever a patient is studied by pneumoencephalography, definite CSF changes occur. For example, an increase in the cell count is seen which only occasionally exceeds 300 cells/ml. There is also fever and moderate meningismus. The leukocytosis is maximal after 10–12 h. At 24 h, the cell count has already dropped by 50%. The onset of the leukocytosis is early, while the procedure is actually being conducted. The degree of elevation is directly proportional to the quantity of air injected and is most marked in the presence of cerebral pathology. Because of this, it is necessary that the cell count be performed on the first specimen of CSF obtained before air injection.

Autonomic complications related to the second phase are to be treated symptomatically. It is important to remember that the severity and duration of accompanying headaches are increased by removing large quantities of CSF.

VI. Complications

The risks of the cisternal puncture have been described above. However, the positive pressure fractional pneumoencephalogram may also be dangerous, particularly when done in the presence of increased intracranial pressure. In situations where increased intracranial pressure is suspected, only a few drops of CSF should be withdrawn since removal of greater quantities increases the risk of tonsillar herniation. It must be emphasized, however, that leakage of CSF through the hole in the dura can continue with signs of herniation appearing much later.

The symptoms of herniation: A "herniation syndrome" can always develop whenever a low pressure spinal system is created through a lumbar puncture. This has already been described above (see p. 184). This danger exists for every case of occlusive hydrocephalus and is especially risky in the marked hydrocephalus of children with closed sutures. Special attention must therefore be given to any suggestion of herniation, such as nuchal rigidity or paresthesias in the shoulders and arms with certain head positions and with transient increases in intracranial pressure (such as with coughing, sneezing, or straining at stool). Pupillary changes are also danger signs. In such situations the risks of pneumoencephalography need to be reconsidered.

Increased intracranial pressure alone is not an absolute contraindication for lumbar pneumoencephalography. However, if clinical signs of impending herniation are present, pneumoencephalography should not be performed. In these cases, the procedure of choice is ventriculography. Ventriculography should also be performed whenever increased intracranial pressure and angiographic evidence of definite hydrocephalus are found together.

For the most part, *tonsillar herniation* can be identified on the lateral pneumoencephalogram. It is seen in a high percentage of cerebellar tumors, less commonly in tumors of the brain stem and frontal lobes. X-ray evidence of tonsillar herniation may also be seen in patients who do not have a space-occupying intracranial process. Consequently, the mere presence of the tonsils below the foramen magnum is not an absolute contraindication for further injections of air. However, no additional CSF should be withdrawn in such cases. Immediate visualization of the position of the tonsils is of the highest priority; X-ray exposure should therefore be made immediately after the first injection of air or, better still, the rising air should be directly observed on a fluoroscope. When tonsillar herniation is present, the procedure should be abandoned and ventriculography performed in its place.

A high percentage of pneumoencephalograms in children are accompanied by EKG changes. Monitoring is therefore indicated particularly in children with known heart disease or with definite evidence of cerebral dysfunction.

The lumbar route of air injection is particularly risky in patients with *marked hydrocephalus.* Because of irritation from the air, there is not infrequently a hypersecretion of CSF with a subsequent additional rise in intracranial pressure. This danger also exists even for ventriculography, however, and is prevented by continuing open ventricular drainage after the study to relieve any pressure increases. Hydrocephalic patients, because of changes in the compressed brain particularly with regard to central regulatory mechanisms, are in a high risk group. That this is so is proven by reports in the literature of deaths in hydrocephalic children following air studies in spite of careful monitoring of respiration, circulatory status, and temperature. In these cases as little air as possible should be injected or, better still, a positive contrast agent should be used instead.

A further complication seen following air studies in patients with space-occupying intracranial processes (glioblastoma, metastases, abscess) is a particular tendency to reactive edema formation. As the cerebral edema intensifies, the intracranial pressure increases, necessitating immediate measures either to lower the pressure or to remove the offending lesion. In cases where this risk exists, prophylactic use of steroids is recommended.

As a result of the pressure changes described earlier (see p. 194), air studies in patients with an *abscess* carry the additional risk that the membrane will rupture. Therefore, when an abscess is suspected, pneumoencephalography should be performed only with special care.

A rare but deadly complication is air embolism. This can occur in pneumoencephalography when a bridging vein is torn and a large portion of the injected air has entered the subdural space, forcing the cortical surface away from the inner table of the skull.

If after several days to several weeks the patient becomes confused or develops a neurological deficit, the possibility of a *subdural hematoma* should be entertained. It can develop after pneumoencephalography particularly when cerebral atrophy is present ("low pressure hematoma"). This results from pulling and tearing of bridging veins as the distance between the cortical surface and inner table of the skull is increased. Subdural and epidural hematomas can also follow ventriculography, particularly in children with massive hydrocephalus where ventricular collapse is followed by tearing of bridging veins.

Serious complications with these procedures are rare, the mortality rate being approximately 0.2%. Higher mortalities have been reported in the smaller series or in association with specific disease entities.

Clinical Syndromes of Herniation. Herniations may be life endangering. The two most pronounced syndromes are:
1) Cerebellar herniations (cerebellar pressure cone), pain and stiffness of the neck, paresthesias in the shoulders and upper extremities – later also bradycardia, vomiting, and arrest of respiration.
2) Mesencephalic herniation (tentorial or temporal pressure cone, rarely also cerebellar upwards herniation), – changes of pupillary size and reaction, homolateral pyramidal signs – later symptoms of decerebration and loss of consciousness.

VII. The Normal Pneumoencephalogram

It is possible to recognize *pathological* changes in the contrast demonstration of the CSF pathways only if one has mastered the study of the normal state and its *physiological variants*. Thus, we will begin with a detailed description of the *normal* ventricular study.

In all our films, the degree of filling is noted as well as the position of the head and angle of projection of the X-ray beams. It is therefore important to correlate which anatomical structures are visualized with each projection and positioning technique (see p. 190 ff.).

We will also now describe the sequence in which individual projections are obtained and how they relate to the position of the patient (sitting, prone, supine, lateral, etc.). Since precise definition of the ventricular system requires simultaneous views of the same structure in two planes – that is, "paired pictures" – both pictures are described one after the other. In the absence of corresponding views in two planes, the relative depth of the contrast image can only be surmised from its shape or the intensity of the projected image, neither of which is reliable. Originally, the CSF pathways were divided into the ventricular system and the subarachnoid spaces. This division will also be employed in the descriptions which follow.

1. The Ventricular System

Ventricular Chambers

The ventricular system consists of both lateral ventricles with their foramina of Monro, the third ventricle, the aqueduct, and the fourth ventricle (Fig. 156). The lateral ventricles are anatomically divided for descriptive purposes into the frontal, occipital and temporal horns. For radiological purposes the frontal horn has been further divided into two parts and the space between the frontal and occipital horns into another two parts, namely the cella media and ventricular trigone. According to the proposals of TORKILDSEN and PENFIELD (1933), each lateral ventricle is thus divided into six sections (Figs. 157, 158).

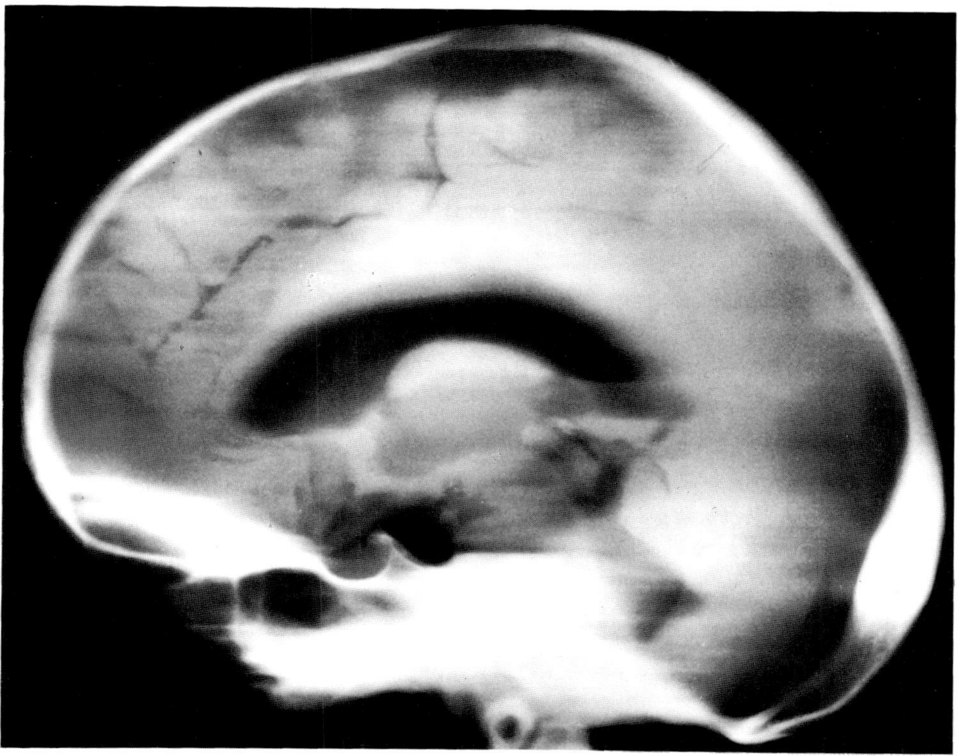

Fig. 156. Lateral tomogram of an air study revealing the fourth ventricle, aqueduct, third ventricle, and both lateral ventricles. Note also the filling of the various cisterns

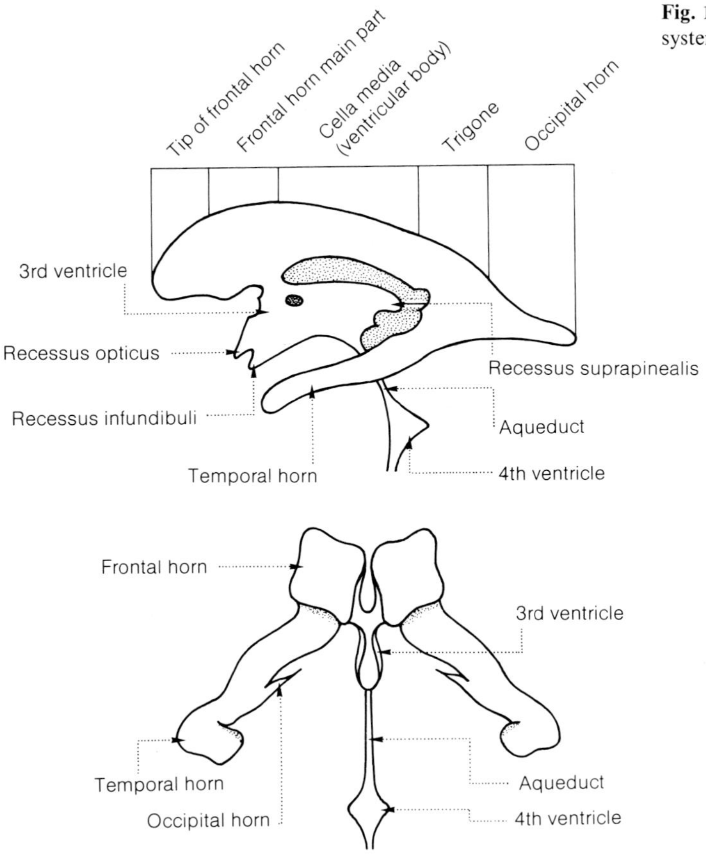

Fig. 157. Lateral and frontal views of the ventricular system with its various segments

1. The frontal horn apex extends from the anterior boundary of the ventricle to the anterior border of the caudate nucleus.

2. The frontal horn body reaches back to the foramen of Monro.

3. The cella media (earlier known as the pars centralis) extends from the foramen of Monro to the anterior edge of the trigone.

4. The three sides of the trigone (or ventricular triangle) border on the cella media, the occipital horn, and the temporal horn.

5. The occipital horn.

6. The temporal horn.

The Ventricular System in the Sitting Position

The fourth ventricle and the aqueduct are the first ventricular structures to be identified after air injection by the lumbar route and are seen on the lateral and half-axial posteroanterior views.

As was noted earlier, the contrast image of the fourth ventricle on the lateral view may be superimposed by enlarged mastoid air cells. In such cases autotomography (see p. 192) or tomography may be employed to correct this problem.

The *fourth ventricle* resembles an isosceles triangle with its base parallel to the clivus and its apex pointing in the direction of the internal occipital protuberance. The length of the base is approximately 3 cm and the height 1.5 cm. The center of the fourth ventricle can usually be transected by a vertical line bisecting Twining's line, which runs from the tuberculum sella to the internal occipital protuberance (Fig. 156). Projecting into the fourth ventricle from below near the apex is the softly defined shadow of the choroid plexus. Because air will usually remain in the fourth ventricle only a short time before passing on, later films are frequently of little value for demonstrating this structure.

The opening into the *aqueduct* is found on the lateral views in the posterior portion of the third ventricle. It originates directly below the suprapineal recess and swings posteriorly and inferiorly in a wide arc (Figs. 152, 156, 159).

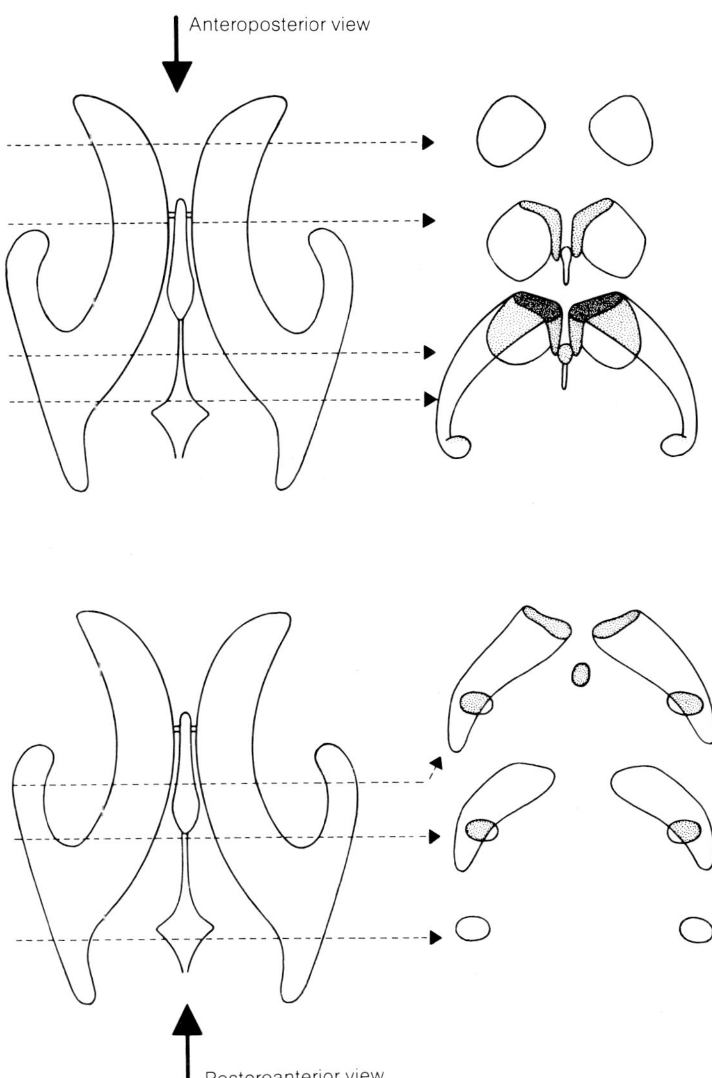

Fig. 158. Diagram of the ventricular system with its various segments. *Right:* schematic representation of various degrees of air filling with the pneumoencephalogram; the anteroposterior view is shown *above*, and the posteroanterior view *below*

The so-called Lysholm line is a coordinate to calculate the expected normal position of the aqueduct. This line runs from the posterior-clinoid process vertical to the clivus as far as the inner table of the parietal skull. The aqueduct crosses this line at a point which is approximately one-third of the distance to the inner table.

The *aqueduct* is occasionally difficult to recognize since the border of the cartilage of the ear is found in the same location and can be confused with it. In such cases tomography or autotomography is recommended. It is also helpful if the ears are first bent forward and held in place with radiolucent tape. While the aqueduct may be readily seen on the routine lateral views, the required anteroposterior view is the half-axial exposure to project the aqueduct above the base of the skull.

The aqueduct is approximately 1.5–2 cm long and has a diameter of 1–3 mm. Normally it runs parallel to the clivus, 3.2–4 cm behind it (Fig. 156). It has two physiological constrictions which are occasionally visible: one at the lower level of the quadrigeminal plate and another below the posterior commissure. Although the course of the aqueduct is generally arched, it can also have a definite angulation which in some cases is accentuated by short, well-circumscribed areas of dilation. Even when no constrictions or dilations are present, the faint angulation is still present as the aqueduct passes between the superior and inferior colliculi. This variant is occasionally so striking that

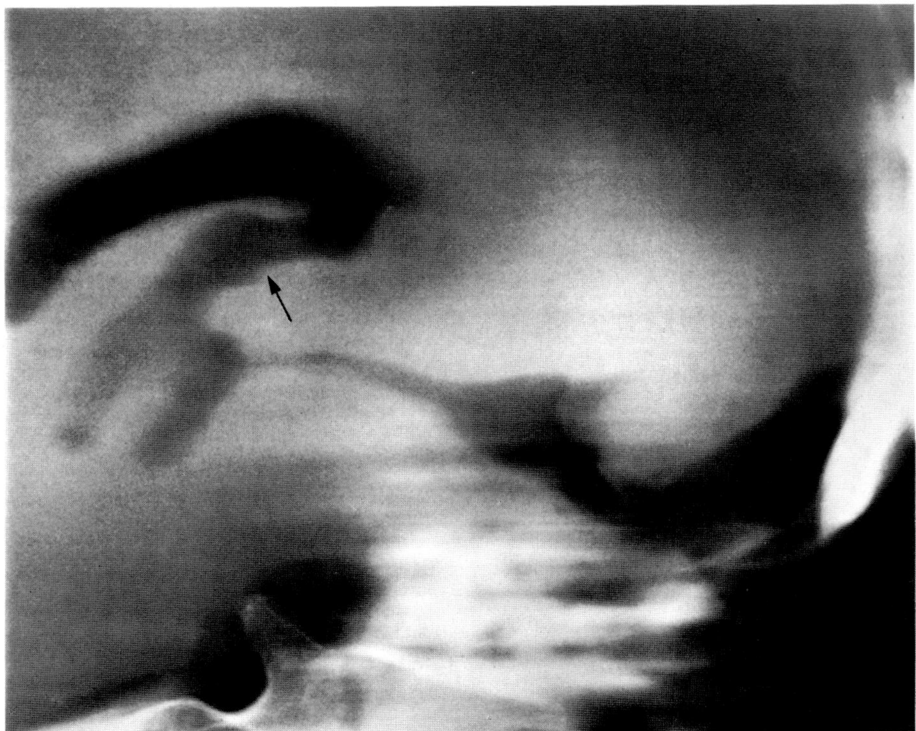

Fig. 159. Midline tomogram demonstrating air filling of a widened suprapineal recess (*arrow*). The cisterna magna looks triangular from this view

it resembles the pathological deformity of the aqueduct seen with certain tumors. A normally situated mid-brain cistern is helpful in establishing the correct diagnosis.

The *third ventricle* appears in the lateral view as a long, rhomboidal structure. The anterior-inferior portion of the third ventricle is not usually seen in the sitting position. There is instead a horizontal air-fluid level.

The *anterior wall of the third ventricle* consists of the lamina terminalis into which the anterior commisure occasionally projects as a small notch directly below the foramen of Monro. In most patients, the *massa intermedia* is found just before the middle of the third ventricle, usually as a round or oval shadow of varying size. With inadequate filling of the third ventricle, this structure can appear to extend to its roof and may be misdiagnosed as a tumor. The massa intermedia is anatomically missing 20% of the time. From a developmental point of view, the massa intermedia is a more or less distinct bridge of thalamic nuclei.

On the *posterior wall of the third ventricle* two extensions are usually found: the longer suprapineal recess and the shorter pineal recess. They are separated by the habenular commissure and the upper portion of the pineal gland (Fig. 152). The suprapineal recess may vary considerably. It is occasionally a few centimeters long and its width and course are extremely variable (Fig. 159). At the lower edge of the pineal recess lies the posterior commissure, below which the aqueduct passes into the posterior cranial fossa.

Remaining views in the sitting position: If air continues to be injected, the lateral ventricles will eventually be visualized on the lateral and anteroposterior views. In this position, the air will rise to the roof of both lateral ventricles, which are formed by the corpus callosum. By varying the head position, this structure can be outlined in its entirety (Fig. 156). In this manner, small invaginations into the ventricle from the corpus callosum can be recognized on the anteroposterior and lateral projections. One such invagination at the upper border of the frontal horn in the shape of a nose consists of radiations of the corpus callosum, and should not be confused with a genuine deformity of the frontal horn by an inwardly projecting tumor (Fig. 160).

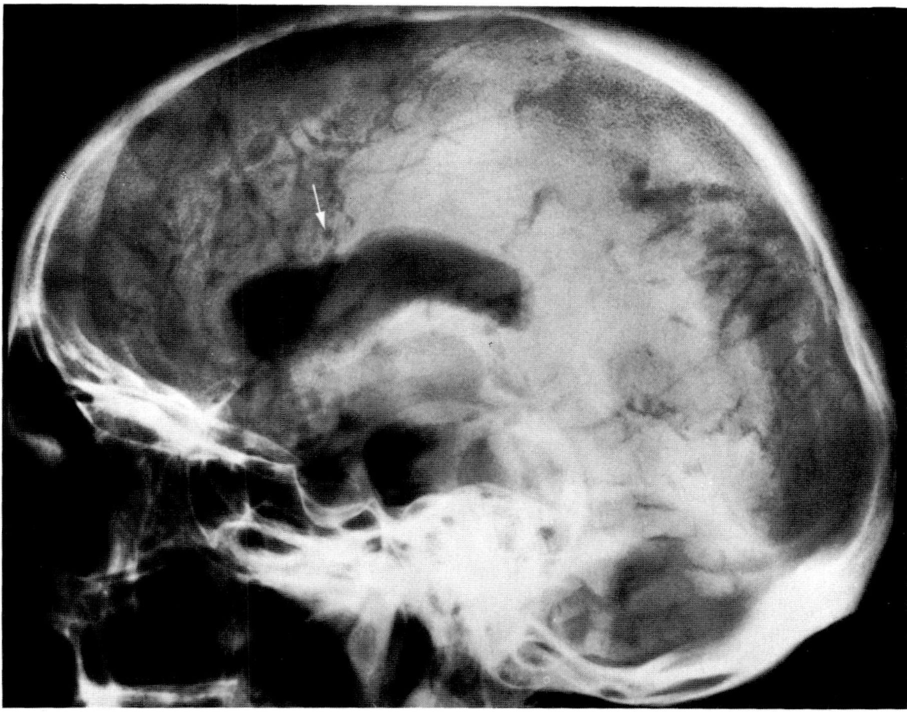

Fig. 160. Frontal horn, lateral view: note the indentations from the roof of the frontal horn corresponding to the normal corpus callosum (radiatio corporis callosi)

The Ventricle in the Supine (Brow-up) Position (Anteroposterior Exposure and Lateral Frontal Horn View)

The apex of the frontal horn: If the anteroposterior view is taken after adequate air filling, the entire frontal horn and cella media may be visualized (see diagrams 1, 2, and 3 in Figs. 157, 158). If the air filling is insufficient, only the frontal horns or even the apices alone may be visible as two rounded images projecting to either side of the midline, 1–2 cm apart. The frontal horn apices are occasionally overlooked when the air filling is minimal. The distance between the two structures is explained by divergent stresses on the frontal horn apices because of their position behind the knee of the corpus callosum and beneath its rostrum. Further posteriorly, the septum pellucidum separates the medial walls of the frontal horn; the inferior medial portions of the frontal horn apices are more separated. The intervening space here consists of the rostrum of the corpus callosum. Laterally the frontal horn apices are bordered by the frontal white matter, and anteriorly and superiorly by the corpus callosum. Posterior to the apex of the frontal horn is the head of the caudate nucleus. It arises from a lateral position and broadly invaginates the ventricle.

On the *lateral frontal horn view* the frontal horn apex has a curved, upwardly convex, fingertip-like shape. The boundary with the body of the frontal horn is marked by the bulge of the caudate head, which impinges on the ventricle from an inferolateral direction (Figs. 157, 158).

Concerning asymmetrical filling, see p. 193.

The body of the frontal horn: With additional filling of the frontal horn the second segment, known as the body of the frontal horn, also becomes visible. It is anatomically bounded medially by the septum, laterally by the caudate head, superiorly by the corpus callosum, and ends at the foramen of Monro (Fig. 161). In the anteroposterior view it lies medial to the weak image of the apex of the frontal horn described above and is shaped like a right triangle whose right angle points medially and superiorly (Figs. 157, 158). The image of the frontal horn body is more pronounced than that of the apex. The lateral ventricular wall has a definite bulge in children so that it sometimes ap-

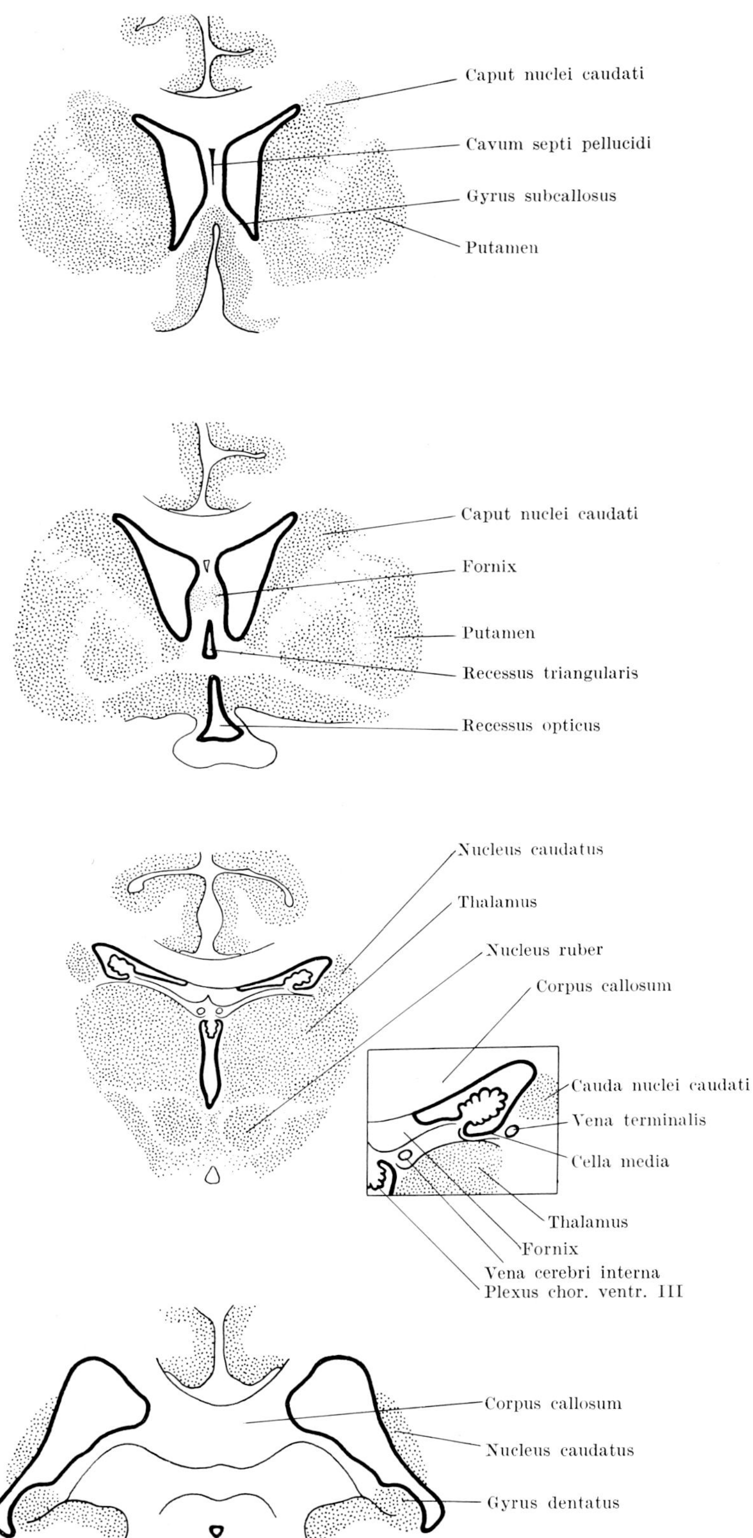

Fig. 161. Topographical limits of the various ventricular segments shown in different anteroposterior views

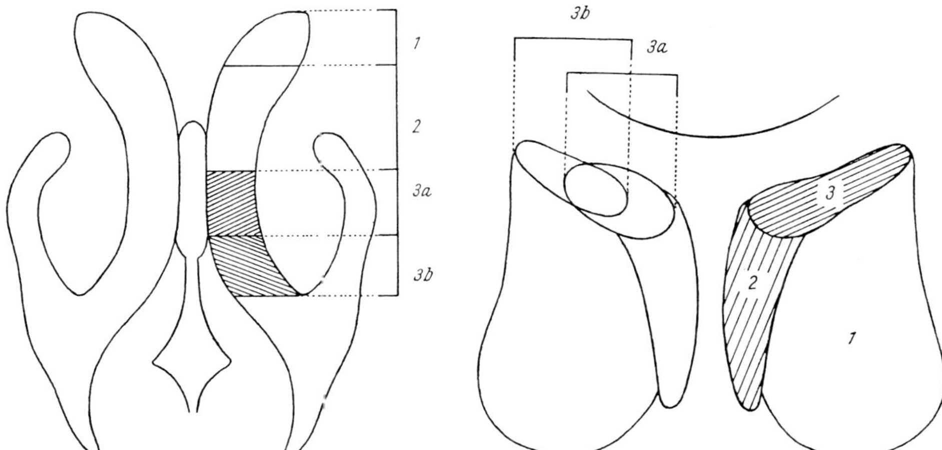

Fig. 162. The cella media (*3 a, 3 b*) is shown in the anteroposterior view as an area of uniform density, but is really made up of two segments which are partly superimposed. Of these, the posterior segment extends farther laterally. Thus, if only the anterior segment is filled on one side, while both segments are filled on the other, an asymmetrical enlargement of the one side when compared to the other will appear to have occurred

pears kinked. The lateral angle of the triangle, the so-called ventricular edge, is drawn out to a point in children (see Fig. 180). The septum, which is the only structure separating the frontal horns of either side, contains a small cleft at this level (Fig. 161).

In the *lateral view,* the combined apex and body of the frontal horn again form a curved, upwardly convex, finger-like structure which is attached to the foramen of Monro at its most posterior and inferior point. As the structure proceeds in the posterior direction, it begins to narrow.

The cella media: With still greater quantities of air, the cella media may also be visualized (Figs. 157, 158). It has the most intense image on the anteroposterior projection because it is superimposed on two other ventricle segments. In this projection it appears to be pear-shaped with its broadest part situated medially.

The cella media is bounded superiorly by the corpus callosum, laterally by the caudate nucleus, and inferiorly by the thalamus. At this level, the choroid plexus begins to project into the ventricle and is often visible as a small inferomedial out-pocketing (Fig. 161). The medial border of the cella media is no longer the septum, but rather the columns of both fornices (Figs. 161, 162), which diverge more as they move posteriorly. Thus, the cellae mediae of either side seem to move away from each other as they proceed posteriorly. Understanding this

principle will help to avoid one of the most common errors of interpretation of the anteroposterior view. If there is a difference in air filling between the two sides, so that more of the cella media is seen on one side, then that side will appear to project further laterally on the anteroposterior view than its counterpart (see Fig. 162). If one fails to appreciate the significance of this unequal filling, it may be erroneously concluded that a pathological asymmetry exists with unilateral ventricular enlargement. In order to avoid this mistake, it is necessary to compare the degree of filling of both sides on the lateral view before interpretating the anteroposterior view.

In the *lateral frontal horn view* the cella media is seen as a posterior extension of the frontal horn body which continues to narrow initially, then begins to expand again in its posterior portion.

Also seen together with the cella media on both anteroposterior and lateral projections is the *anterior part of the third ventricle.* In the anteroposterior view it has the appearance of a vertical pear with its broad part situated between the lower edges of the frontal horn body and with its narrow part pointed downward. If the anterior part of the third ventricle is instead round, it must be considered enlarged. Its diameter varies according to age, but the greatest diameter when employing a ventricle-film distance of 90–100 cm should be 8 mm. As a result of parallax distortion, this value is approximately 25% higher than its actual anatomical dimension. One should, however, not confuse the third ventricle with the more irregular, smaller, and more intense image of the cistern of the lamina terminalis which is also midline in location but extends more in a basal direction.

On the lateral frontal horn view, two cone-shaped projections are seen to extend from the anterior-inferior segment of the third ventricle in the direction of the sella. Together, these projections remind one of an open "fish mouth", with the optic and infundibular recesses constituting the jaws and the optic chiasm the mouth (see Fig. 175).

Films taken in the *supine* (brow-up) position may also show the air-filled apices of the *temporal horns*. They are seen on the *anteroposterior view* as crescent-shaped, medially concave structures projecting within the orbits or on each orbital roof. This shape results from the indentation of the hippocampus, which lies on the floor of the temporal horn. The apices of the temporal horns embrace the hippocampal digitations from above. Variations in shape on the lateral view results from differences in the morphology of the hippocampal uncus. On the *lateral view* the temporal horn has the appearance of a spout with its tip bent slightly downward above and behind the sella. Normally, the tips of the temporal horns point toward the dorsum sella.

In the *anteroposterior half-axial projections* the ventricular chambers are represented obliquely. With extreme air filling they may be visualized throughout their length. Likewise, the third ventricle will be seen on this view. This projection permits especially good recognition of pathological indentations into the ventricle from either side.

Ventricular Views in the Prone (Brow-Down) Position (Posteroanterior Projection and Lateral Occipital Horn View)

The occipital horn: Pneumoencephalograms obtained with the patient on his abdomen (brow-down) also vary depending on the degree of air filling present. With lesser amounts of air only the occipital horns and trigones are visualized.

Of all the ventricular segments, the *occipital horn* shows the greatest degree of variability. In a *lateral view* it can be sharply pointed or

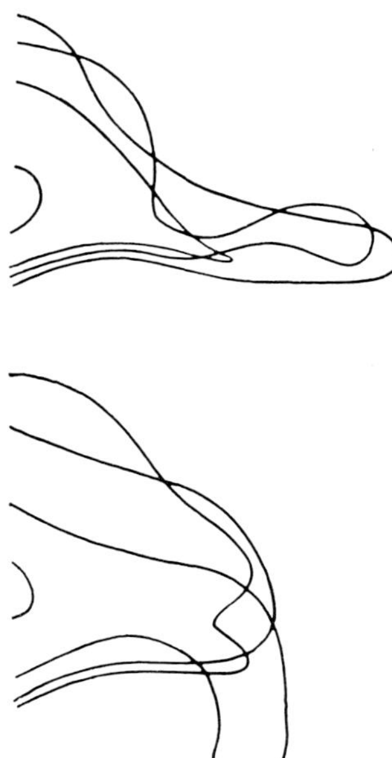

Fig. 163. Various shapes of the occipital horn, some of which are seen with ventricular enlargement. All of these and many more similar shapes may occur as physiological variants (DYES 1937)

blunted or hook-shaped. In the latter case, the hook may point up but usually points down. The occipital horns can occasionally appear as thin finger-like extensions reaching nearly to the occipital pole. This variant is most common on the left side (Fig. 163). The occipital horns can also be absent. This anomaly should therefore not be misinterpreted as indicating the presence of a tumor.

In the *posteroanterior projection*, the beams penetrate the long axis of the occipital horns so that they are represented only as round or oval, approximately penny-sized structures, somewhat medial to the trigone, which they partially overlap. The intensity of the contrast image may also vary considerably. On the lateral occipital horn view, their actual shape with all its variations is apparent, although superimposition with the other side does occur. The diversification of occipital horn images can be confusing and frequently leads to misdiagnoses.

If a better picture in the posteroanterior projection is desired, the half-axial posteroanterior view is recommended (Fig. 164). Anatomically, the occipital horns are surrounded by the white matter of the occipital lobes.

The trigone: The trigone is seldom seen on *anteroposterior views* because of the quantity of

Fig. 164. Schematic representation of a pneumoencephalogram showing the anterior and posterior ventricular segments in the half-axial and reverse half-axial views

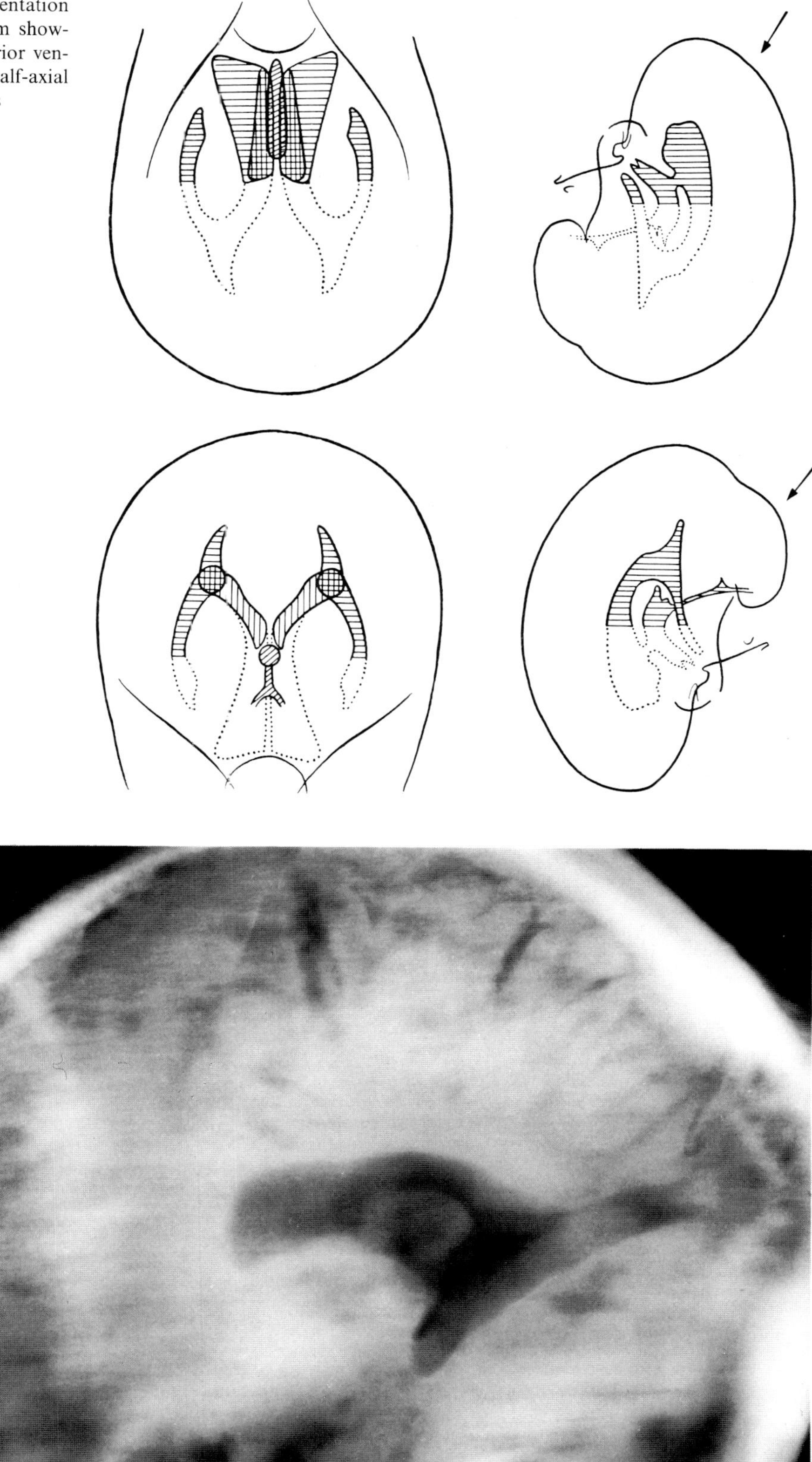

Fig. 165. Enlarged glomus of the choroid plexus

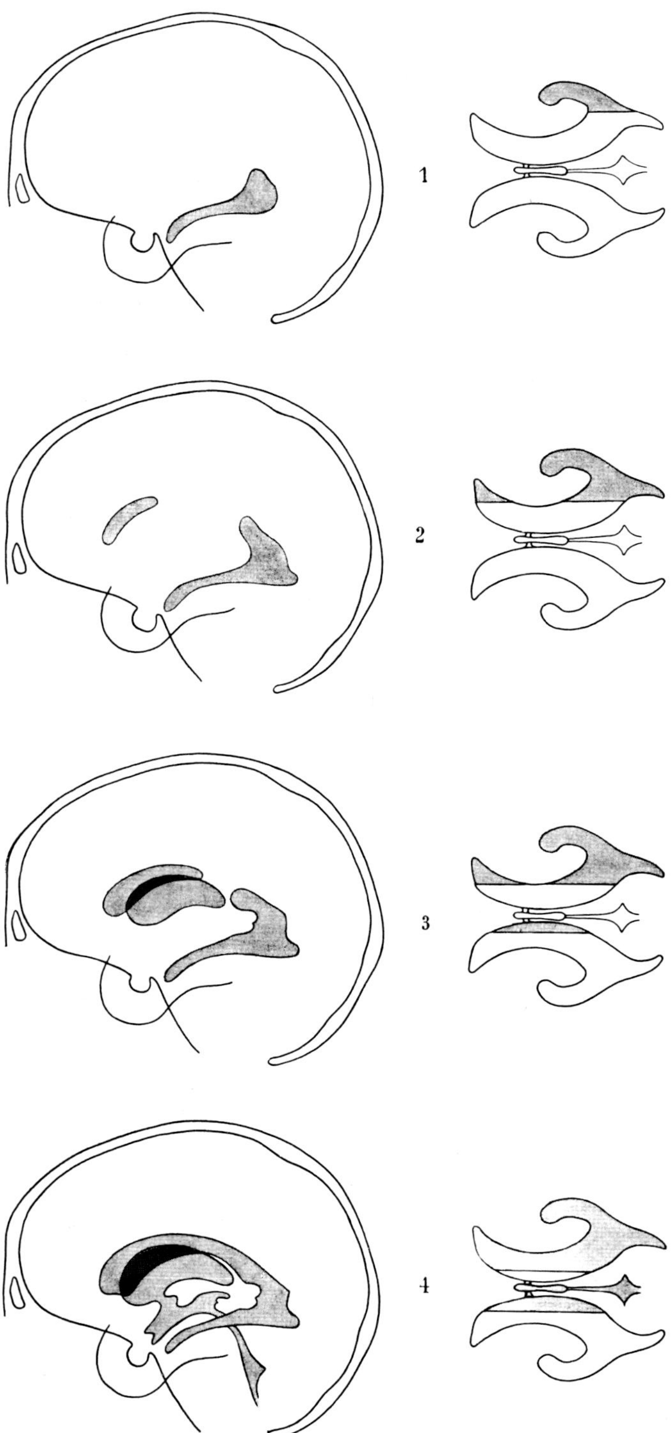

Fig. 166. Schematic representation of the lateral pneumoencephalogram with various degrees of ventricular filling

air required to fill it. On the other hand, it is regularly visualized on the posteroanterior projection, where it is found on either side of the midline as an obliquely placed, finger-like structure forming an angle of 60° with the horizontal. There is a slight angulation present in its midpart. On the posteroanterior projection, each trigone diverges from its partner as it courses inferiorly. The most medial superior edge of the trigone represents its point of juncture with the cella media. At this point the distance between trigones is approximately 2–3 cm. Somewhat medial to and beneath the trigone shadow is found the image of the occipital horn (Figs. 157, 158). Along the medial border in the upper half of the trigone, the glomus of the choroid plexus is frequently seen. This structure is sometimes enlarged and may be cystic (Fig. 165) or calcified.

On the *lateral occipital horn view* the trigone has a characteristic triangular form. The three ventricular horns – including the cella media – form the three corners of the triangle. Anatomically, the trigone is bounded superiorly by the corpus callosum and medially and inferiorly by the fornix and thalamus (Fig. 161). The lateral wall consists of parieto-occipital white matter, particularly the optic radiations and the inferior longitudinal fasciculus.

It is important to keep in mind two special structures: at the transition of cella media to trigone a "knotty defect" is often found in the anterior ventricular shadow, consisting of the choroid glomus mentioned above (Fig. 165). At the point of transition from trigone to posterior horn, a second structure is frequently found projecting into the ventricle from a posterior-inferior direction, corresponding to the eminentia collateralis (calcar avis). It is even more apparent when the occipital horn is aplastic. When present, these structures should not be confused with pathological changes.

On the lateral occipital horn view, the posterior portion of the third ventricle and aqueduct are often well-defined, but only if the air does not flow back into the spinal canal. On the other hand, the fourth ventricle is for the most part covered over by bony structures. Occasionally, portions of the temporal horn are also demonstrated.

On the posteroanterior projection, the caudal and occipital portions of both cellae mediae are also often seen, which are represented as diagonal oval images, 1–2 cm apart. Between and somewhat below these, the posterior portion of the third ventricle is frequently found, appearing as an almost circular shadow in this projection. Its diameter averages 5 mm, although in the elderly it can reach 8 mm (see above pp. 203, 204, projection in comparative sizes). With incomplete air filling one may see only a small round shadow, namely the suprapineal recess of the third ventricle. Sometimes the pineal gland is projected into the third ventricle in such a way that it divides the posterior portion into two halves, one above the other.

In order to judge the exact position of the aqueduct and fourth ventricle on the posteroanterior projection, it is necessary to obtain *a half-axial posteroanterior exposure* which projects the base of the skull away from these structures (Fig. 164).

The Ventricular Picture in the Lateral Position

In the right or left lateral position, the highest portion of the ventricle, the temporal horn, will fill preferentially. Therefore, the lateral position is preferred if that structure is to be studied. This technique is seldom employed today, however, since the temporal horn pictures obtained in the sitting, prone, and supine positions, as well as the special views cited earlier, are usually adequate. Occasionally, an almost complete picture of the lateral ventricle is obtained with the lateral position. In such a case, however, there is frequently some superimposition of air from the opposite lateral ventricle. Since it is unlikely that all air will successfully exit through the foramen of Monro, considering its position, it is inevitable that some air remains trapped within the lower lateral ventricle. This means that the lateral parts of the higher ventricle and the medial parts of the lower ventricle will be superimposed (Fig. 166).

The temporal horn: On films taken in the *sagittal projections* (anteroposterior, posteroanterior, half-axial), the temporal horns are usually only partially filled unless one employs a special technique (see p. 191). It has already been pointed out that in the anteropostererior projection (with the chin elevated) the temporal horn tips are projected into the orbits.

Anatomically, the temporal horn is bounded superiorly by the white matter of the temporal lobe, superomedially by the tail of the caudate nucleus, inferomedially by the hippocampus, and laterally by the temporal white matter.

In the *lateral view,* the temporal horn projects from the lower margin of the trigone as a diminishing shadow in the general direction of the posterior clinoid. It is slightly upwardly concave in the vicinity of the trigone, while its terminal segment is for the most part downwardly concave. At its tip a hook-shaped process is often found pointing inferiorly toward the posterior clinoid process. This hook can at times be heavily contrasted (see above). The temporal horn can be quite variable in shape and may also vary in the proximity of its tip to the temporal pole (normal distance 2–3 cm).

2. The Subarachnoid Pathways

For the analysis of air studies of the subarachnoid pathways, it is necessary first to review mentally CSF flow patterns through these spaces (KEY and RETZIUS, 1875; SPATZ and STROESCU, 1934; LILIEQUIST 1959). For practical purposes, we have adopted the designations of LILIEQUIST in order to achieve uniformity with respect to nomenclature (see Figs. 167–176 and p. 8).

The cisterns: From the cisterna magna the CSF flows along the anterior side of the brain stem through the cisterns of the medulla oblongata and pons to the interpeduncular cistern, then farther to the remaining basal cisterns, and finally to each Sylvian fissure. From here the CSF passes over the convexities. Another pattern of flow is that which runs anteriorly through the chiasmatic cisterns and the cistern of the lamina terminalis to the cistern of the corpus callosum. From here the CSF flows posteriorly over the corpus callosum to the pineal region (Fig. 167).

An additional path to the pontine cistern from the fourth ventricle is by way of the lateral recesses. From the basal cisterns the CSF flows to either side of the midbrain in the ambient cisterns, which join together in the pineal region. This same point may also be reached from the cisterna magna by CSF flowing superiorly over the midline vermis.

Cisterna magna cerebellomedullaris: The bow-shaped cisterna magna is depicted in the pneumoencephalogram as a collection of air between the bony posterior limits of the posterior cranial fossa and the posterior inferior surface of the cerebellum. It is approximately 2×3 cm wide. The cistern lies at the point of exit of the foramen of Magendie, behind and below the tonsils and over the brain stem. It is best recognized on the lateral projection and takes the shape of a triangle in this view (Fig. 159). Its size can vary considerably. Both tonsils extend into the cistern from their anterior-superior location, where they are usually readily recognized. Physiological variants are occasionally seen in which the tonsils extend so far inferiorly as to project beneath the rim of the foramen magnum.

Impressive dilations of the cisterna magna can be seen as normal variants. They may, however, also represent atrophy of the adjacent cerebellum. Whenever an enlarged cisterna magna is encountered, delayed ventricular filling should be anticipated.

For recognition of the vallecula, the deep midportion of the cisterna magna, the *half-axial posteroanterior projection* is most often employed. The vallecula lies normally in a midposition between the two tonsils. It can undergo a significant displacement in association with a laterally placed tumor within the posterior cranial fossa. With the appropriate head position and quantity of air, the *cisterna medullaris* may be outlined. It lies ventral to the medulla oblongata and can only be demonstrated in the sitting position by the half-axial posteroanterior projection (Fig. 170), or on the lateral views by tomography. The lateral extensions of this cistern consist of the cerebellopontine angle or pontocerebellar cisterns (see Figs. 169, 170).

The *paired pontocerebellar cisterns* communicate with the pontine, ambient, and medullary cisterns. They are found on either side of the midline within the cerebellopontine angle. Normally, the pontocerebellar cisterns on each side are similar in length and appearance. Small variations can occur as a result of an asymmetrical development of the skull, particularly with respect to the height and size of the petrous pyramids. On the half-axial posteroanterior exposure, the petrosal vein may be recognized in the lateral corner of the cistern surrounded by air. Through the medial portion of the cistern runs the trigeminal nerve, which in individual cases may be recognized on the sagittal projection.

The following points describe the three different variations of the normal cistern as outlined by LILIEQUIST (1959):

a) The pontocerebellar cistern ends near the internal acoustic meatus and the outer boundary of the ambient cistern.

b) The pontocerebellar cistern ends lateral to the internal acoustic meatus and appears to be widened toward the end.

c) The cistern extends farther laterally. Its extension is so thin that a definite determination of its limits is no longer possible.

The *pontine cistern* is best demonstrated in the lateral sitting position (Fig. 167). Here it is represented as a plate-like collection of air anterior to the pons. Its width from the dorsum sellae to the ventral surface of the pons measures 8 mm. However, in the sitting position

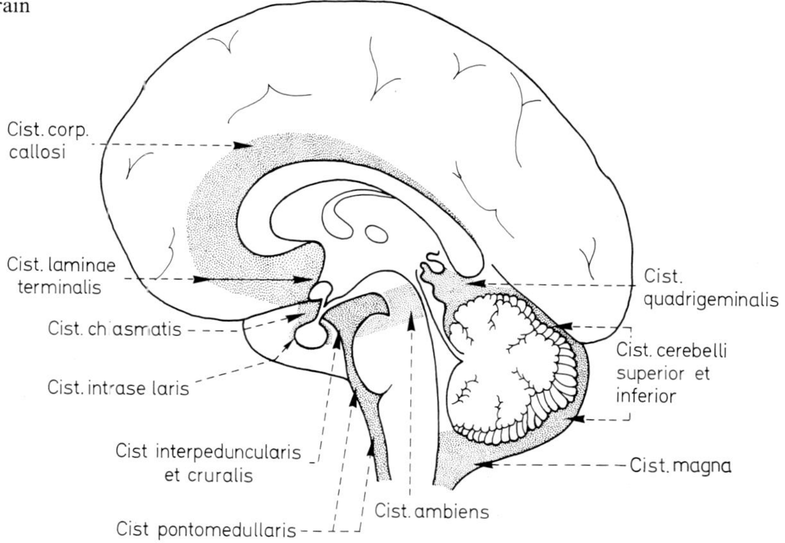

Fig. 167. The major cisterns of the brain in the mid-sagittal section

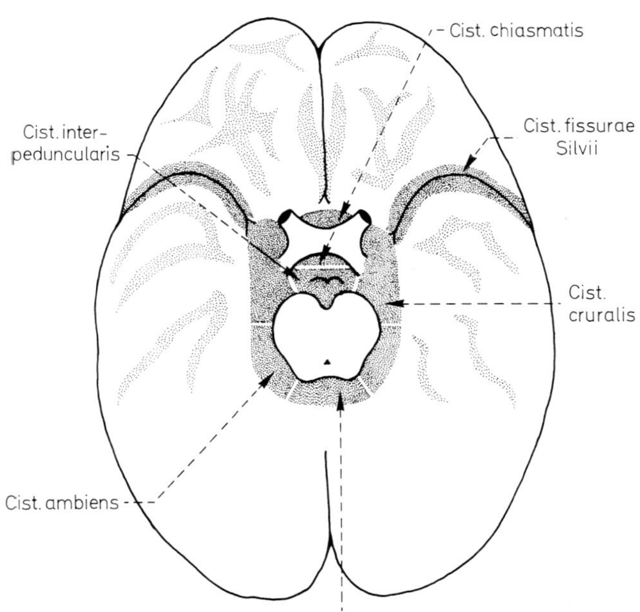

Fig. 168. Schematic representation of the basal cisterns

with the head flexed forward the brain will tend to slide forward somewhat with the result that this distance may be narrowed. When present, such narrowing should not be interpreted as pathological. The basilar artery is almost always apparent within the pontine cistern and is seen particularly clearly on midline tomography (Fig. 171).

The pontine cistern communicates above with the *interpeduncular cistern,* which lies between the peduncles and reaches the posterior margin of the pituitary stalk. From above and anteriorly, the mamillary bodies project into this cistern. Anteriorly, a thin membrane is found (LILIEQUIST, 1959) which in many instances impedes the passage of the air into the chiasmatic cistern.

Within the interpeduncular cistern, the oculomotor nerve is sometimes seen on the lateral view. With adequate air filling, the basilar artery (and its bifurcation) will also be clearly apparent. Occasionally, the origins of the poste-

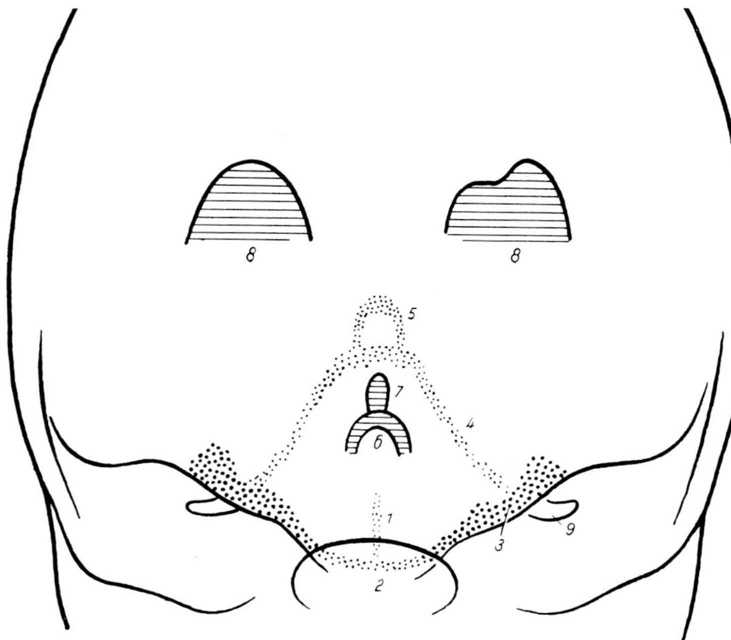

Fig. 169. Schematic representation of the cisterns of the posterior cranial fossa in the half-axial view. Air is seen in the vallecula (*1*), pontomedullary cisterns (*2*), pontocerebellar cisterns (*3*), ambient cisterns (*4*), quadrigeminal cisterns (*5*), within the fourth ventricle (*6*), within the third ventricle (*7*), and in the trigone and occipital horns (*8*). The internal auditory meatus is numbered (*9*)

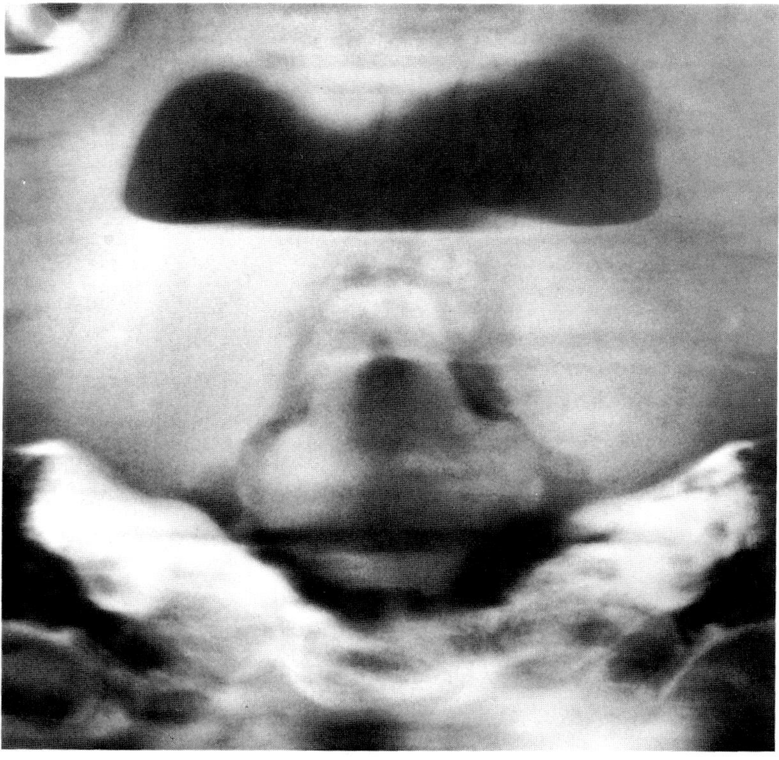

Fig. 170. Half-axial tomogram of the air-filled brain stem and cerebellopontine angle cisterns

rior cerebral and superior cerebellar arteries are visible as well, but tend to project in the direction of the incident X-ray beam.

In the half-axial posteroanterior projection, the picture of the interpeduncular cistern in combination with the bilateral *crural cisterns* forms the "crown of three peaks". The crural cisterns lie to either side of the anterior cerebral peduncle and comprise the lateral "peaks". They then continue as the ambient cisterns. The middle "peak" consists of the interpeduncular cistern (Fig. 172).

Fig. 171. Pontine cistern (*arrow*)

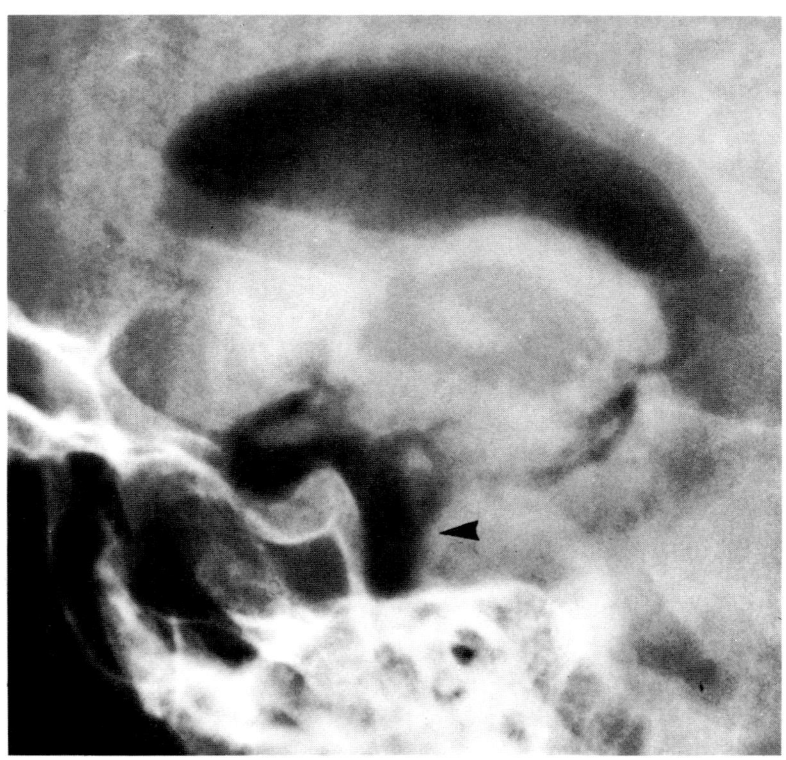

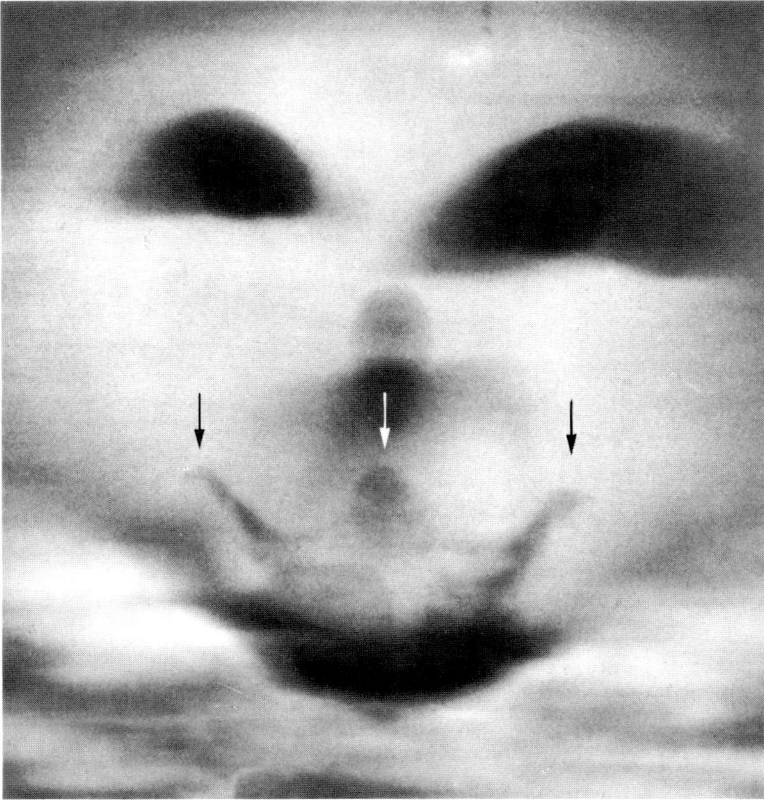

Fig. 172. Interpeduncular and crural cisterns (the so-called crown of three peaks)

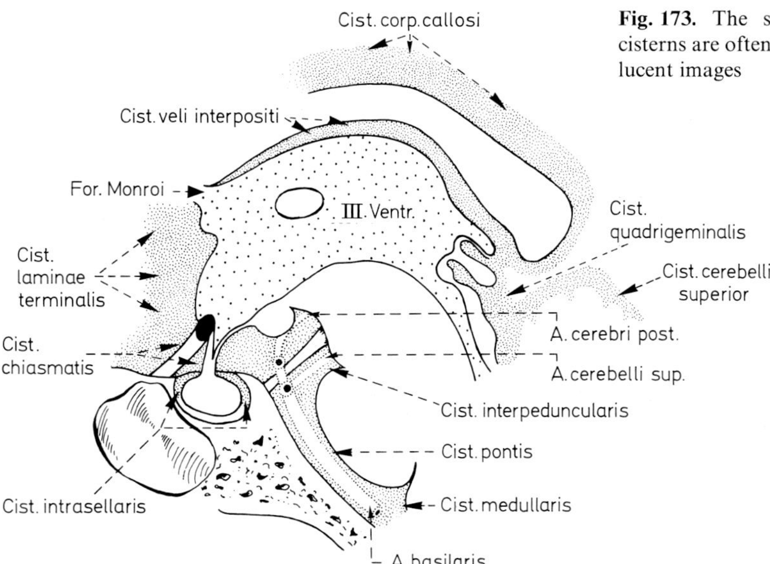

Fig. 173. The structures shown here traversing the cisterns are often recognizable in cisternograms as radiolucent images

Anterior to the pituitary stalk is found the *chiasmatic cistern,* which sits above the sella and totally embraces the optic nerves throughout their subarachnoid course. This cistern is separated from the interpeduncular cistern by the previously described thin arachnoid membrane of LILIEQUIST. It consists of two sections, the prechiasmatic and the postchiasmatic. It borders anteriorly with the cistern of the lamina terminalis (Fig. 167).

Although the chiasmatic cistern is clearly seen on the *lateral view,* it can only be demonstrated on the anteroposterior projection through tomography. A number of additional structures may also be seen passing through in well-contrasted studies (chiasm and optic nerves, internal carotid arteries) (Fig. 173).

Beneath the chiasmatic cistern, an *intrasellar cistern* is occasionally demonstrated which, when enlarged, constitutes the "empty sella". It can extend deep within the confines of the sella (Fig. 173).

Anterior and superior to the chiasmatic cistern is found the *cistern of the lamina terminalis.* This cistern extends superiorly to the rostrum of the corpus callosum. Because it is frequently superimposed on the anterior portion of the cistern of the Sylvian fissure, its precise boundaries may be difficult to determine. It is, however, clearly seen on the anteroposterior view (see p. 204, Fig. 174).

The cisterns of the Sylvian fissures: These cisterns are well portrayed on the sagittal (an-

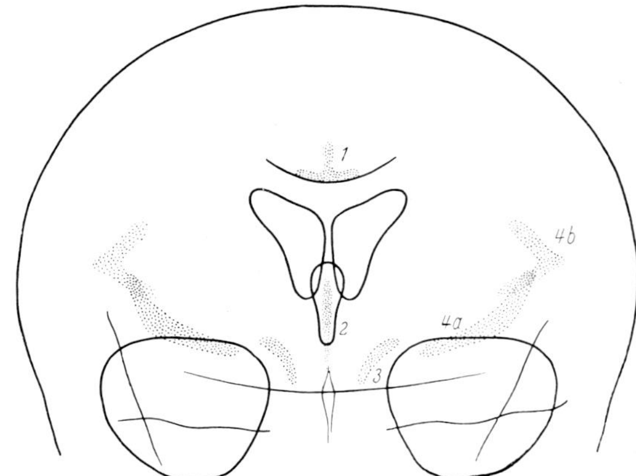

Fig. 174. Schematic representation of the various cisterns as seen in the anteroposterior pneumoencephalogram: cistern of the corpus callosum (*1*); cistern of the lamina terminalis (*2*); olfactory sulci (*3*); sphenoid wing segment of the Sylvian fissure (*4a*); and insular segment of the Sylvian fissure (*4b*)

teroposterior) projection. They extend bilaterally from the chiasmatic cistern in a medial concave curve in an outward and upward direction. From the peak of the curve a short laterally directed process extends to the convexity. The cistern is readily apparent as a light shadow on all views, if one first mentally traces the expected course of the middle cerebral artery. When the cisternal image is more intensely portrayed, the beginnings of atrophy of the adjacent brain are probably present (Figs. 174, 176). In the lateral view the cistern is represented as large individual furrows.

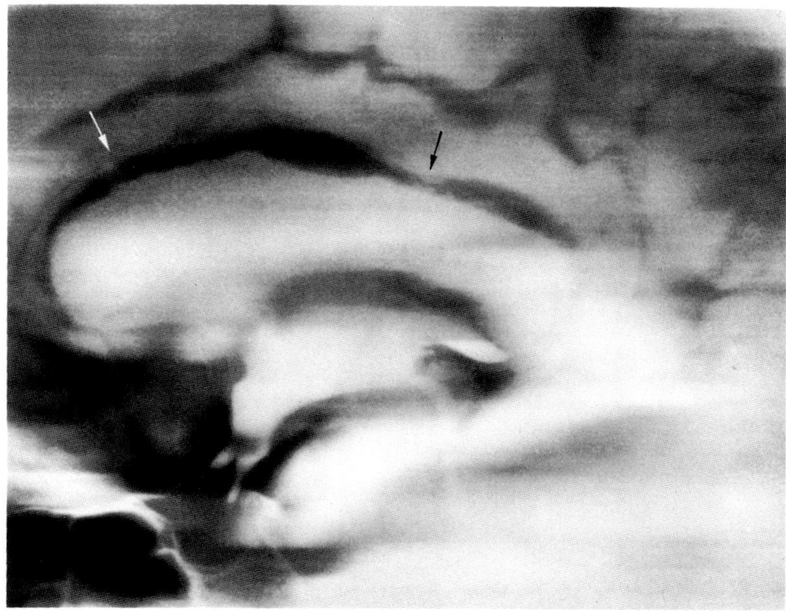

The *cistern of the corpus callosum* (the cistern of the interhemispheric fissure): This cistern has such a characteristic appearance that it cannot be missed on the lateral view. It sits above the curved surface of the corpus callosum and can be divided into three sections: an anterior section, above the genu of the corpus callosum; a middle section, above the body itself; a posterior section, above the splenium. At its posterior limit, the cistern of the corpus callosum communicates with the quadrigeminal cistern. Anteriorly, it is in communication with the cistern of the lamina terminalis (Fig. 175).

If the curve of the callosal cistern is exaggerated, one can assume – as with a similar deformity of the pericallosal artery – that hydrocephalic enlargement of the lateral ventricles is present. This is because the corpus callosum forms the roof of the lateral ventricles (Fig. 167).

On the sagittal view, the cistern of the corpus callosum is equally characteristic, forming an anchor-shaped shadow above the corpus callosum (Fig. 174).

The *quadrigeminal cistern* (cistern of the great vein of Galen) lies above the quadrigeminal plate. The superior and inferior colliculi appear at the base of the air-filled cistern as two round indentations (Fig. 156). The quadrigeminal cistern should always be demonstrated on the pneumoencephalogram in order to determine the precise border of the quadrigeminal plate. This is best accomplished by means of a lateral film taken with the patient sitting. Projecting anteriorly is the *cistern of the velum interpositum* (see Fig. 202), which lies above the roof of the third ventricle. This structure is more often seen in children and rarely in adults, primarily in association with pathological states (see p. 243). The quadrigeminal cistern communicates above with the *cistern of the corpus callosum* and below with the *superior cerebellar cistern,* lying over the upper vermis. Inferiorly, it inserts itself between the anterior surface of the cerebellar vermis and the more anteriorly situated roof of the fourth ventricle. At this level the cistern is separated from the fourth ventricle only by the thin anterior medullary velum. Because of this, a communication between the ventricle and the cistern may erroneously be thought to exist.

The colliculi of the quadrigeminal plate are also clearly seen on the half-axial posteroanterior projection. The upper portion of the cistern tends to extend over the third ventricle in this projection and permits good visualization of the communication of the quadrigeminal cistern with both ambient cisterns.

Of all cisterns, the *ambient cisterns* are most frequently seen on the pneumoencephalogram (Figs. 168, 169, 170). They are paired and extend around the midbrain from the crural cisterns on each side to the pineal region, where they join the quadrigeminal cistern. The ambi-

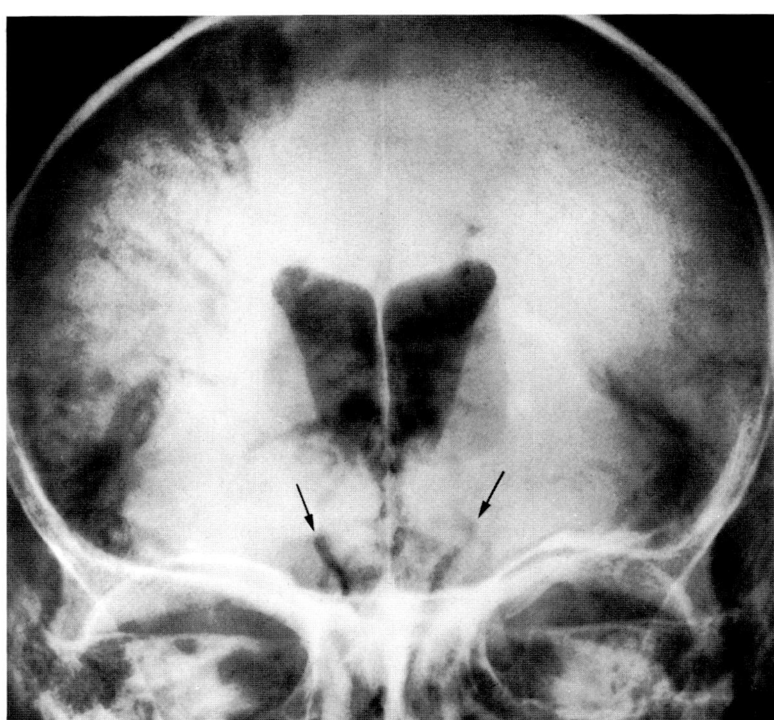

Fig. 176. Dilation of the ventricular system and the cisterns of the Sylvian fissure. Air is also seen in the olfactory sulci (*arrow*)

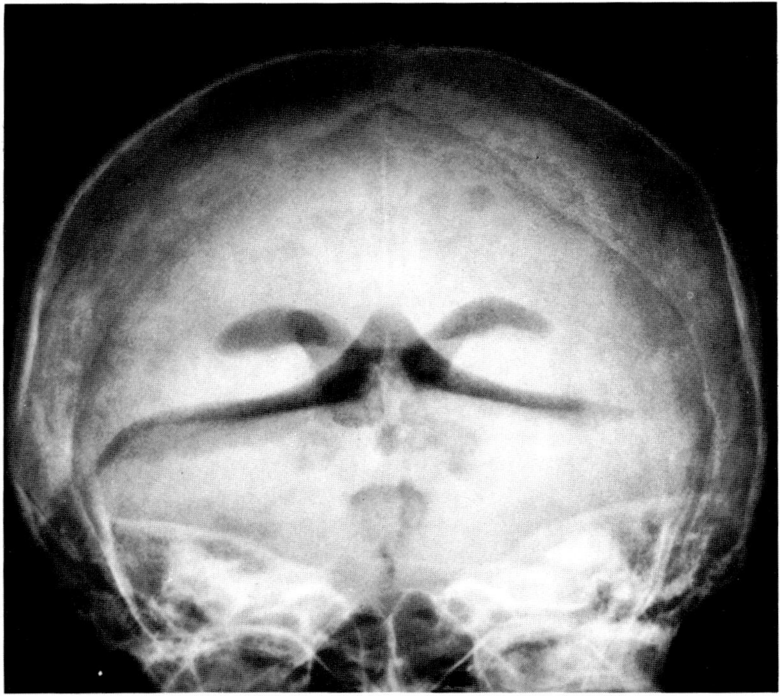

Fig. 177. Anteroposterior air study with filling of the subdural space below the tentorium as well as the ventricular system

ent cisterns send two processes anteriorly and laterally on each side which embrace the pulvinar like a wing (ala) ("ambient wings", "retropulvinar cisterns"). Extending into the ambient cisterns from either side are the sharp edges of the tentorium. They divide the cistern into supratentorial and infratentorial sections. In the half-axial posteroanterior exposure, these sections are projected one on top of the other. Thus, the cistern may appear wider in this view than it actually is. Situated laterally from the rather pronounced image of the ambient cisterns is the weaker image of both wings, which are easily overlooked.

On the lateral projection, only the wings of the ambient cisterns are visible. These bilateral wings – representing the retrothalamic (retropulvinar) spaces – look like commas lying on top of each other, pointing in the direction of the interpeduncular cistern. Superiorly, the ambient wings project toward the middle of the quadrigeminal plate or somewhat beneath it.

The sulci: With pneumoencephalography in a normal brain the sulci are usually quite thin. They become more pronounced with the beginning of involutional atrophy (in the frontal and parietal lobes) or with diffuse brain atrophy (see Figs. 212, 213). Therefore, the sulci of the three frontal gyri, the postcentral gyri, and the medial cortex are all usually prominent. With the help of an atlas of anatomy, identification of these is not difficult.

The olfactory sulci are found on the basal surface of each frontal lobe between the gyrus rectus and the orbital gyri. They extend posteriorly as far as the olfactory trigones. Both sulci lie near the midline and diverge upward. Posteriorly, they communicate with the chiasmatic cistern. Air within the olfactory sulci is only visible on the anteroposterior view of supine (brow-up) patients. Each sulcus is approximately 1 cm high and they are steeper and closer to the midline than the crural cistern, so that confusion between the two should not exist (Fig. 176).

Subdural air: If some air gets into the subdural space on the pneumoencephalogram, this can be recognized by its predilection for certain sites. Also its sharp, smooth contours tend to distinguish it easily from subarachnoid air. Subdural air may be encountered beneath the tentorium (in which case the tentorium may be represented in its entirety on the posteroanterior view, Fig. 177), in the interhemispheric space near the falx, adjacent to the frontal and occipital poles, and less commonly anterior to the pons.

VIII. General Rules for the Interpretation of Pneumoencephalograms

In the evaluation of the pneumoencephalogram, one must keep in mind normal variants and the limitations of the technique (particularly inadequate air filling and improper positioning) before drawing any conclusions. *Otherwise, false interpretation of pathological change may be made.*

Before concluding that pathological findings are present, certain preliminary questions must be posed and answered in each case: *Are the films obtained technically correct and how do they compare with known normal variants?* In the sagittal view (anteroposterior or posteroanterior) the orbitomeatal line should always be perpendicular to the film plane. Then the upper border of the petrous pyramid will be projected into the middle or lower third of the orbit. Each pyramid should be of the same height unless there is a pre-existing anomaly with respect to the base of the skull. The "height" of the ventricular chambers and their shape on the anteroposterior and posteroanterior views depend to a large extent on the direction of the incidental beams, as Fig. 178 shows. In *the sagittal* plane the positioning is correct if the distance between the outer rims of the orbit (or the mandibular rami or mastoid processes) and the outer border of the skull is the same on both sides (Fig. 179). In the presence of head rotation, the true determination of any lateral ventricular displacement is impossible.

The correct projection for the *lateral view* has been achieved only when the contours of both orbital roofs and those of the mandibles are superimposed. This of course will not be possible in the event of cranial anomalies such as those seen with infantile spastic cerebral hemiplegia.

Furthermore, the following questions must be clarified: *Which ventricular parts are filled and which should have filled considering the position of the patient and the technique employed? What is the diagnostic merit of this particular view?* We must first determine the relative filling of each comparable ventricular chamber. On the anteroposterior and posteroanterior projections alone it is often possible to estimate comparative filling by considering the contour and intensity of the image obtained on each side. Such a determination is especially important in comparing the frontal horns and cellae mediae of both sides. In this respect the lateral projections will provide the answer (lateral frontal horn and lateral occipital horn views). If this determination has not been correctly made, comparison of the relative width of the lateral ventricles in the posteroanterior and anteroposterior views will result in a false impression of *unilateral ventricular dilation,* since the side with the greatest air filling will seem to be larger. This is because the side with enough air to fill out the cella media will appear wider than the side where only the frontal horn is filled (see left-hand upper part of Fig. 154, and Fig. 162). It is also important in evaluating lateral films to determine beforehand (by considering the sagittal view) which side has the greatest air filling (see p. 203).

In comparing each cella media on the sagittal projection, it is important to keep in mind that they are mirror images of one another since they diverge sharply as they proceed posteriorly. One must also remember in making these comparisons that the *pneumoencephalogram is not a tomographic representation of a single plane, but rather a composite picture of an air-filled ventricular system with air pockets lying in the direction of the anteroposterior beams superimposed upon each other.*

Finally, it is frequently difficult to tell "where normal ends and abnormal begins" even under the best of conditions, because there is no prior determination of "normal" for a given patient. Individual variations are common and are dependent upon the shape of the skull and the age of the patient (Fig. 180). Nor do we know anything yet about potential "cyclic variations" in venticular size which may occur depending upon the time of day.

Each evaluation must take into consideration the *age of the patient* since a progressive enlargement of the CSF pathways has already begun by the end of the 3rd decade. The brain weight from this point on begins to decrease. The width and diameter of both cellae mediae and the third ventricle begin to enlarge in the fifties (Fig. 180). Moderate and marked widening is found by the age of 60. Cortical atrophy also becomes more impressive with advancing age. This is not to say that the degree of cerebral atrophy will be the same for everyone in a given age group, rather that the highest age

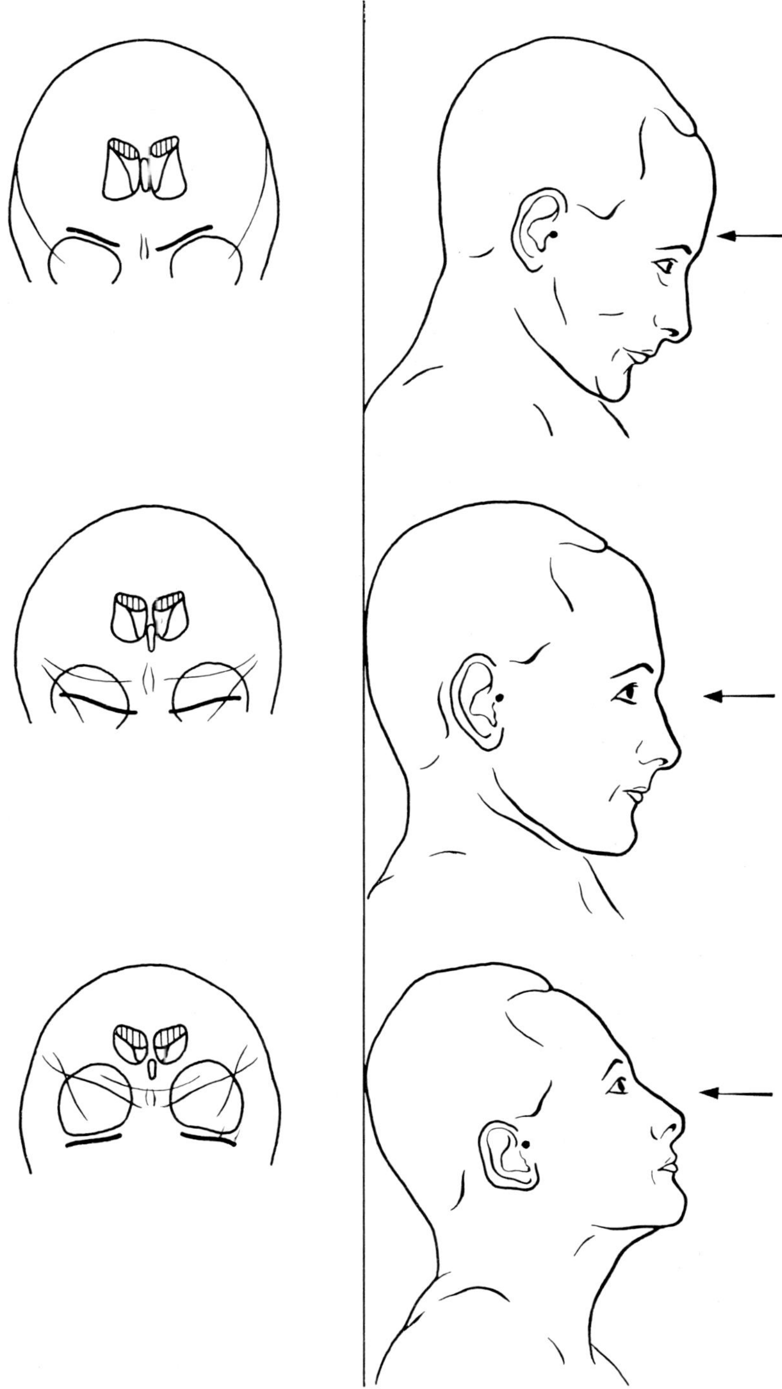

Fig. 178. Schematic representation of the expected ventricular shapes depending upon projection. *Middle:* correct head position with the orbito-meatal line horizontal. Here the upper borders of the petrous pyramids are projected into the orbits

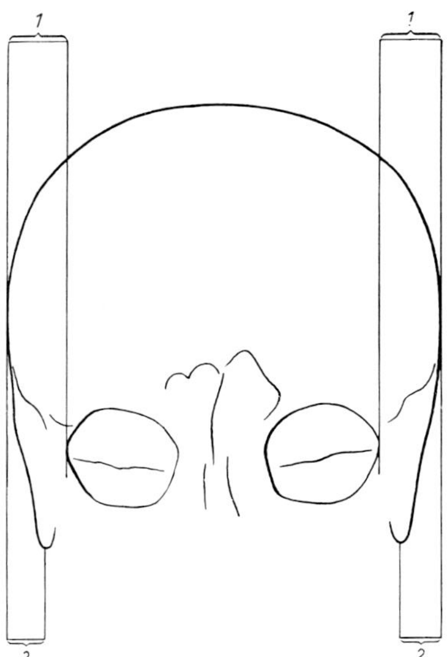

Fig. 179. To eliminate rotation, the correct anteroposterior or posteroanterior head position is confirmed by comparing the distance between the lateral margin of the skull and the outer border of the orbit (*1*) or mastoid process (*2*) on each side. In addition, the upper border of the petrous pyramid should be level and projected into the middle of each orbit

groups will have, relatively speaking, the greatest number of cases of advanced atrophy and ventricular enlargement.

In addition to the "physiological" aging process, consideration must also be given to the countless "normal" variants possible, which were described earlier.

The beginner should therefore accustom himself to review automatically the various sources of error presented in this chapter before deciding that definite pathology exists.

The objective measurement of ventricular size: It would be most useful if there were a method for *calculating ventricular size "objectively" using measurements* obtained from the sagittal and lateral exposures, in order to avoid the subjective inaccuracies of varying interpretations from different observers. A variety of such methods have already been described, but none has been uniformly accepted. The simplest and most reliable method utilizes a single measurement of the third ventricle (SCHIERSMANN 1952, HUBER 1957, etc.). One such method is the measurement of the ventricle in the anteroposterior view by drawing a line from its superomedial edge to its waist. This gives an estimate of the ventricular width. However, this method is still inaccurate since the measured value is not adjusted for variations in the width of the skull.

When ventricular size is smaller than the lowest limits of normal, there is said to be *ventricular hypoplasia.* It should be distinguished from secondary ventricular compressions such as those seen in association with cerebral pathology, particularly cerebral edema (for pseudotumor cerebri, see p. 250).

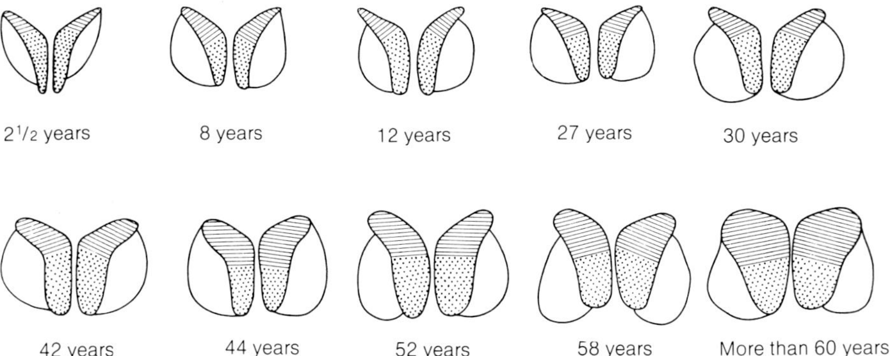

Fig. 180. Variations in ventricular size and shape depending on age, as seen in the anteroposterior projection (from actual air studies)

IX. The Pathological Pneumoencephalogram

If definite abnormalities are present after reviewing the pictures in the manner previously described and excluding inadequate studies and normal variants, these are further categorized as to their pathological significance. Abnormalities may take the following forms: (a) *a displacement or a deformity of the ventricle or subarachnoid space;* (b) *a definite filling defect within the ventricle;* c) *a pathological accumulation of air at the site of a disease process;* or (d) any *combination* of the above. All these changes can be seen with space-occupying processes and are also quite common with the atrophic processes. They can usually verify the position, the shape, and occasionally also the type of the disease process present.

1. Space-Occupying Processes

In analyzing pneumoencephalograms we can distinguish three large groups of space-occupying processes: tumors of the *cerebral hemispheres, midline tumors* in a position to block the flow of CSF, and *paramedian* tumors lying between the above two groups. As a result of their position, paramedian tumors contain many of the radiological findings of the other two groups mentioned (see p. 231).

Tumors of the *cerebral hemispheres* reveal their location through the direction of the displacement of the ventricular system which accompanies them – laterally, inferiorly, or superiorly (see Fig. 181).

Tumors *along the axis of the brain* lead to narrowing of the ventricular pathways and to a secondary enlargement of the proximal ventricular chambers (see Fig. 192). In such cases one attempts to define the superior and inferior limits of the space-occupying process. With tumors at *the base of the brain* a precise investigation of the cisterns is also mandatory since any deformities noted will serve to locate the site of the tumor and may even indicate its shape.

Also indirect evidence for the presence of a tumor may be found, for example, through widening of the cisterns of the velum interpositum and corpus callosum as a result of oc-

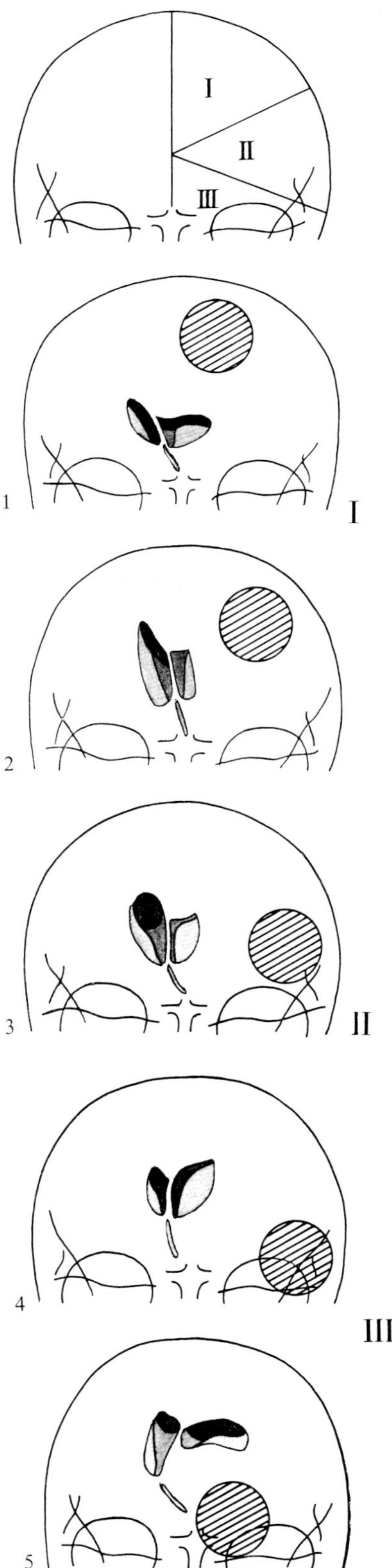

Fig. 181. Schematic anteroposterior views of the ventricular displacement and distortion expected with tumors in the various zones: *I*, dorsal location; *II*, lateral location; *III*, basal location (the most heavily contrasted areas are black)

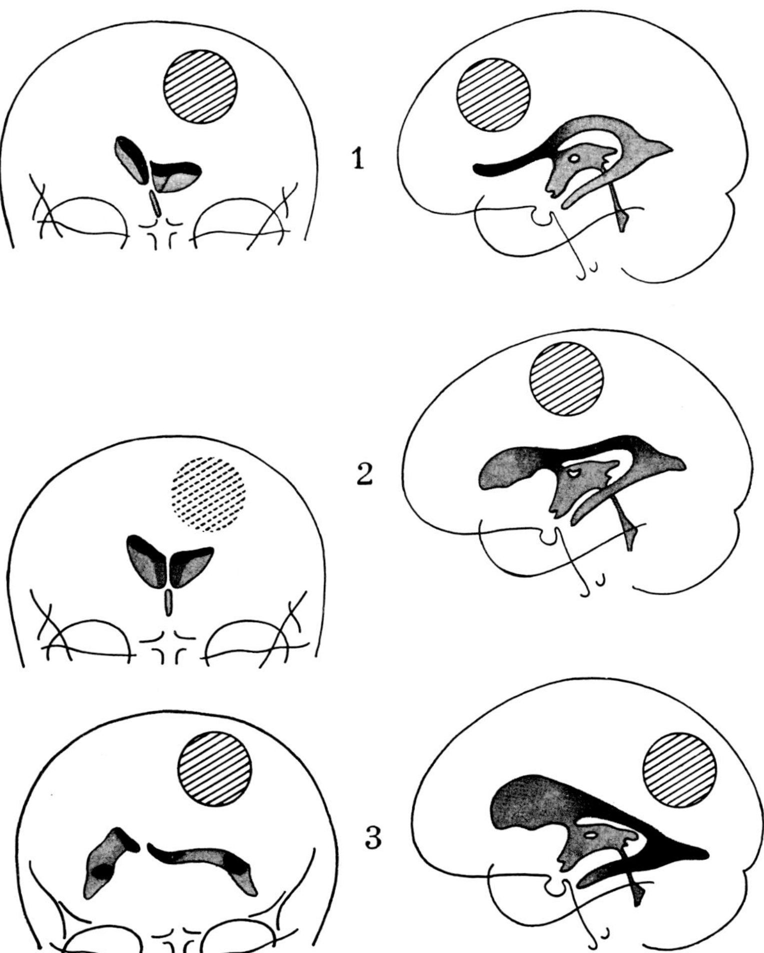

Fig. 182. Various dorsal (parasagittal) tumors with the expected ventricular changes as seen in schematic anteroposterior, posteroanterior, and lateral projections: *1*, anterior location; *2* middle location; *3* posterior location

clusion of the fourth ventricle or through tamponade of the basal subarachnoid spaces with the dorsal pathways remaining open (see p. 18), particularly in children.

a) The Hemispheric Processes

General Survey: Anteroposterior and Posteroanterior Views

In the analysis of pneumoencephalograms with cerebral hemisphere pathology we first determine on the anteroposterior view whether a mass displacement to the left or right across the midline has occurred, since any shift will result in a corresponding displacement of the ventricular system. This will indicate the side of the space-occupying process. Furthermore,

the height of such a lesion above the horizontal level of the base of the skull is important. An attempt is made to determine whether the disease process – in relation to a frontal cut – lies at the level of the lateral ventricular wall (lateral), above it (dorsal), or below it (basal). Consequently, we divide the frontal cut of the cerebral hemispheres into three sections (Fig. 181). Depending on the direction of displacement of the ventricular chamber, the tumor position is indicated as *dorsal* (paragasittal), *lateral,* or *basal.* The direction of the displacement is, however, not dependent solely on the pressure of the space-occupying process in the involved section; rather, it will be further modified by special individual characteristics of the displaced brain parts. There are, however, certain basic rules for displacements which apply to all regions of the brain (see p. 3ff.) and

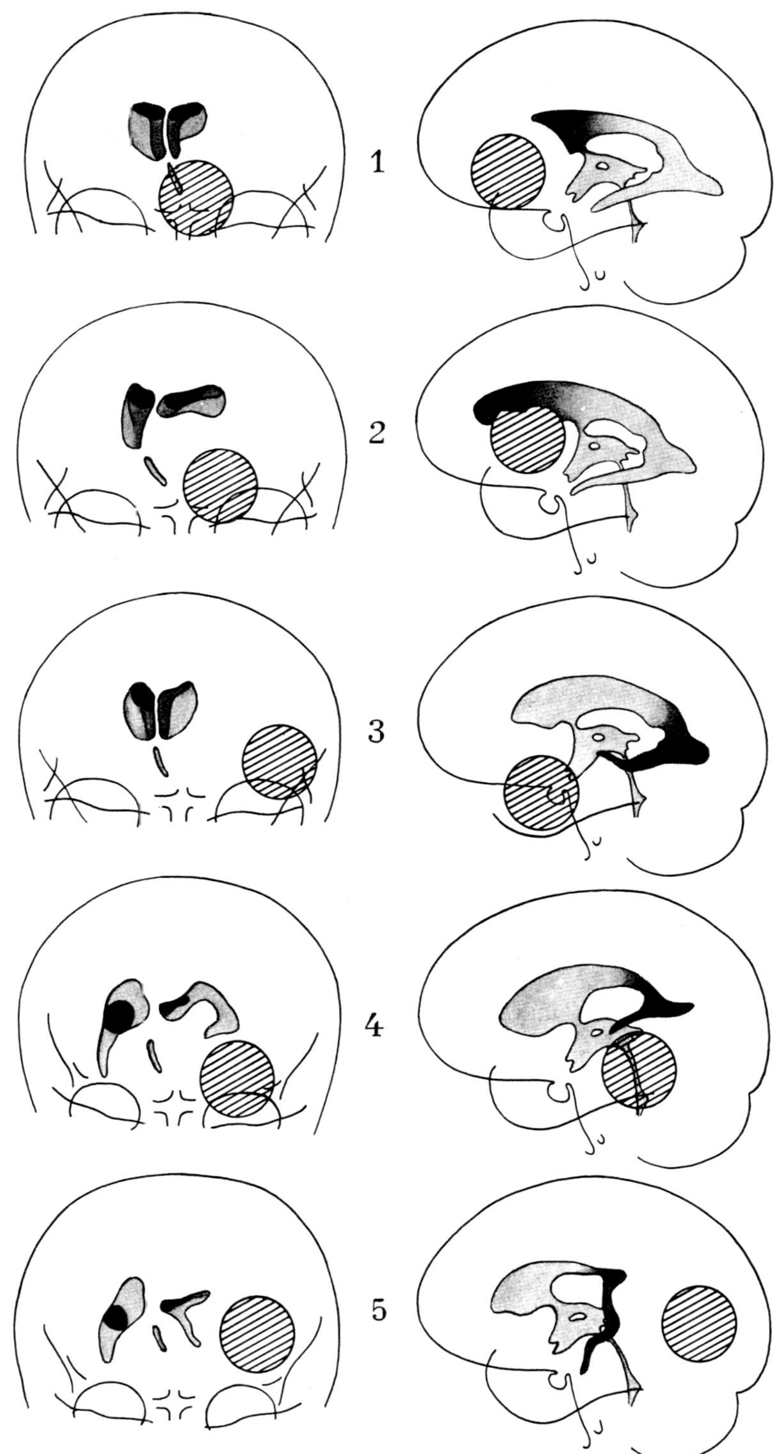

Fig. 183. Schematic representation of expected ventricular changes as seen with various lateral and basal tumors in the anteroposterior, posteroanterior and lateral views: *1,* anterior frontobasal; *2,* posterior frontobasal; *3,* temporal pole; *4,* mid-temporal; *5,* lateral occipital (Figs. 181–183 are taken from similar illustrations by SCHLESINGER 1937)

which are essential for an accurate interpretation of pneumoencephalograms (see pp. 6, 216).

The corpus callosum with its radiating fibers (corona radiata) to the centrum semi-ovale on both sides is a most impressive fiber bundle which at the same time forms the roof of the lateral ventricles. In its frontal region it is surrounded by cerebral tissues which are easily displaced. From the displacement of these tissues and its effect on the corpus callosum, it is possible to determine from which direction the main lateral pressure force is being applied in a space-occupying process. Both lateral ventricles – at least the frontal horns – will understandably be affected by any displacement of the corpus callosum. From the height of both lateral ventricles we can determine the position of the corpus callosum, which for the most part is the best indicator of the existence and site of a space-occupying process in air studies. *A slightly sloping position of the corpus callosum with depression of the lateral ventricular shadow is indicative of a space-occupying process even when other changes are absent.*

If the corpus callosum with its corresponding lateral ventricle on either side is markedly depressed, then the space-occupying process must lie *dorsal* to it (Fig. 181/I); if it is only moderately depressed and yet is strongly displaced horizontally, the lesion must lie *dorsolateral* (Fig. 181/II). On the other hand, if the ventricles remain at the same level and are only horizontally displaced, the direction of the pressure must be from the *lateral* or *laterobasal* position. *Basally* situated processes can even elevate the involved ventricular chamber with its overlying corpus callosum (Fig. 181/III).

The Dorsal Group (Parasagittal)

The more dorsal that a space-occupying process lies, that much stronger will the involved half of the corpus callosum and its underlying ventricle be depressed (Figs. 181, 182). If the ventricular system is simultaneously displaced to the opposite side, then the septum pellucidum will have an oblique position. On account of the easier displaceability of the frontal corpus callosum, the horizontal displacement of the ventricle is bound to be stronger with a frontal tumor location then with a parietal location (see p. 226 ff. and Figs. 4, 167, 181). Corresponding to this division is the relative obliquity of the septum (see p. 226). The upper part of the third

ventricle is likewise displaced laterally with the result that this upper part will be tilted to the normal side. In doing so, the third ventricle remains parallel to or in line with the obliquely tilted septum, referred to as tilting of the "septum-third ventricular line" (Fig. 181).

The Lateral and Basal Groups (Fig. 183)

The more the site of the space-occupying process moves from dorsal to lateral, that much less is the septum tilted even if the lateral displacement is considerable (Fig. 181). With dorsolateral lesions, the septum and third ventricle usually remain parallel or in a straight line (see Fig. 181/I). With laterally placed lesions, the septum remains vertical, while the third ventricle is tilted to the normal side (Fig. 181/II). With basolateral sites, the septum can even be inclined somewhat to the abnormal side, and with basomedial sites of pathology this is regularly the case (Fig. 181/III). Because of that, this tumor group causes a curvature of the "septum-third ventricular line" so that the third ventricle is bent like a sickle. The roof of the lateral ventricle on the affected side, which in dorsal processes is very depressed, remains at a constant distance from the base of the skull in lateral processes. In basal tumors this distance may even be increased on the involved side as the ventricle and its roof are pushed upward by the underlying lesion. The uninvolved roof will thus be lower in such cases (Fig. 39). The "septum-third ventricular line", so important for the localization of tumors within the "various sectors" in the anteroposterior view (Fig. 14), can also give information about the site of the process with regard to the frontal/occipital direction as well. In the sagittal projection the septum and third ventricle appear to lie on top of one another, though the septum is actually anterior to the third ventricle. Local pressure changes will affect the relative position of these structures depending on the site of the lesion and other circumstances. A *frontal* space-occupying process as a rule displaces the *septum* more than the third ventricle, while a more *posterior* tumor (parietal, temporal, or occipital) will displace the *third ventricle* more (Fig. 184). The usual situation in the sagittal exposure of a continuous "septum-third ventricular line" will not only be tilted (as with dorsal processes) and curved (basolateral processes), but will also be separated or

Fig. 184. Typical pneumoencephalogram of a temporobasal extracerebral tumor (sphenoid wing meningioma)

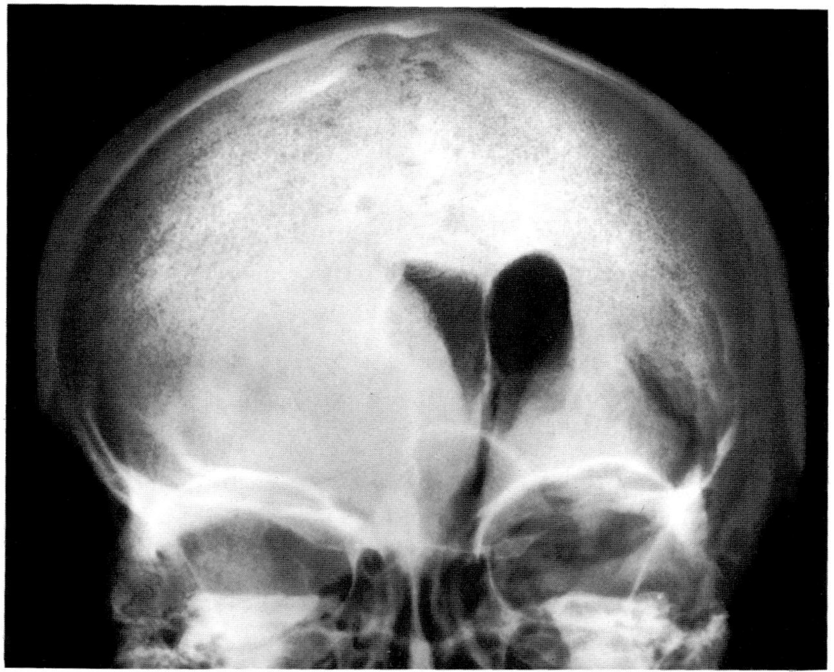

Fig. 185. Indentation into and displacement of a lateral ventricle secondary to a parietal tumor (glioblastoma multiforme)

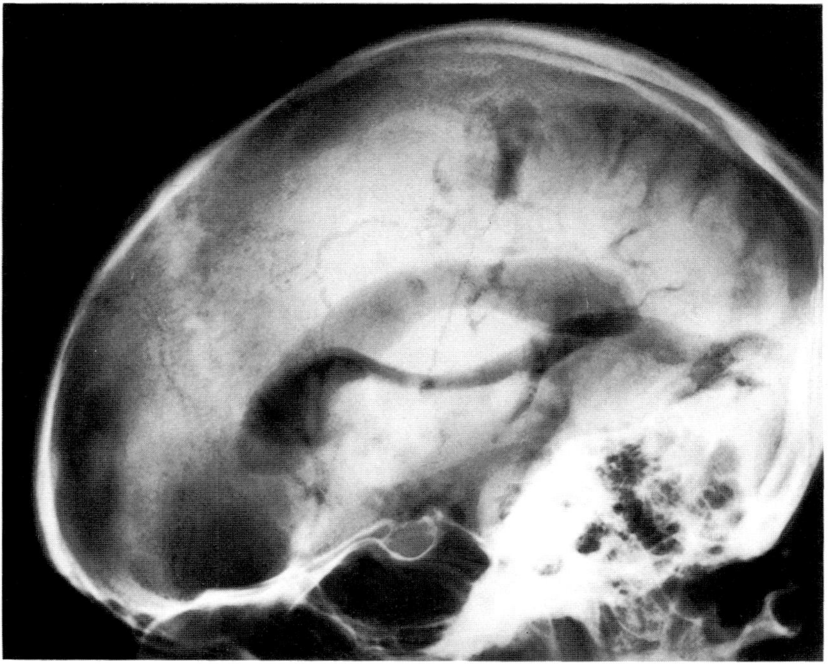

dissociated the more anterior or posterior the lesion is: the septum will then be found to have been pushed lateral to the third ventricle or vice versa. Both, however, remain approximately parallel. Thus, just by observing the character of the "septum-third ventricular line" in the anteroposterior view, it is possible to conclude much about the site of a space-occupying process.

Obviously, additional information can be gained by comparing the anteroposterior view with the posteroanterior view. Supplementary exposures may also be made in the half-axial projection which would give a better proof of localization in terms of the frontal/occipital axis.

Finally, one more point remains to be emphasized (see p. 16, and Fig. 9/III). In occipital space-occupying processes, a horizontal displacement is not possible unless mass displacement has first taken place in an anterior (sagittal)direction because of fixation of the falx to the tentorium posteriorly. In occipital as well as parietal space-occupying processes, horizontal displacements across the midline below the free edge of the falx first require the corpus callosum to be displaced downward, away from the falx. This displacement will be especially marked if the lesion is dorsally situated (see Figs. 15a, b, and 186).

The Lateral Exposure

If the X-ray films in the sagittal projection already indicate a tumor in the frontal/occipital axis, the lateral views will serve to confirm this. With dorsal lesions, the precise position of the tumor in the long axis is not difficult to recognize from the point of maximum depression of the ventricle. Frontal tumors involve primarily the frontal horns, parietal tumors involve the cellae mediae, and parieto-occipital tumors involve the occipital horn or trigone (Fig. 185). *However, only with lateral views in the sitting position are these findings dependable.*

Frontolateral and frontobasal tumors also predominantly affect the frontal horn on the lateral view. The frontal horn is compressed from the side or is pushed posteriorly and/or superiorly from below (Fig. 183/1 and 2). Also with basal tumors, the third ventricle can be displaced in a similar fashion. In temporal tumors, the temporal horn is displaced medially, superiorly, or posteriorly (Fig. 183/3 and 4). In many cases the temporal horn is totally compromised and then does not fill with air. Farther posteriorly, small occipital tumors primarily displace the occipital horn medially. With larger tumors the displacement is more in an anterior direction.

Tumors of Individual Lobes of the Cerebral Hemispheres

Frontal Tumors (see Figs. 181–183)

General signs: It is characteristic of all frontal tumors to affect predominantly the frontal horn. The more posterior ventricular areas are largely unaffected unless there is considerable cerebral edema in the neighboring white matter which can act as an additional space-occupying mass. In the anteroposterior view, the most marked displacements across the midline occur with unilateral tumor involvement. This is also well demonstrated in the half-axial projection. The frontal horn is more depressed if the tumor is situated dorsally or is quite large. The farther lateral the tumor sits, the more the subsequent displacement approximates that seen with temporal tumors (Fig. 181). These effects will be described later. With basal and particularly medial basal tumors, horizontal displacements may well be absent, the displacement occurring predominantly in a superior and posterior direction. This may be apparent only on the lateral frontal horn view (Fig. 183). The lateral or inferior aspects of the affected frontal horn will be compressed or indented. The septum in such cases is always more medially displaced than the third ventricle unless a marked degree of cerebral edema has caused enlargement of the entire hemisphere.

The frontal horn apex may even indicate the side of the tumor on the lateral frontal horn view as, for example, when a dorsally situated tumor forces it inferiorly (Fig. 182/1). In the lateral lesion, the frontal horn apex can remain approximately in its original position, while it is elevated with basal tumors. The foramen of Monro and the third ventricle (often also the brain stem) are displaced posteriorly and inferiorly in accordance with the "axial" displacement process (see also pp. 6, 10).

Frontodorsal tumors (meningiomas of the anterior third of the sagittal sinus, cystic astrocytomas, glioblastomas, see p. 29): With the meningioma in this location, the falx is definitely tilted to the opposite side. In the anteroposterior view the involved frontal horn is markedly depressed, is often compressed nearly to a horizontal slit, and is displaced to the opposite side. On the other hand, the frontal horn of the normal side is elevated, is very small, and is nearly vertical. The two ventricles occasionally form a right angle to one another. In the lateral frontal horn view, the frontal horn apex is depressed posteriorly and inferiorly, so that it is almost perpendicular to the orbital base line of the skull. It is also displaced posteriorly against the body of the frontal horn. The more posterior a tumor lies, the less will be the posterior displacement of the frontal horn, but the more it will be displaced inferiorly. In glioblastomas, the changes are similar, as have been described in general, except that frequently a hydrocephalus of the opposite side is seen as a result of the mass effect compressing and occluding the foramen of Monro (see p. 29).

Frontomedial tumors (oligodendrogliomas, astrocytomas, falx meningiomas, see p. 29): On the lateral frontal horn view, a characteristic "amputation" of the involved frontal horn is commonly seen. Astrocytomas – rarely limited just to the frontal lobes – can grow in an occipital direction and can enlarge the septum whereby this structure pushes against both frontal horn apices. The ventricular contour remains rather flat with astrocytomas, while the oligodendroglioma indents the ventricular wall with numerous projections into it. Gliomas can also displace the foramina of Monro, leading to a bilateral hydrocephalus. In such cases the anteroposterior view is often difficult to evaluate. The *unilateral* falx meningioma (see p. 29) presents with findings similar to the glioma. Frequently, however, these are bilateral and show findings which will be discussed in detail later with the bilateral frontal tumors. On the other hand, there are no signs of infiltrating growth with the meningiomas (smooth ventricular wall contour!).

Frontobasal (subfrontal) tumors (meningiomas and glioblastomas, also the rare "cylindromatous (adenoid cystic)" carcinomas, as well as carcinoma of the ethmoid sinuses, see p. 29): The frontobasal olfactory groove meningiomas elevate both frontal horn apices equally in midline tumors, or will indicate the most involved side if one is more elevated than the other. With unilateral tumors, there is also horizontal displacement which is mostly absent in the bilateral tumors. Usually the third ventricle takes part in the upward movement of the anterior ventricular chambers. The tumors indent the frontal horn inferiorly and anteriorly, which is readily apparent on the lateral frontal horn view: the ventricular contour forms a half-moon cap over the tumor. Also the foramina of Monro are usually posteriorly and outwardly displaced, but are less commonly blocked, so that the resultant hydrocephalus is mostly minimal or absent.

With good filling of the basal cisterns a crescent of air may be seen around the tumor. This makes possible the diagnosis of an extracerebral tumor location.

Very similar are the changes with the cylindromatous carcinoma or other carcinomas of the base of the skull. The tumors situated immediately in front of the sella are discussed with the midline basal tumors.

With glioblastomas the dorsal displacement is less, but there is often an invagination into the frontal horn from below as a result of direct tumor invasion (see lateral frontal horn view). Also, the apices of the frontal horns are often pushed away from each other (anteroposterior view).

Frontolateral tumors (oligodendrogliomas, astrocytomas, glioblastomas, meningiomas of the third frontal convolution, see p. 29): Frontolateral tumors displace the entire ventricular system horizontally to the opposite side. In the anteroposterior view the involved corpus callosum is only slightly depressed or is horizontal. The involved ventricle may be slightly smaller than the normal side, or they may be equal in size. The septum remains vertical. This displacement picture is similar to that seen with temporal lobe tumors (see Fig. 15a), except for two differences. If the tumor lies above the Sylvian fissure, the temporal horn on the lateral frontal horn view remains in normal position or is depressed somewhat inferiorly, the hook-shaped tip being somewhat stretched. Also, in frontolateral tumors, the third ventricle is less displaced than the septum, while with temporal lobe tumors the relationship is usually reversed (see p. 226). In both there is a dissociation of the "septum-third ventricular line". Simultaneously in these cases the temporal horn is either markedly displaced or is absent.

Because of the additional mass effect from secondary cerebral edema, glioblastomas compress and markedly depress the involved frontal horn in the anteroposterior view, depress the corpus callosum until it assumes an oblique position, and cause a more marked horizontal displacement. A similar picture is seen with large meningiomas involving the third frontal convolution.

Bilateral frontal tumors (parasagittal or falx meningiomas, see p. 29): These tumors are described more accurately because of their midline position on p. 228.

Tumors of the Central Gyri (Cystic Astrocytomas, see also Meningiomas of the Middle Third of the Sagittal Sinus and Parietodorsal Tumors; pp. 30, 227)

Small astrocytomas in this area result in early clinical symptoms while the corresponding pneumoencephalogram is still unremarkable. The angiographic picture may as well be negative. The changes seen are basically those of the frontal tumors, though less marked. The most important sign is a slight horizontal displacement of the ventricular system at the level of the body of the frontal horn. The corpus callosum is always slightly inclined as a result of depression of the involved ventricle, while the septum may be inclined to the opposite side or may remain vertical. The exposures taken in the sitting position always show an indentation into the frontal horn or cella media from above (not to be confused with the normal indentation produced by the radiation of the corpus callosum, see pp. 200, 201!).

Temporal Tumors (see Fig. 181/3, 4, 5)

General signs: The body of the frontal horn and cella media on the side of the tumor are displaced to the opposite side on the anteroposterior view with their dorsal border (represented by the corpus callosum) remaining horizontal. When hydrocephalus of the opposite side exists, the roof of this ventricle will often sit higher than that on the side of the tumor. The tumor-compressed ventricle is thus smaller and indented through advancement of the basal ganglia and thalamus. The lateral ventricular edge on the involved side is often drawn out to a point (Fig. 181/III). The septum remains vertical and may even be inclined to the side of the tumor with large, basally situated lesions. The third ventricle is regularly displaced more than the septum (Fig. 181/III). Frequently the "septum-third ventricular line" "wraps itself" to a certain extent around the tumor (see p. 222).

These changes in the sagittal exposures are most characteristic. It is important, however, to demonstrate well the temporal horns in the various projections in order to determine through their displacement the precise position of the tumor within the temporal lobe itself. The temporal horn tip can be displaced me-

dially and elevated in the anteroposterior projection, while the lateral projection shows it pushed more posteriorly or superiorly. The entire temporal horn may also appear to be amputated, in which case it is necessary to guard against errors in technique mimicking filling defects and to employ tomography whenever necessary.

It is apparent that contralateral hydrocephalus with temporal lobe tumors is primarily due to constriction of the foramen of Monro or of the aqueduct (herniation into the ambient cistern). Hydrocephalic enlargement of the ventricle on the tumor side is prevented by the mass effect of the tumor itself.

Temporal pole tumors: anterior temporolateral tumors (glioblastomas, see p. 31): These tumors with their associated marked volume increases result in an overtilting of the septum to the normal side. The involved frontal horn frequently remains somewhat higher than the uninvolved side. It is usually very narrow and the ventricular edge seems to point laterally. In the lateral view the entire frontal temporal horn is either absent or is displaced a long way posteriorly and superiorly.

Posterior temporolateral tumors (oligodendrogliomas, astrocytomas, glioblastomas, meningiomas, see p. 31): With laterally situated tumors, the opposite ventricle is usually wider than the involved side because of displacement of the basal ganglia and thalamus into it. The third ventricle is also markedly displaced to the opposite side and is curved, while the septum remains vertical. In the lateral frontal horn view, either the tip or the entire temporal horn is missing, or it is displaced medially and superiorly. Glioblastomas exhibit the same signs to an exaggerated degree. They may even affect the trigone which, depending on the tumor site, can be displaced superiorly and medially. This results from the associated, often marked, cerebral edema.

The temporobasal tumors (anterior: frontotemporal sphenoid wing meningiomas; posterior: basal meningiomas; see p. 31): Large spherical meningiomas produce a mixture of frontal and temporal signs with the latter predominating (Fig. 184). As a result, the frontal horn is elevated, the septum tilted to the side of the tumor, and the badly bowed third ventricle displaced far to the uninvolved side. The "septum-third ventricular line" forms a semi-circle which surrounds the tumor. The temporal horn is ele-

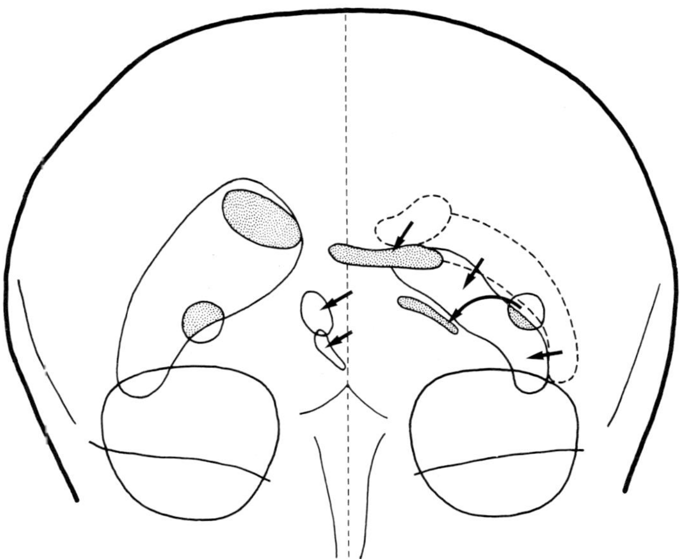

Fig. 186. Semischematic representation of a pneumoencephalogram in a parietal lobe tumor. The *dotted lines* depict the normal position of the cella media and the trigone, with *arrows* showing the direction of the displacement to the expected position. Note the displacement of the occipital horn and midline third ventricle as well

vated. Much more difficult is the recognition of the flat, plate-like, basal meningioma (meningioma-en-plaque). The most definitive signs here are the raising of the temporal horn apex in the anteroposterior and lateral frontal horn views and the eventual encroachment on the basal cisterns seen in frontal tomograms. Another typical temporal lobe tumor in the younger age groups is the cystic gangliocytoma, which is usually speckled with calcium deposits and is found in a temporomedial location.

Parietal Tumors (see Figs. 182/2, 3, 186)

General signs: At first glance the anteroposterior view of these tumors appears to be similar to that of the frontal lobe lesions, and yet a distinct difference exists with respect to the type of displacement of the "septum-third ventricular line" to the opposite side. Here there is less lateral displacement of the septum than the third ventricle, similar in this respect to temporal lobe tumors. If this sign is present, other characteristic changes should be looked for. In the posteroanterior view there is a very typical deformity of the ventricle: the cella media on the involved side is more or less depressed and forms a flat, basal convex bowl (Fig. 186). The trigone in particular in the posteroanterior view is displaced medially, inferiorly, and to the opposite side. In the lateral views in the sitting position, the depression of the cella media and especially of the trigone are both equally well demonstrated (Figs. 182/2, 3, 185).

The parietodorsal tumors (meningiomas of the middle third of the sagittal sinus, astrocytomas, glioblastomas, see p. 30): These parasagittal tumors invaginate and compress the parietal white matter from above and depress the splenium of the corpus callosum. This depression creates a space between the free edge of the falx, permitting posterior subfalceal herniations to the opposite side (Fig. 186). The cella media is markedly displaced to the opposite side, is flattened, and appears as a flat horizontal band; it now straddles the midline. In the posteroanterior view, the most medial part corresponds to the most anteriorly displaced portion. The described band-like shadow flows into the trigone, which is also medially and inferiorly displaced. This contour is very characteristic of parietal lobe tumors (see Fig. 186).

If the parietodorsal tumors lie more anteriorly near the postcentral gyri, they are associated with early neurological symptoms. Consequently, the air study will take place earlier when mass displacements and ventricular deformities are minimal.

The depression of the cella media on both the sagittal (anteroposterior and posteroanterior) and lateral projections will be best seen in the *sitting position.* In this position mild indentations into the lateral ventricles from above will be appreciated more. These indentations into the ventricle are very characteristic of the larger, more posteriorly situated tumors (saddle-shaped indentations, Fig. 185). They occasionally result in an apparent bisection of the cella media into two parts (lateral views can be very deceptive!).

The parietolateral tumors (oligodendrogliomas, astrocytomas, see p. 30): In the posteroanterior view, the cella media is depressed, but the horizontal displacement is less marked than with the dorsal tumors since the corpus callosum remains in its original position just beneath the free edge of the falx. The principle distortion involves the trigone (in the posteroanterior and lateral views), which is displaced inferiorly and toward the uninvolved side.

The frontotemporoparietal tumors (mostly large cystic ependymomas or cylindrical glioblastomas, see p. 31): It is characteristic of these tumors to cause a marked displacement of the entire ventricle to the opposite side. The septum on the anteroposterior view is markedly displaced and tilted to the opposite side, as is the entire third ventricle (it is, however, not curved, only mildly bent!). Noteworthy is the marked depression of the cella media, which is more involved than the body of the frontal horn. The lateral ventricle of the opposite side is usually moderately hydrocephalic. These changes are similar to those seen with subdural hematomas.

The Occipital Tumors

Glioblastomas, meningiomas (see Fig. 183/5): These tumors involve predominantly the trigone and occipital horn, which are displaced anteriorly and either superiorly or inferiorly (Fig. 183/5). Therefore, the changes are apparent only in the prone (brow-down) position. When the occipital horn is clearly seen on the posteroanterior view, it may be displaced toward or away from the side of the tumor depending on its position with respect to the ventricle. The trigone is usually pushed medially and inferiorly, and it is elevated only by basally situated meningiomas (tentorium). The cella media of the involved side is pushed downward from above and is displaced medially, while the third ventricle is tilted slightly to the opposite side.

Still more informative is the lateral occipital horn view, where the occipital horn and trigone are displaced anteriorly and anterosuperiorly. The result is that the angle between the temporal horn and cella media is definitely more blunted than normal, the temporal horn often assuming a perpendicular position both with respect to the base of the skull and with respect

to the trigone and cella media (Fig. 183/5). Dorsal lying tumors depress primarily the cella media and trigone including the occipital horn, while lateral tumors displace particularly the proximal temporal horn medially and superiorly. The displacement process in larger tumors involves the entire hemisphere and even extends frontally, so that there is a slight displacement of the frontal horn to the opposite side with depression of the involved body of the frontal horn. The septum remains vertical or is somewhat tilted to the opposite side. This sometimes leads to errors in interpretation in that the tumor appears to be more anteriorly situated than it actually is.

The Bilateral Tumors

Mostly meningiomas, less commonly gliomas (see pp. 29, 32, 33): Tumors with bilateral extensions exhibit certain peculiarities in the air study. The horizontal displacement of the ventricular system can be minimal if both extensions are equally large, in which case the indentation into the ventricular chambers would be equally on both sides.

Meningiomas occur everywhere in the long axis from the anterior margin of the falx (olfactory groove meningiomas) to the posterior margin of the tentorium (meningiomas of the posterior third of the sagittal sinus or posterior falx meningiomas). Bilateral gliomas are found to involve particularly the corpus callosum and septum (butterfly gliomas). There may be combinations between frontal or parietal tumors and the corpus callosum types.

Meningiomas, depending upon their position, displace individual segments of the lateral ventricle to different degrees. Frontobasal tumors involve primarily the frontal horn and anterior third ventricle by displacing them posteriorly. Tumors at the frontal pole depress both apices of the frontal horns and also lead to a posterior displacement. Tumors of the sagittal sinus as it runs posteriorly indent the adjacent portion of the lateral ventricle from above, while occipital tumors displace the trigone anteriorly and inferiorly. These findings are well demonstrated on the lateral view with the patient sitting with his head appropriately positioned. Falx meningiomas show these displacements to an exaggerated degree and result in a bowl-like distortion of the frontal horn in the anteroposterior view.

Fig. 187. Air study of a butterfly glioma
– anteroposterior view

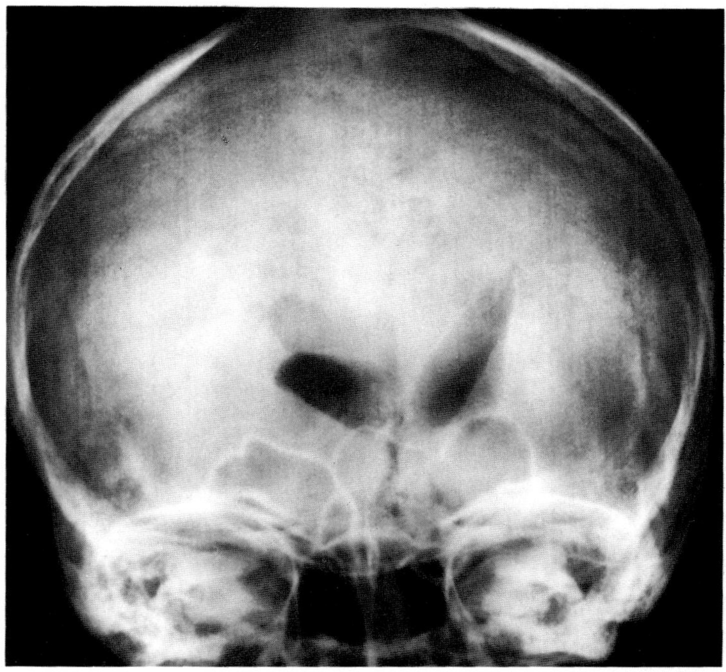

Meningiomas and gliomas can often be differentiated on the basis of the ventricular contour alone, since this will be changed by the infiltrating growth of the glioma which forms bumps and mounds on the wall itself. Falx meningiomas show deeper indentations into the lateral ventricle than those tumors which lie more laterally to the sinus. The differential diagnosis between a falx meningioma and the glioma of the corpus callosum lies in the shape and position of the cistern of the corpus callosum (see pp. 213, 222) or from angiographic findings.

Tumors of the Anterior Corpus Callosum

So-called butterfly gliomas, usually glioblastomas, less commonly oligodendrogliomas, rarely lipomas (see p. 32): The changes with infiltrating tumors of the corpus callosum are shown particularly well on the anteroposterior view. As a result of pressure from above, both frontal horn bodies appear to be depressed and assume a ring-shaped contour. Through widening of the upper septum into which the tumor regularly grows, they are pushed apart from one another. With abundant air filling in the sagittal axis, the tumor of the corpus callosum will occasionally cause a very characteristic double contour of the frontal horn on the anteroposterior projection: the frontal horn apices and the immediately adjacent frontal horn bodies are less depressed and remain higher than the remaining frontal horn bodies and cellae mediae, which are more depressed (Figs. 162, 187, 188). In this manner two oblique segments of the same lateral ventricle come to lie on top of each other. Thus, with suspected tumors of the corpus callosum it is extremely important to obtain anteroposterior and lateral exposures in the sitting position as soon as possible. The direction of the beam should be in line with the long axis of the corpus callosum. On the other hand, this same picture with the double contour may occasionally be seen as well with falx meningiomas and lipomas of the corpus callosum; however, here there is no infiltration of the septum. The differential diagnosis of anterior corpus callosum tumors from bilateral falx meningiomas depends, therefore, on infiltration of the septum and the ventricular wall: the contour of the wall appears uneven and gnarled (Fig. 187), the upper septum is widened, and the lower septum is not involved.

The rare genuine septum tumors show a large filling defect in the hydrocephalic ventricles consisting of a wide, irregular, swollen septum. These tumors can also extend into the third ventricle as well (see p. 260).

With the closed septum pellucidum cyst (see Fig. 189), the septum is markedly and sym-

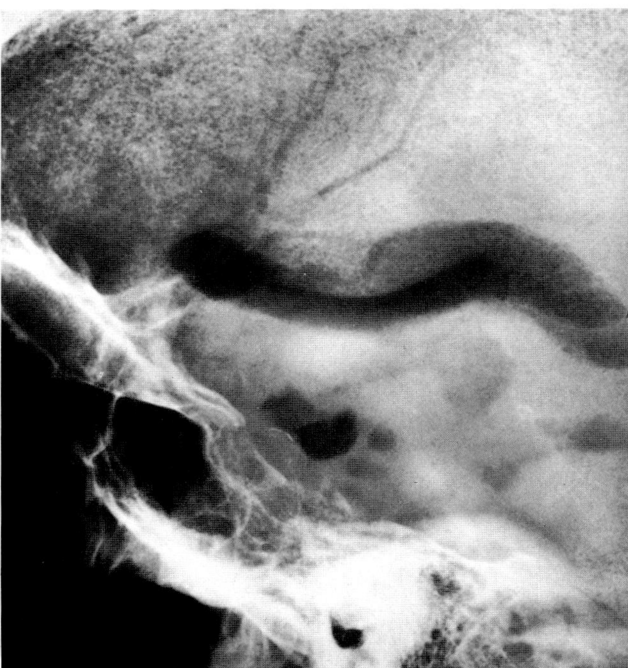

Fig. 188. Air study of a butterfly glioma – lateral view. Note the dorsal indentation into the frontal horn

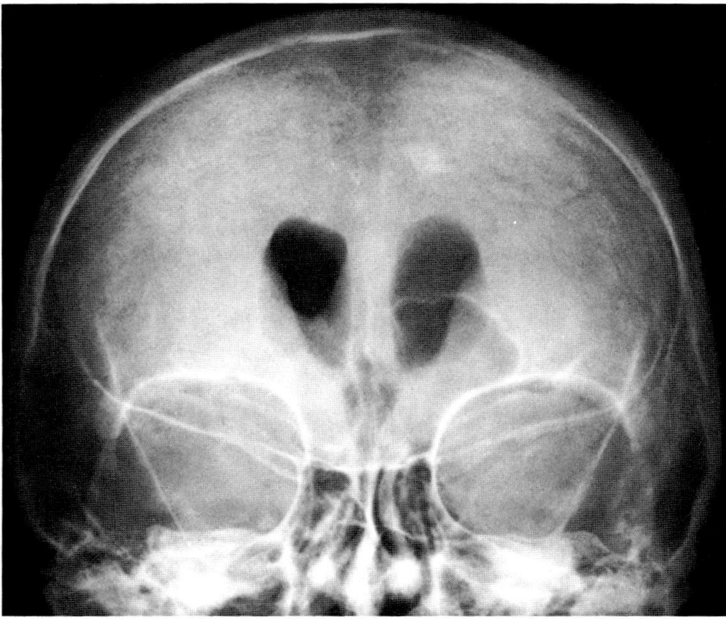

Fig. 189. Closed septum pellucidum cyst with separation of the frontal horns – anteroposterior view

metrically enlarged, both lateral ventricles are pushed laterally apart, but there is no ventricular depression. Changes in the contour of the ventricular wall are also lacking (Fig. 189).

With tumors in the corpus callosum which are beginning, the demonstration of the cistern of the corpus callosum is of prime importance. This cistern is elevated with tumors of the corpus callosum. An air-filled cistern situated be-low the tumor practically always excludes a tumor of the corpus callosum. It speaks instead for an overlying process, e.g., a deep-seated falx meningioma.

Oligodendrogliomas and lipomas can be calcified.

Tomography in the sagittal plane is of particular value from a diagnostic standpoint for all tumors of the corpus callosum.

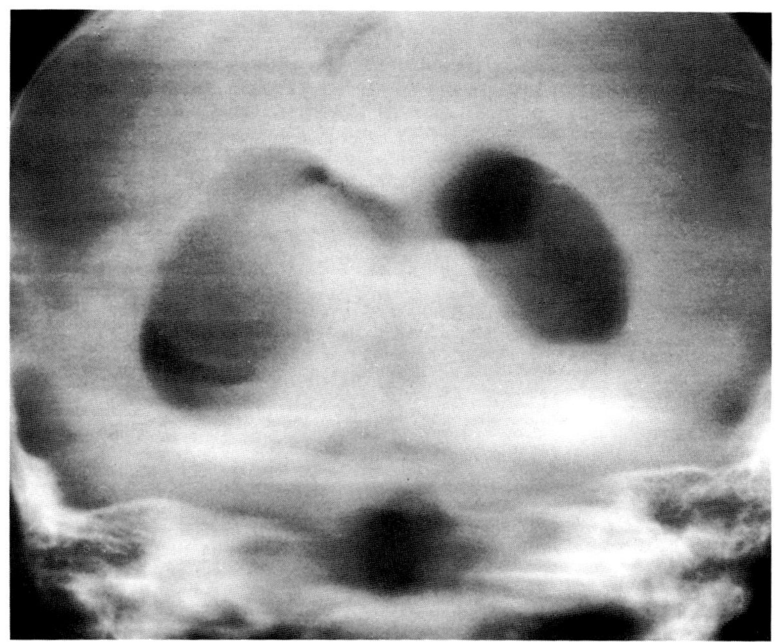

Fig. 190. Tumor shadow of an intraventricular meningioma. Anteroposterior tomogram (see Fig. 18/53)

Tumors of the Posterior Corpus Callosum

Glioblastomas: The picture of the posterior corpus callosum tumor is much less characteristic than the varieties described above, especially since these tumors often extend into one or the other occipital lobes. On the posteroanterior view both cellae mediae and trigones are displaced inferiorly, are compressed, and are pushed apart. On the lateral occipital horn view the posterior portion of the third ventricle is indented posteriorly and superiorly. Nevertheless, on account of the massive changes also present in the lateral ventricles (compression of the trigones), this picture should not be confused with a quadrigeminal plate tumor! Important information in the latter case can also be gained from demonstration of the cisterns.

Changes in the Subarachnoid Spaces with Hemispheric Processes

Intracranial space-occupying processes can also be recognized by changes in the subarachnoid CSF pathways. The absence of filling of the subarachnoid spaces on the side of a tumor over the entire hemisphere or over individual lobes can point to a localized pressure effect with compression of the sulci, if the lack of filling is not due to technical error. Around many tumors of the convexity (meningiomas, mushroom-shaped oligodendrogliomas) a circular or crescent-shaped rim of air is occasionally seen. With nonfilling of the ventricles, mass displacements across the midline can sometimes be demonstrated by changes in the cistern of the corpus callosum.

b) Tumors of the Lateral Ventricles, Basal Ganglia, and Thalamus

General signs (see Fig. 190): Initially, lateral ventricular tumors invaginate the ventricular lumen like polyps. They soon impede the flow of spinal fluid leading to hydrocephalus of the blocked, choroid plexus-containing ventricular segment. Nevertheless the blockage is usually not complete and some air will frequently find its way into the obstructed portion behind the tumor. Large tumors of the trigone can moreover compress and distort the aqueduct, causing obstructive hydrocephalus proximal to this structure. These factors cause the air study findings to vary with individual tumors, but difficulties with differential diagnosis arise only from secondary invasion of an adjacent ventricle. When this happens, there is initially a mild indentation in the ventricular wall or later a wartlike involvement of the ventricular wall with tumor nodules. There are only a few primary tumors of the lateral ventricle and their sites of predilection are well established.

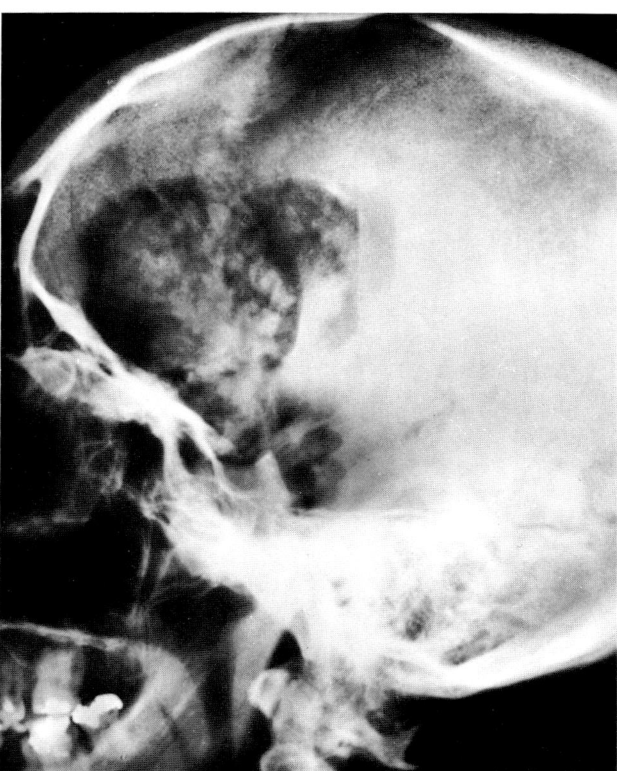

Fig. 191. Typical appearance of an intraventricular epidermoid with speckled pockets of air apparent within the tumor itself

The meningioma of the trigone (see Fig. 190): These rare meningiomas originate from the glomus of the choroid plexus. The temporal horn is usually dilated, as are the trigone and occipital horn, depending on the position of the tumor. Later, the tumor pushes against the aqueduct and third ventricle with a further hydrocephalic enlargement of the proximal ventricular system. In the presence of this marked hydrocephalus, a good air study in the various projections will totally outline the tumor sitting between the foramen of Monro and the trigone. Similar changes accompany the rare, generally calcified, *plexus papilloma.*

The epidermoid of the lateral ventricle (trigone and temporal horn): The epidermoid usually extends from the trigone toward the temporal horn, rarely toward the frontal horn. Because of this, it is associated with the same type of mass displacement seen with large posterior tumors of the temporal lobe. However, the epidermoid has one pathognomonic finding – an air study will reveal speckled pockets of air within the tumor itself between the masses of solid material (Fig. 191).

The ependymoma of the lateral ventricle (at the foramen of Monro): This is associated with the early appearance of significant hydrocephalus on the involved side caused by blockage of the foramen of Monro. The tumor pushes the septum far to the opposite side, which is easily recognized on the anteroposterior view. The cella media of the opposite side sits as a small triangle displaced superiorly and laterally at the upper end of the swollen septum, since the tumor will extend well over to the opposite side in addition. If air enters the frontal horn of the involved side, the tumor will appear on the lateral frontal horn view as a large filling defect between the frontal horn and cella media. Otherwise, the frontal horn will be completely obliterated.

Ventricular tumors in association with tuberous sclerosis: These tumors lie basally in the frontal horn and occlude both foramina of Monro when they are large enough. In such cases, bilateral hydrocephalus ensues which distinguishes this tumor type from the ependymoma. Small tumors can be found anywhere on the ventricular wall and are mostly calcified.

Tumors of the thalamus (glioblastomas, astrocytomas, oligodendrogliomas, see p. 33): In contrast to the tumors described above, thalamic tumors are not true ventricular tumors. They do, however, border on both the cella media and the wall of the third ventricle, which is why they will be described here.

Through occlusion of the aqueduct a proximal hydrocephalus results similar to that seen with meningiomas of the trigone. The enlarged thalamus displaces and compresses the third ventricle, the cella media, and the trigone. This is seen especially clearly in the posteroanterior or anteroposterior views on which the displaced third ventricle is wrapped around and outlines the tumor. The cella media is pushed upward and is converted to a small crescent, while the trigone is horizontally displaced and curves around the tumor margin as well. As a prolongation of this ring of ventricular segments, the origin of the temporal horn is occasionally seen. On the lateral occipital horn view or on other lateral views with good air filling, the tumor will be apparent as a knotty invagination into the hydrocephalic lateral ventricle. Thalamic tumors in children (oligodendrogliomas) are – on account of the elastic, growing skull – symptomatic later and thus larger in size at the time of the study than the thalamic tumors of later years (astrocytomas and glioblastomas), which may even be bilateral.

c) Occlusion of the Midline Ventricular Pathways (Third Ventricle, Aqueduct, Fourth Ventricle)

The most important consequence of occlusion of the midline ventricular pathways between the foramina of Monro and the foramen of Magendie is a symmetrical hydrocephalic enlargement of the proximal ventricular system (see Fig. 192). In spite of this, the blockage is not always complete. Frequently, there is only a constriction or displacement, as from a tumor. The various disease processes which can cause ventricular obstruction have a typical site of predilection and usually a typical shape. To identify these processes is the goal of the procedure. This goal can be accomplished through lumbar pneumoencephalography or through ventriculography. The purpose of the examination is certainly to demonstrate the proximal ventricles, i.e., the dilated ventricular system as far as the obstructing tumor as well as the distal ventricular system on those occasions when the blockage is incomplete. In the latter situation the extent of the tumor is frequently out-

lined by the narrowed or displaced ventricular segment. In so doing it is important not to be satisfied with anything less than the sharp definition of the CSF pathways adjacent to the tumor (Figs. 192, 201). By proper positioning of the patient, the injected air should be brought to the dilated ventricular segment and then used to outline the upper margin of the obstructing lesion. Here tomography is of proven value for the clear demonstration of the relationships present (see p. 192), as is the use of positive contrast agents (see p. 187).

The decision as to which route of injection will be employed – lumbar or ventricular – is dependent to a certain extent on the clinical findings and on the results of other procedures, such as angiographic demonstration of enlarged ventricles. Ventriculography is preferred if a complete occlusion of the ventricular pathways is suspected. Here an attempt should be made to pass a catheter through the frontal horn into the foramen of Monro to arrive at the anterior portion of the third ventricle (see p. 187ff.). It is better to employ a small amount of air or positive contrast in outlining the third ventricle, aqueduct, and fourth ventricle in order to minimize the risk of herniation and strangulation of the brain stem (see p. 7ff.). If instead an incomplete occlusion is suspected, as is seen in pontine lesions and tumors in the vicinity of the sella, visualization of the proximal ventricular system can be attempted first by the lumbar route. If necessary, ventriculography may be employed as a second procedure in such cases. This combination is particularly useful if one is attempting to demonstrate the upper and lower limits of an obstructing process as, for example, an aqueductal stenosis. Fluoroscopy during the procedure will greatly simplify these determinations. The following is a detailed analysis of a typical study: For lumbar pneumoencephalography the goal of the investigation is to outline the pathological process with the injected air. To accomplish this, air must pass by the lesion which cannot be completely obstructing the CSF pathways. If the air does not pass by the obstruction to the proximal dilated ventricular segments, pneumoencephalography should be abandoned and ventriculography substituted. If the air passes by the obstruction without sufficiently outlining it, additional air should be injected to fill the dilated ventricular system better (approximately 30–40 ml). Finally, the lumbar needle is re-

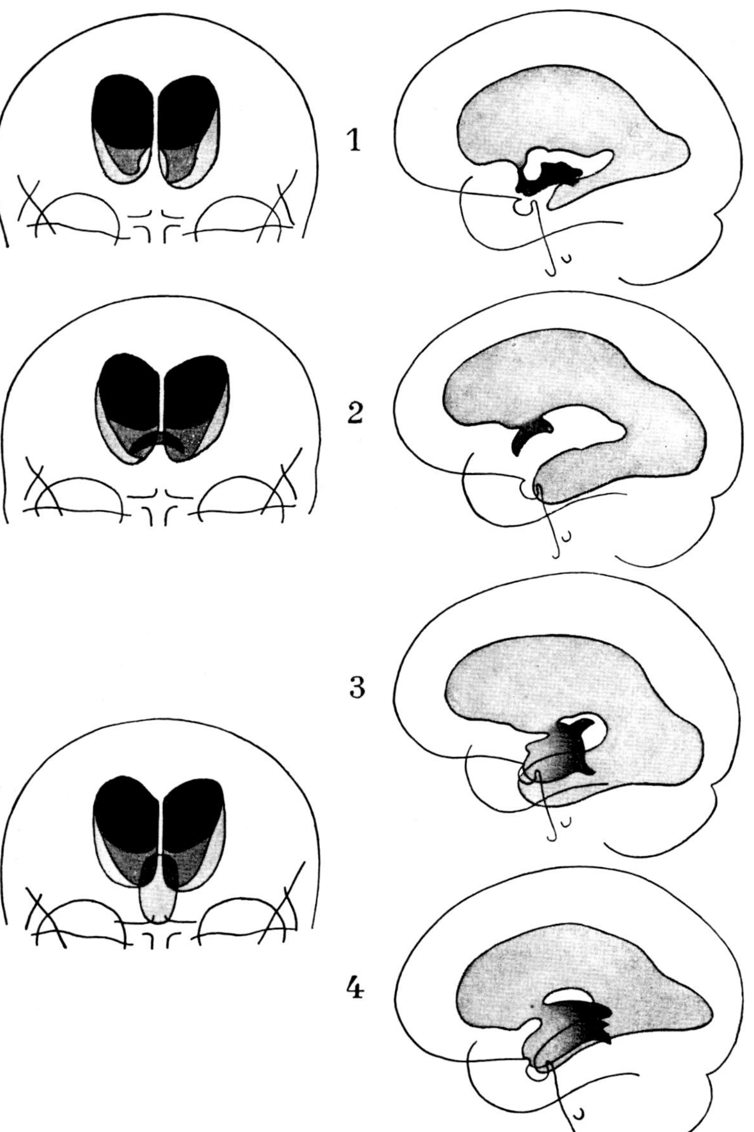

Fig. 192. Schematic illustration of the expected anteroposterior and lateral ventricular changes with various tumors of the third ventricle and aqueduct: colloid cyst of the foramen of Monro (*1*); anterior third ventricular tumor, complete obstruction (*2*); posterior third ventricular tumor (*3*); obstruction at level of aqueduct (*4*)

moved and X-rays made in the supine (brow-up) position with the head hanging back. In this position the anterior part of the third ventricle with the foramina of Monro is the uppermost ventricular part. If the channels here are open, air must flow into the third ventricle. If this does not occur and the technique has been correctly performed, one can presume a partial obstruction at the level of the foramina of Monro or involving the anterior portion of the third ventricle (Fig. 192/1 and 2).

If the anterior part of the third ventricle fills normally, then the posterior portion is investigated. This requires a change to the prone (brow-down) position or the "lateral occipital horn view". If a space-occupying process resides in the posterior portion of the third ventricle or in the pineal region, the anterior border of the tumor will be brought into view (Fig. 192/3).

A technical difficulty in the study of the third ventricle should, however, be mentioned. The required change in position from supine to prone will occasionally cause the air to re-enter the lateral ventricles. To avoid this one must take special care always to keep the foramina of Monro the highest point of the lateral ventricles (see pneumoencephalographic technique, p. 184ff.). If the air does re-enter the lateral ventricle during this part of the procedure, it will be necessary to resume the supine hanging head position to force the air back into the anterior third ventricle before trying again. The change in position is carried out with assistance while the head of the patient is held down. In children it is possible to perform a reverse somersault to accomplish this goal.

If the posterior portion of the third ventricle is also hydrocephalic and intact, the point of obstruction must be still more distal and the study will proceed to outline the aqueduct. To achieve this, the lateral occipital horn views and the half-axial posteroanterior views are used. The obstruction may be intrinsic to the aqueduct itself ("primary" stenosis, Fig. 192/4) or it may be a secondary phenomenon and result from kinking of this structure. This is the case in tumors of the cerebellar region, particularly when the vermis is involved (Fig. 201/1 and 3, see also p. 184ff.).

If the air injection is performed by *ventricular puncture*, there are two possible methods for visualizing the ventricle. With the catheter in the third ventricle the patient is turned onto his abdomen (brow-down) and a lateral X-ray is made while approximately 5 ml air is being instilled. This usually results in a good representation of the open CSF pathways as far as the cervical cord. Subsequently, films are also taken in the sagittal plane and with tomography, additional air being injected as needed.

If the pictures obtained are still unsatisfactory, the patient is placed on his back and the procedure is repeated with a positive contrast agent (now almost exclusively Metrizamide) which is heavier than the CSF and tends to sink. By contrast, the air is lighter and rises. With such agents, exposures obtained in this fashion are always optimal.

It is, however, quite another matter if the catheter is lying in the lateral ventricle and a positive contrast agent is employed. Here the patient is positioned as for pneumoencephalography except that the maneuvers are reversed when demonstrating the various parts of the ventricle; thus, the brow-down (prone) position is used to portray the anterior third ventricle and the brow-up (supine) position for portrayal of the posterior third ventricle, aqueduct, and fourth ventricle.

If the determination of ventricular size is important, still more air may be required.

The Degree of Hydrocephalus

Less severe grades of hydrocephalus begin with a rounding off of the edges of the lateral ventricles on the anteroposterior view. Because of this, the basal ganglion portion of the frontal horn is spread out. With more severe hydrocephalus the original shape of the ventricular chamber becomes more and more altered. In some children with hydrocephalus the ventricles are completely round and have the appearance of air-filled balloons. In the most extreme cases only a few millimeters of cortical mantle will remain. When an obstructive hydrocephalus is restudied a sufficient interval after operative intervention (tumor removal, shunt procedure), a very definite recession is frequently seen in the degree of hydrocephalus. In such cases the brain tissue which had previously been compressed by the dilated ventricles under the pressure of CSF secretion will even regain its former shape, with familiar convolutions and sulci returning. An unusual picture occasionally arises when massive hydrocephalus in children is studied: the air can show numerous round shadows of varying size which obviously correspond to bubbles (Fig. 193). They have no pathognomonic significance and are possibly related to protein in the CSF. In such cases the air/fluid interval is also quite wavy.

After these general remarks regarding midline obstructions of the ventricular pathways, individual syndromes will now be described in greater detail.

Third Ventricular Tumors: Upper Anterior Group

Occlusion of the Foramina of Monro

Ependymal (colloid) cysts of the foramen of Monro (see p. 32): These cherry-sized cysts produce a very characteristic block of the foramina of Monro. Their half-circular contour between the bodies of the frontal horn and eventually the third ventricle can be seen in the anteroposterior view (Fig. 194). The demonstration is significantly improved when the same exposure is made in the half-axial projection. If both lateral ventricles and the third ventricle are filled with the contrast agent (either by the lumbar or ventricular approach), the cyst in its entirety may occasionally be outlined in the lateral frontal horn view (192/1). Less commonly,

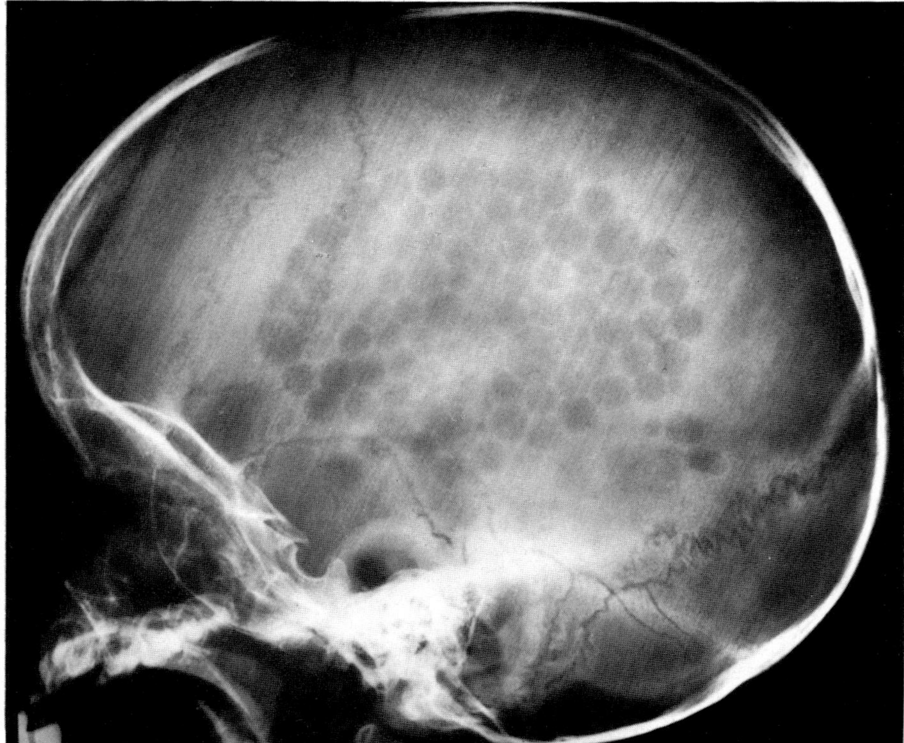

Fig. 193. Air study in an infant with obstructive hydrocephalus; note the air bubbles

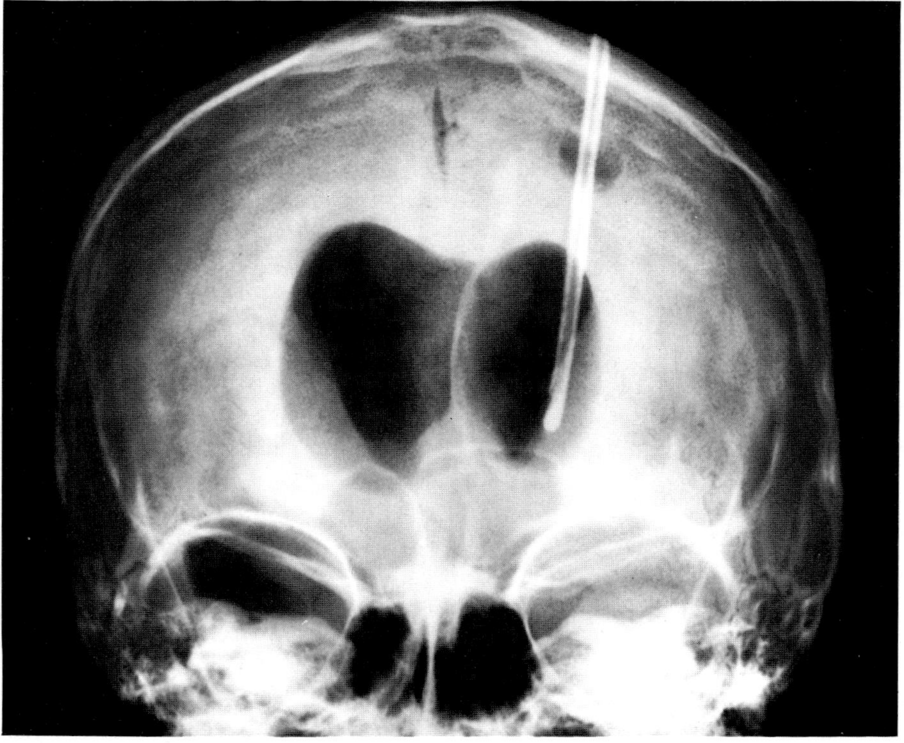

Fig. 194. Ventriculogram of a patient with an ependymal (colloid) cyst at the foramen of Monro (see Fig. 192/*1*)

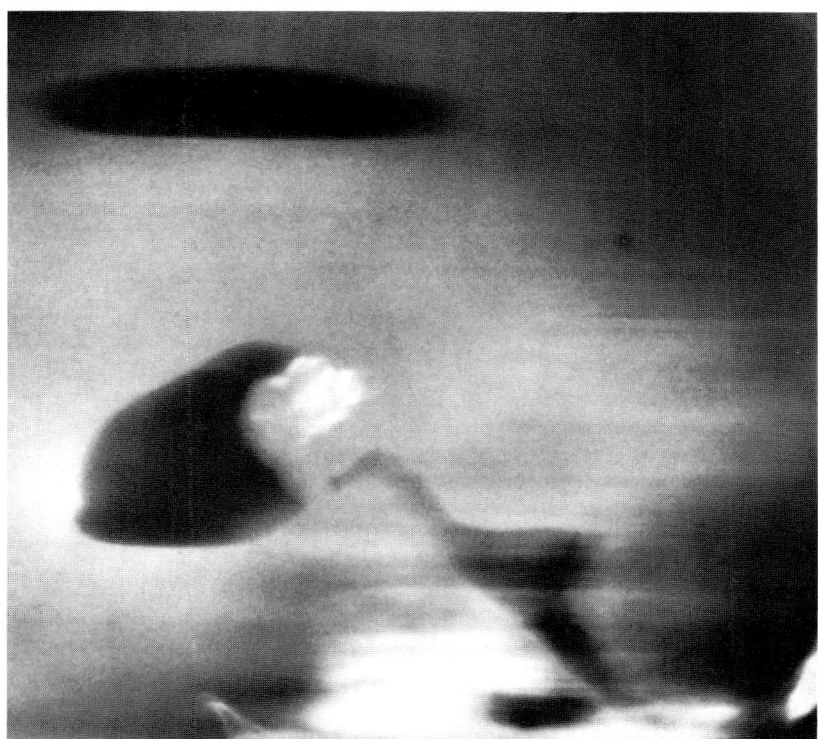

Fig. 195. Lateral tomogram of a patient with a pinealoma. Note the tumor invagination into the posterior third ventricle and the kinking of the aqueduct

the cyst is offset to one side, resulting in an unilateral enlargement of the involved ventricle.

Other tumors in the rostral portion of the third ventricle include choroid plexus papillomas, intraventricular craniopharyngiomas without involvement of the sella, and the pilocytic astrocytomas; all of these may also lead to a block of the foramina of Monro, but differ from the colloid cyst by their more expansive growth.

Third Ventricular Tumors: Upper Posterior Group

"Pineal Region Tumors"

Pinealomas/germinomas, teratomas of the pineal, ependymomas of the third ventricle, pilocytic astrocytomas of the quadrigeminal plate (see p. 34): We have chosen to group these tumors under the inclusive term "pineal region" or posterior third ventricular tumors because the air study of each is almost always the same regardless of their precise site of origin.

Tumors from the pineal region extend into the posterior third ventricle in such a fashion that the smooth or irregular rounded surface of the advancing mass gives the posterior limit of the dilated third ventricle a concave contour (Fig. 192/3).

With complete obstruction of the ventricular pathways at midbrain level, the dilation of the third ventricle can achieve considerable proportions with this structure being converted into a paper-thin bubble. This results in pressure changes in the sella as well as the clinical hypothalamic/chiasmal syndrome.

Pinealoma/germinoma: In the majority of cases these expand in an anterior direction (Fig. 195), since they will encounter the relatively resistant buttress of the corpus callosum and falx superiorly. In the air study they are recognized as an irregular, sizable filling defect occupying the posterior third ventricle. Ependymomas often have a similar appearance. Pinealomas/germinomas may often be heavily calcified in their early phases of growth.

The remaining "pineal region" tumors (teratomas, ependymomas, ependymal and arachnoid cysts; see p. 34): Teratomas, pilocytic astrocytomas, meningiomas of the tentorial hiatus, and arachnoid or ependymal cysts all present with a smooth advancing surface. Also, the venous aneurysms of this region may simulate tumors and usually have a smooth surface. In such cases angiography will confirm the correct diagnosis (Figs. 196, 197).

Tumors of the quadrigeminal plate itself (infiltrating pilocytic astrocytomas): These "pineal tumors" result initially in a thickening of the plate, especially in the upper portion, which leads to a deformation or an obstruction of the quadrigeminal cistern. As the tumor enlarges, it begins to indent also the dorsal portion of the third ventricle, as mentioned above. Eventually, changes in the aqueduct will occur mostly through growth of the tumor. At the same time the aqueduct is displaced from above, inferiorly. If the walls of the aqueduct are infiltrated with tumor, their contour on the air study will be irregular. When the distance between the aqueduct and the quadrigeminal cistern is definitely widened, it is possible to make the diagnosis of a true glioma, particularly with smaller tumors. It is important to consider the differential diagnosis between the various primary causes of aqueductal stenosis, tumor invasion of periaqueductal tissues, inflammatory processes, and membrane formation.

The Midline Tumors

Basal Group

These consist of the sellar and parasellar tumors because of their tendency to invade the third ventricle and the chiasmatic and interpeduncular cisterns. They may be further divided into median and paramedian groups.

General characteristics: With tumors in this region the third ventricle is invaginated from below and may be displaced horizontally. In addition, the chiasmatic cistern may also be displaced or compressed by the advancing tumor. The diagnostic evaluation of these tumors should also include angiography, since this often gives important information not available with the pneumoencephalogram. Neither study is, however, sufficient without the other. Pneumoencephalography, for example, more clearly defines the margins and the size of the tumor.

Median Group

Tumors of the chiasmal region (pituitary adenomas, craniopharyngiomas, meningiomas of the tuberculum sella, chiasmal/hypothalamic pilocytic astrocytomas, gangliocytomas, and finally, medially situated supraclinoid internal carotid artery aneurysms, see p. 32).

With tumor extension above the sella there may follow secondarily an obstructive hydrocephalus because of invasion of the anterior third ventricle. In such cases the floor of the ventricle is elevated (Figs. 198, 199) until the flow of the CSF out of the foramina of Monro is occluded. This is particularly true of the suprasellar craniopharyngioma.

In neurosurgery it is important to differentiate the suprasellar type of craniopharyngioma, which leaves the pituitary fossa intact, from the "intrasellar" type which will also extend into the suprasellar region, similar to a pituitary adenoma.

Despite invasion of the anterior third ventricle by large tumors, a small communication from the foramina of Monro to the aqueduct will usually persist for an extended period. In these cases the lateral ventricles may be only slightly dilated. At the same time the tumor will extend anteriorly and superiorly into the chiasmatic cistern, with the result that an impression of tumor contour can also be gained through cisternography (Fig. 198).

On the survey film in the lateral view, air may appear to reside in the suprasellar region which, in reality, is lateral to the midline tumor. This can lead to the mistaken impression that no suprasellar mass is present or that the mass is small. Tomography in such cases will permit precise location of the air. The differential diagnosis is often between a glioma of the hypothalamus and an extracerebral tumor of the sellar region. The optic nerve glioma, which can also involve the chiasm, will likewise be identified by cisternography. To confirm the suprasellar extension of a tumor, excellent visualization of the entire third ventricle is imperative. Special hanging head views will reveal indentations into the third ventricle anteriorly and inferiorly (Fig. 198).

Large craniopharyngiomas and pituitary adenomas can compromise not only the third ventricle, but may also extend over the chiasm into the frontal lobe and, less commonly, into the temporal lobe or midbrain.

Paramedian Group

To the paramedian mediobasal tumors belong parasellar chondromas, epidermoids, trigeminal neurilemmomas, supraclinoidal and infra-

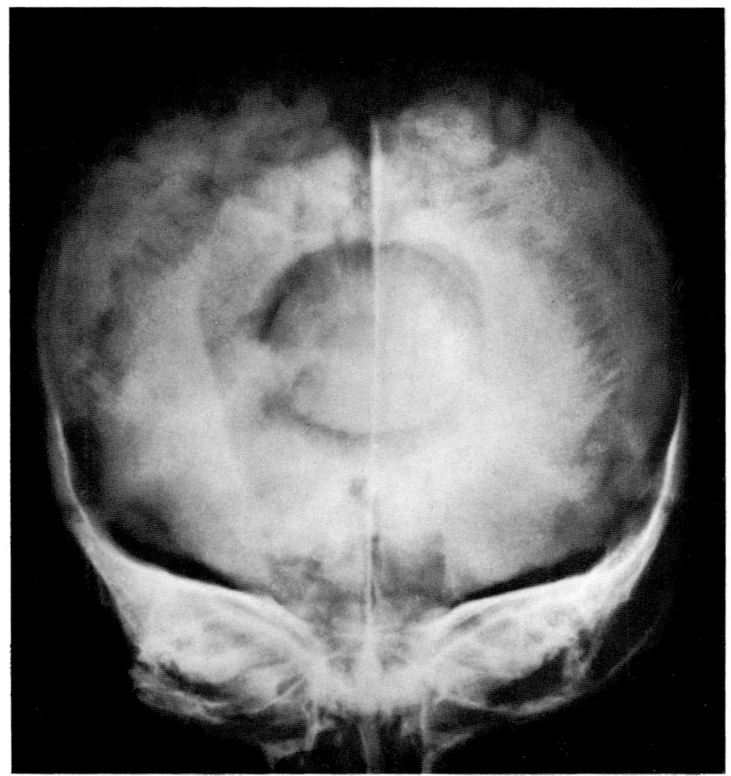

Fig. 196. "Aneurysm" of the vein of Galen. Pneumoencephalogram

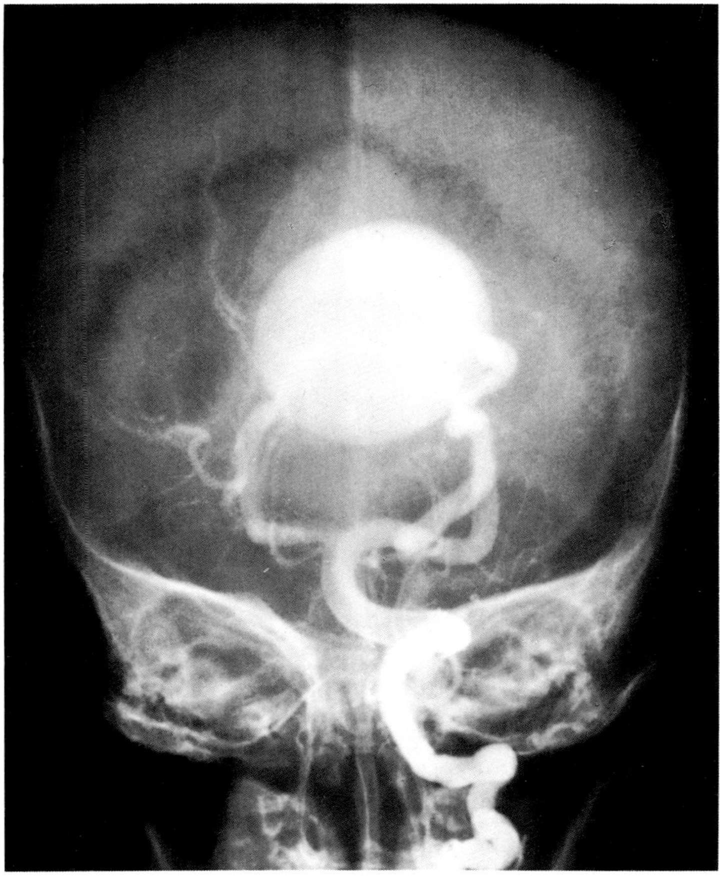

Fig. 197. Angiographic study of the same patient as in Fig. 196

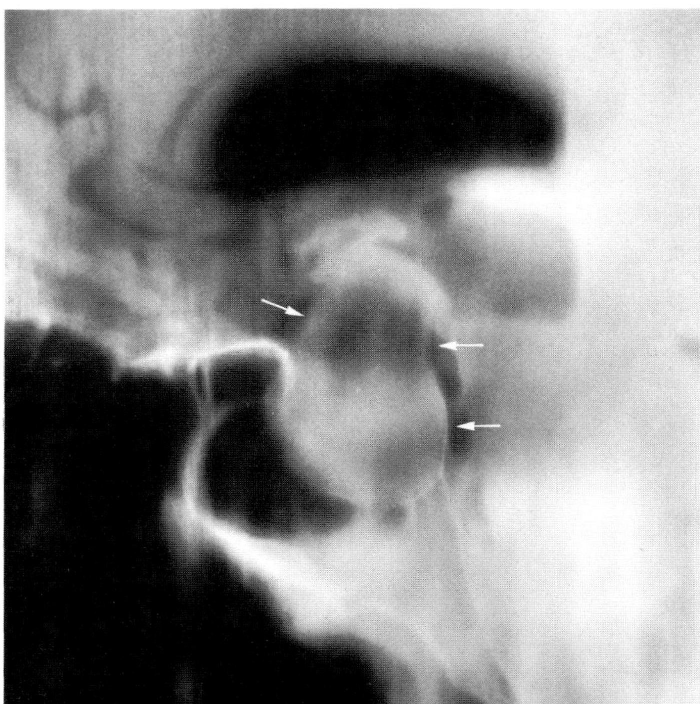

Fig. 198. Cisternogram of a pituitary tumor (*arrows*) with suprasellar extension. Note the cisternal distortion and the tumor invagination into the anterior basal third ventricle

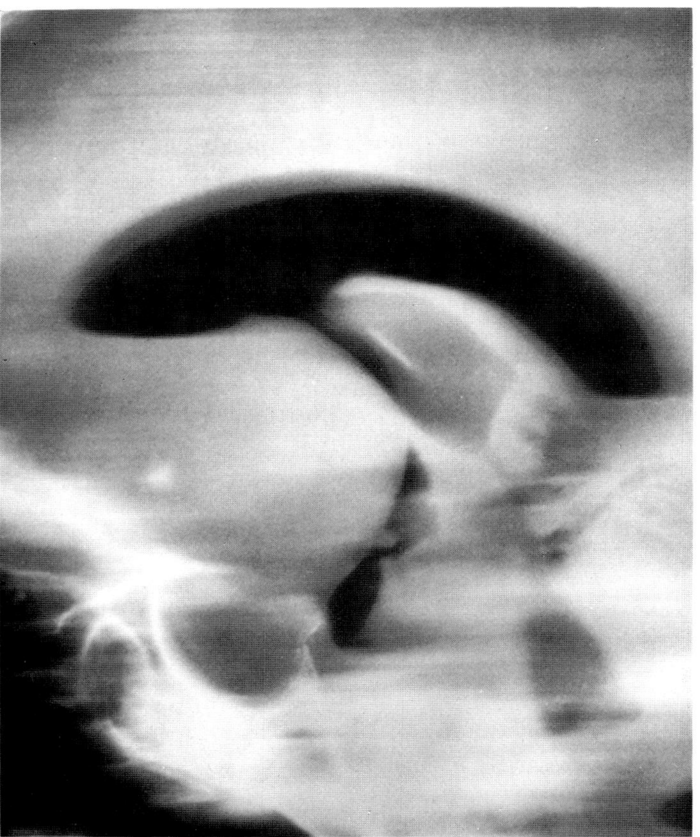

Fig. 199. Lateral tomogram of an air study which shows a craniopharyngioma from the pituitary region indenting the third ventricle. Note the calcium deposits in the anterior portion of the tumor

clinoidal aneurysms of the internal carotid artery, meningiomas, teratomas, and asymmetrically growing pituitary adenomas (see p. 32, 42): Here, the same investigative procedures are performed as for the evaluation of the chiasmal region. Also with these tumors it is important to obtain a precise definition of the fourth ventricle, aqueduct, and third ventricle, as well as of the basal cisterns and particularly the midbrain cistern, since this is frequently displaced to one side or the other by the tumor mass. For this purpose, tomography is again essential.

The Aqueductal Stenoses

In aqueductal stenosis, distinction is made between primary and secondary types. *Primary* aqueductal stenosis can be congenital (as with a malformation, such as the Arnold-Chiari syndrome, or with fetal inflammations), it can result from aqueductal tumors (pilocytic astrocytomas, rarely ependymomas), or it can be seen in later life following inflammatory processes (such as chronic ventriculitis).

Complete occlusions of the aqueduct are rare. Even if no air appears to pass, CSF flow may continue on an intermittent basis ("valve-like occlusion"). It is often advisable to demonstrate the upper and lower limits of the obstruction by a combination of ventriculography and pneumoencephalography respectively.

Secondary aqueductal stenoses occur as a result of the mass displacement of neighboring tissues with secondary distortion of the aqueduct.

Congenital occlusions are usually proximally situated, that is, the stump of the aqueduct is seldom longer than 2–3 mm. As a result, this blind stump is cone-shaped, but may also be club-shaped (Fig. 200).

In order to determine from pneumoencephalography whether the aqueductal stenosis is primary or secondary and what disease process is occurring, it is again necessary to portray the quadrigeminal cistern. If the contour and position of the cistern are normal, primary aqueductal stenosis is likely. In such cases the suprapineal recess is frequently blown up like a large balloon. It can also (see above) occasionally present below the tentorial hiatus as a large cyst compressing the cerebellum. Significant enlargement of the suprapineal recess

speaks for a primary aqueductal stenosis of long duration since tumors of the posterior cranial fossa with their resultant upward cerebellar herniation will offer resistance to the type of expansion of the suprapineal recess described above, and particularly the infratentorial component.

Tumors in the Region of the Fourth Ventricle

Tumors of the posterior cranial fossa result in an obstructive hydrocephalus involving the lateral ventricles, the third ventricle, the aqueduct, and that portion of the fourth ventricle proximal to the occlusion (Fig. 201). The position and shape of the aqueduct and fourth ventricle vary depending on the site and dimensions of the tumor. The demonstration of the aqueduct is therefore of utmost importance. This shows that tumors of the posterior cranial fossa share with other tumors the tendency to displace and compress cisterns and adjacent ventricular segments and, by so doing, to use up the reserve CSF spaces. Not only do such tumors displace the aqueduct and distort the fourth ventricle, they also compress or fill up the pontine and pontocerebellar cisterns as well as the cisterna magna. Tumors of the posterior cranial fossa exert their mass effect in all directions equally. In the superior direction the tentorium provides a resistent barrier to expansion, so that *upward cerebellar herniation* can only occur through the tentorial hiatus (see Fig. 10).

Because of *downward* (tonsillar) *herniation,* fractional pneumoencephalography is unsuccessful in tumors of the posterior cranial fossa, failing to fill the ventricles and aqueduct (see Fig. 10). In such cases the cisterna magna and the foramina of Magendie and Luschka are all displaced and compressed. This lack of filling, in itself, can point to a tumor of the posterior cranial fossa. Displacement and compression of the appropriate cisterns can also contribute to the diagnosis and the precise position of the tumor. Additional information of value can be gained from displacement of the vallucula, unilateral obliteration of the pontocerebellar cistern, and also unilateral obliteration of the ambient cistern when this is associated with preservation and enlargement of the supratentorial retropulvinar "wings".

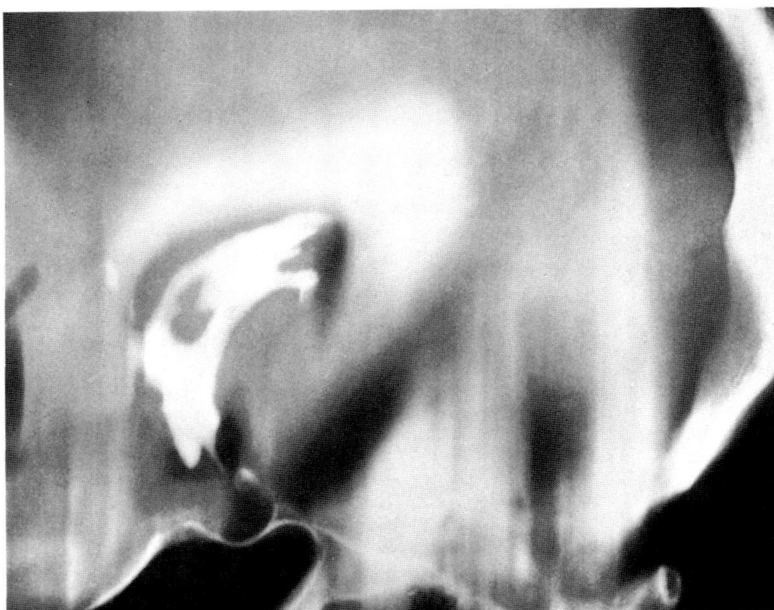

Fig. 200. Occlusion of the aqueduct – lateral positive contrast ventriculogram

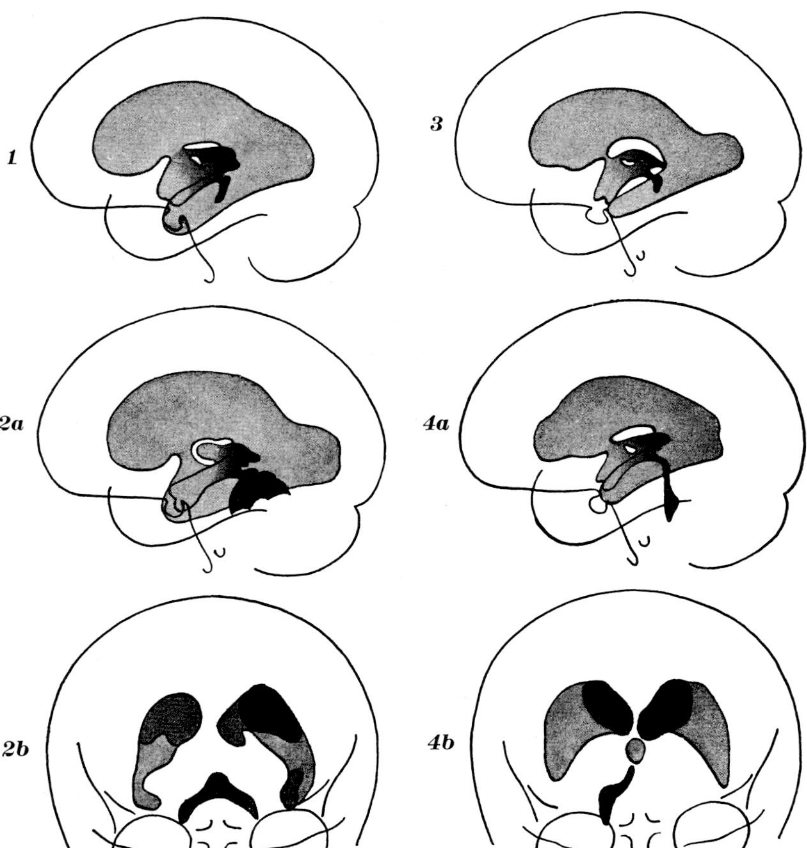

Fig. 201. Schematic representation of possible changes in the air study with two posterior fossa tumors. *Left,* midline position; *right,* lateral position

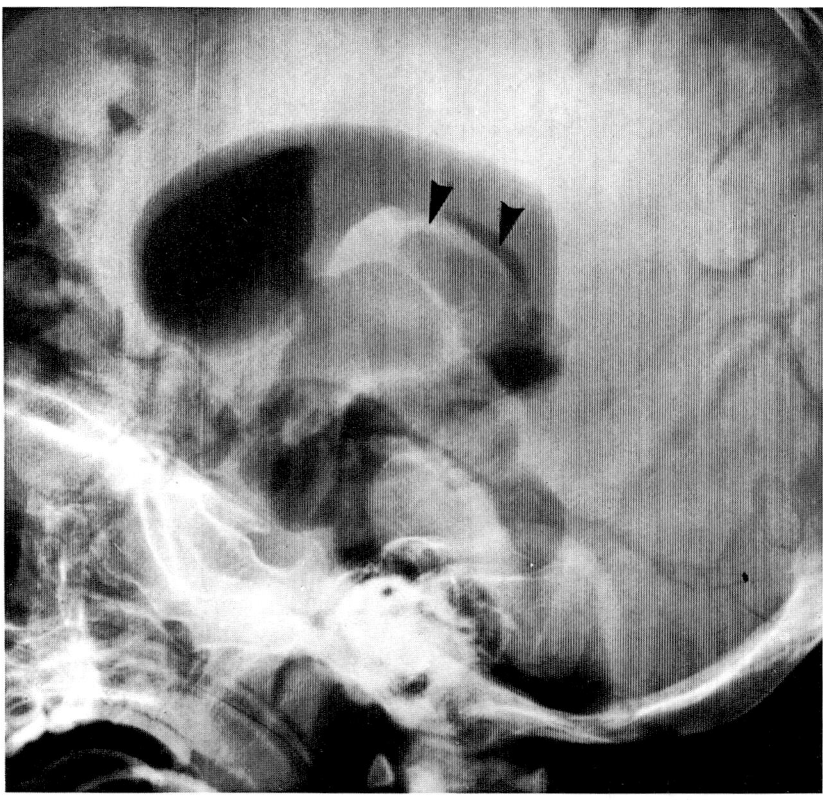

Fig. 202. Demonstration of the cistern of the velum interpositum in a normal infant

Even changes in the supratentorial cisterns may be used to advantage in diagnosing infratentorial tumors, e.g., when the median and paramedian supratentorial cisterns are enlarged. In such cases there is often a collection of air seen in the vicinity of the anterior third ventricle, which represents the markedly enlarged cistern of the velum interpositum (Fig. 202). The cistern of the corpus callosum may also be enlarged, which will form an unusual "rabbit-ears" image in the sagittal views. These changes are brought about by an occlusion of the basal CSF pathways, while those passing above the cerebellum remain open.

Pontine tumors (pilocytic astrocytoma, see p. 35): Pontine tumors primarily displace the CSF pathways in the region of the fourth ventricle and aqueduct (Figs. 203, 204), both of which are elevated and arch around the enlarged pons. The posterior third ventricle can also be indented by the expanding mass. Early pontine tumors may only cause subtle changes in the pneumoencephalogram, for example, reduction in the anteroposterior diameter of the fourth ventricle alone with no other abnormalities present. Measurements performed at this stage will also show that Twining's point is now below the fourth ventricle.

Twining's point bisects the line connecting the tuberculum sella with the internal occipital protuberance and normally lies within the fourth ventricle.

In the half-axial posteroanterior projection the fourth ventricle will appear to be widened since it is indented and spread out from below by the actions of the tumor (Fig. 204).

In pontine tumors visualization of the cisterns is of prime importance. The pontine cistern is markedly narrowed and may be totally occluded. Similarly, the interpeduncular cistern may be missing as a result of mass displacement and upward herniation. The ambient cisterns are widely separated in an upward/downward direction and appear to encircle the ventral aspect of the enlarged brain stem in a wide curve. If the quadrigeminal cistern is also visualized, it will be found displaced superiorly. The proximal hydrocephalus with this tumor is usually minimal. Differentiation from extrapontine tumors (for example, the clivus meningioma) may require angiography.

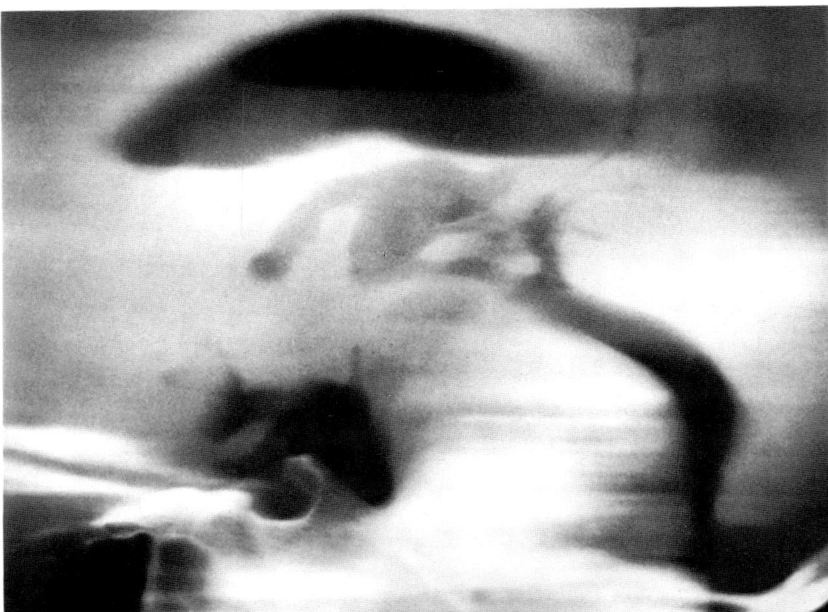

Fig. 203. Displacement of the fourth ventricle with a pontine glioma. Lateral tomogram

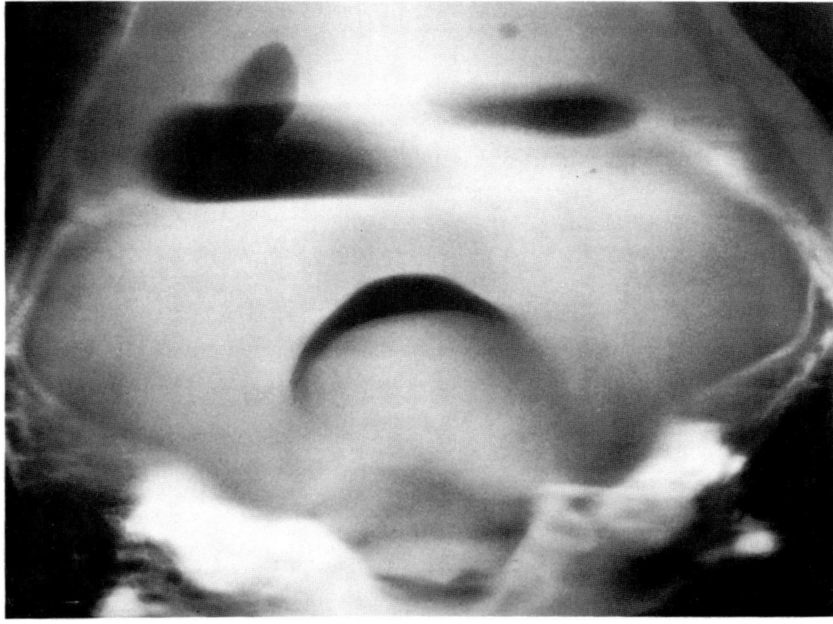

Fig. 204. Same patient as in Fig. 203. Anteroposterior tomogram showing the arch-like image of the fourth ventricle which outlines the tumor

The cerebellar vermis tumors (medulloblastoma, pilocytic astrocytoma): With midline cerebellar tumors, the aqueduct will show a distinct kinking about 5 mm distal to its origin from the third ventricle. This results from mass displacement of the brain stem and anterior cerebellum in the direction of the tentorial hiatus, which pushes up the distal portion of the aqueduct. The greater the mass effect present, the more acute will be the aqueductal kinking until the angle formed is quite pointed (Figs. 201, 205).

The cerebellar hemisphere tumors (pilocytic astrocytoma, see p. 35): If the tumor is situ-

Fig. 205. Positive contrast ventriculogram with a posterior fossa tumor. Note the kinking (*arrow*) of the aqueduct

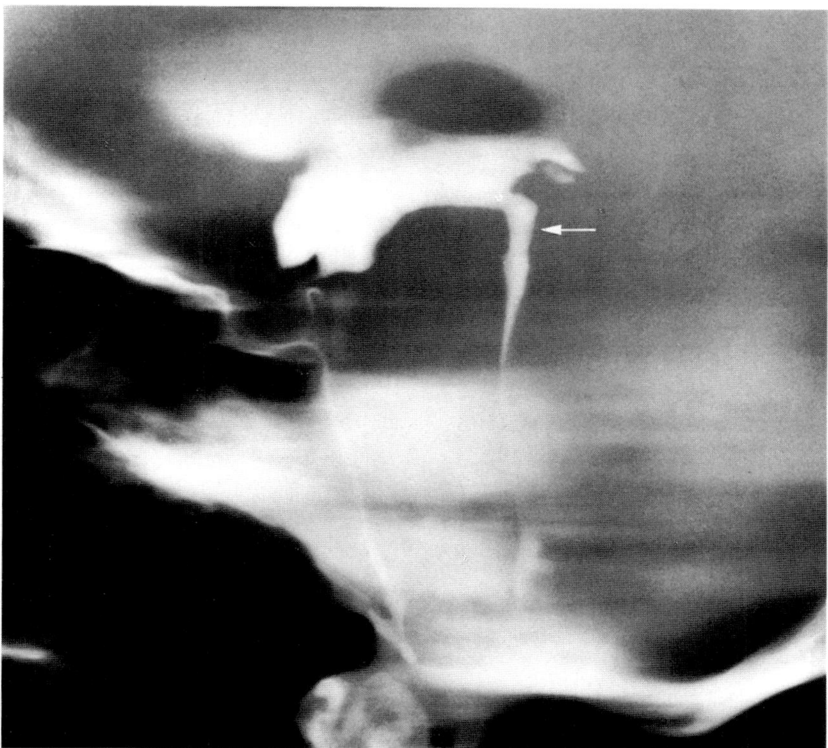

ated laterally in one of the cerebellar hemispheres, the aqueduct is again pushed upward, but not so much forward as before. The kink is less marked, tending to resemble a horse's tail (Fig. 201/3) and the blockage less pronounced. Simultaneously, the aqueduct and the compressed fourth ventricle are displaced to the opposite side, as is apparent on the half-axial posteroanterior exposure (Fig. 201/4). This change is especially important for the recognition of small hemangioblastomas which initially may not produce a significant aqueductal kinking.

The tentorium meningioma: Meningiomas originating from the tentorium show changes similar to the tumors of the intracerebellar vermis and hemisphere. They can be diagnosed with certainty on the air study only when there are both infratentorial and supratentorial extensions (dumbbell tumor), the latter causing distortion of the trigone, temporal horn, or occipital horn. Filling abnormalities with respect to the subarachnoid spaces can also confirm the extracerebellar location of this tumor. Angiography in such cases can be helpful as well, revealing hypertrophy of the tentorial arteries (see Fig. 34).

Tumors of the Fourth Ventricle

Proximal: plexus papilloma and pilocytic astrocytoma; distal: ependymoma and, rarely, hemangioblastoma (see p. 35): Tumors which originate within the fourth ventricle lead to a hydrocephalic enlargement of the proximal portion of the fourth ventricle (Fig. 201/2). The rostral tumor border is usually round (Fig. 206) and may be recognized on either the half-axial posteroanterior projection or lateral tomography.

Also many cerebellar vermis tumors (particularly the medulloblastoma) invaginate the fourth ventricle from above. If the tumor is situated somewhat more distally, both the aqueduct and the enlarged proximal portion of the fourth ventricle will be seen. Here the fourth ventricle will embrace the tumor in the shape of a bowl, its caudal limit being determined by the positon of the tumor. Either the half-axial posteroanterior view or the lateral view can be used to verify these findings.

Occlusion of the Foramen of Magendie

Arachnoid scarring, high cervical cord tumors: When a blockage occurs at the outlet of the

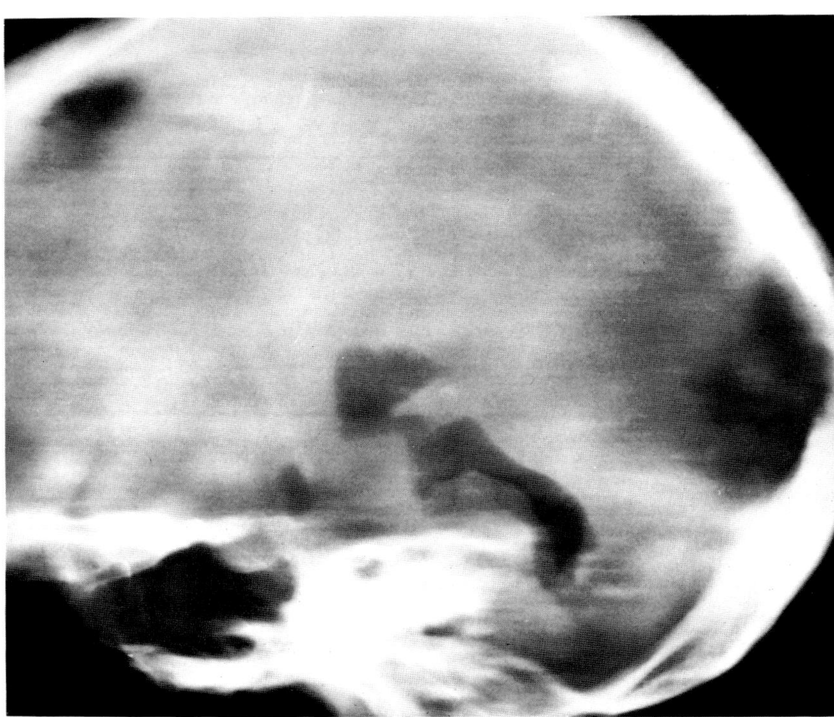

Fig. 206. Another posterior fossa tumor which is indenting the air shadow of the fourth ventricle

fourth ventricle and the entire fourth ventricle is enlarged, arachnoidal scarring with occlusion of the foramen of Magendie should be suspected. Various types are possible: either the obstruction involves the foramen itself, in which case the enlarged fourth ventricle displaces the cerebellum into the cisterna magna, or the obstruction lies at the outlet of the cisterna magna. In the latter situation, both the fourth ventricle and the cisterna magna are enlarged together, which is apparent on the air study (ventriculogram). In the final stages, these two forms cannot be differentiated. A further possibility is a combined occlusion of the foramen of Magendie and the rim of the cisterna magna. In this case the enlarged cistern forms an enormous cyst, which acts as a space-occupying mass in the area of the former cistern. Since it is a closed cyst, it will appear on the air study only as a space-occupying process. Finally, the tonsils themselves may (rarely) be involved in the scarring process to such an extent that they are stuck to the floor of the ventricle preventing its expansion and giving the appearance that the distal third of the ventricle has been cut off.

Occlusion of the foramina of Magendie and Luschka can also be congenital (*Dandy-Walker syndrome*). This anomaly is caused by a developmental defect involving the fourth ventricle and cerebellum. The markedly enlarged fourth ventricle fills practically the entire posterior cranial fossa and can also extend into the upper cervical region. The cerebellar hemispheres are extraordinarily small and are displaced laterally and anteriorly. The anterior third of the vermis is also displaced, but in an anterior and superior direction, while the remaining vermis undergoes pressure atrophy and becomes membranous. The occipital skull is very thin and the posterior cranial fossa enlarged and flattened. At the same time the position of the transverse sinuses and torcular are higher than normal, which is pathognomonic for the Dandy-Walker syndrome.

Because of the occlusion of the foramina mentioned above, pneumoencephalography will not be successful. Ventriculography will show an enlarged ventricular system and an enormous fourth ventricle which fills nearly the entire posterior cranial fossa. Angiography will demonstrate the high position of the torcular and the transverse sinuses.

In contrast to the congenital occlusion found in the Dandy-Walker syndrome, that which is caused by scarring secondary to arachnoiditis results in a generalized increased intracranial pressure and does not cause increase in the size of the posterior cranial fossa or flattening and thinning of the occipital skull. The position of the transverse sinuses is also normal. Ventriculography will reveal a generalized enlargement of the ventricular system. The fourth ventricle, however, is never so markedly enlarged as with the Dandy-Walker syndrome.

Also cervical cord tumors can extend superiorly, displacing and occluding the foramen of Magendie and causing a secondary hydrocephalus.

d) Cerebellopontine Angle Tumors

Acoustic neurilemmoma, meningioma, ependymoma, glomus tumors, epidermoids, chondroma of the apex of the petrous pyramid (see p. 34): A technically satisfactory contrast study with air, or more particularly with a positive contrast agent, will permit precise identification of cerebellopontine angle tumors and their relationship to the internal acoustic meatus. Not uncommonly it is possible to diagnose an acoustic neurilemmoma in its infancy, provided it has not extended too far beyond the internal acoustic meatus.

Cisternography with Air

The air study is performed in the sitting position by the fractional lumbar positive pressure technique. The head position is particularly important in order to insure that the air enters the cisterns, rather than the ventricular system. Also, the air injection itself may proceed faster than when ventricular filling is desired. Since only a certain amount of air can enter the ventricular system within a given time frame, the excess air will enter the subarachnoid spaces. With a small tumor in this location, ventricular shape and position will be normal, and attention can be turned to the demonstration of the *pontocerebellar cisterns.* If a small tumor is present, the pontocerebellar cistern may be somewhat enlarged. The border of the tumor can then be completely outlined by the air (Fig. 207), which will define the full extent of the mass. Larger growths will show more marked changes, such as deformity of the pons, which is indented from laterally and inferiorly. The pontocerebellar cistern on the opposite side is often compressed through mass displacement into it (Fig. 208).

Diagnostic difficulties can arise when there is primary enlargement of the cistern or when adequate visualization of the pontocerebellar cistern cannot be achieved. In the former instance, complete air filling of an enlarged cistern is difficult and air/fluid levels may persist. To correct this problem, it is necessary to turn the head farther to the uninvolved side in order to drain off more CSF, then to inject more air.

If the cistern does not fill with air, it can be assumed that a tumor is present which is completely filling it. It is, however, also possible that a technical error has occurred. The neck should then be strongly extended and the head turned to the opposite side. The air injection is then repeated. In our experience, with a correct head position and a technically correct air injection, visualization of the cistern is always possible. However, it should be mentioned that previous surgery or a pre-existing inflammatory condition involving the pontocerebellar cistern can lead to a closed arachnoid cyst which will hinder filling of the cistern.

Ambient Cistern

With a cerebellopontine angle tumor, the ambient cistern on the involved side is often enlarged, especially when the pontocerebellar cistern is obstructed. It may also appear to be cut off from below.

Fourth Ventricle and Aqueduct

If tumor size cannot be determined by cisternography, it is often necessary to visualize the fourth ventricle in addition. Here, a deformity of the lateral recess will almost always be found. If the tumor has spread between the pons and the clivus, the fourth ventricle will be displaced posteriorly and to the opposite side. Simultaneously, the pontine cistern will be compressed. The pneumoencephalogram will show the same picture in this case as in a unilateral extensive pontine glioma.

The diagnosis of *cerebellopontine angle tumors* with pneumoencephalography is satisfactory for tumors which have grown out of the internal acoustic canal into the intracranial space. However, the tumor must have reached a certain size before it will be adequately diagnosed on the cisternal air study.

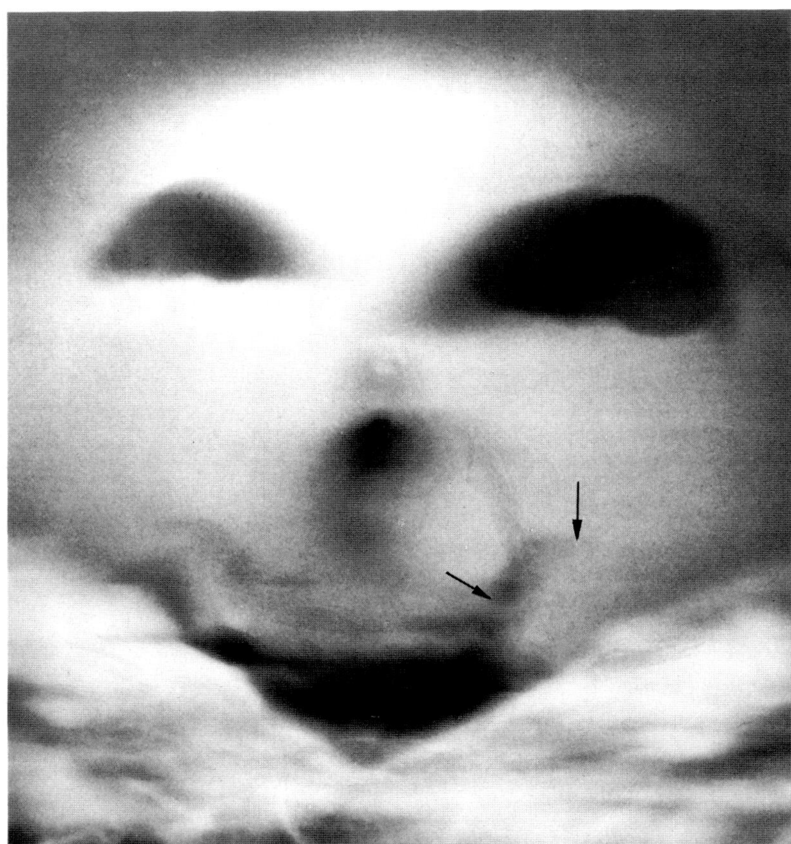

Fig. 207. Anteroposterior tomogram of an air study, outlining a left cerebellopontine angle tumor (acoustic neurilemmoma)

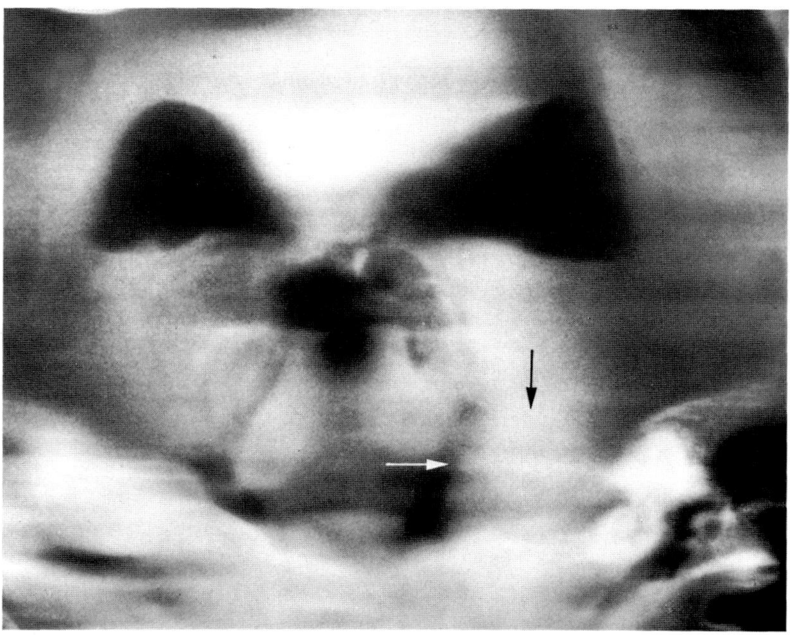

Fig. 208. Anteroposterior tomogram showing a large acoustic neurilemmoma. The left pontocerebellar and ambient cisterns are blown up and the adjacent pons is displaced

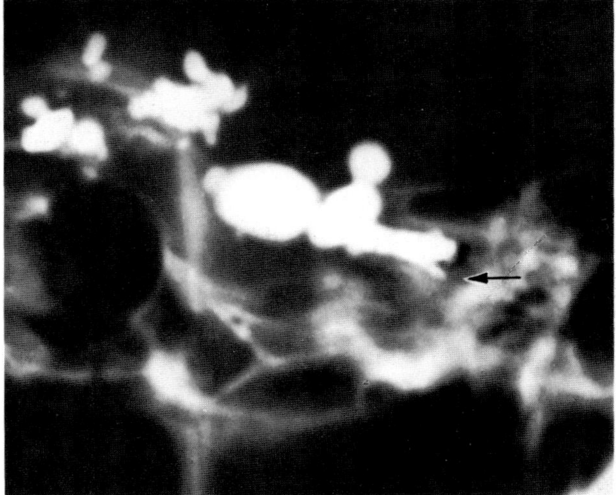

Fig. 209. Positive contrast cisternogram with normal filling of the internal auditory meatus. Note the falciform crest

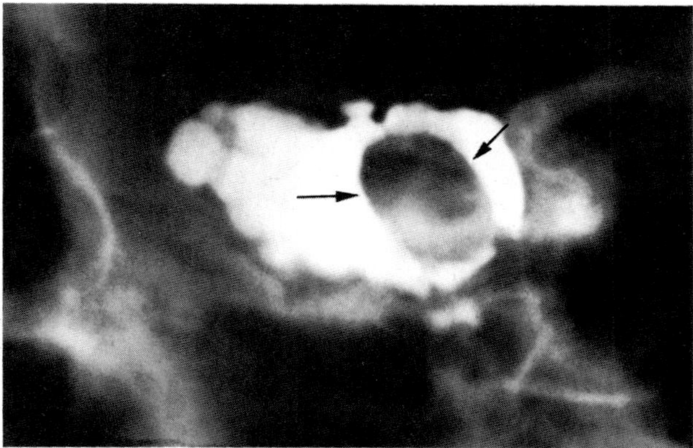

Fig. 210. Positive contrast cisternogram showing a cerebellopontine angle tumor

It is, however, desirable to diagnose the acoustic neurilemmona as early as possible, i.e., before it has left the confines of the internal acoustic canal and when otological symptoms first appear. In such cases, positive contrast cisternography has a definite role. It is invaluable in the diagnosis of early cerebellopontine angle tumors, particularly and specifically the acoustic neurilemmoma.

Technique of Positive Contrast Cisternography

After lumbar puncture in the sitting position, 1–1.5 ml of Pantopaque is injected. The patient is placed in the recumbent lateral position on a tilt-adjustable X-ray table on the side of the suspected tumor. For 3 min the table is placed at 35° with the head of the patient down. A restraint is required to prevent the patient sliding off the table at this point. While this position is held, the contrast medium flows from the spinal canal to the intracranial cerebello-pontine cistern and to the internal acoustic meatus. After 3 min, the table is returned to the horizontal and the head positioned for a Stenvers view. With the head fixed in this position, a tomogram is made of the pyramid. The X-rays will show the contrast medium in the cerebellopontine angle cistern and in the internal acoustic canal. The filling of the internal acoustic canal with contrast is usually clearly seen on the films obtained. Finally, one can turn the head and upper body of the patient and permit the contrast medium to pool in the opposite pontocerebellar cistern and internal acoustic canal. Thus, with a single study both sides can be portrayed, one after the other (Fig. 209).

Normally, the positive contrast agent will enter and fill the internal acoustic meatus and canal. In the majority of cases the falciform crest is recognizable along with the medial portion of the pontocerebellar cistern and trigeminal nerve (which stands out as a circumscribed negative image). In the presence of pathological findings, the contrast medium will either not enter the canal at all or fill it incompletely. There is then a tumor shadow in the region of the internal acoustic meatus, usually including the canal itself. In most cases the tumor shadow is semicircular (Fig. 210).

A similar finding can, however, also be seen with arachnoiditis or swellings in the region of the eighth nerve. In such cases, however, the contrast image is irregularly formed and does not have a typical tumor configuration.

Advantages of the Various Methods

If a small tumor in the region of the 8th nerve is suspected (purely otological symptoms; otherwise, no neurological deficit), one should immediately proceed with positive contrast cisternography. On the other hand, the presence of other neurological symptoms makes pneumoencephalography with cisternal filling the procedure of choice, since this method will permit visualization of the ventricular system and identification of lesions involving the cerebellum and brain stem as well. The question may be posed whether pneumoencephalography is truly indicated in the presence of precise neurological findings and plain film changes suggestive of an extrinsic angle tumor. In such cases, however, it is recommended that pneumoencephalography be performed anyway, since the addition of positive contrast cisternography will serve to complement the air study, each providing important and necessary information. For the early diagnosis of the beginnings of cerebellopontine angle tumors, however, positive contrast cisternography remains the procedure of choice.

A further possibility for the early diagnosis of cerebellopontine angle tumors is occasionally provided by air filling of the internal acoustic canal. This technique, which is carried out via the lumbar approach with the patient in an oblique position (so that air will enter the appropriate cistern and internal acoustic canal), appears to be relatively more difficult to perform and the X-ray pictures more difficult to interpret. Tomography is therefore essential so that the walls of the air-filled internal acoustic canal can be identified with certainty.

e) The Normal Air Study in Space-Occupying Processes

Every tumor passes through an early phase in which significant mass displacement with local distortion of the adjacent ventricle has not yet occurred. The air study in such cases may not show any definite changes. In the presence of neurological deficit pointing to a specific location (for example, the precentral and postcentral gyri), the discrepancy between clinical findings and the neuroradiological study may be due simply to the small size of the lesion.

Even large mass displacements may not be apparent on the air study if there is a co-existent diffuse cerebral atrophy with enlargement of the subarachnoid spaces. This is especially true in the elderly, where the mass effect is initially compensated for by local changes and the diagnosis thereby complicated. Prior to the advent of CT these "senile tumors" were often misdiagnosed for long periods as cerebrovascular insufficiency. The differential diagnosis in those cases where definite neurological symptoms were present included a space-occupying necrotic cerebral infarct. In both situations secondary mass displacements would be present. Angiography (in the absence of CT) will usually help by confirming the presence of tumor. The isotope brain scan can also be valuable when it shows a progressive increase in uptake – usually after a week's interval – in an area of infarct. When the repeat isotope scan shows an extension of the area of activity, the possibility of a tumor is heightened. To clarify further the diagnosis in later stages, pneumoencephalography is recommended since it will show a local increase in atrophy at the site of an infarct.

f) Multiple Tumors, Pseudotumor Cerebri

The pneumoencephalographic diagnosis of *multiple tumors* (metastases, multiple meningiomas with or without von Recklinghausen's disease) or of bilateral subdural hematomas (in cases where other indications for pneumoencephalography were present) can present special difficulties. Sometimes the mass effect of one tumor is so pronounced that it masks the effects of other tumors. On the other hand, the individual mass effects of many small tumors on opposite sides can balance each other or lead to an unintelligible air study. In the case of a contrast study with "paradoxical" findings or absent pneumoencephalographic changes with increased intracranial pressure, the diagnosis of multiple tumors should always be entertained.

Finally, there does exist a syndrome of increased intracranial pressure without a co-existent space-occupying process. This syndrome was first described by Nonne (1904, 1937), who called it "pseudotumor cerebri". Here the cause of the generalized increased intracranial pressure is not even clarified by the contrast study and one finds only narrowed ventricles secondary to the generalized volume increase.

Certainly, such a state could reflect a subacute diffuse cerebral edema (intracellular or extracellular) of undetermined etiology, which still can subside later (metabolic disturbances, interruption of steroid therapy in children, birth control pills in women). These symptoms can also follow spontaneous or intentional (intraoperative) sinus thrombosis, or occlusion of a large cerebral venous channel. The differential diagnosis here also includes multiple tumors, which of course is not reversible. Findings suggestive of pseudotumor cerebri can also be found in countries where cysticercosis is endemic through a diffuse, generalized involvement of the brain which leads to a significant inflammatory reaction with edema. Only later (after healing) do these calcify and become apparent on the plain X-ray. Should the cysticerci involve the ventricular wall, the air study is frequently misleading and may suggest an invasive tumor. With the racemose form, a displacement of the basal cisterns may occasionally be seen.

g) Specific Diagnosis of Space-Occupying Processes from the Air Study

For the diagnosis of specific space-occupying intracranial processes, pneumoencephalography is of limited value. There are very few findings on the pneumoencephalogram which are as specific as the finding of tumor vessels on an angiogram. Only the intraventricular epidermoid (cholesteatoma) with its evenly distributed air pockets amid the tumor flakes and clumps is truly pathognomonic (Fig. 191). This results from the breakdown of the flimsy surrounding capsule and the introduction of air into the tumor mass during the pneumoencephalogram. In other cases the site and contour of the tumor mass are sufficient to render an accurate diagnosis as, for example, the round cherry-sized colloid cyst which is found between the foramina of Monro (Fig. 194). Intraventricular ependymomas and the ventricular tumors

of tuberous sclerosis may also fit these qualifications, but much less commonly. Also characteristic is the picture of an extracerebral convexity meningioma with its surrounding sickle of air.

In some of the cases, the diagnosis may be based upon site and age, although this combination is more variable. For example, tumors within the trigone are much more frequently meningiomas than choroid plexus papillomas, large thalamic tumors in the young are usually oliogodendrogliomas, large cystic hemisphere tumors in the young ependymomas, etc. Also the growth characteristics and biological peculiarities of certain tumors can suggest specific diagnoses which, however, should only be considered rules-of-thumb: in this category one finds only pinealocytomas or germinomas of the pineal region metastasizing to the infundibulum. Similarly, a calcified suprasellar tumor may be presumed to be a craniopharyngioma. In the differential diagnosis between meningiomas and glioblastomas, one must consider the width of the ventricular system. With glioblastoma there is frequently a hydrocephalus of the opposite side, since this rapidly growing tumor elicits considerable cerebral edema and causes early obstruction of the ventricular pathways. With meningiomas, on the other hand, the ventricular system does not usually expand since tumor growth is slow, there is little surrounding edema, and deformities of the ventricular pathways are gradual.

The relationship to the ventricular wall can also be helpful. Changes in ventricular contour caused by meningiomas are usually smooth bordered and semicircular. If, however, a glioma (such as an oligodendroglioma) invades the ventricular wall, there follows a knobby indentation into the ventricle. Also, regressive changes in the tumor may be accidentally portrayed on the air study and can be most helpful: if one accidentally punctures and outlines a tumor cyst in performing ventriculography, it will usually turn out to be an ependymoma in the younger age groups, an astrocytoma in the middle aged, and a metastasis or glioblastoma in the elderly.

2. Atrophic Processes

The air study with the cerebral atrophies can be interpreted with relative ease if one is familiar with the morphological changes of a particular disease process and can infer how these changes will affect the adjacent CSF pathways. It must be emphasized, however, that the air study is rarely diagnostic of a specific atrophic process. This is because a variety of pathological processes affect the CSF pathways in a similar fashion. The various atrophic processes differ in the air study only with regard to their sites of predilection and the magnitude of their effect, which combination offers certain diagnostic possibilities. One can describe a continuous series of changes beginning with the generalized cerebral atrophies and ending with the circumscribed atrophy of a particular disease process.

a) Generalized Cerebral Atrophies

One uniform characteristic of the generalized cerebral atrophies is enlargement of the ventricular system – internal hydrocephalus. It is therefore important to recognize and distinguish the various causes of hydrocephalus, as follows:

1) Hydrocephalus from impairment to CSF outflow (occlusive hydrocephalus with obstruction in the ventricular system)

2) Absorptive hydrocephalus with impairment at the site of primary resorption or with blockage in the subarachnoid pathways (as, for example, after arachnoidal hemorrhage or normal pressure hydrocephalus)

3) Hypersecretory hydrocephalus (for example, with a plexus papilloma)

4) Hydrocephalus from atrophic cerebral processes (e vacuo)

Recent advances have made it possible to carry out studies of CSF dynamics by means of radioactive isotope tagging.

A variety of pathophysiological mechanisms are known to result in *generalized* cerebral atrophy (Figs. 211–214). These include presenile dementia, arteriosclerosis, hypertension, thrombangiitis obliterans and other similar vascular diseases (for example, syphilis), the encephalitides (especially Rocky Mountain spotted fever, progressive paralysis, or toxoplasmosis), encephalitic reactions to infectious diseases, fetal illnesses as well as perinatal and infant brain injuries, poisonings (especially by carbon monoxide), the various traumatic processes, hypoxic injuries (including asphyxia at birth), hyperglycemic and hypoglycemic shock,

other metabolic disturbances, illnesses associated with hypotensive shock, the dystrophies of infancy and old age, the specific and diffuse cerebral atrophies (after Alzheimer), and other rare encephalopathic cerebral processes, such as multiple sclerosis. All these disease processes result in diffuse cerebral atrophy involving the white matter, or both the gray *and* white matter, with secondary enlargement of the ventricular and subarachnoid pathways.

There is usually a certain correlation between the distribution of the atrophy (white matter versus gray matter) and the major CSF pathway involved (ventricles versus subarachnoid spaces), which should be considered only as rule-of-thumb (Zülch and Eschbach 1965). Thus, the pneumoencephalogram with trauma shows a definite marked enlargement of the ventricular system, usually through damage to white matter by edema, with lesser involvement of the subarachnoid spaces. After *arachnoidal hemorrhages,* including those of traumatic etiology, there commonly follows an absorptive hydrocephalus through blockage of the subarachnoid pathways over the convexities or at the cisternal level. Following *brain injuries in infancy,* the pneumoencephalogram will often reveal enlargement of both the ventricular and subarachnoid spaces. In cases of *seizures* of uncertain etiology, there is again a uniform enlargement of both CSF pathways. *Intoxications* and *metabolic disturbances* predominantly injure the white matter through edema and correspondingly cause primary ventricular enlargement. The senile and presenile *dementias* primarily involve the gray matter, but also the white matter. Correspondingly, they cause a marked enlargement of the subarachnoid spaces with less ventricular dilatation. *Multiple sclerosis* and the other *encephalitides* result in equal involvement of both pathways. The situation during and after *meningitis* predisposes primarily to ventricular dilatation on an absorptive basis.

Internal hydrocephalus e vacuo begins (similar to obstructive hydrocephalus) in the region of the frontal horns and gradually spreads to involve the remaining segments of the lateral ventricle. The temporal horns are usually the last and the least involved. With enlargement of the subarachnoid spaces, there is enlargement of individual sulci, primarily in the frontal, temporal, and parietal regions (Figs. 212, 213). The atrophy involves *the base of* the fron-

Fig. 211. Obstructive hydrocephalus with symmetrical dilation of the ventricles

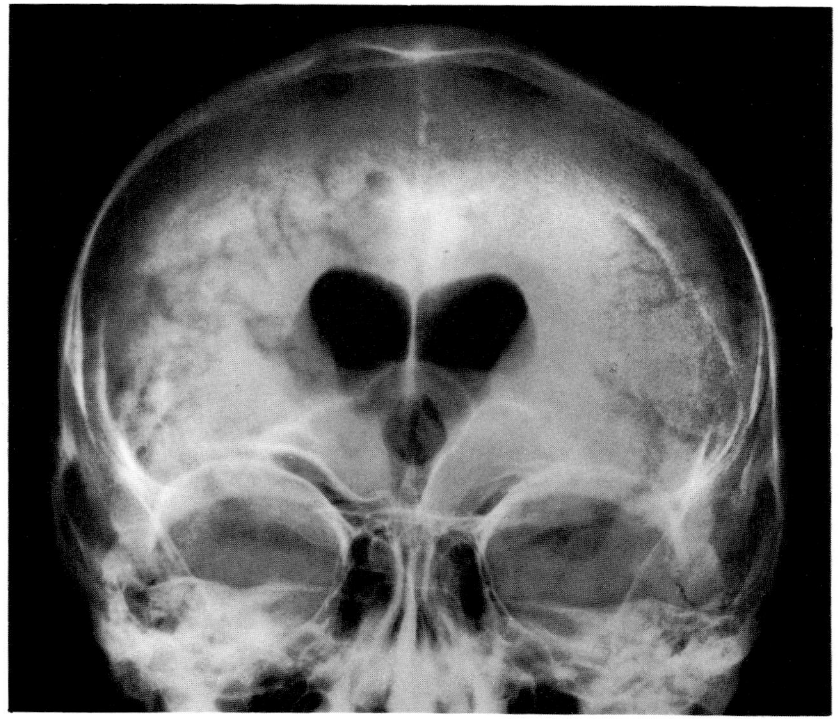

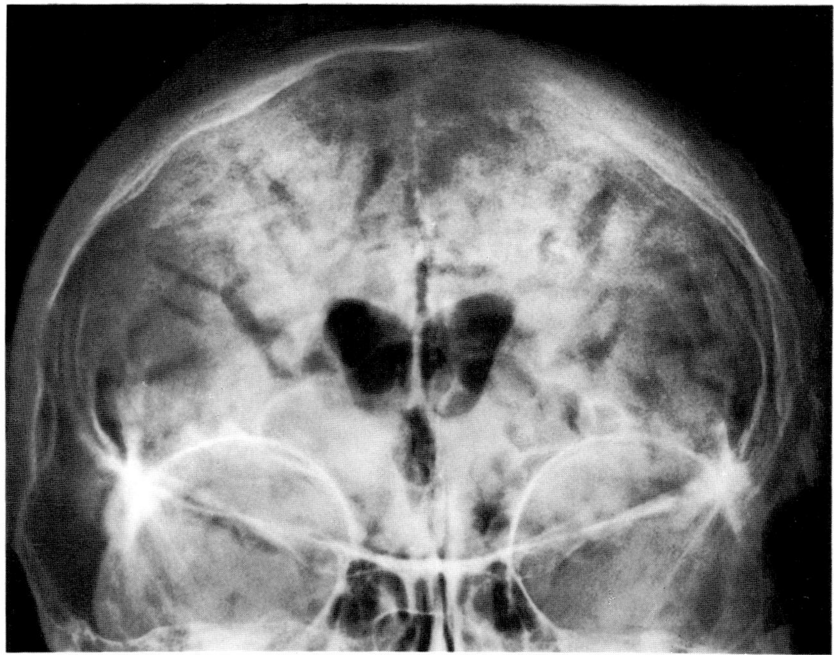

Fig. 212. "Communicating" hydrocephalus with enlargement of both the ventricles and the subarachnoid pathways (anteroposterior view)

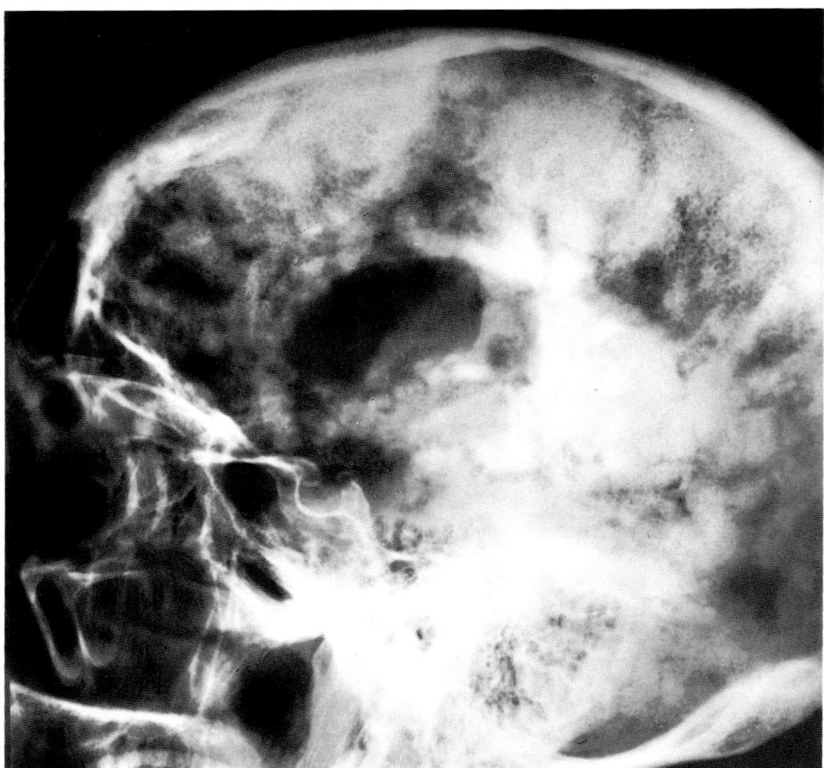

Fig. 213. Similar problem as with Fig. 212 – lateral view

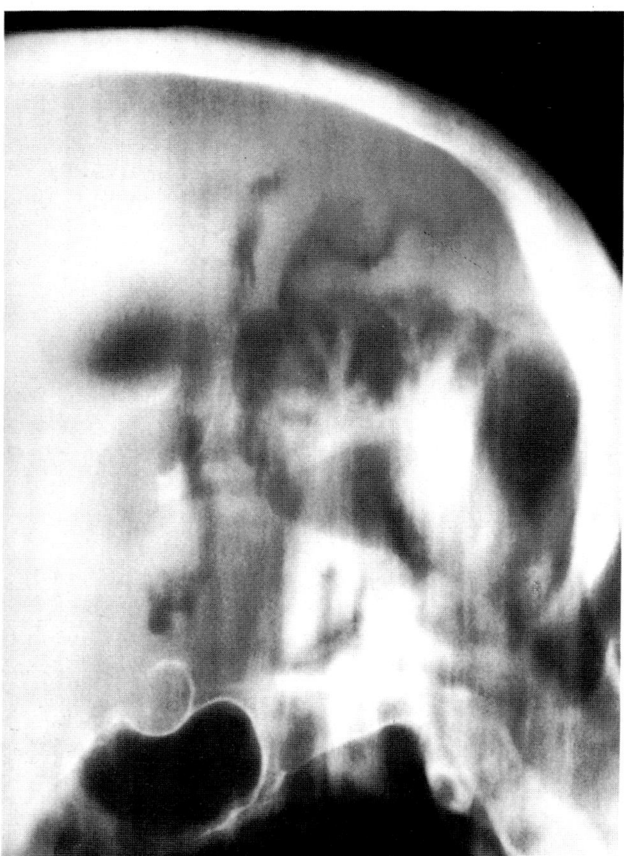

Fig. 214. Lateral tomogram of an air study showing cerebellar atrophy

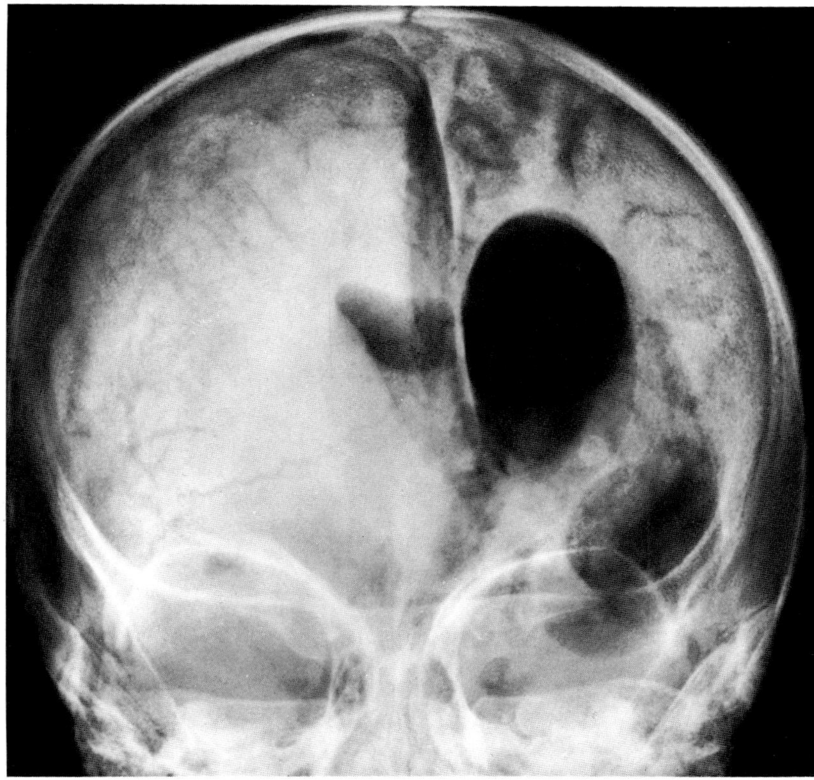

Fig. 215. Anteroposterior air study of a patient with an old left hemisphere brain injury. Note the marked ventricular dilation on the left with displacement of the ventricular system to the side of the injury. The atrophic convolutions are prominent and have the appearance of a cock's comb

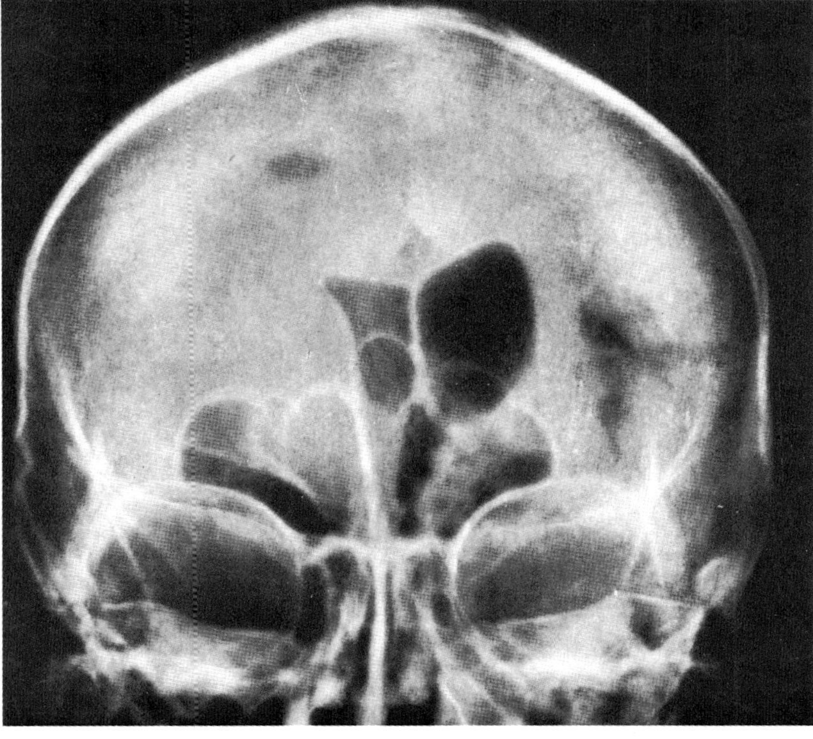

Fig. 216. Typical unilateral cerebral atrophy with "ventricular migration" to the side of an old carotid occlusion (secondary to a gunshot injury). Note the dilation of the cistern of the Sylvian fissure

tal lobes only in Pick's disease, while the occipital lobe is rarely involved. The generalized atrophies result in an early enlargement of the Sylvian fissures secondary to atrophy of the surrounding tissues, with preference for the insula: a particularly prominent insular cistern on the air study is therefore one of the earliest and most reliable signs of generalized cortical atrophy. It is clearly seen on the anteroposterior view (less commonly on the posteroanterior view) and is most characteristic when present.

b) Unilateral Atrophic Processes

Unilateral cerebral atrophy is frequently associated with AVMs, after vascular occlusions (particularly carotid occlusions) and after trauma (including birth injuries). Here the asymmetry of the ventricular system is the impressive feature (Figs. 215, 216, 218) while unilateral enlargement of the entire lateral ventricle, particularly the cella media and trigone, characterizes this type of injury. There is often an associated cystic structure ("porencephalic cyst") in the territory of supply of the middle cerebral artery, which may not fill in every air study. It is therefore important to carry out the study of the subarachnoid spaces and cisterns with care in order to demonstrate this abnormality. The picture seen with unilateral carotid clamping and thrombosis in the older age groups is usually associated with less marked changes than in the very young brain, where the tendency to total cystic transformation is greater. Occasionally there is a marked deformity of the ventricle on the involved side (Figs. 215, 216), as well as enlargement of the subarachnoid spaces (particularly the Sylvian fissure). Moderate enlargement of the opposite ventricle may also be seen.

In literature it is frequently stated that enlargement of the third ventricle may be seen in association with injury to the diencephalon. Based upon anatomical investigation, however, it would appear that dilation of the third ventricle predominantly follows atrophy of the adjacent cerebral structures which form its lateral walls.

Migration of the entire ventricular system to the involved side secondary to unilateral cerebral atrophy can mimic the displacement caused by a *space-occupying process* on the opposite side (Fig. 216). The differential diagnosis will be more carefully considered below (see p. 255).

c) Atrophy of Lobes

Atrophy of individual lobes is especially typical of the systematic atrophies of Pick. Depending on their localization ("frontal Picks's disease", "temporal Pick's disease", or combinations of both), an enormous collection of air is found over the atrophic convolutions, particularly the basal frontal lobe which, in the usual atrophic process, is either never involved or involved very late. The adjacent ventricular segments are also markedly enlarged.

Under the localized "systematic" atrophies, the cerebellar cortical (Purkinje cell) or cerebellopontine (olivopontocerebellar) atrophies are most frequently encountered (Fig. 214). In the former, one sees a coarse enlargement of the sulci normally present between the cerebellar folia, especially in the region of the upper vermis, early on. Later, this atrophy will spread to involve the entire vermis and the hemispheres. Then the cisterna magna and fourth ventricle will also be considerably enlarged.

With olivopontocerebellar atrophy, the atrophy of the pons and olive is much more impressive than the less-involved Purkinje cell dropout. Here one sees, *in addition,* significant enlargement of the pontine, pontocerebellar, and medullary cisterns.

d) Local Circumscribed Atrophies

A local, circumscribed loss of cerebral substance is usually the result of a small vessel infarct or other localized insult (contusion, laceration, repeated ventricular punctures in infants). If a small vessel occlusion is at fault, the area of atrophy will usually lie near the cortical mantle and will be seen on the air study as a cystic collection of air within the brain substance or in open communication with the subarachnoid space. Large vessel infarcts (for example, of the middle cerebral artery) and more extensive contusions usually cause a significant loss of white matter with a resultant enlargement of adjacent ventricular chambers. Specific changes on the air study with cerebral trauma will be described later (see pp. 255, 257ff.). It should be pointed out, however, that even with large subcortical defects (as, for example, following forceps injuries at birth) routine pneumoencephalography will frequently fail to fill the cyst and may require special cisternographic techniques to do so.

Attention should also be paid to the existence of cystic enlargements of the ventricle following hemorrhage with decompression into the ventricular system (as with AVMs) or following trauma with deep lacerations in the white matter, which is particularly common with frontobasal trauma.

3. Changes After Trauma to the Skull and Brain – Expert Legal Testimony

Acute brain injuries usually require angiography if CT is unavailable (see pp. 46ff., 118ff.). The long-term consequences of brain trauma will be discussed in detail, since they often form the basis for expert legal testimony. Although in head injuries disturbances in the cerebral tissues can theoretically occur in any place and have many manifestations, there is a definite predilection for the site and the type of the resultant pathological change, i.e., for the ensuing brain atrophy. The following classification lists the most frequent changes seen with pneumoencephalography (Fig. 217).

a) *Local ventricular changes* most frequently take the form of a tenting, or more pointed enlargement, or a drawing out of the roof of the ventricle toward a scarred, circumscribed area of injury (Fig. 218).

b) *Large cystic outpocketings of the lateral ventricles* are seen especially in trauma, which locally affects the large white matter masses, i.e., involving the frontal or temporal or occipital horns. Initially, these large areas of contusion go through a space-occupying phase. Later, there is resolution of this process and a removal of damaged tissues. Occasionally these areas will communicate with the CSF pathways resulting in club-shaped, cystic outpocketings of the ventricle. In children these cysts often assume large proportions and not infrequently follow forceps injury at birth. At this point, consideration should also be given to the "growing" skull fracture of childhood (with an underlying dural laceration) with its intracranial consequence of ventricular dilatation.

c) *Diffuse enlargement of a ventricular segment* is most apparent at the apices of the frontal, temporal, or occipital horns and is most certainly a consequence of diffuse cortical damage following edema or hypoxia.

d) *Diffuse enlargement of an entire ventricle* follows generalized damage to the white matter of the entire hemisphere. The subarachnoid spaces on the involved side may be obliterated if, after bleeding into the area, a significant inflammatory reaction occurs.

e) *A generalized enlargement of the ventricular system* can also be seen in the "normal pressure hydrocephalus" syndrome.

f) It is difficult to prove that *asymmetrical enlargement of a lateral ventricle* on the air study is a pathological finding related to trauma. The problem becomes even more complex if one considers the great number of technical errors which can lead to a misdiagnosis of unilateral ventricular dilatation (see p. 216ff.).

Assuming the technique to be flawless, there are many nontraumatic causes of ventricular enlargement. Furthermore, it should be noted that the left ventricle is frequently slightly larger than the right as a normal physiological variant, although the reverse may be seen as well. There are also a variety of pre-existing traumatic events possible as, for example, a perinatal or early childhood injury. To the "traumatic" changes should also be added the development of ventricular diverticuli following repeated ventricular punctures for therapeutic or diagnostic purposes and obstructive hydrocephalus in early infancy.

g) An additional consequence of trauma is *aerocele* or *pneumocephaly*. Such an intracranial collection of air can arise whenever there is a communication between the intracranial space and the adjacent sinuses (Fig. 219). In the majority of cases these follow fractures in the region of the cribriform plate, less frequently following fractures of the frontal or maxillary sinuses. By this means, air can be brought to an extracerebral location (epidural, subdural, and subarachnoid) as well as intracerebral (extraventricular or intraventricular). Combinations of the above are likewise possible. Although this condition nearly always has a traumatic etiology, a similar communication between the intracranial and extracranial spaces can also be seen with tumors of the anterior cranial fossa or sellar region, as well as with generalized increased intracranial pressure.

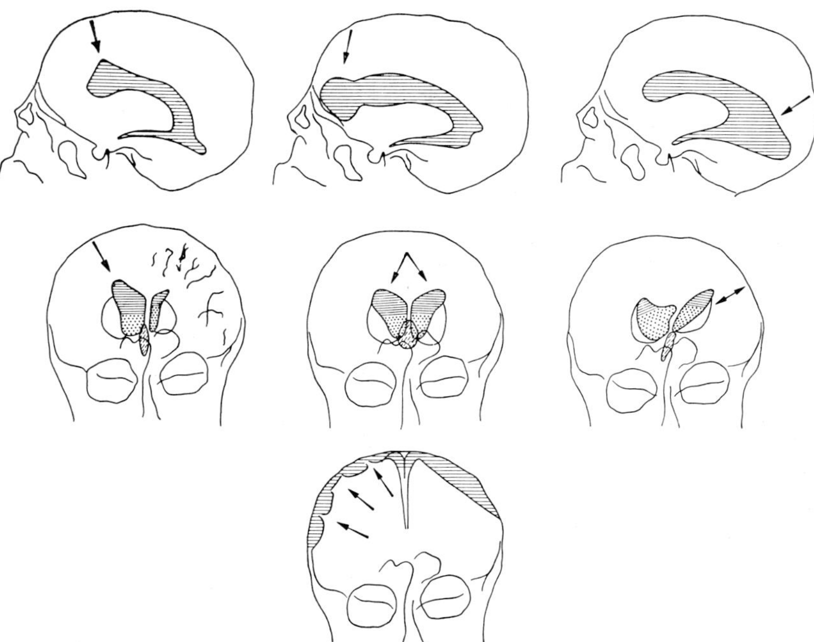

Fig. 217. Schematic representation of the most common ventricular changes seen following open or blunt craniocerebral trauma. Above: *left*, ventricular "tenting" or "pointing"; *middle*, cystic dilation in the frontobasal area; *right*, enlargement of a ventricular segment with minimal alteration in shape. Middle: *left*, unilateral ventricular dilation with adhesions and obliteration of the subarachnoid spaces; *middle*, generalized hydrocephalus; *right*, distortion and migration of the entire ventricular system to the side of the impact. Below: subdural contrast study with tent-like adhesions between the brain and dura

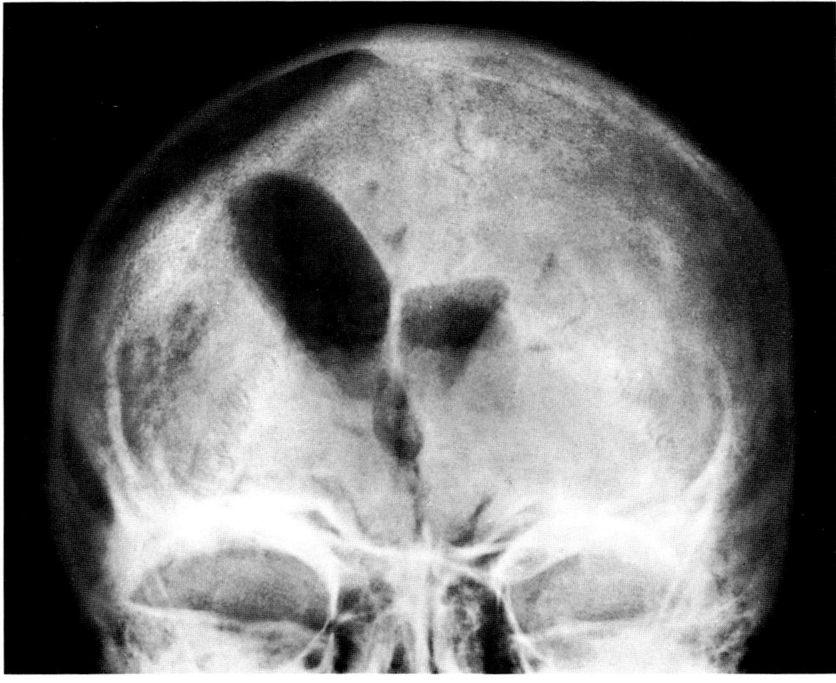

Fig. 218. Posttraumatic asymmetrical ventricular dilation with migration of the entire ventricular system to the affected side

Fig. 219. Pneumocephaly showing communication between the ventricular system and the large cyst

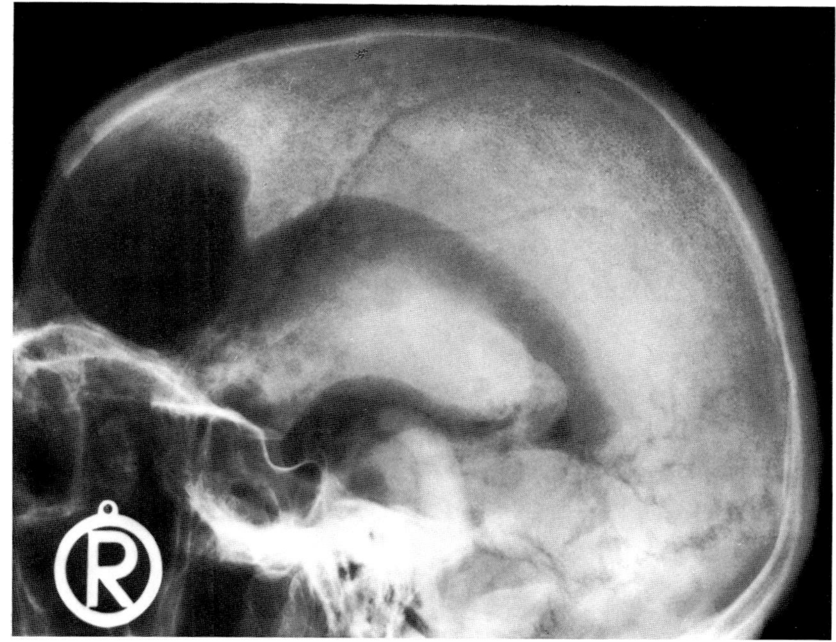

Fig. 220. Ventricular displacement away from an intracerebral abscess caused by a gunshot wound

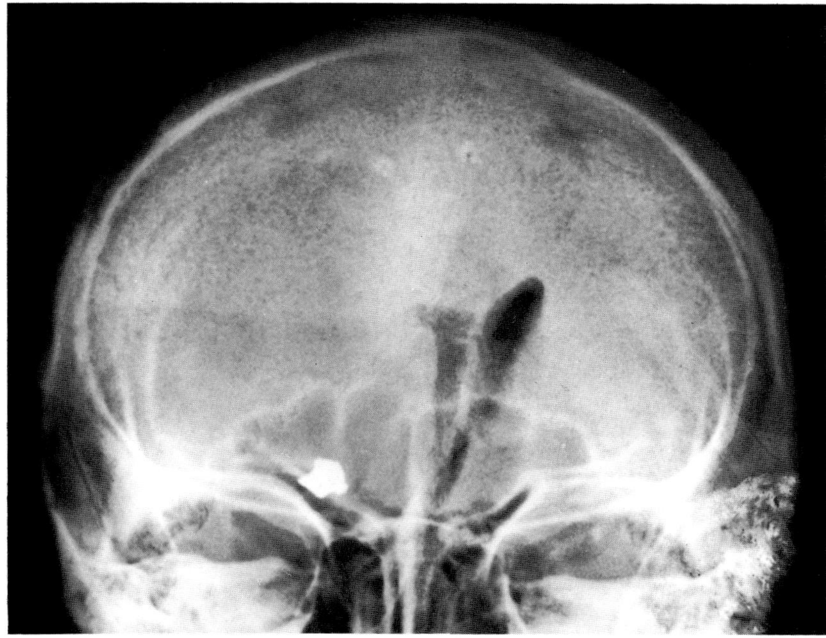

h) *Subdural hematomas* displace the ventricular system to the opposite side, which is indicative of a space-occupying intracranial process. Conformation that the lesion present is in fact a subdural hematoma usually requires CT or angiography. Delayed abscesses, however, can also lead to a similar ventricular displacement (Fig. 220).

Testimony about trauma to the skull and brain with regard to neuroradiological findings: The pneumoencephalogram has considerable merit as a means of verifying morphological changes following brain injury. It must, however, be accompanied by competent critical analysis. Thus, it is not permissible simply to point out a change in the air study and to infer automatically that this change is causally related to the earlier traumatic event. Rather, it is necessary to demonstrate by the appropriate history and clinical findings that the change seen correlates with the findings observed. A great number of additional possibilities have already been considered (see p. 252 ff.).

For similar reasons it is just as difficult to correlate a clinical symptom – for example, a convulsion – with an abnormality on the pneumoencephalogram without justifying the relationship. The radiological picture confirms only that a certain pathological change exists, usually not the cause for the change or the clinical consequences. Although a schematic listing of the most frequent posttraumatic changes seen on pneumoencephalography has already been given, very few are so specific as to be unquestionably related to trauma without further proof. Thus, the diagnostic precision of this procedure is limited. To this is added the fact that a negative air study may be found in the presence of a major posttraumatic neurological deficit. In fact, such deficits are frequently difficult to demonstrate on radiological studies, particularly when they are secondary to brain stem injuries. It is also possible to suffer a definite traumatic injury as a result of a noncompensatory illness (for instance, a fall during a seizure).

These introductory remarks show that pneumoencephalographic findings are only one of a variety of methods available for determining a causal relationship between a traumatic event and a neurological deficit, the proof of which requires consideration of all the available evidence (history, clinical findings, EEG, brain scan, CT, angiography, etc.).

The most frequent question asked with respect to legal testimony is as follows: When are ventricular asymmetries or local deformities so great that they must reflect pathological change (see p. 216 ff.)? This decision cannot be made on the basis of any measurement and usually comes only from personal experience. In borderline cases, therefore, expert opinions will often be divided. Similarly, opinions will also vary with respect to the determination of "generalized enlargement" of the ventricular pathways, as well as for the upper limits of the physiological atrophy in old age (see p. 218).

4. Malformations

a) The Septum Pellucidum Cyst

The most frequent of the visible malformations on air studies are the enlargement of the cavum septi pellucidi (the so-called septum pellucidum cyst) and the cavum Vergae cyst, which is situated in the posterior part of the septum. These cysts have no pathognomonic significance and are found in 5% of all autopsies. Earlier, it was assumed that there were two types of septum pellucidum cyst: the "open" (in free communication with the ventricles) and the "closed". Since both types are readily apparent on the pneumoencephalogram, this distinction has been questioned in recent years.

In the air study, the "closed" septum pellucidum cyst (on the sagittal exposure) appears as a smooth-walled widening of the normal septum up to approximately 10 mm. As a result of this, the distance between both lateral ventricles is increased symmetrically. If the cyst is "open" (Fig. 221) it appears as a collection of air between the frontal horns, from which it is separated by a thin membrane. The differential diagnosis in such cases is between a closed septum pellucidum cyst and a tumor of the corpus callosum which has invaded the septum. The cyst is favored when there is symmetrical enlargement of the entire septum, when its walls are smooth, and when there is an absence of any change in the corpus callosum itself, i.e., when there is a smooth contour to the ventricular roof (see p. 229 and Fig. 189).

The cavum Vergae cyst should also be considered here since it is occasionally seen in combination with a septum pellucidum cyst. Only

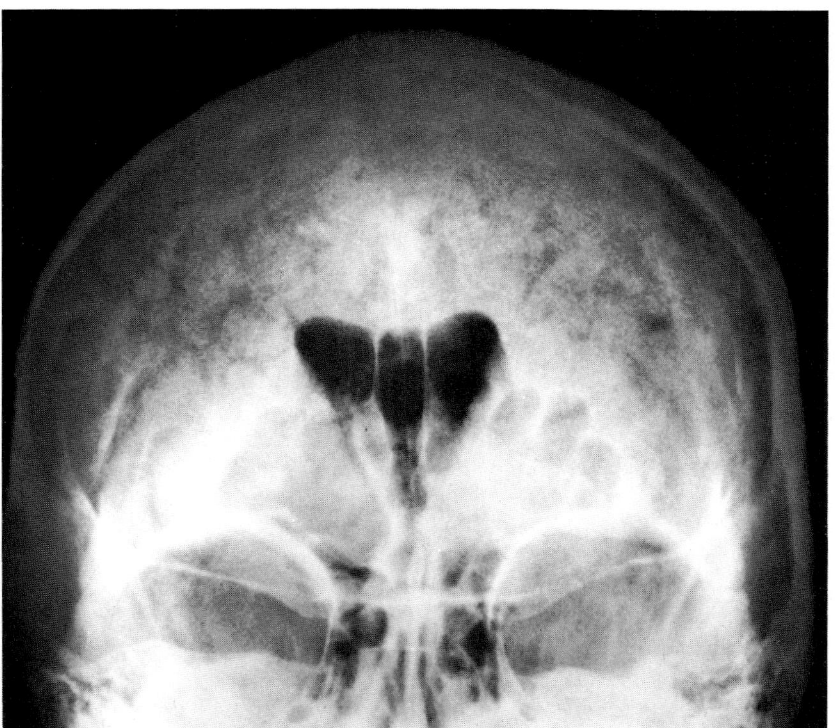

rarely is it found as an independent structure. It lies posterior to the cavum septi pellucidi and is best seen in the brow-down lateral and posteroanterior projections. If both cysts are filled with air, they are portrayed on the lateral view as an hourglass, with the waist representing the border between them. An enlarged cavum Vergae cyst can obstruct the aqueduct and result in a proximal hydrocephalus.

b) Agenesis of the Corpus Callosum

A complete or partial aplasia of the corpus callosum results in a type-specific deformity of the ventricular system. In the anteroposterior view, the frontal horns are widely separated and swing out like a pair of steer horns. Their normal point of contact, the septum, is absent. The third ventricle lies higher and is frequently positioned between the lateral ventricles (Fig. 222). This anomaly is occasionally seen in association with other malformations, for example, with lipomas. Since it is commonly encountered as an incidental finding in studies performed for other reasons, it has no pathognomonic value.

c) The Unpaired, Cyclops Ventricle

"Cyclopia" is frequently encountered in association with the arrhinencephalies. In such cases, the anterior forebrain fails to divide into cerebral hemispheres because of abnormal development of the olfactory region. The frontal horns and the cellae mediae of the lateral ventricles then form a single unpaired ventricular chamber (Fig. 223). The trigones and temporal horns, on the other hand, usually remain paired.

d) Arachnoidal Cysts

Arachnoidal cysts can be found in a variety of locations involving the peripheral cortex. These may be divided into primary and secondary cysts. Congenital cysts are, as a rule, found in association with asymmetry of the skull – for example, a bulging temporal bone – secondary to the local effect of the underlying cyst. They are relatively rare, show definite sites of preference (for example in the region of the Syl-

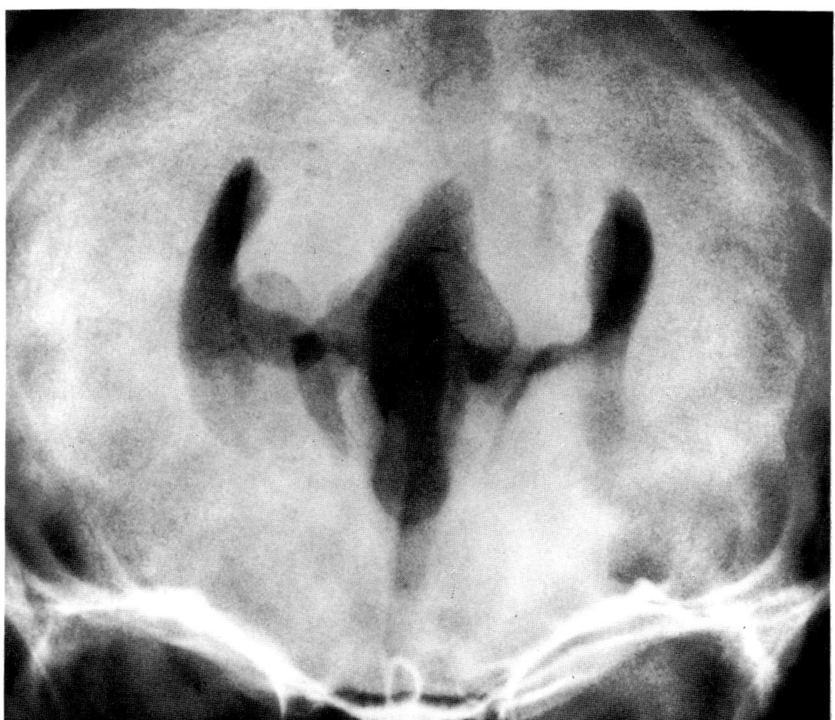

Fig. 222. Typical "steer horn" ventricle in aplasia of the corpus callosum – antero-posterior view

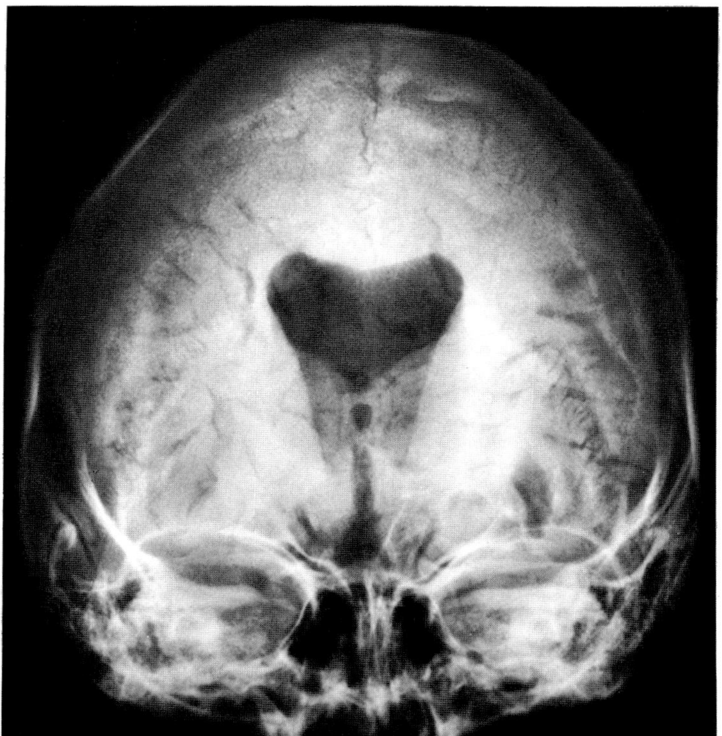

Fig. 223. Typical demonstration of the so-called Cyclops ventricle

vian fissure) and are often difficult to diagnose with pneumoencephalography. If communication exists between the cyst and the subarachnoid space, it may be recognized by the abnormal collection of air. However, if no communication exists, the cyst will present as a space-occupying mass lesion. Such a cyst in the temporal fossa with associated absence of the anterior temporal lobe will present as a foreshortened temporal horn, which is mildly displaced posteriorly and superiorly. The pneumoencephalogram is therefore not characteristic.

Porencephaly arises as a result of a circumscribed, deep-seated brain injury. It develops following resorption of an area of necrotic brain, which can be caused by thrombosis, hemorrhage, or trauma. The porencephalic cyst is usually found in the cortex and may communicate with the ventricular system, although such communication can also be lacking.

For literature, see: Azambuja et al. (1956a), Decker (1960), Kunze (1974), Liliequist (1959a/b), Lindgren (1954), Ruggiero (1974), Soyka (1969), Taveras and Wood (1964, 1976).

X. Indications and Contraindications for Angiography and Pneumoencephalography (or Ventriculography) in the Absence of CT

Neuroradiological contrast procedures (and/or CT when available) are always indicated

1) If the clinical picture is suggestive of a space-occupying or atrophic process

2) Whenever an aneurysm, an AVM, or other intrinsic arterial abnormality (such as stenosis or occlusion of a large vessel) is suspected

3) When the clinical picture is confusing, in order to demonstrate the cerebral anatomy and to reveal any pathological changes

4) When confirmation of "brain death" is desired

It would be incorrect to think of pneumoencephalography (or ventriculography) and angiography as concurrent methods, for the two procedures probe different realms of the brain. The information gleaned from one may complement that of the other, but the indications for each are different.

Nevertheless, in some cases the diagnosis can be made equally well with either procedure, while in other cases one procedure may be clearly inferior to the other or may not be useful at all. In still other instances, the information from both may be needed. In such situations it is not unimportant which method is chosen *first*. The question to be raised, therefore, is not only *"whether"* a particular procedure is indicated, but also *"when"* it should be employed.

In this regard it is imperative that the least dangerous method be used first. If this criterion does not provide a clear-cut choice, then consideration should first be given to that procedure which will provide the *most useful information* and which may make the use of a second diagnostic procedure unnecessary.

Absolute rules for the choice of pneumoencephalography, ventriculography, or angiography which will cover every case cannot be given. The site, type, vascular pattern, and stage of development (risk of herniation) of the suspected pathological process will determine in each individual case the appropriate method of choice.

The following scheme can be used as a guideline:

I. In suspected space-occupying processes:
   a) For cerebral hemisphere lesions: angiography
   b) For ventricular or brain stem lesions: pneumoencephalography or ventriculography
   c) For tumors of the posterior cranial fossa: angiography or, especially in children, ventriculography or pneumoencephalography
   d) For intracranial processes of uncertain localization with increased intracranial pressure: angiography

II. In suspected intrinsic vascular lesions or primary atrophic processes:
   a) For AVMs, aneurysms, infarcts, and spontaneous hemorrhages (subarachnoid hemorrhage, etc.): angiography
   b) For secondary atrophy from occlusion of a major vessel: angiography, also pneumoencephalography
   c) For atrophic processes secondary to trauma or to undetermined factors: pneumoencephalography

III. In case of uncertain cerebral pathology with no sign of increased intracranial pressure: pneumoencephalography

IV. For the confirmation of "brain death": angiography

Relative contraindications:

1) Angiography:
   a) Proceed with caution in elderly patients with coronary or vascular disease and uremia!
   b) Proceed with caution in patients with a history of multiple allergies!
2) Pneumoencephalography:
   a) Proceed with caution if the intracranial pressure is raised!
   b) Proceed with caution in children with intracranial anomalies and/or massive hydrocephalus!

It should be emphasized that papilledema is not the only sign of increased intracranial pressure. Equally important in this regard are alterations in the conscious state, the "beaten silver" skull, spreading sutures, erosion of the sella, headache and neck pain, transient paresthesia in the shoulders and extremities, vomiting, and any sign of impending herniation (see p. 196).

In addition, it should be emphasized that these guidelines should only be taken as general rules for the initial selection of a procedure. *Be careful of the tendency to view these as routine procedures.* Each case should be handled individually. The following considerations may be helpful.

I. In every case in which a *space-occupying process* is clinically suspected and CT is unavailable, angiography is the procedure of choice particularly if signs of increased intracranial pressure already exist. In these cases angiography can simultaneously confirm the presence of a tumor, reveal its position, and occasionally give information as to its histology – all with only one procedure and in the shortest time possible. Moreover, there is no danger of a catastrophic rise in intracranial pressure as so often happens after pneumoencephalography. In those cases in which angiography has not provided sufficient data to proceed with surgery, there is at least time for further diagnostic procedures and no necessity for immediate operative intervention. If angiography has demonstrated an inoperable tumor, the ultimate sad outcome of the disease has at least not been hastened by the diagnostic procedure.

On the other hand, it should be pointed out that many tumors of the cerebral hemispheres are difficult to visualize on the angiogram and the diagnosis may remain in doubt. Such is the case with *tumors* of the *corpus callosum,* which may not be visualized on angiography but are readily apparent on the pneumoencephalogram. Similarly, *frontal lobe tumors* are also sometimes not identified well enough to warrant surgical exploration. This is particularly true for "avascular" tumors which are therefore not readily apparent on the angiogram, such as tumors of the corpus callosum, of the septum pellucidum, and of the thalamus and basal ganglia. The addition of pneumoencephalography in such cases may even be necessary as adjuncts to CT and radionucleotide scanning if these fail to give the desired information. In other areas, angiography (or CT) is clearly the procedure of choice, e.g., when a tumor lies within the watershed zone of the middle cerebral artery. In these cases, angiography can reveal whether the tumor in question has arisen in the frontolateral area and has expanded temporally, or has originated in the anterior temporolateral location and has extended frontally. Thus, *anterior temporal lobe tumors* are beauti-

fully demonstrated angiographically, while the pneumoencephalography requires difficult manipulations to position air within the temporal horn.

Parietal lobe tumors are again excellently depicted on the pneumoencephalogram (and CT scan) but are less well recognized by angiography. In the parieto-occipital location they are occasionally not seen at all on the angiogram, which is also the case with *occipital lobe tumors.* The latter lie exclusively in the distribution of the posterior cerebral artery and are frequently missed on the carotid study, particularly when the tumor is small and no shift of the middle cerebral artery occurs. In these cases, *vertebral angiography* will often provide the diagnosis. Otherwise, the addition of pneumoencephalography will be necessary.

Angiography is of particular value for the differentiation of *subdural* and *epidural hematomas* (see pp. 118–125). However, in the lateral view they are often hardly recognized at all and may even escape recognition in the anteroposterior view when situated frontally or occipitally. In such cases tangential views are necessary in order to confirm the presence of the hematoma (see Fig. 75 b).

Angiography is also of great value in the diagnosis of *brain abscess.* Here the risk of rupture of the capsule makes pneumoencephalography undesirable. Since angiography is not usually associated with intracranial pressure changes, it is the procedure of choice. However, vessel displacement with a brain abscess may be less marked than it would be with a tumor of the same size. This results from tissue breakdown, tissue removal, and subsequent scarring which can take place in the vicinity of an abscess and which can offset the co-existing mass effect of the abscess itself. This is true only for some of the abscesses; others are accompanied by marked cerebral edema and a significant mass effect. Occasionally, the capsule of the abscess may appear as a delicate, vascularized marginal zone.

Whenever a mass-producing intracerebral process is suspected, but the *affected side is not yet diagnosed,* it is advisable to proceed with cerebral angiography. If the displacement of the anterior cerebral artery shows that the incorrect side has been examined, the correct side may then be studied without further delay.

If the anteroposterior view of the angiogram demonstrates no displacement, but evidence of hydrocephalus is apparent on the lateral view, it is safe to conclude that a *midline obstructing lesion* is present somewhere between the third ventricle and the foramen of Magendie. An air study – usually ventriculography – can be carried out either immediately in conjunction with the angiogram or at some later time, and provides more valuable information than angiography when the lesion is situated within the lateral ventricles, the corpus callosum, the third ventricle, aqueduct, or fourth ventricle. An exception to this rule is the lesion lying within or close to the pituitary fossa. In this case, angiography is of considerable value due to the characteristic displacement of the internal carotid artery and its major branches. It should also be emphasized that aneurysms have a particular predilection for this area as well.

Differentiation of the previously mentioned median and paramedian lesions from tumors in the lateral ventricles and basal ganglia or thalamus can be difficult. While these lesions may clinically simulate an intrahemispheric tumor because of the secondary hemiparesis, the presence of hydrocephalus on the angiogram should lead to the correct diagnosis. *Vertebral angiography* is most helpful in the diagnosis of *tumors* involving the *midbrain* and *posterior fossa,* as is cisternography.

II. An absolute indication for angiography exists for those patients who are clinically suspected of having had a subarachnoid hemorrhage from either an *AVM* or *aneurysm*. In such cases, no other diagnostic procedure will suffice. Because of the possibility of multiple aneurysms, it is advisable to complete the study (both carotids and the vertebral) even after the demonstration of *one* aneurysm. This is particularly true when the clinical symptoms do not correspond to the localization of the aneurysm demonstrated. Similarly, it is important to remember that AVMs are often fed by more than one arterial system and all should therefore be demonstrated.

In addition, angiography is of prime importance in distinguishing between *vascular occlusions* (or *stenoses*), *subdural hematomas*, and *intracranial tumors*, all of which may mimic one another. Occasionally it is possible to exclude a tumor with certainty or to identify the site of a vascular occlusion. The indications for "four vessel angiography" have been described elsewhere (see p. 137), as have sites for predilection of vascular occlusive disease. Small vessel occlusions cannot always be diagnosed, even when special magnification techniques are employed. Indirect evidence is frequently provided by the location of the collateral vascular supply.

When an atrophic process of traumatic or uncertain origin is suspected, pneumoencephalography is the procedure of choice in the absence of CT. When this demonstrates unilateral hemispheric or lobar atrophy or a localized dilation of the ventricle, angiography should then be carried out to exclude the possibility of an underlying AVM.

III. In case of a suspected *cerebral lesion of undetermined type and location* and with no signs of increased intracranial pressure, pneumoencephalography used to be our procedure of choice. It permits bilateral visualization of both the supratentorial and infratentorial spaces at the same time, and has the additional merit of demonstrating the atrophic processes as well as space-occupying lesions. If a tumor is suspected, it can easily be followed by angiography for further clarification.

IV. For the confirmation of "brain death", angiography alone is of value.

XI. Comparison of the Indications for Conventional Neuroradiological Procedures and for CT

Guidelines for the application of conventional neuroradiological procedures have been established over the years (see p. 264). However, since the second edition of this book was published, the rapid development of CT has substantially altered these indications in certain situations, making many of the conventional studies unnecessary and outmoded. The advantage of this method is that it is safe, pleasant, and noninvasive, and gives a wealth of information about the intracranial, intraorbital, and intraspinal spaces.

CT is recognized today as the single most important tool in the diagnostic armamentarium of the neuroradiologist and has become the initial procedure of choice in the differential diagnosis of all space-occupying intracranial processes. By this method, tumors are recognized with an accuracy approaching 98%, are correctly localized, and are even characterized as to histological type and malignant potential with a fair degree of accuracy. Similarly, hemorrhages are readily apparent as such and cerebral edema is easily distinguished from both tumors and hemorrhage. Thus, the line of distinction between a primary lesion and its surrounding peripheral edema – which in combination comprise the total volume of the mass lesion – is recognized without difficulty, as are secondary displacements of adjacent cerebral tissues. Furthermore, multiple lesions are diagnosed with ease and serial studies can be carried out in order to follow the growth of a tumor, the relative extent of its peripheral edema and mass effect, and its eventual regression following radiotherapy and/or chemotherapy.

Even so, the full potential of CT will not be realized for some time, since technical advances continue to be made. In addition, the cost of purchasing and maintaining the computers is still so high that many years will pass before they are routinely available at every hospital or even at major centers in poorer countries.

The CT scan functions by calculating the relative density of different points on a "slice" of brain several millimeters thick. These densi-
ties are determined by the relative absorption of thousands of X-rays sent through the slice from many different angles. The computer rapidly analyzes these data and assigns density values to hundreds of points on the slice. After completion of a series of such slices, precise information is given about the position, size, and shape of the CSF pathways, of normal brain tissues, of tumors, of hematomas, and of cerebral edema with corresponding mass displacements and midline shifts.

Many indications for pneumoencephalography and some indications for angiography have been supplanted by the CT scan. The initial procedure of choice in the differential diagnosis of all space-occupying processes today is, without question, CT. However, even when the space-occupying process has been identified, operative intervention is rarely undertaken without the addition of angiography to show the position of the arteries and veins, as well as the precise location and relative vascularity (or neovascularity) of the lesion.

Angiography is also still necessary to demonstrate intrinsic disease of the arteries, veins, and sinuses (such as arteriosclerotic changes, AVMs, aneurysms, and venous and sinus thromboses). The CT scan is able to give some broad information about vascular lesions and particularly their sequelae, but does not match the precision afforded by angiography which is frequently able to demonstrate the responsible lesion, as well as any available collateral blood supply.

On the other hand, much new information never before available has been learned through CT, including absolute confirmation of hematomas, of cerebral edema and/or cerebral necrosis, and of cysts. It is the only neuroradiological procedure necessary in many cases of craniocerebral trauma, intracranial hemorrhage, degenerative diseases, malformations, atrophic changes, and inflammatory disorders. In other instances, it is used in association with air or some water-soluble contrast agent injected into the subarachnoid space. This combination has merit in demonstrating the cisterns about the base of the brain and has been used to great advantage in the diagnosis of small or intracannulicular acoustic neurilemmomas, frequently obviating the need for additional diagnostic studies.

Pneumoencephalography and positive contrast ventriculography have been almost completely supplanted by CT except for the identification of small lesions adjacent to dense bony structures, as often occurs in the parapituitary region, along the clivus, or at the foramen magnum. Although positive contrast ventriculography is of value in demonstrating the precise configuration and position of the ventricular system, its use in evaluating tumors which indent these structures – important in previous years – is of limited value today.

In addition to being the procedure of choice in space-occupying lesions, CT has become the procedure of first choice in evaluating almost any pathological condition affecting the brain. It is also an invaluable tool in the evaluation of orbital disease, having supplanted both arteriography and venography in this area. Detailed studies of the spinal cord are now becoming possible, but additional myelography has retained its position for the moment, at least. Because it is a superb diagnostic tool, easy to operate and free of complications, it is imperative that it be made available to all centers where neuroradiology is practiced.

With the unparalleled value of CT so apparent, the question may well be raised as to whether pneumoencephalography and ventriculography should be performed at all. In defense of these studies, it need only be re-emphasized that the expense of purchasing and maintaining CT limits their availability. In addition, the knowledge obtained from pneumoencephalograms and ventriculograms, as well as from angiograms, is invaluable in correctly interpreting the computed tomograms themselves. For those centers where CT is available, the following table may serve as a guide to the disease processes best suited to it:

Table 2. Course of investigations in neurological and neurosurgical diseases

Diagnosis	Methods of investigation leading to a final diagnosis
Atrophic processes	CT
Infarcts and hemorrhages	CT, Angiography prior to operative therapy
Vascular malformations	CT and angiography
Degenerative and inflammatory vascular processes	CT and angiography
Inflammatory diseases of the brain (space occupying)	CT
Degenerative diseases of the brain	CT
Malformations of the brain	CT
Injuries of skull and brain (acute and chronic)	CT (angiography only in cases of carotid cavernous sinusfistulas
Brain tumors	CT and mostly angiography
Tumors of the cerebellopontine angle	Combination of CT and air-cisternography
Orbital diseases	CT, ultrasound, possibly additional venography of the orbit

E. Myelography

I. History

In 1919 air myelography was introduced by DANDY as a radiologic diagnostic procedure (see p. 183). Initially, the results were unsatisfactory, considering the state of X-ray technology at this time. It was thought that the deficiencies of air myelography might be overcome with the help of a positive contrast agent and indeed SICARD and FORESTIER, who had developed *Lipiodol* – an iodized poppy seed oil – for bronchoscopy, used it in 1922 to carry out the first positive contrast myelogram. After the injection of the contrast medium into the cisterna magna in quantities up to 2 ml, information about the spinal canal could be obtained by allowing the oil to flow through it. Smaller pathological processes, which did not completely block the flow of the oil, generally went unrecognized. A further disadvantage came from the fact that the Lipiodol was not resorbed and sometimes led to foreign body granulomas or to chronic adhesive arachnoiditis. Similar problems accompanied the use of Iodipin, an iodized sesame seed oil.

In 1944 *Pantopaque* was introduced as a positive contrast medium for myelography by RAMSEY, FRENCH, and STRAIN. This was a mixture of isomeric ethyl iodine esters. Similar preparations were *Myodil*, *Ethiodan*, and *Duroliopaque*. The advantages of these preparations compared to iodized oils were their reduced tendency to foaming, their reduced viscosity (20 times less), and their greater cohesiveness. However, these agents had their disadvantages as well. Consequently, attempts were made to replace them with water-soluble preparations. To this end ARNELL and LINDSTROM developed a 20% sodium salt of monoiodine-methane sulfuric acid in 1931 which, however, could only be used in lumbar myelography after the area had been thoroughly anesthetized. It was marketed under the names of *Abrodil, Methiodal, Contrast U,* and *Skiodan*.

In recent years, these contrast agents have been replaced by preparations which can be used without lumbar anesthesia. Of these preparations, *Dimer-X* – a 60% solution of a methyl glucaminic salt of iocarminic acid – was best tolerated. Its use, however, was limited to visualization of the lumbar and lumbosacral spinal canals. It could not be used for the myelographic examination of the thoracic and cervical spinal areas, since it irritated the spinal cord and led to muscle spasms in the lower extremities.

Meanwhile other authors, some independent of Dandy, had begun to use air as a contrast medium for myelography (BINGEL 1921; JACOBÄUS 1921; WIDERÖE 1921). However, it was LINDGREN in 1939 who first developed a method of investigation, using tomography, which was readily applied to the study of the cervical and thoracic regions. Further modifications of the technique were described in subsequent years by MURTAGH et al. (1955), JIROUT (1956–1966), and DECKER (1957).

In 1969 at the suggestion of ALMEN, the laboratories of Nyegaard and Company developed a new water-soluble contrast agent – *Amipaque*. It is extremely well tolerated and in fact performs better than all known water-soluble contrast media in this regard. It is a molecular solution and thus is not dissociated into ions. Since its specific weight is heavier than that of spinal fluid, it can be injected via the lumbar route and will flow toward the cervical region with appropriate tilting of the X-ray table (for a comprehensive list of references, see GREPE 1974).

II. Technique

1. Myelography Using Water-Insoluble Positive Contrast Media

The examination is carried out by means of *fluoroscopy* and a tilt table; this combination permits ready positioning of the patient for erect, horizontal, and reverse tilt film exposures. An image intensifier with a television screen should also be available for posteroanterior and anteroposterior viewing. Recently, similar equipment has been developed for screening in the lateral plane. Video-recording of the fluoroscopy has been shown to have considerable merit.

The contrast medium is injected into the subarachnoid space by *lumbar puncture*. This is usually carried out with the patient lying recumbent on the table, either on his side or prone, so that the contrast medium may be visualized as it is injected. Alternatively, the puncture and injection may be accomplished with the patient sitting erect. The cannula is then left in position after injection so that the contrast medium can be withdrawn following the examination. Withdrawal is most successful when the puncture is as far caudal as possible, i.e., at the level of L-4/5 or L-5/S-1. However, this benefit is outweighed by the disadvantages of needle artefact in cases where a lumbar disc herniation is suspected at either of these two levels. In such cases, an L-2/3 or L-3/4 puncture site is preferable.

In general, 10 ml of *contrast medium* is sufficient for a complete analysis of the spinal canal. However, 15–20 ml of contrast medium can be used when necessary. When the clinical examination or manometry at the time of the procedure leads one to suspect a complete block to contrast flow, 2–3 ml of contrast medium will usually suffice.

When space-occupying lesions in the upper portion of the lumbar spine completely obstruct the passage of CSF, the removal of only a few drops of spinal fluid can result in extreme root pain. The same symptoms will recur during injection of the contrast medium. When this occurs, the presumption of a complete block may already be made and only a minimal amount of contrast medium should be injected, being exchanged drop for drop with the CSF.

After injection of the contrast medium into the subarachnoid space, the patient is carefully placed in the *prone (brow-down) position,* if not already in that position, without disturbing the cannula. Shoulder braces and foot rests are essential, while handles for gripping give the patient an additional feeling of security at the extremes of table tilt. To prevent flow of the contrast medium into the intracranial space, the chin is placed on padding in order that the cervical spine may be maximally extended.

The flow of the contrast medium cephalad can be impeded by a lumbar intravertebral disc protrusion as well as by marked kyphotic deformity of the thoracic spine, as occurs in Scheuermann's disease. In such cases it is necessary to increase the amount of contrast medium used to 20 ml in order to obtain adequate filling of the subarachnoid space. Under continuous fluoroscopic control, the cephalad flow of the contrast medium is carefully monitored while the table is being tilted and spot films are being made of various segments of the spinal canal. These are later arranged in sequence so as to permit visualization of the entire subarachnoid space as a unit. As the contrast passes through the thoracic and into the cervical canals, it is important to observe not only the *shape* of the *advancing column,* but also the character of its pulsations.

Lateral views with the horizontal beam are also routinely made in the cervical region. Here, it is advisable to pull the arms of the patient caudally in order to avoid superimposition of the shoulders on the lower cervical canal. With elevation of the head of the table the reverse flow of the contrast medium is again carefully monitored and appropriate X-ray exposures made.

With the patient in the prone position, it is very difficult and sometimes impossible to outline the thoracic canal and its dorsal kyphosis with a continuous column of contrast medium. This difficulty can occasionally be overcome by employing the Queckenstedt maneuver as follows: the contrast is first collected within the cervical canal; the head of the table is then elevated so that the contrast will flow caudally; as the lower pole of the contrast column approaches the apex of the kyphus, the jugular veins are compressed, and the column is forced over the kyphus intact. Careful fluoroscopic monitoring and appropriate spot films will permit detailed analysis of this difficult area.

It must be mentioned at this point that myelography with water-insoluble contrast media can also be put to use to study the *cerebrospinal fluid dynamics,* especially in the region of the lumbar spinal canal. The test is carried out by having the patient strain or cough while observing the effect on the contrast column. Such analyses demonstrate that the shape and width of the lumbar dural sac, and the surrounding epidural space, vary considerably.

The extradural space consists of fatty tissue and venous plexuses which show considerable individual variation. These veins communicate with the paravertebral venous plexuses and possess no valves. During straining, coughing, or sneezing, blood will flow out of the paravertebral veins into the extradural venous plexus, with resultant venous engorgement and compression of the dural sac. This compression may be sufficient to force most of the CSF and con-

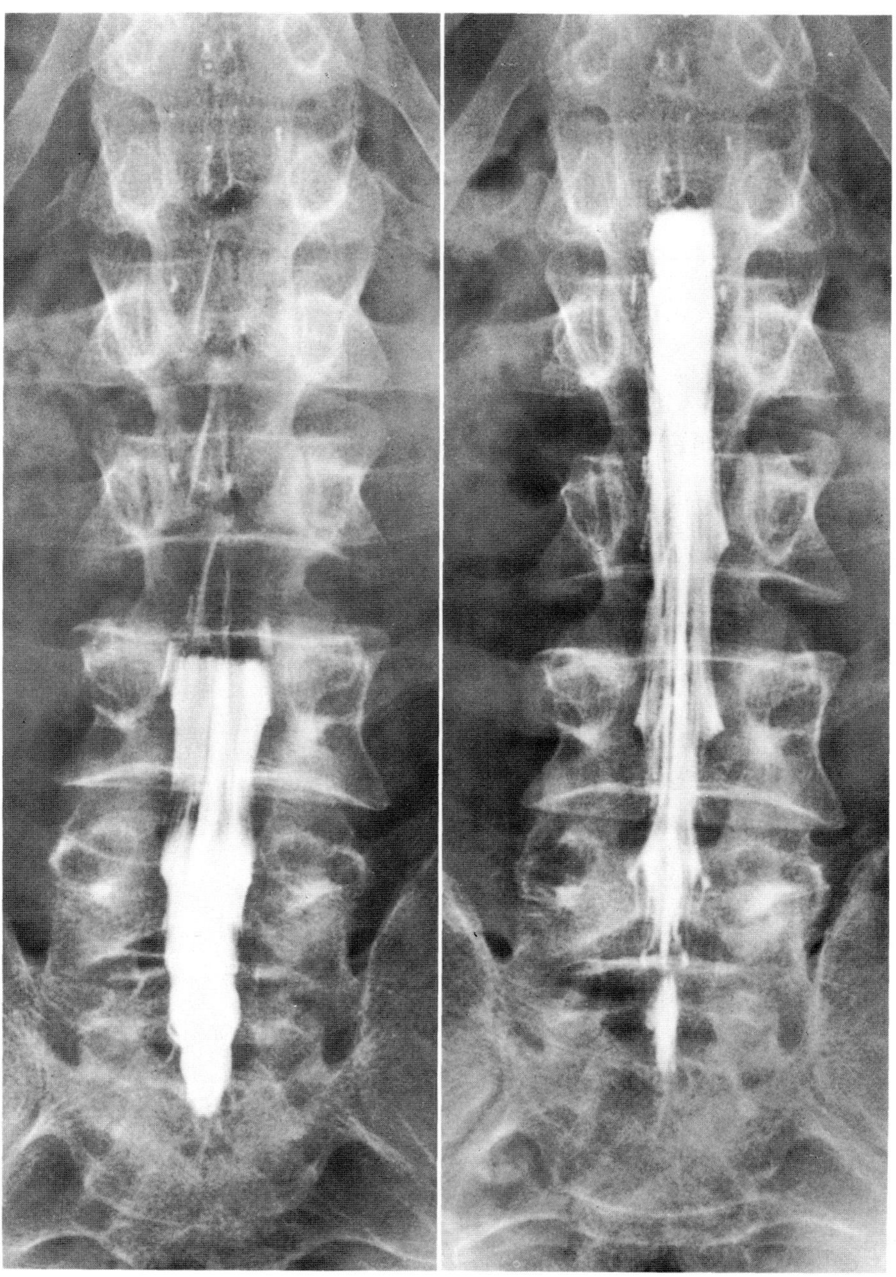

Fig. 224a, b. Positive contrast myelogram showing: a Contrast filling of the lumbosacral area with 6 ml of contrast medium – erect position. b By having the same patient strain, the dural sac is compressed and the contrast medium is forced to a higher level

trast out of the lumbar region to higher levels (Fig. 224a and b). In such a situation, the dural contents will consist almost exclusively of the roots of the cauda equina.

If the examination in the prone position gives the desired information, the contrast medium is then *withdrawn* by means of the cannula which was left in position. At this point lateral screening with a horizontal beam will reveal the precise position of the canula tip within the canal, as well as its relationship to the contrast column, and will facilitate contrast removal. If a few drops still remain in the cervical or thoracic region of the spinal canal with the patient upright, coughing will frequently loosen these and permit them to flow caudally where they can be removed.

If further examination in the *supine (brow-up) position* is deemed necessary, the cannula must first be removed before the patient is positioned on his back. It should be noted that precautions are necessary to prevent the contrast from entering the intracranial space with the head of the table tilted down in this position as with the prone position. This is accomplished by placing a pillow under the head and flexing the neck (see above).

With removal of the cannula, contrast medium and CSF will flow into the extradural space via the hole in the dura mater. In this case, the picture seen will resemble that which occurs when a small amount of contrast medium is injected extradurally. To prevent this *needle-hole leakage,* the cannula should be as thin as possible.

If one wishes to demonstrate the extent of a *complete block,* it is necessary to insert contrast medium above as well as below the lesion. Only with cisternal or high cervical instillation of contrast medium will demonstration of the upper border of the lesion be possible. This is particularly important when the clinical level is higher than the demonstrated myelographic block. Usually 1–2 ml of injected contrast medium will suffice.

2. Myelography Using Water-Soluble Positive Contrast Media

Of the water-soluble contrast media available, Amipaque almost exclusively used today. The most common indication for an Amipaque myelogram is lumbar disc herniation. In the description which follows, the technique for identification of a herniated disc is used. For demonstration of tumors in this region, additional oblique views are required.

The examination is again carried out under fluoroscopy on a *tilt table* which has the additional capacity for obtaining lateral films using a *horizontal X-ray beam* and a grid cassette. The patient is premedicated with an intramuscular injection of 10 mg of Valium. The lumbar puncture may be performed with the patient either sitting or recumbent. If the sitting position is employed, the patient is then carefully placed in the lateral recumbent position on the affected side without disturbing the cannula. If the recumbent position is used initially, the lateral position with the affected side down is again employed. The puncture site is determined in part by the clinical symptoms, but is normally done at the L-3/4 level since most intervertebral disc prolapses are found at the L-4/5 or L-5/S-1 levels. If the clinical examination suggests the possibility of an L-3/4 disc herniation, the puncture site is made at L-2/3.

A lumbar anesthetic is generally not necessary when using Amipaque. If the pain due to an acute intervertebral disc prolapse is so severe that the patient is unable to lie on his side, lumbar puncture is first performed in the sitting position following which a lumbar anesthetic is given at a dose which is approximately 10% of that required for total lumbar anesthesia. For this purpose, we use 0.2–0.3 ml of 5% Xylocaine. This relatively small dosage of anesthesia is sufficient to permit a painless examination to be carried out without producing motor paralysis. Thus, the patient will be able to help position himself throughout the procedure. After the head of the table is elevated some 15°–20°, CSF flow from the needle should be sufficient to permit collection of a specimen for analysis. The concentration for Amipaque varies from 170–190 mg/ml for lumbar myelography to 280 mg/ml for cervical myelography. The diluted contrast medium is then injected into the subarachnoid space over a period of 10–20 s. When the injection time is longer, mixing is poor and stratification tends to occur with contrast outlining only portions of the caudal dural sac, particularly when this is enlarged. On the other hand, if the injection time is too rapid, the contrast medium will spread out and mix with such a large volume of CSF

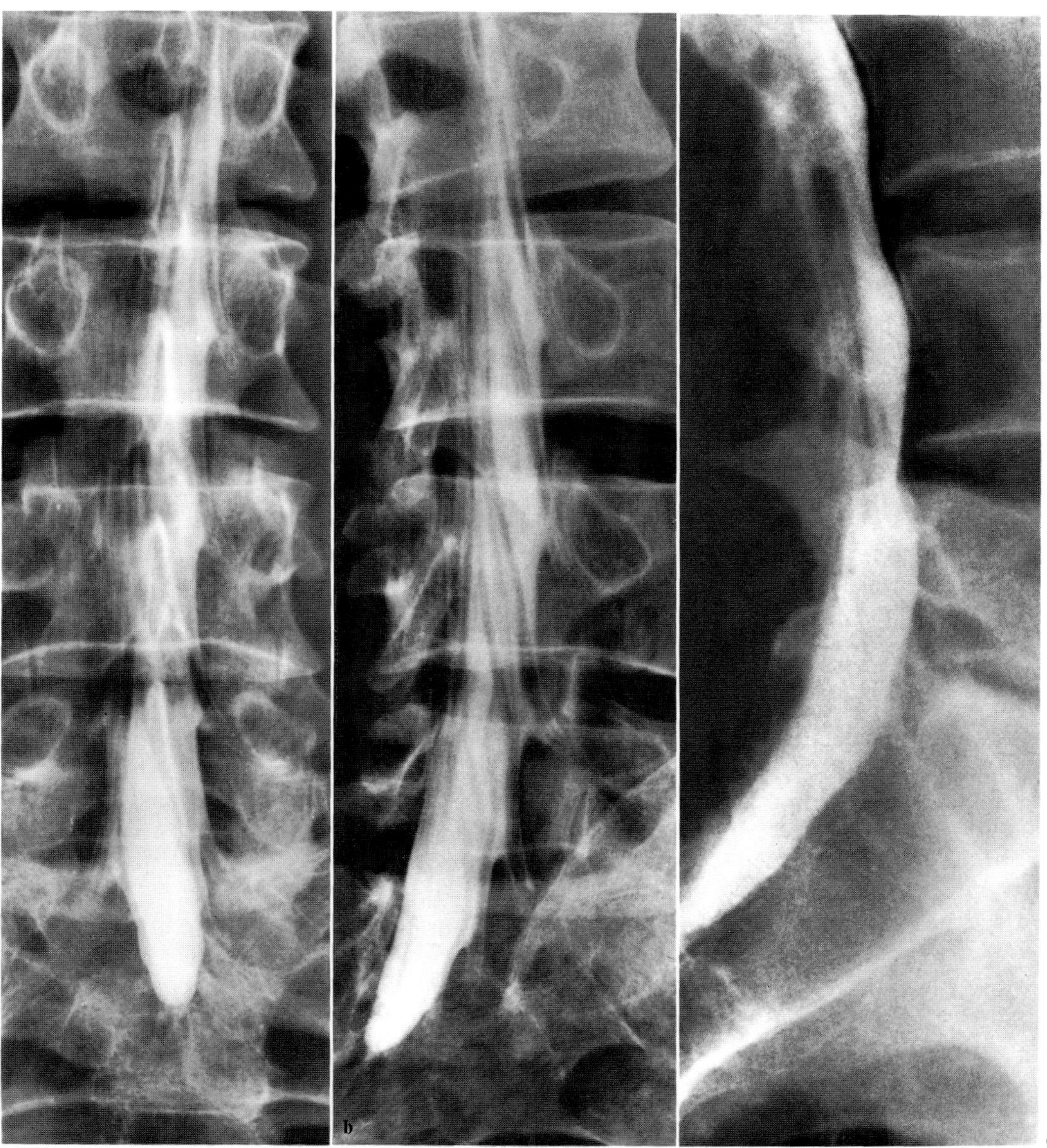

Fig. 225a–c. Normal positive contrast myelogram using a water-soluble agent: **a** Horizontal (anteroposterior view) exposure with the patient in the lateral position. **b** Horizontal exposure with the patient oblique. **c** Horizontal (lateral view) with the patient prone

that its contrast density will be considerably reduced. The injection can be monitored under fluoroscopy and the rate of injection altered as needed to obtain the desired column size and density. X-ray exposure can also be made with the horizontal beam in this position to confirm that the column is adequate. In cases with large caudal sacs, an additional injection of contrast may well be needed.

The first X-ray film exposure is made in the anteroposterior or posteroanterior projection using the horizontal beam with the patient still on the affected side. Here it is particularly important to cone down the X-ray field to enhance resolution. The second film is an oblique view, again using the horizontal beam with the patient being turned 15°–20° toward the prone position. The third picture is also an oblique view, but with the angle increased to 30°–35°. The final film is a lateral view taken with the patient in the prone position. As noted, all films are taken with the horizontal beam (Fig. 225). In patients with bilateral symptoms, both sides are examined in sequence. This technique has the advantage of demonstrating the root sleeves better than alternative methods (such as, fluoroscopy with spot films). If the column of contrast obtained proves to be too short, this deficiency may be overcome by reducing the head-up tilt of the table and by compressing the abdomen until the contrast column reaches the desired level.

At the termination of the procedure, it is essential that the upper torso of the patient remains elevated at 15° to the horizontal for 6–8 h to prevent flow of the contrast medium into the thoracic canal, while avoiding the excessive leakage of CSF from the puncture site and the "low pressure" headache which would result from a more upright position. As thin a spinal needle as possible should be employed to reduce CSF leakage. For similar reasons, the patient should be instructed to avoid coughing or straining as much as possible.

Cervical myelography: It is recommended that the contrast medium be injected directly into the cervical CSF spaces in order to get adequate visualization of this region with the smallest possible amount of contrast agent. With the patient in the prone position the spinal subarachnoid space is entered laterally between C-1 and C-2 under fluoroscopic control. After penetration through the dura – the resistance of which is easily felt – the stylette is removed and CSF flow noted. A bolus of 5–8 ml of Amipaque (270 mg/ml) is then injected with fluoroscopic monitoring.

Amipaque may be also injected by the lumbar route and the flow of contrast medium cephalad followed by fluoroscopy. With this method, visualization of the lumbar and thoracic segment of the spinal canal may be accomplished if the patient is cooperative and the contrast agent sufficiently concentrated. Minimal patient motion and rapid performance are also essential preconditions.

3. Myelography with Negative Contrast Media

Air is generally the agent of choice for negative contrast myelography. Three different methods for air myelography are commonly employed:

Technique of LINDGREN (1939): The technique described by Lindgren permits demonstration of the spinal canal throughout its entire length and permits ready recognition of neoplasms and degenerative changes. It is also useful in determining the diameter of the spinal cord.

Injection can be accomplished by the lumbar, high cervical, or cisternal routes. For a cisternal puncture, the patient is placed in the lateral recumbent position (for technique see p. 186) and the head of the table lowered approximately 15° from the horizontal, in order to prevent air from entering the intracranial space. Approximately 10 ml of CSF is removed and 10 ml of air injected in the manner described earlier. At this point a mixture of air and CSF will flow from the cannula. Pains behind the ears or involving the temples indicate that air has begun to enter the intracranial subarachnoid space. Then another 20 ml of air is injected so that a positive pressure will be maintained within the spinal canal. This is necessary to insure that the entire subarachnoid space is expanded. Only in this manner will space-occupying lesions in the extradural space be identified. In adults, 100 ml air is usually required to outline the complete spinal canal including the cervical region.

It is also possible to fill the entire canal successfully by means of a *lumbar puncture*. The lateral recumbent position is again employed with the patient horizontal and the head hanging over the shoulder. In this fashion, air will be prevented from entering the intracranial space after injection. Lumbar puncture is then performed and an air/fluid exchange accomplished as before until the air and CSF mixture is seen. Here again a slight positive pressure within the canal is required. At this point, both the thoracic and lumbar region are available for radiologic survey. Finally, the head is raised to the horizontal position permitting air to flow into the cervical region as well.

A modification of this technique requires two needle punctures, similar to the "double Queckenstedt maneuver". To accomplish this, the patient again assumes the lateral recumbent position with the head down and both lumbar and cisternal punctures are performed. After injection of the air via the lumbar route, CSF will flow from the cisternal needle. The air/CSF interchange is continued until no more CSF flows from the upper needle. The cisternal needle is then closed and additional air injected via the lumbar route until a positive pressure has been obtained, insuring full expansion of the subarachnoid space. This method also permits identification of the upper pole of an obstructing lesion when the block is complete by allowing air injections to be made via both the cisternal and lumbar routes.

Technique of MURTAGH et al. (1955): This technique uses the fact that an air bubble in a liquid medium will remain intact and will rise to the highest point available. By manipulating the position of the patient, an air bubble of 40–50 ml is sufficient to demonstrate sequentially the different regions of the spinal canal.

Technique of JIROUT (1958): For the demonstration of the cervical spinal cord, Jirout's method is especially advantageous. The patient is placed in the sitting position with his head maximally extended so that the cervical canal is the highest point of the CSF space. After lumbar puncture, 20–40 ml of air is exchanged with CSF. Lateral films of the cervical spine in this position will show the dorsal portion of the cervical subarachnoid space, the occipito-cervical boundary, the cisterna magna, and the fourth ventricle. With a sufficient air/fluid interchange, the ventral border of the cervical cord should also be apparent. If this latter border is not clearly seen, the patient should be repositioned and repeat X-rays made with the body supine and the head held down lower than the neck. This method is particularly useful in identifying ventrally situated cervical disc herniations and in assessing the mobility of the spinal cord under various conditions.

The value of the information gained from air myelography is dependent not only on X-ray technique, but also on the experience of the examining physician. Because of the relative weakness of air as a contrast agent, the air/spinal cord boundaries are not always distinct and film interpretation is not easy.

The *radiological technique* of choice for air myelography is always tomography. Optimum exposure techniques are extremely important. To accomplish this, a high kV/low mA technique is recommended. X-rays are then made after measuring the level of the necessary cuts. In the lateral position, a tomographic cut is made at the level of the spinous process. Two additional cuts are made 0.5 cm above and 0.5 cm below the first. If the films thus obtained are satisfactory, the patient is placed in the supine position and anteroposterior tomography is carried out. The level of each tomographic cut must be measured again since they vary depending on patient size. In the anteroposterior view, the cervical and the upper thoracic spinal cord are both superimposed by the air-filled trachea. Therefore, in these regions it is only necessary to obtain lateral and oblique views. Oblique films are also required whenever intervertebral disc herniations are suspected.

Air myelography can also be performed *on children* depending on their age, but should only be done via lumbar puncture. Children must be adequately sedated or, better still, fully anesthetized.

For literature, see: JIROUT (1969).

III. Complications and Errors

Complications in myelography may begin with the lumbar or cisternal punctures. The error of injecting a *water-insoluble contrast agent* into the extradural or subdural spaces can be largely avoided if the medium is injected under fluoroscopic control. With injection into the extradural space, the contrast medium forms irregular deposits which do not pulsate and which fail to flow as a single bolus cephalad or caudad when the table is appropriately tilted.

After a *lumbar extradural* injection, the contrast medium will distribute itself superiorly and inferiorly and will tend to follow the nerve roots into the paravertebral spaces. After a period of days, linear strips of contrast can be found extending into the true pelvis. Eventually this contrast medium is resorbed or otherwise removed so that it is no longer apparent some months later. *Subdural* contrast injections form thin-walled cylinders of the root sleeves, represented as fine parallel lines in the sagittal exposure extending only a few millimeters distal to the foramina. More proximally, the contrast coalesces to form little pockets at the level of the roots. Subdurally and extradurally injected contrast media cannot be removed by aspiration to any significant degree.

Difficulties in puncture can be experienced when this is attempted adjacent to a large medially herniated disc. Since in these cases the tip of the cannula will reside in the midst of densely compressed nerve roots, painful sensations can be experienced. Moreover, the CSF may flow very slowly or not at all. If such a position of the cannula is suspected, the contrast medium should be injected only under fluoroscopic control. Withdrawal of the contrast agent from this site will usually prove to be impossible and will thus require a second puncture for the removal. This puncture site should be chosen to place the cannula tip within the greatest pooled volume of contrast seen.

The fear that the esters (Pantopaque and others) may lead to arachnoiditis can be refuted by large controlled studies.

In myelography with *water-soluble contrast media,* it is especially important to perform a successful puncture of the lumbar subarachnoid space on the first try. After repeated punctures a collection of CSF may form within the extra-dural space simulating a disc herniation. This problem, however, is a diagnostic pitfall common to all forms of myelography. One must pay careful attention to the positioning of the patient as described above in order to prevent the contrast medium from running into the thoracic area. Moreover, the patient should avoid excessive coughing or sneezing since this will lead to transient CSF pressure increases with secondary dispersion of the contrast agent. It should be emphasized that withdrawal of large quantities of CSF by the lumbar route in cases where a spinal (or posterior fossa) tumor has caused a complete or nearly complete block to contrast flow may result in changes in the CSF dynamics sufficient to increase the neurological deficit. Even when smaller initial amounts of CSF have been removed, subsequent leakage via the needle puncture hole may increase the cumulative loss over a period of hours with similar dire consequences. Under these conditions, immediate surgical intervention following the myelogram may be desirable. Alternatively, a lateral C-1/C-2 tap with insertion of contrast above the lesion will not only outline the superior pole of the tumor, but may also help reduce the CSF pressure upon it.

Hypersensitivity reactions to the contrast agents have been experienced in individual cases. Consequently, means of resuscitation must be immediately available, as with all examinations employing water-soluble contrast media. If a hypotensive crisis ensues, appropriate pressor drugs must be administered.

Similar precautions are to be observed during *air myelography* as well, although such occurrences should not be expected if the indications and contraindications for lumbar or suboccipital punctures are followed. An immediate reaction is a transient root pain in the expected segmental distribution similar to that which accompanies a tumor or a herniated disc. If an extradural injection of air follows, false findings compatible with an extradural tumor may result (as when the same space is filled with CSF) or the study may be inadequate. If an irregularity at the site of the needle puncture compatible with an extradural mass remains after needle withdrawal, an iatrogenic epidural hemorrhage should be suspected. This, however, is quite rare. If the spinal cord seems to be stuck to the wall of the spinal canal, arachnoiditis may be erroneously diagnosed. However, in such cases exposures done in varying positions will show that the position of the cord varies as well.

Diagnostic difficulties are to be expected in patients with marked scoliosis. In these patients it is not always possible to depict the entire length of the spinal canal even with tomography.

IV. Indications

The myelography technique may be varied to suit the particular needs (localization, tumor type) of the lesion in question. Occasionally, no one technique is clearly indicated, or one technique may complement another. It is generally accepted that positive contrast myelography, because of its density, is simpler to analyze than the air myelogram. Air myelography is also more complicated in that tomograms are usually required, effectively lengthening the examination time and adding to the discomfort of the patient.

Naturally, air myelography is not associated with hypersensitivity reactions to the contrast media or with remnants of residual contrast. This latter complication can occur with the water-insoluble agents despite good technique and careful attempts at removal. This is particularly true for examinations of the craniocervical junction where contrast medium can easily enter the basal cisterns. Failure to remove all the contrast media is currently not a serious complication, but may impede later examination.

Only in children or with large meningoceles is air myelogram preferred in this region.

V. The Normal Myelogram

The anatomical relationships of the bony spinal canal, the dural sac and its contents, and the extradural space all play an important role in shaping the column of contrast medium. These relationships vary considerably from one region of the spinal canal to the next and, consequently, the individual characteristics of each region (cervical, thoracic, and lumbar) must be considered before a correct myelographic interpretation is rendered.

A complete myelographic study of the *cervical subarachnoid space* is only possible when it is demonstrated in its entirety by a continuous column of contrast. This is obtained using the method described above.

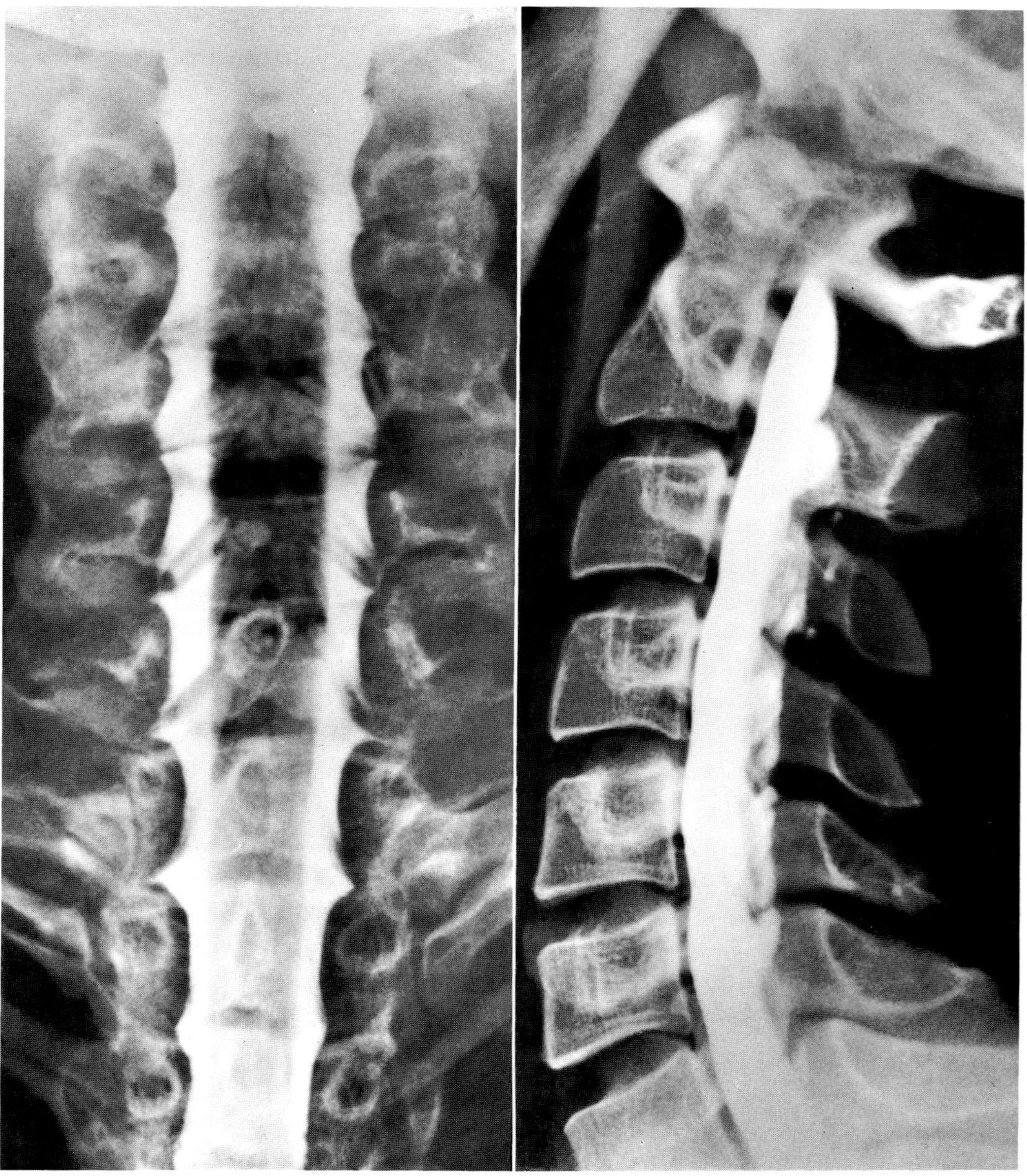

Fig. 226a, b. Normal positive contrast cervical myelogram using a water-insoluble agent: **a** Anteroposterior view: the central radiolucent band in the contrast column corresponds to the spinal cord, while the smaller linear lucent areas running obliquely to each root sleeve are the individual nerve roots. **b** Lateral view: the small radiolucent impressions in the dorsal column of contrast here correspond to the exiting posterior nerve roots

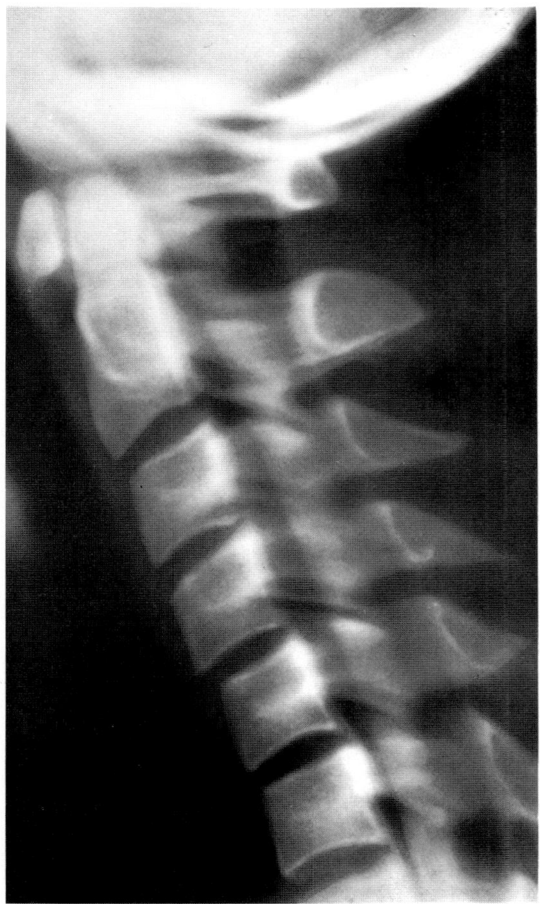

Fig. 227. Normal air myelogram of the cervical region

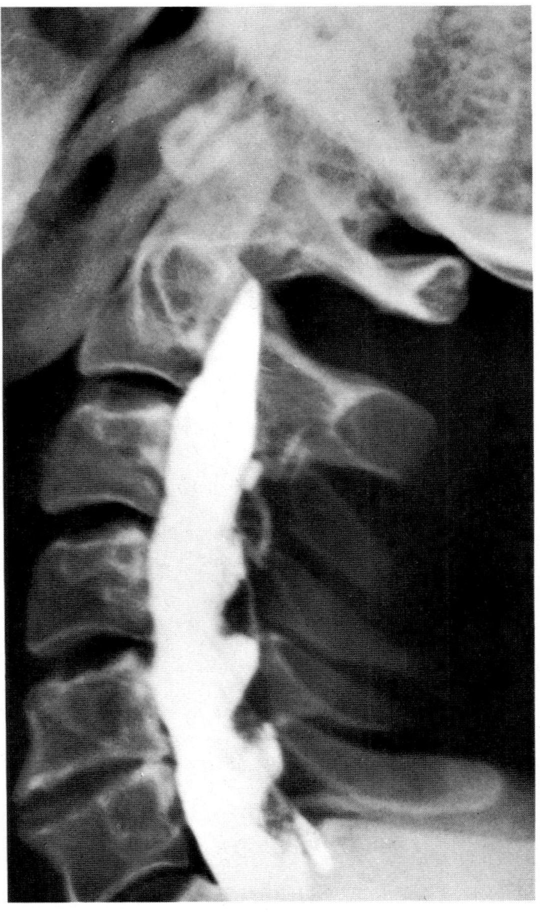

Fig. 228. Normal lateral view of a positive contrast cervical myelogram using a water-insoluble contrast agent. The segmental indentations into the dorsal column of contrast are caused here by infolding of the ligamentum flavum

In the *anteroposterior view* of a cervical myelogram, the spinal cord appears as a transparent central band within the positive contrast image of the canal, or a dense band if air is used. With adequate filling of the subarachnoid space using a positive contrast medium, the cervical root sleeves reveal themselves as short, stumpy out-pockets of contrast on either side of the column, directed caudally. One or two transparent bands traverse each stump, corresponding to the individual nerve roots (Fig. 226).

Lateral views of the air myelogram (taken in the sitting position with the head extended) generally permit good visualization of the dorsal cervical subarachnoid space, the cisterna magna, and the ventral subarachnoid space when sufficent air is injected (Fig. 227).

One can also outline the ventral extradural space using a positive contrast agent in a lateral view with the patient prone. It is usually about 1 mm wide, but increases to 2–3 mm at the level of C-2 (Fig. 226b). As will be seen later, the width of the space has considerable diagnostic significance. With maximum extension of the neck, dorsal indentations into the column of contrast are readily identified when water-insoluble positive contrast agents have been used and represent folds of the ligamenta flava (Fig. 228), which tend to disappear when the neck is in a neutral or flexed position. When this condition is exaggerated and superimposed upon cervical degenerative disease, a disc prolapse, or congenital spinal stenosis, cervical cord compression will result. In acute hyperextension injuries of the cervical spine, in particu-

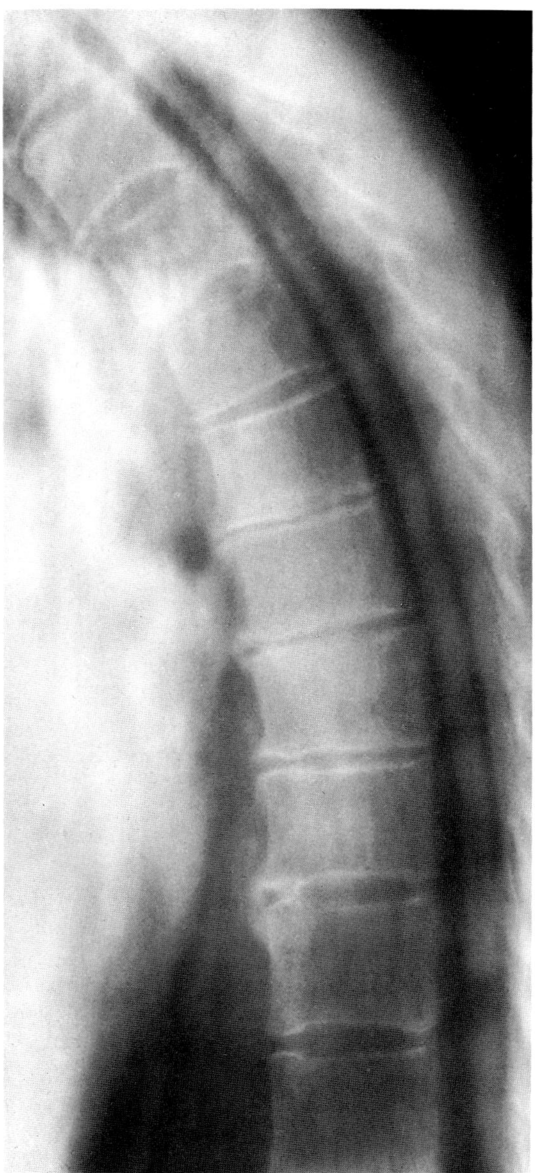

Fig. 229. Lateral tomogram of an air myelogram in the thoracic region. Note the excellent visualization of the spinal cord throughout its length

lar, these conditions lead to cord injury by means of a "pincer-like" effect.

The *thoracic spinal canal* is also well demonstrated throughout its entire length in an adequate air myelogram (Fig. 229), or another technique. The thoracic root sleeves are very short while the width of the dorsal and ventral extradural spaces (as seen on the lateral view) are fairly constant at 1 mm. This is the distance between the anterior and posterior borders of the bony canal and the adjacent column of contrast.

The width of the *lumbar dural sac* exhibits considerable individual variation. This is due not only to variations in the width of the bony canal, but also to variations in the size of the extradural space which will even fluctuate in a given individual depending upon the state of engorgement of the epidural venous plexus (see p. 273). The dural sac will usually taper to a point caudally anywhere from the last lumbar vertebra to approximately S-2. The roots of the cauda equina exit from both sides, running diagonally in an inferolateral direction. At the level of their exit from the dura, they are enveloped for a short distance by their root sleeves and then leave the confines of the spinal canal just below the appropriate pedicle. Better visualization of the lumbar and sacral root sleeves is obtained with water-soluble contrast media than with the viscous oil-based agents. In air myelography these structures are barely discernible.

It is important to remember that the relative size of the extradural space can be increased by any maneuver which increases the engorgement of the epidural venous plexuses, i.e., any maneuver which increases the intra-abdominal pressure, such as coughing, sneezing, straining, and even flexion or extension of the lumbar spine.

VI. The Pathological Myelogram

Similar to the radiologic analysis of other contrast-filled channels in the body, myelographic abnormalities tend to take one of two forms: either a narrowing or a widening (circumscribed or diffuse) of the contrast column.

In analyzing the myelogram one must keep in mind that the contrast is in reality filling a cylinder, which is wrapped around the spinal cord and spinal roots and which is bordered by the arachnoid and dural membranes. Narrowing of the cylindrical column of contrast may result either from a space-occupying lesion or from abnormalities of the meningeal coverings (such as adhesions). The space-occupying lesions are generally divided into intramedullary, intradural/extramedullary (juxtamedullary), or extradural lesions.

Widening of the contrast column, on the other hand, may result from either a congenital deformity or an acquired bulging of the dural sac. Unanticipated congenital deformities are most typical of the meningocele group, while acquired deformities usually follow trauma or (less commonly) surgical intervention.

1. Intramedullary Space-Occupying Lesions

Every intramedullary space-occupying lesion, regardless of type (see p. 42), leads to an enlargement of the spinal cord with narrowing of the surrounding cylinder of contrast. In the anteroposterior view, the contrast shadows on either side of the cord will be gradually thinned, eventually to disappear as the cord pushes against the pedicles (Fig. 230). Similar changes occur on the lateral view. Eventually, as the lesion grows, the enlarged cord will completely fill the confines of the canal resulting in a localized block to contrast flow. Of the intramedullary tumors, ependymomas, pilocytic astrocytomas, and hemangioblastomas achieve the greatest length. They may involve ten or more vertebral segments and may include multiple elongated cysts. A high cervical or cisternal myelogram may be required to verify the upper margin of the tumor. Lateral views in such cases are essential since enlargement of the cord may be simulated by compression and flattening of

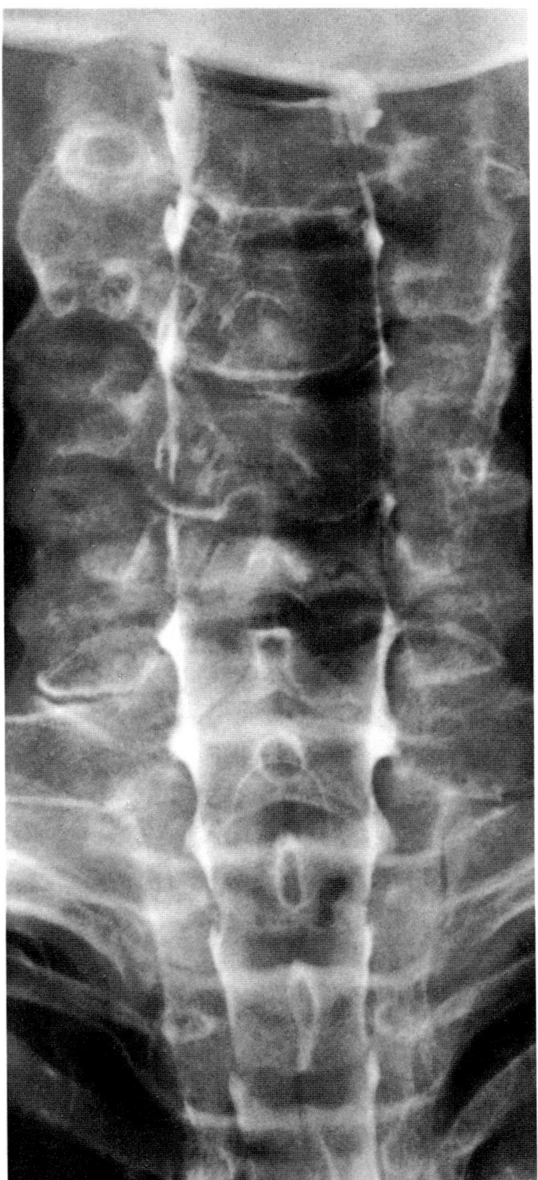

Fig. 230. Positive contrast myelogram showing an intramedullary tumor. Note the enlargement of the spinal cord in the cervical and upper thoracic regions. Here the subarachnoid space has been nearly obliterated, leaving only a fine line of contrast in each lateral gutter

the cord from a ventrally or dorsally situated extradural mass, in which case the cord shadow will be displaced anteriorly or posteriorly. Myelitis, cord edema, or an intramedullary granuloma may all mimic an intramedullary tumor on the myelogram.

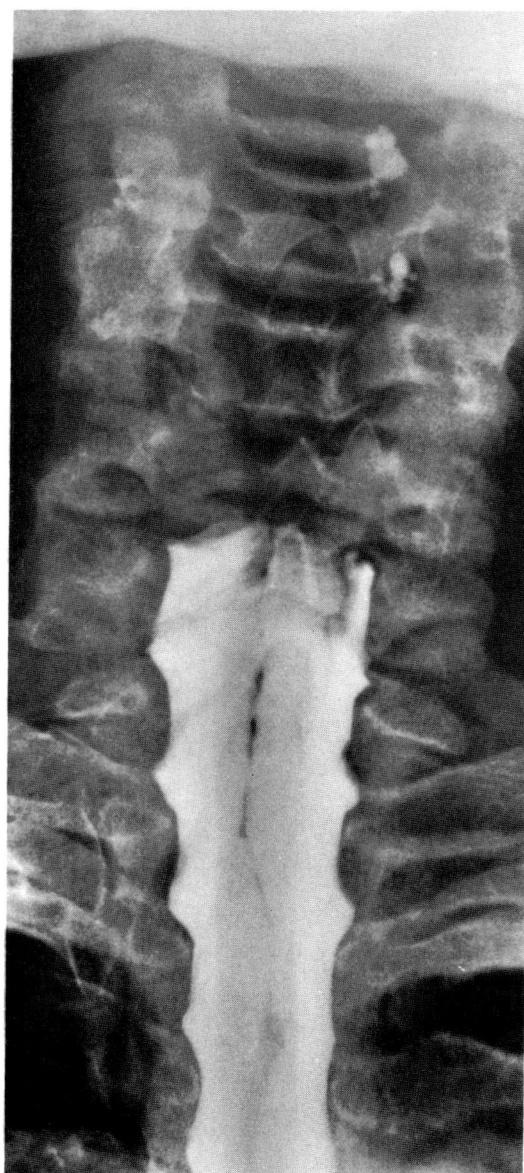

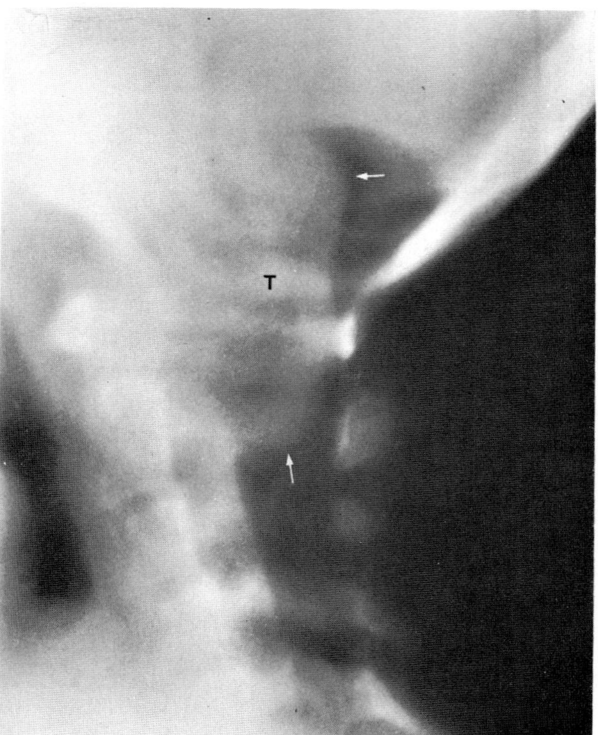

Fig. 232. Air myelogram demonstrating a lipoma at the craniospinal junction

◁

Fig. 231. Extramedullary intradural tumor with a complete block to contrast flow. The cervical cord is displaced to the left so the width of the dense zone of contrast is wider on the right than the left. Note the translucent bands of some nerve roots. The curved upper border of the contrast column corresponds to the inferior pole of the tumor

2. Intradural, Extramedullary Space-Occupying Lesions

The spinal cord is forced to the opposite side by an extramedullary space-occupying lesion. Consequently, the subarachnoid space above and below the lesion will be widened and the contrast shadows indented in concave fashion by the upper and lower poles of the lesion. The displaced cord may be identified as a transparent band in the contrast shadow (Fig. 231). Meningiomas and neurilemmomas are by far the most common tumors in this group. Much

less frequently, epidermoids, dermoids, teratomas, lipomas, and cysts are found (Fig. 232). The meningiomas are mostly lobulated and irregular, while neurilemmomas are generally recognized by their smooth outline (Fig. 233). When the tumor reaches sufficient size to fill the intraspinal space completely at a given segment, a complete block to contrast flow will ensue. It is, however, important to emphasize that closed manometrics (as determined by the Queckenstedt test) are not always confirmed as complete myelographic blocks. Sometimes contrast will overcome the predicted obstruction and will pass the lesion in small amounts. When

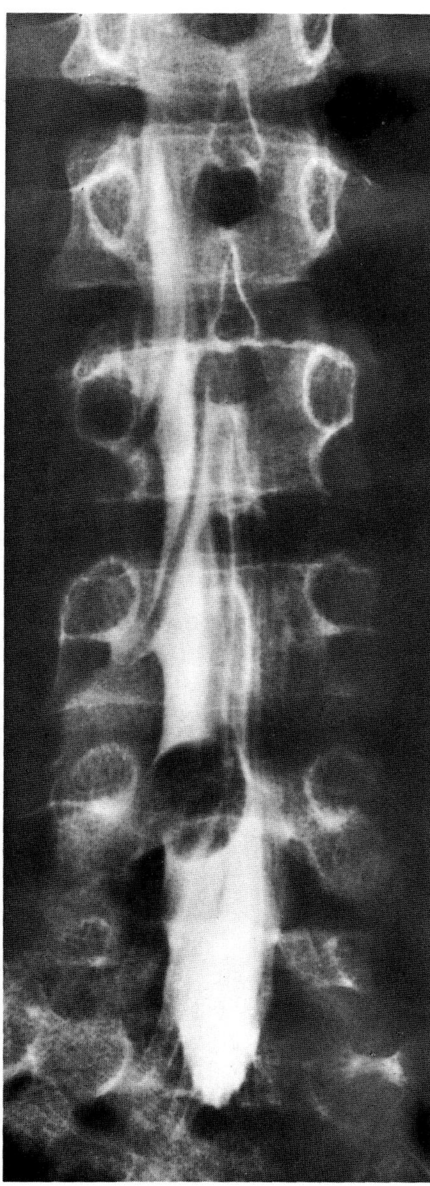

Fig. 233. The cherry-sized radiolucent defect in this water-soluble contrast myelogram is a neurilemmoma of the right L-5 root

myelographic blocks are present, contrast must be instilled above and below the lesion to verify its limits.

3. Extradural Space-Occupying Lesions

Extradural space-occupying lesions displace the dural sac away from the lesion, so that the extradural space appears widened. Lesions of the vertebral bodies or herniated discs will displace the column of contrast posteriorly, lesions of the lamina and ligamentum flavum will displace it anteriorly, and lesions of the pedicle laterally. It is characteristic of lesions in this location that the displaced column of contrast gradually resumes its normal position above and below the level of the abnormality (Fig. 234).

Extradural neurilemmomas can cause pressure erosion of the adjacent vertebral body and pedicle with subsequent enlargement of the corresponding intervertebral foramina ("hourglass" tumor). Through precise analysis of the involved bone architecture, it is possible to distinguish between hemangioblastomas of the vertebra, chondromas, and giant cell tumors.

Teratomas can also be recognized as such when they contain bone elements. Plasmacytomas and the highly invasive chordomas, which can be found as extradural space-occupying lesions, are usually recognized on plain X-ray films as malignant processes because of the bony destruction they cause. This is also true for spinal metastases where diagnosis is possible even in the face of an unknown primary due to the presence of multiple areas of destruction. Relatively common are epidural malignant "lymphomas", such as reticulum cell sarcoma.

Epidural empyema constitutes a special type of extradural space-occupying lesion in that the dura is compressed from all sides simultaneously. This results in thinning of the contrast columns to either side of the cord shadow and eventually to a complete myelographic block. In such cases, inflammatory changes occur within the dura as well as in the extradural space. Similar changes are seen in association with extradural infiltration by myeloid leukemia (Fig. 235).

Another special type of extradural space-occupying process which can be diagnosed by myelography is the herniation of an intravertebral disc into the spinal canal.

Midline cervical disc herniations, as well as the posterior osteophytic ridging of the vertebral margins adjacent to degenerated cervical discs, are both recognizable on the cervical myelogram as anterior indentations into the contrast column. When air is used as a contrast agent, the subarachnoid space is more completely outlined and the size of the protrusion more apparent (Fig. 236). With positive contrast media, these abnormalities are portrayed as horizontal bands of decreased density in the

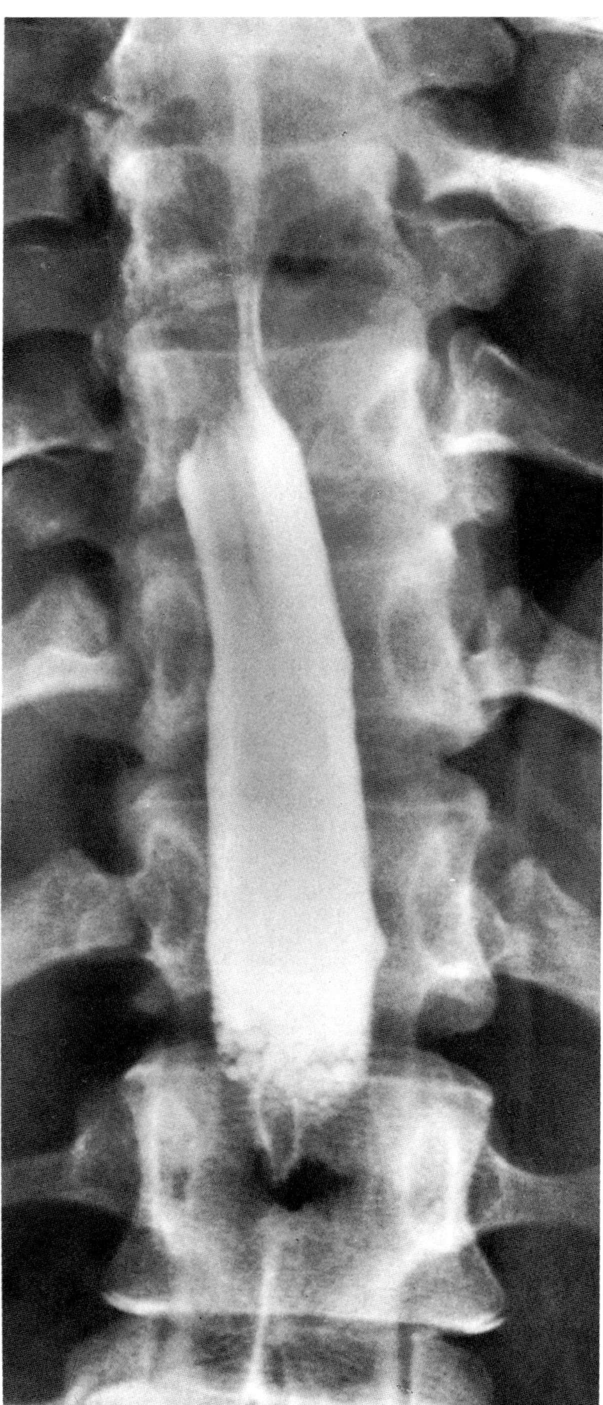

Fig. 234. Complete block with an extradural tumor: the dural sac and spinal cord (T-10, T-11) are being pushed away from the pedicles on the left at the level of the block (primary extradural melanoma)

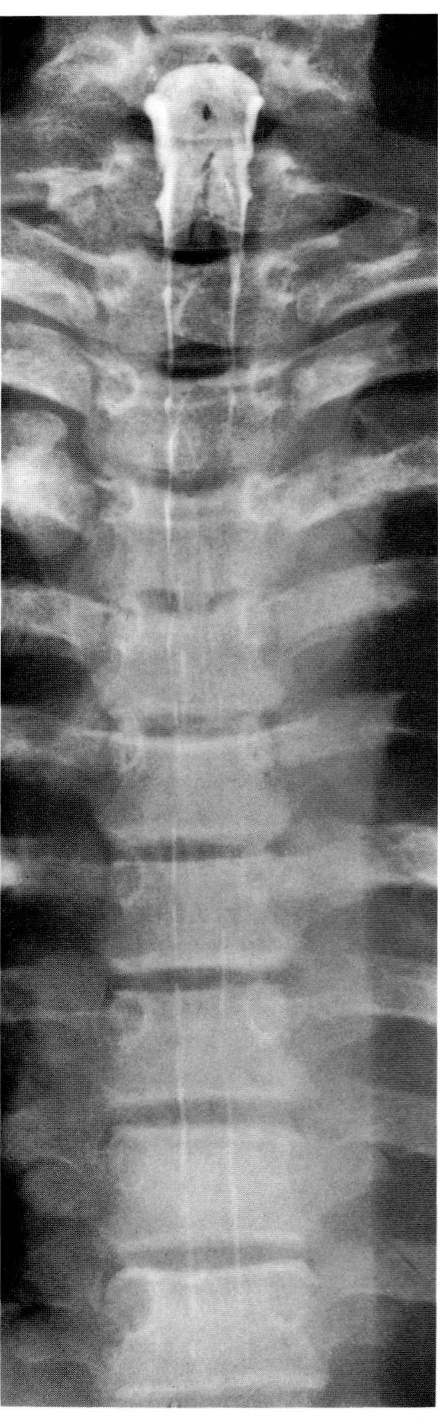

Fig. 235. Displacement of the column of contrast away from the lateral margins of the spinal canal on both sides with extradural infiltration in a case of myelocytic leukemia. Note the thin lines of contrast throughout the thoracic region

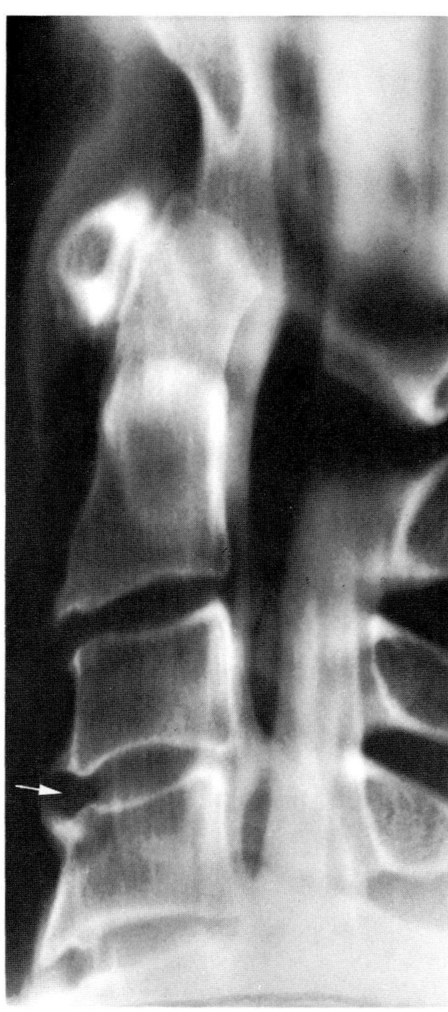

Fig. 236. Midline herniation of an intervertebral disc (C-3/4) as demonstrated on a lateral air myelogram using tomography. The column of air between the spinal cord and the vertebral body is interrupted at the level of the lesion

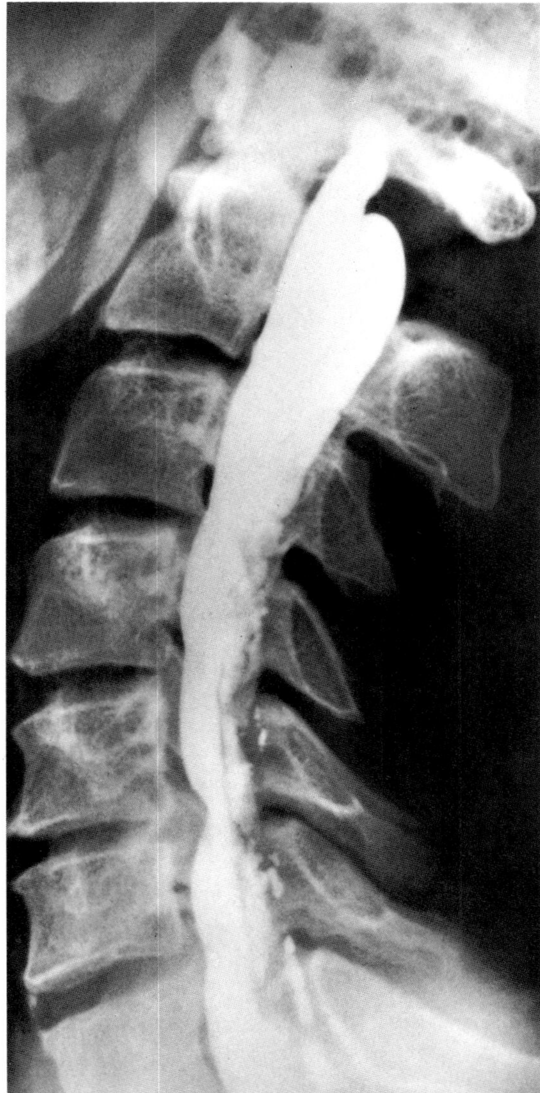

Fig. 237. Pantopaque myelogram showing midline bulge with posterior herniation of an intravertebral disc (C-5/6). Note the definite "pincer" effect on the spinal cord at this level

contrast column or complete interruptions of the column at the level of the pathology. With hyperextension of the cervical spine, the previously described *pincer mechanism* (see pp. 281, 282) can, in narrowed spinal canals, result in a complete block to contrast flow. This block can be relieved by bringing the head to a neutral or flexed position (Fig. 237). The changes described are commonly seen with *myelopathy* secondary to cervical degenerative disease.

Posterolateral cervical disc herniations lead to deformity of the corresponding root sleeves, a defect which is apparent only on positive con-

trast myelograms. Smaller protrusions lead to shortening and widening of the root sleeves, while large prolapses cause complete obliteration of the root sleeves and even indentations into the adjacent column of contrast (Fig. 238).

Intervertebral disc herniations in the *thoracic region of the spinal canal* are seldom seen. In the majority of these cases, the middle third of the thoracic spine is affected, i.e., the area of maximum thoracic kyphosis. In examinations with the patient in the prone position, the positive contrast medium will usually stop at the level of the bulging disc until the examina-

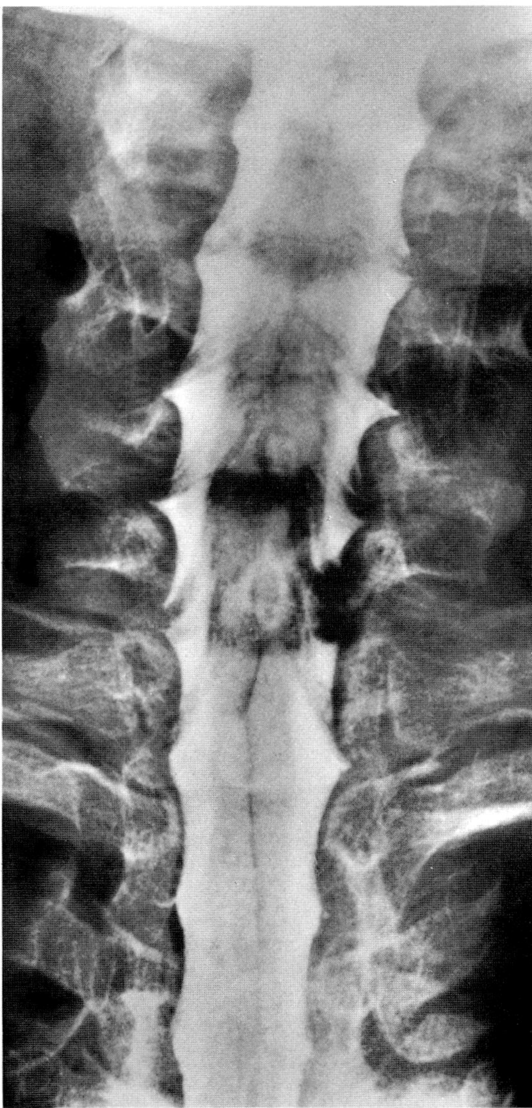

Fig. 238. Lateral intervertebral disc herniation (C-7/T-1, left)

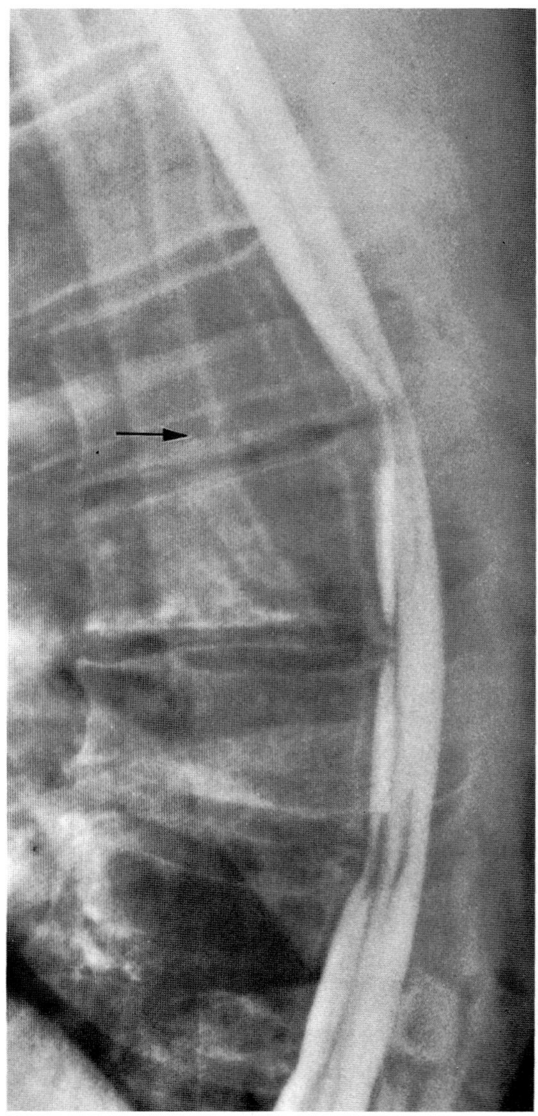

Fig. 239. Indentation (*arrow*) of the column of contrast by a T-8 disc prolapse

tion table is tilted sufficiently to allow it to pass, at which point it will rush on to a higher level. Similar difficulties arise when attempts are made to outline the defect from above. To overcome this problem, it is recommended either that air be used or that the positive contrast examination be performed with the patient on his back (supine) and with the needle out (see Fig. 239). In this position, the lowest point should be the area of dorsal kyphosis, which the heavier contrast medium will readily fill permitting more detailed analysis of the prolapsed disc.

Water-soluble contrast agents are most frequently used for the demonstration of a ruptured lumbar disc. Posterolateral prolapses are best seen on oblique films. Depending on the size of the herniation, there may only be obliteration of the corresponding root sleeve or, in addition, a large indentation in the adjacent column of contrast (Fig. 240). On the other hand, if the prolapse is limited to the extreme lateral position, the sole myelographic finding – if there is one at all – may be asymmetrical shortening and widening of the involved root sleeve (Fig. 241), while midline or central disc hernia-

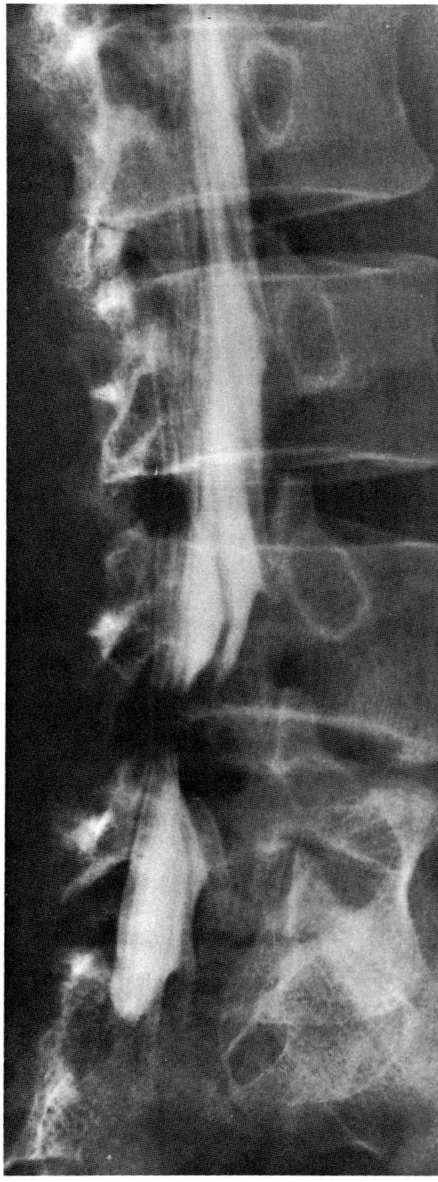

Fig. 240. Positive contrast myelogram with a water-soluble agent showing a prominent defect in the contrast column secondary to an L-4 lateral disc prolapse

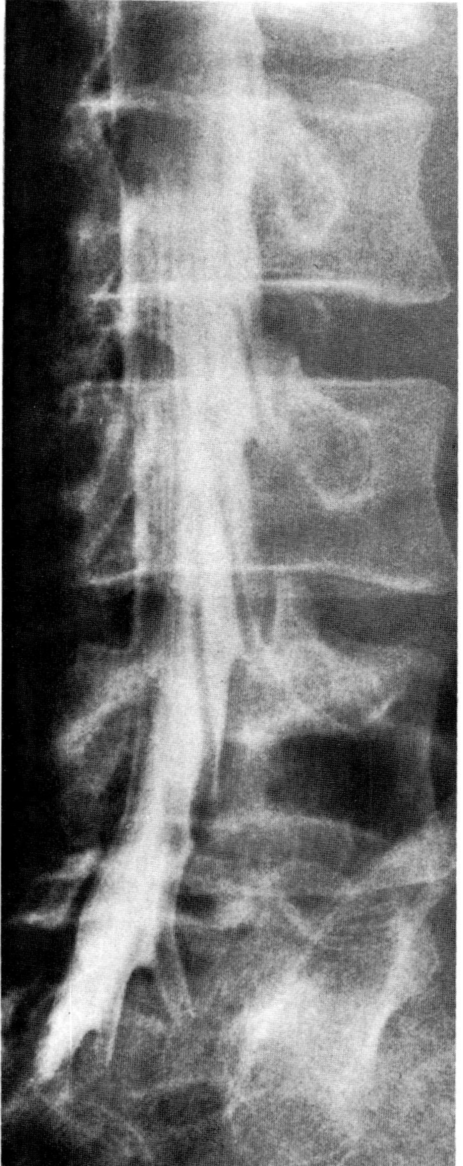

Fig. 241. Amputation of the L-5 root sleeve in another example of an L-4 lateral disc prolapse

tions may simply displace the column of contrast posteriorly without affecting the root sleeves on either side.

Massive herniations have been known to obstruct contrast flow completely, in which case the differential diagnosis will have to include other obstructing extradural mass lesions as well (Fig. 242). Lateral views usually reveal that the mass of disc material is situated anterior to the column of contrast adjacent to an intervertebral space.

Myelographic interpretation following disc surgery is complicated by the fact that postoperative scarring and adhesions can mimic a recurrent prolapse. However, this interpretation should be made only when the changes are limited to the column of contrast itself (irregular borders, narrowing) and do not affect the root sleeves at all. Finally, it should be emphasized that lumbar disc herniations with nerve root entrapment can be present in spite of a perfectly normal myelogram, and may be

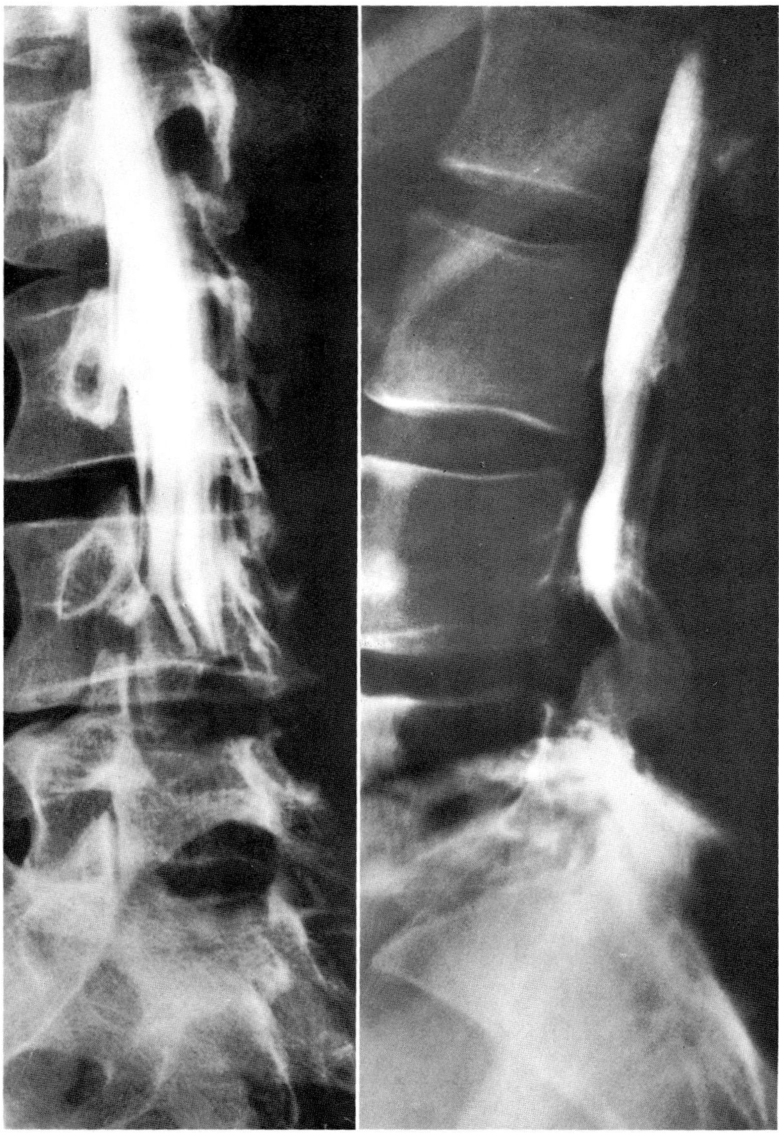

Fig. 242a, b. Complete block of contrast flow (inferiorly) secondary to a large midline disc herniation: **a** oblique view; **b** lateral view, prone position

absent in spite of an abnormal myelogram. In the latter situation, hypertrophic changes in the adjacent facet joints are frequently found at surgery.

4. The Spinal Arteriovenous Malformations

Arteriovenous malformations (AVMs) of the spinal cord are similar to AVMs of the brain in that there is persistence of an anastomotic network of large primitive vessels between the arterial and venous systems in place of the usual capillary system. The hypertrophied feeding arteries and draining veins can involve several vertebral segments and lie, for the most part, on the surface of the cord where they are readily identified as serpiginous defects with the positive contrast myelogram (Fig. 243). The examination is best performed in a supine position. Air myelography, on the other hand, is seldom satisfactory in this condition and should not be used here.

In the initial stages of the procedure, when the diagnosis is unknown, contrast flow in the area of the lesion will be slower than normal

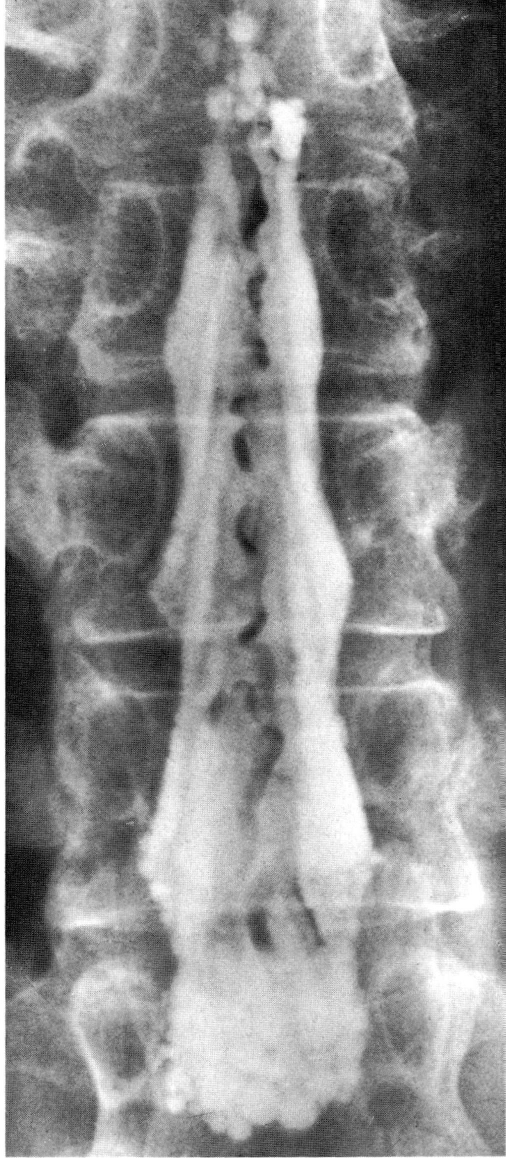

Fig. 243. Positive contrast myelogram showing a spinal cord AVM. Note the worm-like vessel images within the column of contrast

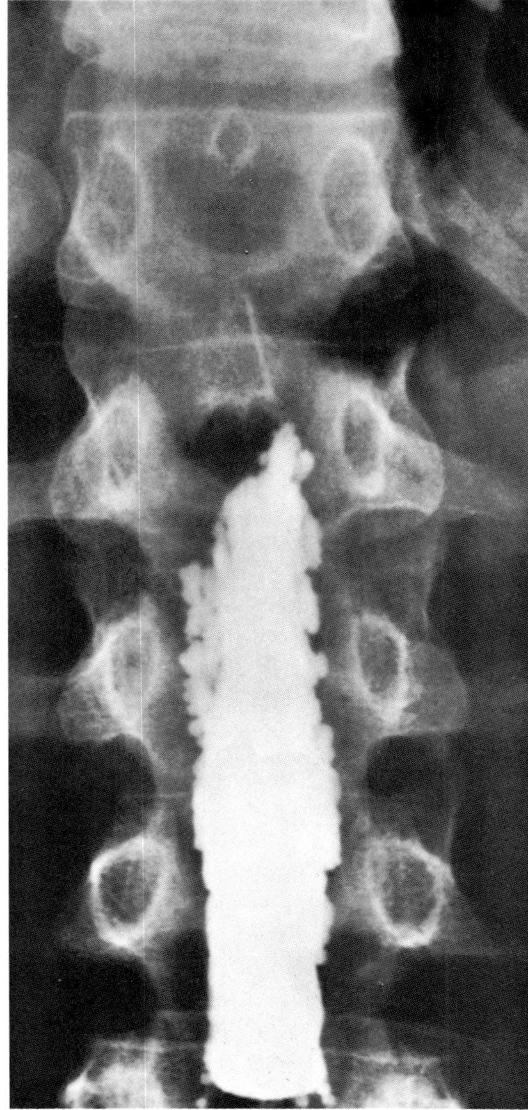

Fig. 244. Complete block to contrast flow in a case with meningeal adhesions. Note the irregular contour of the contrast column

and will serve to direct attention to the pathology. The aforementioned serpiginous defects (representing the engorged blood vessels) may also be clustered together in such a fashion that strings of pearl necklaces come to mind. The intramedullary portion of the AVM can distort the spinal cord in the same way as any other intramedullary space-occupying lesion and results in similar myelographic findings. The angiographic characteristics of the spinal angioma are described on p. 298 ff.

5. Meningeal Adhesions and Arachnoiditis

Adhesions of the meninges including arachnoiditis can be diagnosed from the myelogram when there is a complete or incomplete obliteration of the subarachnoid space at the level involved. There may be a complete block to contrast flow or an incomplete block, but the positive contrast findings are characteristic enough (ragged margins and odd-shaped pockets of retained contrast) to avoid confusion with an obstructing mass lesion (Fig. 244). This picture is caused by random adhesions of the meninges and formation of cysts which may or may not communicate with the contrast-filled subarachnoid space. Communication is assured when pockets of contrast appear, but these may be difficult to empty. Occasionally, manipulation of the patient and the table – as well as the aid of a timely cough – are required before successful emptying of the pockets is realized. Following meningitis, the entire subarachnoid space is so affected by adhesions that successful lumbar puncture may be impossible. Lesser degrees of involvement are readily recognized because the cord is not displaced despite obliteration of the surrounding subarachnoid spaces.

6. Posttraumatic Changes

Meningeal injuries following trauma to the vertebral column are caused by displaced bone fragments and by hemorrhage, which is a common cause of meningeal adhesions. Prolonged continuous compression of the dural sac is a further cause of adhesions familiar to the surgeon. Traumatic disc herniations are most common in the lumbar region and are usually associated with fracture of the posterior margin of the adjacent vertebral body. Traumatic cervical disc herniations are less frequently seen.

On the other hand, *nerve root avulsions* are fairly common in the *cervical* and *upper thoracic* regions, but rarely involve the lumbosacral roots. The myelographic diagnosis is made when the positive contrast agent is seen to leak out of the torn root sleeves into pockets both within and outside the spinal canal. In the latter case, the contrast flows via the intravertebral foramina to accumulate in the paravertebral space (Fig. 245). Occasionally, the contrast medium will even find its way as far laterally as the brachial plexus from where it cannot be retrieved. Otherwise, appropriate positioning of the patient will generally result in successful retrieval of most of the contrast medium from the extradural and paravertebral pockets. Cystic enlargement of the cervical root sleeves is an anatomical variant which should not be confused with root avulsion.

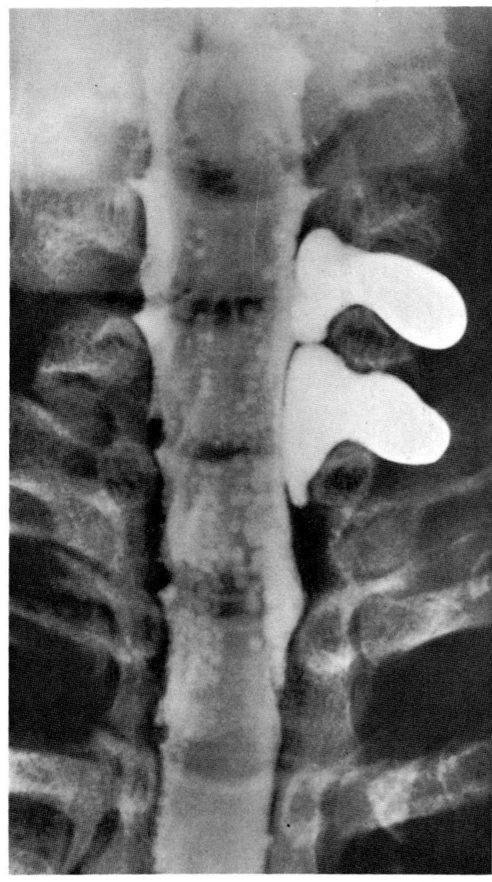

Fig. 245. Positive contrast myelogram showing posttraumatic avulsion of the left C-7 and C-8 roots with escape of contrast into finger-like pockets. The deformities of the T-1 and T-2 root sleeves on the same side, though less dramatic, are likewise indicative of root avulsion

7. Spinal Cord Atrophy

Circumscribed or generalized atrophy is best demonstrated with water-soluble agents, which are exclusively employed for this condition. In syringomyelia, the myelographic picture is characteristic in that the cord will be seen to bulge in some areas and to shrink in others. Bulges are typically found in the cervical cord, while atrophy is usually restricted to the thoracic cord. In any event, the thickened portion always lies superior to the thinned portion. When changes are limited to cord thickening, the differential diagnosis must include an intramedullary tumor. If the cystic syrinx, which lies within the thickened cord, communicates with the fourth ventricle by way of the central spinal canal, it may be emptied of its contents by lowering the patient's head.

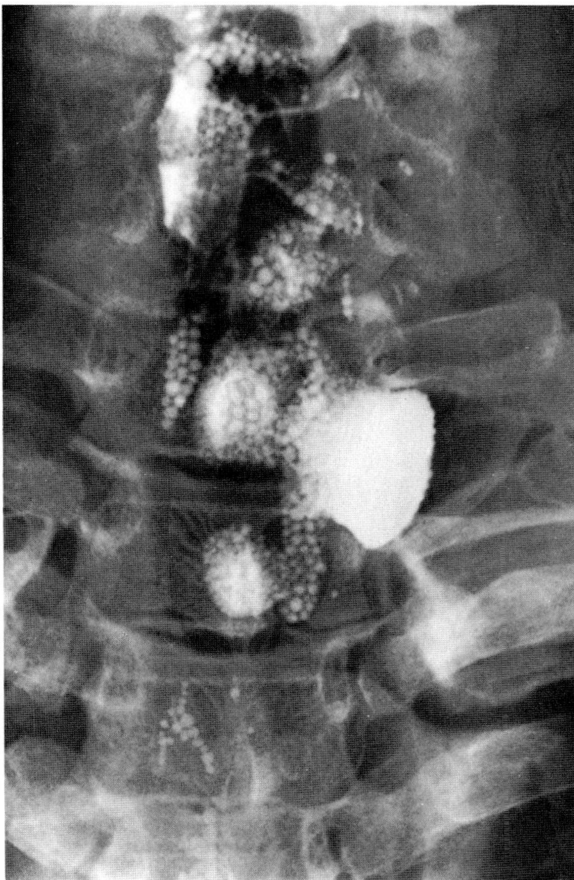

Fig. 246. Positive contrast myelogram demonstrating a meningocele at T-1/2 on the left

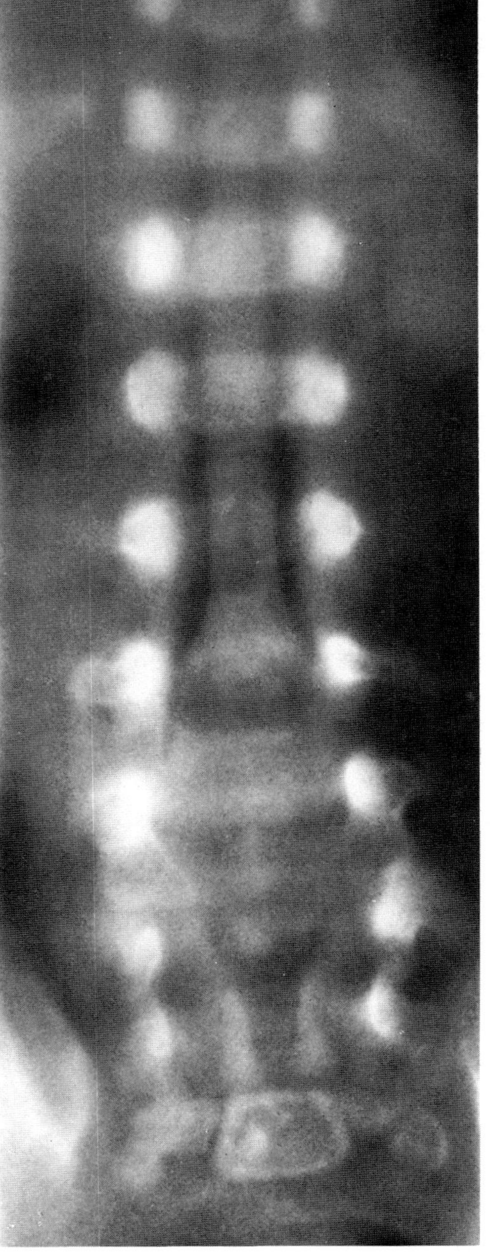

Fig. 247. Air myelogram showing tethering and enlargement ▷ of the spinal cord shadow with a fibrolipoma. Note the widened interpedicular distances in the lumbar region as well as the low position of the enlarged conus

8. Congenital Malformations of the Spine and Its Contents

The most common congenital malformation likely to be encountered on the myelogram is the *meningocele*. This condition is distinct from the open myelomeningocele (spina bifida cystica) with its attendant clinical consequences. Meningoceles occur in the lateral, dorsal, and ventral positions. The ventral meningocele is most frequently found in the sacral region, while the lateral and dorsal meningoceles are rare accompaniments of von Recklinghausen's disease. With the lateral type, the dural sac will be seen to protrude through the intervertebral foramen (Fig. 246). Occasionally, ventral and lateral meningoceles occur in combination. If the communication with the meningocele is of a "ball-valve" type, it may prove to be impossible to retrieve the contrast medium. Consequently, air or a water-soluble contrast agent

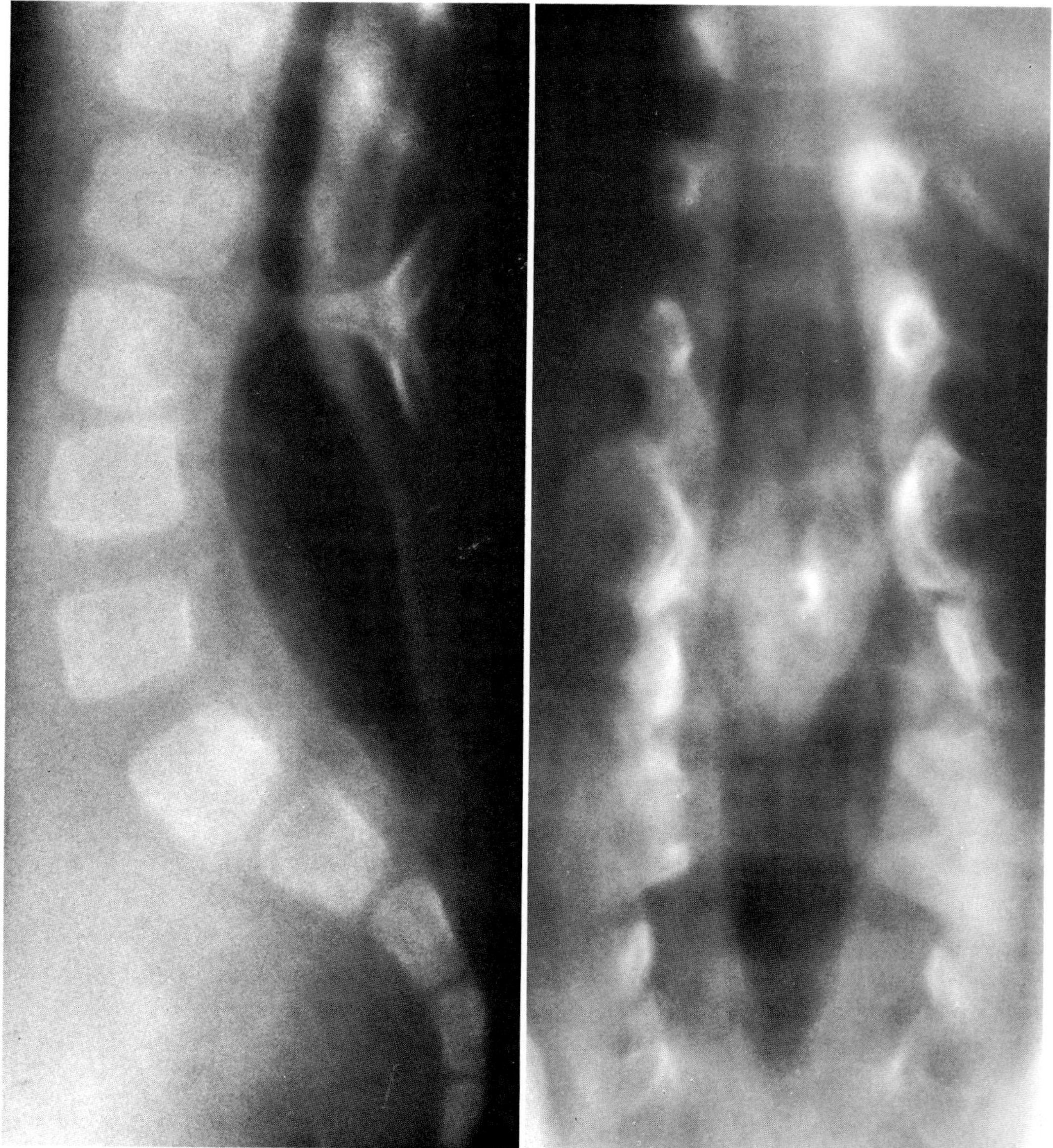

Fig. 248. Air myelogram with diastematomyelia. The cord has been split into two parts and fixed by a bony spur

is recommended whenever this diagnosis is entertained.

Another characteristic malformation apparent on the myelogram is seen with tethering of the spinal cord secondary to a shortened *filum terminale*. (Fig. 247). In such cases, the lower end of the spinal cord will extend as far as the lower lumbar or sacral segments. Myelography will verify the low position of the conus medullaris and the nerve roots will be seen running horizontally to their respective intervertebral foramina rather than diagonally downward.

Occasionally, a diffuse enlargement of the caudal dural sac will be seen as a variant of normal, or the caudal sac may taper to a small opening which then communicates with a larger cystic pocket at the very end of the sac.

Diastematomyelia is characterized by division of the spinal cord into two parts which surround a bony or cartilaginous spur, or a fibrous partition (Fig. 248).

For discussion of positive contrast cisternography with reference to the diagnosis of acoustic neurilemmomas, see pp. 247–250.

F. Spinal Angiography

With spinal angiography, visualization of normal and abnormal spinal cord vessels, particularly AVMs, is possible. This examination was not performed for many years as a result of difficult access to and the small caliber of the supplying segmental arteries. Technical advances were also needed to permit radiographic visualization of these vessels due to superimposition of the vertebral structures and adjacent soft tissue masses.

I. History

Demonstration of an AVM of the spinal cord by arteriography was first reported by HENSON and CRAFT in 1956, the technique having been developed 3 years earlier. In the succeeding years HÖÖK and LINDVALL (1958) and MORRIS (1960) successfully opacified cervical AVMs via vertebral angiography, while RAND and RAND (1960) were able to demonstrate thoracolumbar AVMs with aortography. DJINDJIAN et al. (1969, 1970) and DICHIRO et al. (1967) perfected the method further so that "selective spinal angiography" is today routinely recommended as the procedure of choice for visualization of spinal AVMs.

II. Normal and Pathological Anatomy of the Spinal Cord Vessels

For successful interpretation of a spinal angiogram, it is imperative that one be familiar with the normal vascular supply to the cord. Developmentally, the arterial supply is initially laid out symmetrically in segments. Later, as described by ADAMKIEWICZ (1881, 1882) and KADYI (1889), many of the segmental arteries become atrophic until only 5–8 of the 22 remaining vessels carry a substantial volume of blood. Of these, two are particularly noteworthy – the branch to the cervical enlargement (at the approximate level of C-5/6) and the largest segmental vessel, the so-called artery of Adamkiewicz. This latter vessel is found at the T-9/11 level in 80% of cases, while it occupies any upper lumbar position in the rest. Between these two major arteries of supply, the feeding vessels are usually of small caliber. The most caudal artery of supply enters the spinal canal at the

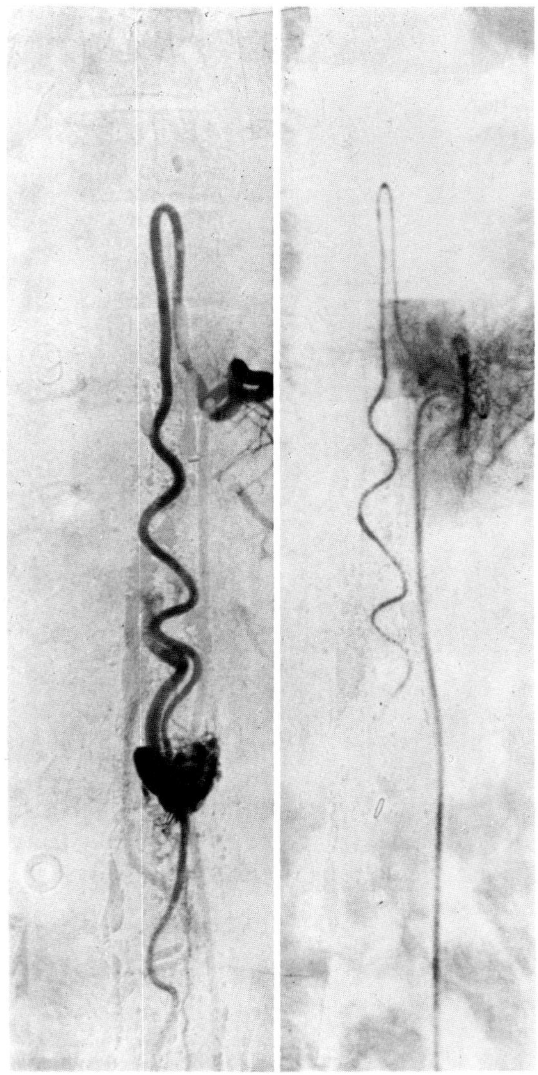

Fig. 249. Extramedullary AVM before and after embolism. Courtesy of the late Professor R. DJINDJIAN, Paris

L-5/S-1 level and travels cephalad to supply the region of the conus medullaris.

This general description of arterial supply to the spinal cord is found in approximately 90% of the population. In the remaining 10%, the blood supply is less than optimal in that there are, at most, two or three segmental vessels feeding the anterior and posterior spinal arteries, while the remaining vessels supply only the roots and peripheral zones of the spinal cord (ZÜLCH 1962, 1976).

The segmental branches to the cervical region as far as T-4 arise from the vertebral arteries, while those to the thoracic and lumbar regions originate directly from the aorta. Impairment of flow by mechanical or hemodynamic

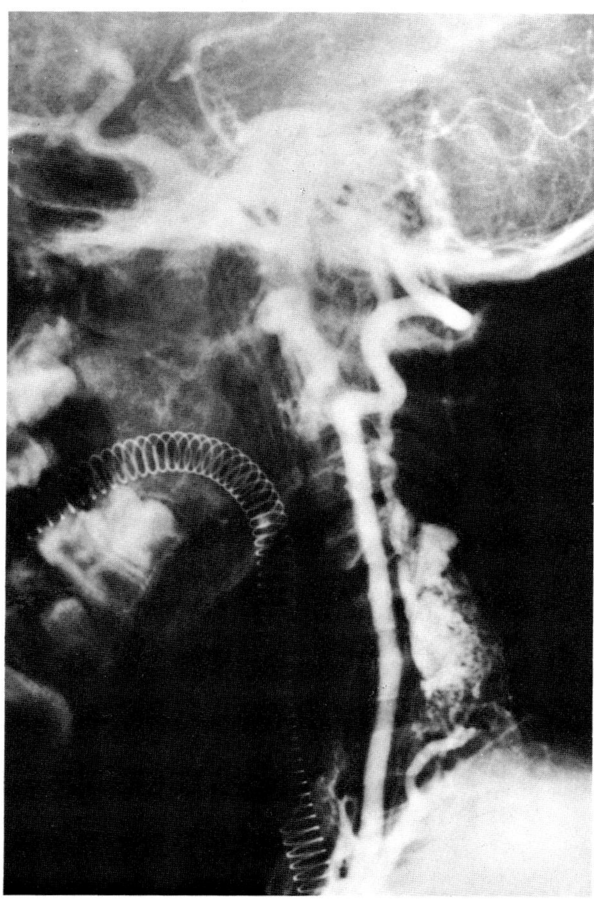

Fig. 250. Demonstration of a spinal cord AVM in the cervical region via retrograde brachial angiography

disturbances may result in ischemic injury to the "watershed" zones, T-4/5 and L-1, for reasons analogous to those outlined in the discussion of similar zones in the cerebral hemispheres.

A third "watershed" zone is found at C-4. However, this entity usually results from high cervical fracture/dislocations which are generally incompatible with survival.

The appearance of the anterior spinal artery, which is frequently the only one seen angiographically, is best described in terms of a linked chain since it is not a continuous vessel. Its segmental feeders, such as the great thoracic radicular artery, tend to split into ascending and descending branches which form the various links of the chain.

The great anterior radicular artery (artery of Adamkiewicz) also divides, but the ascending branch is thinner than the thick descending branch (Fig. 249). The anterior spinal artery and both posterior spinal arteries then form a segmental circumferential network of vessels which supply the corresponding segment with perpendicular perforating branches (ZÜLCH 1976).

An understanding of the "watershed" zones is critical since paraplegia can be caused by hemodynamic disturbances without any apparent regional pathology. Complications of angiographic demonstration of the aorta, for example, are most likely to involve these areas.

As noted in the section on myelography, AVMs of the spinal cord consist of an anastomotic network of large primitive vessels between the arterial and venous systems instead of the usual capillary system.

Clinically these malformations may result in recurrent hemorrhage and ischemic disturbances of the adjacent spinal cord. Although the association of cutaneous angiomas with other spinal anomalies is extremely rare, such an association may occasionally occur with AVMs of the spinal cord. Thus, the finding of a cutaneous angioma may suggest an underlying spinal anomaly. Such patients may also harbor vascular pathology in other organ systems – for example, aneurysms and arteriovenous shunts of the lung, liver, or kidney.

On the basis of anatomical studies and angiographic findings, *AVMs of the spinal cord may be divided into three distinct groups:* (a) a relatively localized cluster of abnormal vessels with slow perfusion, reminiscent of the glomus tumor (Fig. 250); (b) a larger lesion comprised twisted vessels and extending over several segments, with a single or multiple feeding vessels and with slow perfusion; and (c) finally, an elongated AVM, especially prevalent in children, with multiple feeders and with high perfusion. This lesion resembles AVMs of the brain.

Sites of predilection for AVMs of the spinal cord are as follows: 10% are found in the cervical region, 30% in the thoracic, and 60% at the thoracolumbar junction. This distribution should be kept in mind when one is deciding which segmental artery to catheterize during angiography.

III. Examination Technique

The examination is begun with femoral catheterization (Seldinger technique). Contrast demonstration of the aorta rarely provides adequate visualization of a spinal cord AVM and, because of the volume of contrast medium employed, is not without considerable risk of complications if the tip of the catheter is positioned near the origin of either the great radicular artery of Adamkiewicz or the upper dorsal radiculomedullary artery. In such cases, large quantities of contrast will enter these vessels and may result in spinal cord ischemia or more permanent cord damage, i.e., transverse myelitis, monoparesis, or the Brown-Séquard syndrome (see DJINDJIAN et al. 1970).

Consequently, aortography has been largely abandoned in favor of the selective angiography of single segmental arteries with small volumes of contrast (2–3 ml). To accomplish this task, selective catheterization of each intercostal or lumbar artery is carried out using a fine catheter with an "S" configuration at the tip. Since subtraction studies are necessary to outline the course of each delicate spinal artery, it is essential that the examination be performed only under general anesthesia to guarantee patient immobility.

In the section which follows, the examination technique will be explained in greater detail.

1. Demonstration of the Anterior Spinal Artery in the Cervical Region

After transfemoral catheterization, the two vertebral arteries are selectively injected using 6–7 ml of contrast medium. In this manner, the descending branch of the anterior spinal artery in the cervical region may be visualized. Since the further supply to the anterior spinal artery in this region is supplied by radicular branches which vary considerably in their origin and course, it is recommended that selective study of the deep and/or ascending cervical arteries as well as the thyrocervical and costocervical arteries of both sides be carried out.

2. Demonstration of the Anterior Spinal Artery at the Thoracolumbar Junction

The thoracolumbar segment of the anterior spinal artery is supplied by the great radicular artery of Adamkiewicz which normally arises from the 8th, 9th, or 10th intercostal artery on the left side. These are selectively catheterized and 2–3 ml of contrast medium injected into each. The appropriate levels are identified by fixing small lead numbers to the skin overlying the corresponding vertebrae before X-rays are taken.

When injection of these vessels does not succeed in filling the artery of Adamkiewicz, the arteries of T-11, T-12, and L-1 on the left side are selectively injected, followed by the arteries of T-8 to L-2 on the right side.

Difficulties are occasionally encountered in older patients because of tortuosity of the aorta, which moves the origins of the intercostal and lumbar arteries to atypical locations. Selective catheterization of the L-1 and L-2 arteries is also difficult due to the flow of blood into the renal arteries which diverts the catheter tip away from the orifice of these vessels.

3. Comparison of Various Methods Available for Spinal Angiography

In addition to the clinical neurological findings, the presence of an AVM can be suspected from the plain spine films whenever there is a widening of the spinal canal, a localized erosion or, occasionally, calcium deposits within the lesion. None of these findings are, however, specific for AVMs. Positive contrast myelography will demonstrate the dilated, often obstructed, twisted vessels of the lesion as defects in the column of contrast (see Fig. 243). Massive AVMs can result in a complete block to the flow of contrast medium. In this situation, the precise identification of the obstruction is impossible since the differential diagnosis must include other intradural space-occupying lesions.

With ossovenography, the diagnosis of AVM is possible only when there is a vascular communication between the bony channels and intraspinal AVM. Such communication is, however, extremely rare.

Vertebral angiography will occasionally demonstrate a cervical AVM. Finally, retrograde aortography may also be used to advantage whenever feeding vessels are visualized. Normally, such studies are inadequate, however, since the opacified aorta will interfere with visualization of the smaller AVMs, which are generally poorly outlined in this study.

Occasionally, lumbar venography with bilateral injection of the lumbar veins will also demonstrate individual portions of an AVM.

The most reliable angiographic method for demonstration of spinal AVMs is, however, "selective" angiography of the anterior and posterior spinal arteries. Occasionally, a "thrombosis" of the anterior spinal artery will be demonstrated, which also supports the clinical diagnosis of AVM.

IV. Complications

Since the first description by ANTONI and LIND-GREN (1949), many serious complications have been reported in association with attempts at spinal angiography (see KILLEN and FOSTER 1966). Both quadriplegia and paraplegia have been described, which were blamed on the suspected neurotoxic effects of the concentrated contrast medium. It seems more likely, however, that in such cases a major segmental branch of supply to the spinal cord arteries was occluded, perhaps as the result of an intramural injection of contrast medium. In any event, it is recommended that selective catheterization of the smaller caliber spinal arteries, as well as high pressure injections, be avoided. Such injections should be done by hand under low pressures.

It is also recommended that interruption of the blood supply to the catheterized segmental vessels be kept at a minimum, particularly when the vessel being studied is a major source of supply to the cord (for example, the artery of Adamkiewicz).

Whenever vasospasm follows aortography or selective angiography of any vessel, it is advisable to terminate the procedure without delay. However, vasospasm is rare following injection of the major segmental feeders to an AVM, since the majority of contrast will then be rapidly taken up by the lesion.

Finally, employment of the Seldinger technique does carry the additional risk of dislodging an embolus from an ulcerated plaque in atheromatous sections of the descending aorta with secondary peripheral infarcts.

If the examination is carried out with great care and attention to detail, the number of complications will be kept so low *that the procedure should be offered to anyone with a suspected diagnosis of spinal cord AVM who would be considered a candidate for angiography elsewhere in the body*. For literature, see: DJINDJIAN et al. (1970).

G. Discography

Discography gives direct information about the shape of the disc and the intervertebral space. At the same time it is possible to assess the type and extent of any disc pathology present.

Discography is employed in various clinics with varying frequency. Lumbar discography is, in fact, rarely performed today. In the cervical region, it is used for diagnostic clarification of nonspecific pain syndromes, root entrapment syndromes, some myelopathies, and especially in the preliminary evaluation for fusion operations.

I. History

In 1931 SCHMORL reported the X-ray analysis of discs after injection of bismuth paste into the nucleus pulposus of cadavers. In 1941 LINDGREN reported injecting Perabrodil into a normal disc in a live patient. Further technical advances were made by LINDBLOM (1941, 1944, 1948). ERLACHER (1950), WITT (1950), and CLOWARD and BUZAID (1952), particularly with regard to the demonstration of lumbar discs.

II. Technique of Cervical Discography

For safety reasons a double cannula technique is used (CLOWARD), in which the shorter outer cannula (5.5 cm) is advanced only as far as the annulus fibrosis. The inner cannula is 1 cm longer (6.5 cm) and it alone perforates the annulus to reach the nucleus pulposus. In this fashion, penetration from the anterior margin of the annulus cannot exceed 1 cm and damage to the spinal cord is virtually impossible.

Preliminary sedation is mandatory since discography is quite painful. The patient lies supine on the X-ray table with the neck extended. The cervical area to be studied is then palpated with the second and third fingers and the adjacent midline structures (thyroid cartilage, trachea, and esophagus) displaced to the opposite side. After skin puncture and first contact of the needle with the vertebral bodies, verification of the desired level is obtained with anteroposterior and lateral X-rays. Following this, approximately 5 ml Novocaine is injected into the periosteum, the anterior longitudinal ligament, the prevertebral fascia, and the anterior margin

of the annulus fibrosis. Only after X-ray confirmation that the shorter cannula is in the correct position is the second needle advanced through the first and into the nucleus pulposus. The needle tip should now lie within the intervertebral space. Injection of 0.5–2 ml of the contrast agent (Renographin 60 or Conray 60) then takes place under direct visualization by lateral fluoroscopy. When one is satisfied that the disc has been adequately outlined, the needle is withdrawn and anteroposterior and lateral films again exposed.

Generally, it is recommended that each session be limited to the study of one disc.

During injection of the contrast medium, the patient should be questioned to ascertain whether or not the disc injection caused exacerbation of pain similar to that experienced before.

III. The Normal Discogram

Discography in adults is rarely completely normal. In addition, variations from normal with respect to the shape and size of the nucleus pulposus is the rule rather than the exception. In the lumbar region, for example, the normal diameter of the nucleus varies from 1 to 2.5 cm (Fig. 251 a).

IV. The Pathological Discogram

Interpretation of the discogram is not difficult. With herniation into the spinal canal, the injected contrast will follow and outline the prolapse as it extends beyond the posterior longitudinal ligament, revealing not only its precise location, but also its size (Fig. 251 b). In a totally degenerated disc which has not yet escaped the confines of the annulus fibrosis, the contrast will be seen to fill the intervertebral space to its peripheral margins in both the anteroposterior and lateral projections. It should be emphasized that contrast injection into a degenerated disc will be painful and will cause severe radicular pain, even in the absence of nerve root compression. This "discogenic" pain will tend to follow the appropriate segmental dermatome.

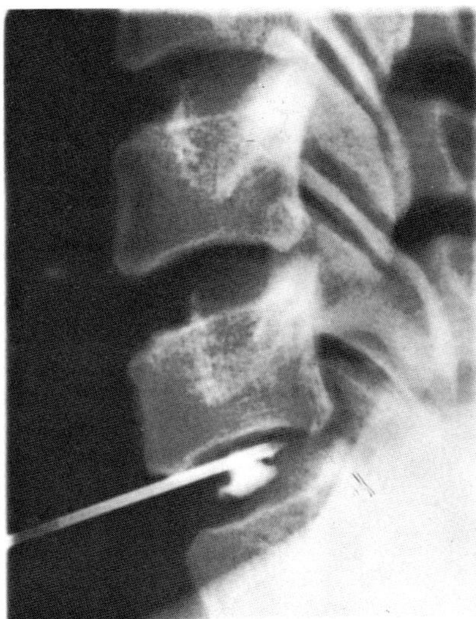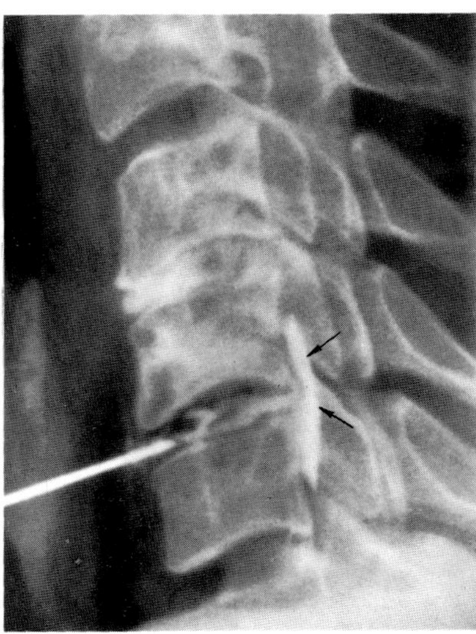

Fig. 251. a Normal discogram. **b** Pathological discogram showing posterior intervertebral disc herniations at C-4/5 and C-5/6. At the level of the lower protrusion there is leakage of the contrast out under the posterior longitudinal ligament (X-rays courtesy of Professor FRIEDMANN, Cologne)

Discography permits direct visualization of the nucleus pulposus in both its normal and pathological states. Disc herniations into the spinal canal and elsewhere are readily recognized and additional information is gleaned from the reproduced pain, even when disc herniation is absent. In contrast to myelography, the CSF pathways are not disturbed and the procedure is simple with no real need for hospitalization during the recovery period. On the other hand, the information obtained is restricted to pathological processes involving the disc being studied. Other causes of similar symptoms cannot be evaluated by this method, a disadvantage which myelography does not share.

V. Complications

Complications of discography include inflammatory changes within the disc or neighboring bone structures. Transient hoarseness and minor swallowing difficulties have been reported, but these have always eventually resolved. A serious complication to be avoided because of the certain risk of infection is perforation of the esophagus by the cannula. To avoid this problem, the patient is warned neither to talk nor swallow during the needle insertion.

For literature, see: CLOWARD (1958), LINDBLOM (1944, 1948).

H. Ossovenography and Epidural Venography

I. History

HENNING (1940) and EHRHARDT and KNEIP (1943) were the first to report injection of contrast medium into bone. In 1952 FISCHGOLD et al. reported that contrast injections into a human spinous process resulted in an outline of the venous plexus of the attached vertebral body. In subsequent years improvements have been made which now permit contrast visualization of the venous plexuses of the entire vertebral axis.

II. Anatomy

The valveless venous system of the vertebral axis includes both the inner (epidural) and outer (extravertebral) venous plexuses. These two systems are interconnected by anastomoses.

The *epidural venous plexuses* consist of two pairs of well-demarcated channels, one anterior and the other posterior to the dura, which are interconnected by a series of circumferential anastomotic rings. The external venous plexuses are likewise organized along similar lines, the anterior plexus lying in front of the vertebral bodies and the posterior plexus encircling the spinous processes. Both communicate with the internal venous plexuses, with venous pathways in adjacent bony structures including the emissary veins of the skull, and with the intercostal veins. In contrast to the other plexuses, the anterior external plexus consists of many fine individual channels.

III. Technique

For this investigation, the patient is placed in the prone position on the X-ray table. A rubber balloon is blown up under the abdomen to compress the inferior vena cava. The spinous process of the vertebral body at the level of the suspected pathology is punctured with a sternal puncture needle using a twisting motion. With correct placement of the needle a low pressure injection by hand should be sufficient to rapidly inject 20 ml of the contrast medium (60% solution). Alternatively, a high pressure automatic injector can also be used.

During the injection, the patient should hold his breath and should strain (Valsalva maneuver) in order that the venous pressure is increased and good contrast demonstration of the veins obtained. Towards the end of the injection, X-ray films are taken in the posteroanterior and lateral projections. Because of difficulty in differentiating individual venous plexuses, simultaneous tomography has been recommended and has proven quite useful (see Angiotomography, p. 64).

For demonstration of the epidural venous plexus in the mid and upper cervical regions, *ventral* puncture of the cervical vertebral body has been used to advantage. The patient lies supine with his neck extended. A carotid puncture needle is advanced to the anterior margin of the 5th or 6th cervical vertebra and lightly hammered into place. Fluoroscopic control during this maneuver is essential.

IV. Results

Intervertebral disc herniations into the spinal canal cause unilateral interruption of the epidural venous plexus at the disc level on the ossovenogram. If the herniation is very large, bilateral interruption of the epidural veins will be seen. On the other hand, a far lateral prolapse may cause minimal disturbance of the internal venous plexus.

Malignant processes involving the *vertebrae* with infiltration into the surrounding soft tissues or epidural space are also recognizable with this procedure as interruptions of the paravertebral venous systems. This infiltration, as revealed by ossovenography, is often more extensive than either the plain X-rays or myelogram are capable of demonstrating.

Both *extradural and intradural tumors* lead to similar changes in the epidural veins. If paravertebral collateral flow is present, the upper or lower margins of the tumor may be determined as well. "Hour-glass" neurilemmomas lead to displacement of the epidural and paravertebral veins with demonstration of the space-occupying lesion. Other *intradural processes* which are not normally space-occupying will not disturb the epidural venous plexus.

Although demonstration of an *angioma* of the *vertebral body* is poorly seen on ossovenography, combinations of epidural and vertebral AVMs with involvement of the adjacent soft tissues and the epidural space are well depicted. *Intradural* AVMs are, however, seldom apparent on this study.

V. Complications and Contraindications

Paravertebral deposition of the contrast agent does occasionally occur, but is harmless and the contrast quickly resorbed. Complications of a permanent nature are not usually seen. Contraindications include the blood dyscrasias as well as local inflammation in the vicinity of the puncture site.

For literature, see: CLEMENS (1961), SCHOBINGER (1960), VOGELSANG (1969).

References

Aaron C, Doyon D, Fischgold DH, Metzger J, Richard J (1970) Artériographie de la carotide externe – étude anatomoradiologique et clinique. Masson, Paris

Adamkiewicz A (1881) Die Blutgefäße des menschlichen Rückenmarks. I. Teil: Die Gefäße der Rückenmarkssubstanz. Sitzungsber Akad Wiss Wien Math Naturwiss Kl Abt 3 84:469–502

Adamkiewicz A (1882) Die Blutgefäße des menschlichen Rückenmarks. II. Teil: Die Gefäße der Rückenmarksoberfläche. Sitzungsber Akad Wien Math Naturwiss Kl Abt 3 85:101–130

Ahlgren P (1969) Lumbale Myelographie mit Conray Meglumin 282. ROEFO 111:270–276

Ahlgren P (1972) Dimer-X. A new contrast medium for lumbar myelography without spinal anaesthesia. Acta Radiol [Diagn] (Stockh) 13:753–761

Alajouanine T, Castaigne P, Lhermitte F, Cambier J, Gautier J-C (1961) Les obstructions bilatérales de la carotide interne. Sem Hôp Paris 35:1149–1161

Amplatz K, Harner R (1962) A new subclavian artery catheterization technic. Radiology 78:963–966

Andersen PE (1963) Angiographic localization of small intracerebral hematomas. Acta Radiol (Stockh) 1:173–181

Antoni N, Lindgren E (1949) Steno's experiment in man as complication in lumbar aortography. Acta Chir Scand 98:230

Arnell S, Lidström F (1931) Myelography with Skiodan (Abrodil). Acta Radiol (Stockh) 12:287–288

Azambuja N, Arana-Iñiguez R, Sande MT, Garcia-Güelfi A (1956a) Central ventriculography. Acta Neurol Lat Am 2:58

Azambuja N, Lindgren E, Sjögren SE (1956b) Tentorial herniations. I. Anatomy. Acta Radiol (Stockh) 46:215–223

Azambuja N, Lindgren E, Sjögren SE (1956c) Tentorial herniations. II. Pneumography. Acta Radiol (Stockh) 46:224–235

Azambuja N, Lindgren E, Sjögren SE (1956d) Tentorial herniations. III. Angiography. Acta Radiol (Stockh) 46:236–241

Bailey P (1932) Cellular types in primary tumors of the brain. In: Penfield W (ed) Cytology and cellular pathology of the nervous system. Hoeber, New York, pp 905–951

Bailey P (1951) Die Hirngeschwülste. Enke, Stuttgart

Bailey P, Cushing H (1926) A classification of the tumors of the glioma group on a histogenetic basis with a correlated study of prognosis. Lippincott, Philadelphia

Bailey P, Cushing H (1930) Die Gewebsverschiedenheit der Gliome und ihre Bedeutung für die Prognose. Fischer, Jena

Balado M (1926) La radiografia del tercer ventriculo. Bol Inst Clin Quir (Buenos Aires) 2:603

Barbieri PL, Verdecchia CG (1957) Vertebral arteriography by percutaneous puncture of the subclavian artery. Acta Radiol (Stockh) 48:444

Bauer RB, Sheehan S, Wechsler H, Meyer JS (1962) Arteriographic study of sites, incidences and treatment of arteriosclerotic cerebrovascular lesions. Neurology (Minneap) 12:689–711

Baumgartner J, Woringer E, Braun JP, Abada M (1963) Phlébogramme cérébral profond de face et ses variations en cas de processus expansifs de l'espace intra-cranien sus-tentoriel. Acta Radiol (Stockh) 1:182–205

Baumgartner J, Braun JP, Caron J, Cécille J, Fischgold H, Gonsette R, Hirsch JF, Legré J, Metzger J (1970) Radiculographie au Dimer-X. Premiers résultats après 630 examens. J Radiol Electrol 51:557–559

Becker H, Radtke F (1949) Eine Methode zur willkürlich steuerbaren Luftfüllung der Ventrikel bzw. peripheren Liquorräume. Nervenarzt 20:442

Belloni G (1941) Pneumographische Passageprüfung der Arachnoidalräume. Zentralbl Neurochir 6:43–48

Bergleiter R, Fekas L (1964) Das Cavum septi pellucidi und Cavum vergae in Klinik und Röntgenbild. Fortschr Neurol Psychiatr 32:361–399

Bernasconi V, Cassinari V (1956) Un segno carotidografico tipico di meningioma del tentorio. Chirurgia (Milan) 11:586–588

Bernasconi V, Cassinari V (1957) Caratteristiche angiografiche dei meningiomi del tentorio. Radiol Med (Torino) 43:1015–1026

Bernstein EF, Greenspan RH, Løken MK (1958) Intravenous abdominal aortography. Surgery 44:529

Bier A (1897) Die Entstehung des Collateralkreislaufs. Teil 1. Bier A (1898) Die Entstehung des Collateralkreislaufs, Teil 2. Arch Pathol Anat 147:256. Arch Pathol Anat 153:306

Biermann HR, Miller ER, Dyrow RL, Dod KS, Kelly KH, Black DH (1951) Intra-arterial catheterization of viscera in man. AJR 66:555

Bingel A (1921) Intralumbale Lufteinblasung zur Höhendiagnose intraduraler extramedullärer Prozesse und zur Differentialdiagnose gegenüber intramedullären Prozessen. Dtsch Z Nervenheilkd 72:359–370

Bingel A (1921/1922) Encephalographie, eine Methode zur röntgenographischen Darstellung des Gehirns. ROEFO 28:205

Birkmayer A (1960) Die Messung der zerebralen Durchblutungszeit mit Radioisotopen. Zentralbl Ges Neurol Psychiatr 158:247

Bogatyrev YV (1961) On the technique of cerebral angiography through the A. temporalis (in Russian). Vopr Nejrokhir 25:40–42

Boulay G du (1963) Distribution of spasm in the intracranial arteries after subarachnoid hemorrhage. Acta Radiol (Stockh) 1:257–266

Bradac GB, Simon RS, Holtz U (1972) Zur Auswertung der venösen Phase des Vertebralisangiogramms. ROEFO 117:630–637

Braun JP, Wackenheim A (1972) Phlébographie mesencéphalique dans les tumeurs du tronc cérébral. Acta Radiol (Stockh) 13:45–53

Bregéat P, David M, Fischgold H, Talairach J (1952) Opacification des vaisseaux orbitaires et de la choroide par l'angiographie carotidienne. Rev Neurol (Paris) 87:549–551

Brismar J (1974) Orbital phlebography. Medical dissertation, University of Lund

Brock M, Schürmann K, Hadjidimos A (1969) Cerebral blood flow and cerebral death. Acta Neurochir (Wien) 20:195–209

Buchtala V, Gerlach J (1954) Mandrinkanülen zur Arteriographie. Zentralbl Neurochir 14:118–120

Bücheler E, Käufer C, Düx A (1970) Cerebrale Angiographie zur Bestimmung des Hirntodes. ROEFO 113:278–296

Bull JWD (1962a) Contribution of radiology to the study of intracranial aneurysms. Br Med J 2:1701–1708

Bull JWD (1962b) The significance of displacement of the internal carotid artery. Br J Radiol 35:801–814

Bull JWD (1971) Myelography. Neuroradiology 2:1–2

Bull JWD (1973) Technique of oil myelography. Br Med J 1:280–282

Castellanos A, Pereiras R (1939) Countercurrent aortography. Rev Cubana Cardiol 2:187

Chiari H (1891) Über Veränderungen des Kleinhirns infolge von Hydrocephalie des Großhirns. Dtsch Med Wochenschr 42:1172–1174

Clar HE, Bock WJ, Grote W, Löhr E (1976) Atlas der Encephalotomographie. Thieme, Stuttgart

Clemens HJ (1961) Die Venensysteme der menschlichen Wirbelsäule (Morphologie und funktionelle Bedeutung). de Gruyter, Berlin

Cloward RB (1958) Cervical diskography. Technique, indications and use in diagnosis of ruptured cervical disks. AJR 79:563

Cloward RB, Buzaid LL (1952) Discography. AJR 68:552

Collins W, Slade H, Lockhart W (1957) Brachial vertebral angiography in adults. J Neurosurg 14:466–468

Courville CB (1967) Intracranial tumors. Notes upon a series of three thousand verified cases with some current observations pertaining to their mortality. Bull Los Angeles Neurol Soc [Suppl 2/2] 32

Cronqvist S (1959) The postoperative myelogram. Acta Radiol (Stockh) 52:45–51

Curtis JB (1949) Rapid serial angiography: preliminary report. J Neurol Neurosurg Psychiatry 12:167–182

Dandy WE (1918) Ventriculography following the injection of air into the cerebral ventricles. Ann Surg 68:5

Dandy WE (1919) Roentgenography of the brain after the injection of air into the spinal canal. Ann Surg 70:397–403

Dandy WE (1937) Carotid-cavernous aneurysms (pulsating exophthalmos). Zentralbl Neurochir 2:77–133, 165–206

Davidoff LM, Dyke CG (1946) The normal encephalogram. Lea & Febiger, Philadelphia

Davidoff LM, Epstein BS (1950) The abnormal pneumoencephalogram. Lea & Febiger, Philadelphia

Decker K (1951a) Technik und diagnostische Möglichkeiten der percutanen Vertebralis-Angiographie. Acta Neurochir (Wien) 2:74–80

Decker K (1951b) Percutane Vertebralis-Angiographie. Nervenarzt 22:32

Decker K (1953) The displacement of the posterior cerebral artery in vertebral angiograms. Acta Radiol (Stockh) 40:91–95

Decker K (1955) Die A. ophthalmica im Karotisangiogramm. ROEFO 82:667–673

Decker K (1957) Encephalographie am Bildwandler. ROEFO 87:707–714

Decker K (1958) Der Schlaganfall als neuroradiologisches Problem. Dtsch Med Wochenschr 83:205

Decker K (1960) Klinische Neuroradiologie. Thieme, Stuttgart

Decker K, Backmund H (1970) Pädiatrische Neuroradiologie. Thieme, Stuttgart

Decker K, Backmund H (1975) Paediatric Neuroradiology. Thieme, Stuttgart

Dejean C, Boudet C (1951) Du diagnostic des varices de l'orbite et de leurs complications par la phlébographie. Bull Soc Fr Ophthalmol 64:374

Denny-Brown D (1951) The treatment of recurrent cerebrovascular symptoms and the question of "vasospasm". Med Clin North Am 35:1457–1474

Denny-Brown D (1953) Basilar artery syndromes. Bull N Engl Med Cent 15:53–60

Di Chiro G (1961) Ophthalmic arteriography. Radiology 77:948–957

Di Chiro G (1962) Angiographic patterns of cerebral convexity veins and superficial dural sinuses. AJR 87:308–321

Di Chiro G (1967) An atlas of detailed normal pneumoencephalographic anatomy, 2nd edn. Thomas, Springfield

Di Chiro G (1971) An atlas of pathologic pneumoencephalographic anatomy. Thomas, Springfield

Di Chiro G, Doppman J, Ommaya AK (1967) Selective arteriography of arterio-venous aneurysm of spinal cord. Radiology 88:1065–1077

Dilenge D (1962) L'angiographie de l'artère carotide interne. Masson, Paris, pp 1–230

Dilenge D, Fischgold H, David M (1965) L'angiographie par soustraction de l'artère ophthalmique et de ses branches. Masson, Paris

Djindjian R, Merland J-J (1978) Superselective arteriography of the external carotid artery. Springer, Berlin Heidelberg New York

Djindjian R, Houdart R, Hurth M (1969) Les angiomes de la moëlle. Sandoz, Paris

Djindjian R, Hurth M, Houdart R (1970) L'angiographie de la moëlle épinière. Masson, Paris

Djindjian R, Merland J-J, Djindjian M, Stoeter P (1981) Angiography of spinal column and spinal cord tumors. Thieme, Stuttgart

Doppman JL, di Chiro G, Ommaya AK (1969) Selective arteriography of the spinal cord. Green, St Louis

Dyes O (1934a) Leitsätze zur Aufnahme und Deutung von Hirnkammerluftbildern. Dtsch Z Nervenheilkd 134:251–266

Dyes O (1934b) Das Röntgenbild der 3. und 4. Hirnkammer. ROEFO 50:230

Dyes O (1937) Die Hirnkammerformen bei Hirntumoren. ROEFO 52:79

Dyes O (1948) Röntgenuntersuchungen des Bandscheibenprolapses. Med Klin 24–25

Ecker AD (1948) Upward transtentorial herniation of brain stem and cerebellum due to tumor of the posterior fossa. J Neurosurg 5:51–61

Ehrhardt W, Kneip P (1943) Die "offene Tür" vom Knochenmark zum Kreislauf. Geburtshilfe Frauenheilkd 5:29

Einsiedel-Lechtape H, Lechtape-Grüter R, Hennemann U (1977) The angiographic diagnosis of occlusions of the posterior cerebral artery. Neuroradiology 14:47–57

Einsiedel-Lechtape H, Zülch KJ (1975) Arteriosclerosis of the brain vessels as an indication to vascular surgery. J Neurosurg Sci 19:23–28

Elsberg CA (1932) The blood supply of the gliomas. Bull Neurol Inst NY 2:210

Erlacher PR (1950) Direkte Kontrastdarstellung des Nucleus pulposus, zugleich ein Beitrag zur Pathologie der Bandscheibe. Z Orthop 80:40

Eskuchen K (1930) Liquoruntersuchung – Lumbalpunktion – Zisternenpunktion – Encephalographie – Ventrikulographie – Myelographie. Urban & Schwarzenberg, Wien Berlin (Neue deutsche Klinik, vol 6, pp 213–271)

Espagno J (1969) La circulation cérébrale du morphologique au fonctionnel normal ou pathologique. Neurochirurgie [Suppl 2] 15

Farinas P (1941) A new technique for the arteriographic examination of the abdominal aorta and its branches. AJR 46:641

Fields WS (1972) Selection of stroke patients for vascular surgery. Z Neurol 201:95–97

Fields WS, Bruetman ME, Weibel J (1965) Collateral circulation of the brain. Monogr Surg Sci, Williams & Wilkins, Baltimore, vol 2, pp 183–259

Finkemeyer H (1955) Verletzungen der A. carotis interna in ihrem intrakraniellen extraduralen Abschnitt. Zentralbl Neurochir 15:65–73

Fischer E (1938) Lageabweichungen der vorderen Hirnarterie im Gefäßbild. Zentralbl Neurochir 3:300–313

Fischer E (1939) Die arteriographische Diagnostik der Stirnhirn- und oralen Stammgangliengeschwülste. Zentralbl Neurochir 4:72–98

Fischer E (1940) Erscheinungsformen und diagnostische Bedeutung der Zisternenverquellungen im Hirngefäßbild. Langenbecks Arch Klin Chir 200:213–226

Fischer-Brügge E (1949) Der persistierende Hirnprolaps nach Schußverletzungen. Zentralbl Neurochir 9:18–45

Fischer E, since 1949 Fischer-Brügge E.

Fischer-Brügge E (1950) Lokalisation von raumbeengenden Prozessen durch Angiographie. Dtsch Z Nervenheilkd 162:23–49

Fischgold H, Adam H, Ecoiffier J, Piquet J (1952a) Opacification des plexus rachidiens et des veines azygos par voie osseuse. J Radiol Electrol 33:37

Fischgold H, Clement J, Talairach J, Ecoiffier J (1952b) Opacifications des systèmes veineux rachidiens et craniens par voie osseuse. Presse Méd 60:599

Fischgold H, David M, Talairach J, Bergeat P (1953) Direct opacifying injections into venous system of the head. Acta Radiol (Stockh) 40:128–139

Fisher CM (1954) Occlusion of the carotid arteries. Further experiences. Arch Neurol Psychiatry 72:187–204

Flügel F (1932) Die Encephalographie als neurologische Untersuchungsmethode. Ergeb Inn Med Kinderheilkd 44:327–433

Foerster O (1925) Encephalographische Erfahrungen. Z Gesamte Neurol Psychiatr 94:512–584

Foix C, Levy M (1927) Les ramollissements sylviens (syndromes des lésions en foyer du territoire de l'artère sylvienne et de ses branches). Rev Neurol (Paris) 34/2:1–51

Frenckner P (1934) Some experiments with venosinusography: A contribution of the diagnosis of otogenous sinus thrombosis. Acta Otolaryngol (Stockh) 20:477–485

Friedmann G, Frowein RA, Wieck HH, Pilka N (1964) Röntgenologische Bestimmung der zerebralen Zirkulationszeit bei intrakranieller Drucksteigerung. ROEFO 100:483–489

Gänshirt H (1961) Messung der Hirndurchblutung mit der Methode Kety-Schmidt bei Schädelinnendrucksteigerung. Acta Neurochir [Suppl] (Wien) 7:451–458

Gänshirt H (1972) Der Hirnkreislauf. Thieme, Stuttgart

Gejrot T, Lauren T (1964a) Retrograde venography of the internal jugular veins and transverse sinuses. Acta Otolaryngol (Stockh) 57:556

Gejrot T, Lauren T (1964b) Retrograde jugularography in diagnosis of glomus tumors in the jugular region. Acta Otolaryngol (Stockh) 58:191

Gejrot T, Lindblom A (1960) Venography of the internal jugular vein and the transverse sinuses. Acta Otolaryngol [Suppl 158] (Stockh) 52:180–186

Gonsette RE (1973) Metrizamide as contrast medium for myelography and ventriculography. Acta Radiol [Suppl] (Stockh) 335:346–358

Gonsette RE, André-Balisaux G (1970) Etude expérimentale et clinique de quelques produits de contraste hydrosolubles en vue de leur utilisation pour la radiculographie, la myelographie et la ventriculographie. J Radiol Electrol 51:19–28

Gould P, Peyton W, French A (1955) Vertebral angiography by retrograde injection of the brachial artery. J Neurosurg 12:369–374

Greitz T (1956) A radiologic study of the brain circulation by rapid serial angiography of the carotid artery. Acta Radiol [Suppl] (Stockh) 140

Greitz T, Sjörgen SE (1963) The posterior inferior cerebellar artery. Acta Radiol (Stockh) 1:284–297

Greitz T, Liliequist B, Müller R (1962) Cervical-vertebral phlebography. Acta Radiol (Stockh) 57:353

Grepe A (1974) Examination of intracranial basal cisterns with water-soluble contrast medium. Medical dissertation, University of Stockholm

Grepe A (1975) Cisternography with the non-ionic watersoluble contrast medium metrizamide. A preliminary report. Acta Radiol [Diagn] (Stockh) 16:146–160

Hackensellner HA, Pape R (1954) Über Meningokelen bei Neurofibromatosis Recklinghausen. ROEFO 81:66–71

Häussler G (1938) Über stereoskopische Arteriogramme der Carotis interna. Zentralbl Neurochir 3:313–316

Hammer B, Scherer H (1972) Choice of contrast medium in lumbosacral myelography. Neuroradiology 4:114–117

Hasse HM, Alexander K (1962) Neue Technik zur Angiographie der A. vertebralis. Z Kreislaufforsch 51:980–986

Hassler O, Saltzman GF (1963) Angiographic and histologic changes in infundibular widening of the posterior communicating artery. Acta Radiol (Stockh) 1:321–327

Hauge T (1954) Catheter vertebral angiography. Acta Radiol [Suppl] (Stockh) 109:1–219

Heiskanen O (1964) Cerebral circulatory arrest caused by acute increase of intracranial pressure: A clinical and roentgenological study of 25 cases. Acta Neurol Scand [Suppl 7] 40:11–57

Henning N (1940) Die intrasternale Injektion und Infusion als Ersatz für die intravenösen Methoden. Dtsch Med Wochenschr 66:737

Henschen F (1955) Tumoren des ZNS und seiner Hüllen. In: Scholz W (ed) Erkrankungen des zentralen Nervensystems III. Springer, Berlin Göttingen Heidelberg (Handbuch der speziellen pathologischen Anatomie und Histologie, vol 13/3, pp 413–1040)

Henson RA, Croft PB (1956) Spontaneous spinal subarachnoid hemorrhage. J Med 25:53

Heubner O (1872) Zur Topographie der Ernährungsgebiete der einzelnen Hirnarterien. Zentralbl Med Wiss 10:817–821

Heubner O (1874) Die luetische Erkrankung der Hirnarterien. Vogel, Leipzig

Hindmarsh T (1973) Methiodal sodium and metrizamide in lumbar myelography. Acta Radiol [Suppl] (Stockh) 335:359–365

Höök O, Lindvall H (1958) Arteriovenous aneurysms of the spinal cord. J Neurosurg 15:84

Holm O (1944) Cinematography in cerebral angiography. Acta Radiol (Stockh) 25:163

Huang YP, Wolf BS (1964) Veins of the white matter of the cerebral hemispheres (the medullary veins); diagnostic importance in carotid angiography. AJR 92:739–755

Huang YP, Wolf BS (1965) The veins of the posterior fossa: Superior or galenic group. AJR 95:808–821

Huang YP, Wolf BS (1966) Precentral cerebellar vein in angiography. Acta Radiol (Stockh) 5:250–262

Huang YP, Wolf BS (1970) Differential diagnosis of fourth ventricle tumors from brain stem tumors in angiography. Neuroradiology 1:4–19

Huber G (1957) Pneumencephalographische und psychopathologische Bilder bei endogenen Psychosen. Springer, Berlin Göttingen Heidelberg

Ingvar DH, Lassen NA (1965) Methods for cerebral blood flow measurements in man. Brit J Anaesth 37:216

Jacobäus HC (1921) On insufflation of air into the spinal canal for diagnostic purposes in cases of tumors in the spinal canal. Acta Med Scand 55:555–564

Jensen JT (1973) Epidural placement of Pantopaque after myelography. Neuroradiology 5:197–201

Jirout J (1956) Changes in the size of the subarachnoid space after the insufflation of air. Acta Radiol (Stockh) 46:81–85

Jirout J (1958) Pneumographic investigation of the cervical spine. Acta Radiol (Stockh) 50:221–225

Jirout J (1966) Neuroradiologie. VEB Verlag Volk und Gesundheit, Berlin

Jirout J (1969) Pneumomyelography. Thomas, Springfield

Kadyi H (1889) Über die Blutgefäße des menschlichen Rückenmarks. Monogr Math Naturwiss Cl Akad Wiss Krakau 1:1–144

Kaplan A, Ford DH (1966) The brain vascular system. Elsevier, Amsterdam London New York

Kazner E, Schiefer W (1966) Die Echoencephalographie bei raumfordernden Prozessen der hinteren Schädelgrube. Acta Neurochir (Wien) 14:177–196

Kazner E, Kubicki S, Kunze S, Schiefer W, Wende S (1969) Die Bedeutung der klinischen Zusatzuntersuchungen für die Differentialdiagnose zerebrale Massenblutung-Hirninfarkt. Fortschr Neurol Psychiatr 37:225–250

Kernohan JW, Sayre GP (1952) Tumors of the central nervous system. Armed Forces Institute of Pathology, Washington

Kernohan JW, Mabon RF, Svien HJ, Adson AW (1949) A simplified classification of the gliomas. Proc Mayo Clin 24:71–75

Key A, Retzius G (1875) Studien in der Anatomie des Nervensystems und des Bindegewebes. Norstedt & Söner, Stockholm

Killen DA, Foster JH (1966) Spinal cord injury as a complication of contrast angiography. Surgery 59:969

Klefenberg G, Saltzman G (1959) Gasmyelographic studies in syringomyelia. Acta Radiol (Stockh) 52:129–138

Krayenbühl H (1958) The diagnostic value of orbital angiography. Br J Ophthalmol 42:180–190

Krayenbühl H (1962) The value of orbital angiography for diagnosis of unilateral exophthalmos. J Neurosurg 19:289–301

Krayenbühl H, Richter HR (1952) Die cerebrale Angiographie. Thieme, Stuttgart

Krayenbühl H, Yasargil MG (1957) Die vaskulären Erkrankungen im Gebiet der A. vertebralis und A. basilaris. Thieme, Stuttgart, pp 1–170

Krayenbühl H, Yasargil MG (1958) Das Kleinhirnangiom. Schweiz Med Wochenschr 88:99–104

Krayenbühl H, Yasargil MG (1965) Die zerebrale Angiographie. Thieme, Stuttgart (1965)

Krayenbühl H, Yasargil MG (1972) Klinik der Gefäßmißbildungen und Gefäßfisteln. In: Gänshirt H (ed) Der Hirnkreislauf. Thieme, Stuttgart, pp 465–511

Krayenbühl H, Yasargil MG, Huber P (1979) Zerebrale Angiographie für Klinik und Praxis. Thieme, Stuttgart

Kubik CS, Adams RD (1946) Occlusion of the basilar artery – A clinical and pathological study. Brain 69:73–121

Kunze S (1974) Die zentrale Ventrikulographie mit wasserlöslichen, resorbierbaren Kontrastmitteln. Springer, Berlin Heidelberg New York

Lang EK (1963) A survey of the complications of percutaneous retrograde arteriography. Radiology 81:257

Lasjaunias P, Michotey P, Vignaud J, Clay C (1975) II. Radio-anatomie de la vascularisation artérielle de l'orbite, à l'exception du tronc de l'artère ophthalmique. Ann Radiol (Paris) 18:181–194

Lazorthes G, Gauazé A (1968) Les voies anastomotiques de suppléance (ou systèmes de sécurité) de la vascularisation artérielle de l'axe cérébro-médullaire. Extrait du "Bulletin de l'association des anatomistes", 53. Réunion, Tours, 7–11 avril 1968. Thomas, Nancy

Lechtape-Grüter H, Zülch KJ (1971) Gibt es einen Spasmus der Hirngefäße? Radiologe 11:429–435

Lemke R (1959) Atlas der Pneumoencephalographie bei Hirntumoren. VEB Verlag Volk und Gesundheit, Berlin

Lie TA (1968) Congenital anomalies of carotid arteries (angiographic study and review of the literature). Excerpta Medica, Amsterdam

Liliequist B (1959a) The subarachnoid cisterns. Acta Radiol [Suppl] (Stockh) 185

Liliequist B (1959b) Pontine angle tumors. Acta Radiol [Suppl] (Stockh) 186

Lindblom K (1941) Eine anatomische Studie über lumbale Zwischenwirbelscheibenprotrusionen und Zwischenwirbelscheibenbrüche in die Foramina intervertebralia hinein. Acta Radiol (Stockh) 22:711

Lindblom K (1944) Protrusion of discs and nerve compression in lumbar region. Acta Radiol (Stockh) 25:195

Lindblom K (1948) Diagnostic puncture of intervertebral discs in sciatica. Acta Orthop Scand 17:231

Lindgren E (1939) Myelographie mit Luft. Nervenarzt 12:57–62

Lindgren E (1948) A pneumographic study of the temporal horn. Acta Radiol [Suppl] (Stockh) 69

Lindgren E (1949) Some aspects in the technique of encephalography. Acta Radiol (Stockh) 31:161

Lindgren E (1950a) Percutaneous angiography of the vertebral artery. Acta Radiol (Stockh) 33:389–490

Lindgren E (1950b) Encephalographic examination of tumours in the posterior fossa. Acta Radiol (Stockh) 34:331–338

Lindgren E (1951) Encephalography in cerebral atrophy. Acta Radiol (Stockh) 35:277

Lindgren E (1954) Röntgenologie einschließlich Kontrastmethoden. In: Olivecrona H, Tönnis W (eds) Handbuch der Neurochirurgie, vol II. Springer, Berlin Göttingen Heidelberg

Lindgren E (1956) Another method of vertebral angiography. Acta Radiol (Stockh) 46:257–261

Lindgren E (1957) Radiologic examination of the brain and spinal cord. Acta Radiol [Suppl] (Stockh) 151

Loeb E, Favale F (1962) Contralateral EEG abnormalities in intracranial arteriovenous aneurysms. Arch Neurol 7:121–128

Loeb E, Meyer JS (1965) Strokes due to vertebrobasilar disease. Infarction, vascular insufficiency and hemorrhage of the brain stem and cerebellum. Thomas, Springfield

Löfgren OF (1958) Vertebral angiography in the diagnosis of tumors in the pineal region. Acta Radiol (Stockh) 50:108–124

Löfstedt S (1950) Intracranial arterial aneurysms; preliminary report. Acta Radiol (Stockh) 34:339–349

Löhr W (1936) Hirngefäßverletzungen in arteriographischer Darstellung. Langenbecks Arch Klin Chir 186:298

Loman J, Myerson A (1936) Visualization of cerebral vessels by direct intracarotid injection of thoriumdioxide. AJR 35:188–193

Lombardi G (1949a) Studio radiologico delle cisterne cerebrali in condizioni normali. Radiol Med (Torino) 35:395–409

Lombardi G (1949b) Studio radiologico delle cisterne cerebrali in conditioni patologici. Radiol Med (Torino) 35:763–790

Lombardi G (1951) Studio radiologico degli angiomi cerebrali. Radiol Med (Torino) 37:1

Lombardi G (1964) Spinal cord diseases. Williams & Wilkins, Baltimore

Lombardi G (1967) Radiology in neuro-ophthalmology; orbit and contrast media. Williams & Wilkins, Baltimore

Lombardi G (1969a) Venography of the orbit: pathology. Br J Radiol 42:184

Lombardi G (1969b) Ophthalmic artery anomalies. Ophthalmologica 157:321–327

Lombardi G, Passerini A (1968) Venography of the orbit: technique and anatomy. Br J Radiol 41:282

Lombardi G, Passerini A, Migliavacca F (1963) Intracavernous aneurysms of the internal carotid artery. AJR 89:361–371

Lorenz R (1940) Differentialdiagnose der arteriographisch darstellbaren intrakraniellen Geschwülste. Glioblastom, Meningeom, Sarkom. Zentralbl Neurochir 4:30–60

Luckett WH (1913) Air in the ventricles of the brain following a fracture of the skull: report of a case. Surg Gynecol Obstet 17:237

Lysholm E (1941) Röntgenologische Diagnostik in der Chirurgie der Gehirnkrankheiten, Bd. III. In: Krause F (ed) Die spezielle Chirurgie der Gehirnkrankheiten. Ferdinand Enke, Stuttgart, pp 2–189

Lysholm E, Ebenius B, Sahlstedt H (1935a) Das Ventrikulogramm. I. Röntgentechnik. Acta Radiol [Suppl] (Stockh) 24

Lysholm E, Ebenius B, Sahlstedt H (1935b) Das Ventrikulogramm. II. Die Seitenventrikel. Acta Radiol [Suppl] (Stockh) 25

Lysholm E, Lindblom K, Sahlstedt H (1935c) Das Ventrikulogramm III. Teil. Acta Radiol [Suppl] (Stockh) 26

Maslowski HA (1955) Vertebral angiography: Percutaneous lateral atlanto-occipital method. Brit J Surg 43, 1–8

McDonald CA, Korb M (1939) Intracranial aneurysms. Arch Neurol Psychiatr 42:298

McDowell F (1966) Indications for arteriography in cerebrovascular disease. Assoc Res Nerv Dis Proc 41:188–195

Metzinger H, Zülch KJ (1971) Vertebro-basilar occlusion and its morphological sequelae. In: Zülch KJ (ed) Cerebral circulation and stroke. Springer, Berlin Heidelberg New York, pp 67–81

Meyer JS, Denny-Brown D (1957) The cerebral collateral circulation. I. Factors influencing collateral blood flow. Neurology (Minneap) 7:447–458

Meyer JS, Waltz AG, Gotoh F (1960a) Pathogenesis of cerebral vasospasms in hypertensive encephalopathy. I. Effects of acute increases in intraluminal blood pressure on pial blood flow. Neurology (Minneap) 10:735–744

Meyer JS, Waltz AG, Gotoh F (1960b) Pathogenesis of cerebral vasospasm in hypertensive encephalopathy. II. The nature of increased irritability of smooth muscle of pial arterioles in renal hypertension. Neurology (Minneap) 10:859–867

Moniz E (1927) L'encephalographie artérielle, son importance dans la localisation des tumeurs cérébrales. Rev Neurol (Paris) 2:72

Moniz E (1933) Tronc basilaire et artères dérivées. Encephale 28:705

Moniz E (1934) L'angiographie cérébrale. Masson, Paris

Moniz E (1940) Die cerebrale Arteriographie und Phlebographie. In: Bumke O, Foerster O, Rüdin E, Spatz H (eds) Monographien aus dem Gesamtgebiet der Neurologie und Psychiatrie, Heft 80. Springer, Berlin (Ergänzungs-Serie II zum Handbuch der Neurologie)

Morris L (1960) Angioma of the cervical spinal cord. Radiology 70:785–797

Murtagh F, Chamberlain WE, Scott M, Wycis HT (1955) Cervical air myelography. A review of 130 cases. AJR 74:1–21

Newton TH, Potts DG (1974) Radiology of the skull and brain. Mosby, St Louis

Nonne M (1904) Über Fälle von Symptomenkomplex "Tumor cerebri" mit Ausgang in Heilung (Pseudotumor cerebri). Über letal verlaufene Fälle von "Pseudotumor cerebri" mit Sektionsbefund. Dtsch Z Nervenheilkd 27:169–216

Nonne M (1937) Über Pseudotumor cerebri. Sitzungsbericht des 22. Treffens der Society of British Neurological Surgeons vom 22. Juni bis 3. Juli 1937 in Berlin und Breslau. Zentralbl Neurochir 2:358

Obrador Alcalde S, Sanz Ibanez J (1955) Tumores intracraniales. Monografia del Instituto Nacional de Oncologia, Madrid

Patterson RH, Goodell H, Dunning HS (1964) Complications of carotid angiography. Arch Neurol 10:513–520

Pendergrass EP (1930) The value and the indications for encephalography and ventriculography. With discussion of the technique. Surg Clin North Am 10:1461

Pendergrass EP (1931a) Encephalography: an explanation of a possible error in technique. AJR 25:754

Pendergrass EP (1931b) Indications and contraindications for encephalography. JAMA 96:408

Penfield W (1927) Principles of the pathology of neurosurgery. In: Nelson's loose leaf surgery. Nelson & Sons, New York, pp 303–347

Penfield W (1931) The classification of gliomas and neuroglia cell types. Arch Neurol Psychiat 26:745–753

Penfield W, Norcross NC (1936) Subdural traction and posttraumatic headache. Arch Neurol Psychiatry 36:75–94

Penin H, Käufer C (1969) Der Hirntod. Thieme, Stuttgart

Peterson HO, Kieffer SA (1972) Introduction to neuroradiology. Harper & Row, Hagerstown

Pfeifer RA (1931) Anastomosen der Hirngefäße, dargestellt am asphyktisch-hyperämischen Kindergehirn. J Psychol Neurol (Lpz) 42:1–173

Pia HW (1954) Die Verquellung der Cisterna basalis und ambiens im Hirngefäßbild. Acta Neurochir (Wien) 3:315–328

Piscol K (1970) Die percutane Katheterisierung der Vena

frontalis zur Darstellung der orbitalen Venen und des Sinus cavernosus. ROEFO 112:56

Poppen JL (1949) Aid of arteriograms in diagnosis and treatment of intracranial aneurysms. Radiology 52:347

Potts GD, Taveras MJ (1963) Differential diagnosis of space-occupying lesions in the region of the thalamus by cerebral angiography. Acta Radiol (Stockh) 1:373–383

Pouyanne H, Caillon F, Leman P, Got M, Salles M, Gouaze A (1960) L'angiographie vertébrale par voie sous-clavière. Neurochirurgia (Stuttg) 3:35–45

Radner S (1947) Intracranial angiography via the vertebral artery. Acta Radiol (Stockh) 28:838

Radner S (1951) Vertebral angiography by catheterization. A new method employed in 221 cases. Acta Radiol [Suppl] (Stockh) 87

Ramsey GG, French JD, Strain WH (1944) Iodinated organic compounds as contrast media for radiographic diagnoses, pantopaque myelography. Radiology 43:236

Rand RW, Rand CW (1960) Intraspinal tumors of childhood. Thomas, Springfield

Ratschow M (1955) Die Perlschnurarterie. Zentralbl Neurochir 15:154–159

Ray BS, Dunbar HS, Dotter CT (1951) Dural sinus venography as an aid to diagnosis in intracranial disease. J Neurosurg 8:23–37

Riechert T (1949) Die Arteriographie der Hirngefäße, 2nd edn. Urban & Schwarzenberg, Munich

Riessner D, Zülch KJ (1939) Über die Formveränderungen des Hirns (Massenverschiebungen, Zisternenquellungen) bei raumbeengenden Prozessen. Dtsch Z Chir 253:1–61

Riggs HE, Rupp C (1963) Variation in form of circle of Willis. Arch Neurol 8:8–14

Ring BA (1962) Middle cerebral artery: anatomical and radiographic study. Acta Radiol (Stockh) 57:289–300

Ring BA, Waddington M (1967) Ascending frontal branch of middle cerebral artery. Acta Radiol [Diagn] (Stockh) 6:209–220

Rio Hortega P del (1945) Nomenclatura y classificacion de los tumores del sistema nervioso. Lopez & Echtegoyen, Buenos Aires

Riverson EA, Zülch KJ (1979) Pineal parenchymal tumours and germinomas (the problem of the so-called pinealomas). Neurosurg Rev 2:3–11

Roberson GH, Llewellyn HJ, Taveras JM (1973) The narrow lumbar spinal canal syndrome. Radiology 107:89–97

Robertson EG (1941) Encephalography. Macmillan, Melbourne

Robertson EG (1946) Further studies in encephalography. Macmillan, Melbourne

Robertson EG (1957) Pneumoencephalography. Thomas, Springfield

Roussy G, Oberling C (1931) Atlas du cancer. Alcan, Paris

Rubinstein LJ (1972) Atlas of tumor pathology. Tumors of the central nervous system, II. ser, fasc 6. Armed Forces Institute of Pathology (AFIP), Washington

Ruggiero G (1957) L'encéphalographie fractionée. Masson, Paris

Ruggiero G (1974) Radiological exploration of the ventricles and subarachnoid space. Springer, Berlin Heidelberg New York

Ruggiero G, Castellano F (1952) Carotid-cavernosus aneurysms. Acta Radiol (Stockh) 37:121

Ruggiero G, David M (1961) Le choix du type de myélographie dans les affections du rachis d'intérêt neurochirurgi-

cal. In: Rajewsky (ed) IXth International congress of radiology 1959. Thieme, Stuttgart, pp 462–465

Russell DS, Rubinstein LJ (1971) Pathology of tumours of the nervous system. 3rd edn. Arnold, London

Salamon G (1971) Atlas de la vascularisation artérielle du cerveau chez l'homme. Sandoz, Paris

Samii M (1974) Pneumoencephalo-Tomographie. Enke, Stuttgart

Schaltenbrand G (1932) Spontane Luftfüllung der Ventrikel bei Zisternenpunktion im Sitzen. Med Klin 28:609–611

Schiefer W (1972) Zwischenfälle bei der Hirngefäßdarstellung. In: Gänshirt H (ed) Der Hirnkreislauf. Physiologie – Pathologie – Klinik. Thieme, Stuttgart, pp 781–796

Schiefer W, Struck G (1957) Serienangiographische Untersuchungen bei diffusen cerebralen Gefäßerkrankungen. Dtsch Z Nervenheilkd 176:595–616

Schiefer W, Vetter K (1957) Das zerebrale Angiogramm in den verschiedenen Altersstufen. Zentralbl Neurochir 17:218–231

Schiefer W, Tönnis W, Udvarhelyi G (1954) Das Glioblastoma multiforme im Serienangiogramm. Acta Neurochir (Wien) 4:76–105

Schiefer W, Tönnis W, Udvarhelyi G (1955) Die Artdiagnose des Meningeoms im Gefäßbild. Dtsch Z Nervenheilkd 172:436–456

Schiersmann O (1952) Einführung in die Enzephalographie. Thieme, Stuttgart

Schlesinger B (1937) Einführung in die Ventrikulographie; eine Diagnostik der Hirngeschwülste. Urban & Schwarzenberg, Berlin Vienna

Schmidt-Wittkamp E, Roscher M (1966) Zur Lagebestimmung des "Angulus venosus" im seitlichen Phlebogramm. ROEFO 105:92–98

Schmorl G (1931) Beiträge zur pathologischen Anatomie der Wirbelbandscheiben und ihre Beziehungen zu den Wirbelkörpern. Arch Orthop. Unfallchir 29:389

Schober R, Bender R (1968) Orbita-Phlebographie. ROEFO 109:345

Schobinger R (1960) Intra-osseous-venography. Grune & Stratton, New York London

Schürmann K (1954) Darstellung der A. vertebralis und ihrer Äste im Angiogramm von der A. carotis externa aus. Zentralbl Neurochir 14:362–365

Schurr PH (1951) Angiography of the normal ophthalmic artery and the choroidal plexus of the eye. Br J Ophthalmol 35:473–478

Scott M, Frederick M, Lapayowker M, Baird RM (1963) Vertebral basilar and carotid angiography by injection of brachial artery. AJR 90:546

Seldinger SI (1953) Catheter replacement of the needle in percutaneous arteriography. Acta Radiol (Stockh) 39:368

Shapiro R (1975) Myelography, 3rd edn. Year Book Medical, Chicago

Shimidzu K (1937) Beiträge zur Arteriographie des Gehirns – einfache percutane Methode. Langenbecks Arch Klin Chir 188:295–316

Sicard JA, Forestier JE (1921) Méthode radiographique d'exploration de la cavité epidurale par le lipiodol. Rev Neurol (Paris) 28:1264

Sicard JA, Forestier JE (1922) Méthode générale d'exploration radiologique par l'huile iodée (Lipiodol). Bull Soc Med Hop Paris 46:463

Sjögren SE (1953) Percutaneous vertebral angiography. A review of 250 cases. Acta Radiol (Stockh) 40:113

Sjöqvist O (1938) Arteriographische Darstellung der Gefäße der hinteren Schädelgrube. Chirurg 10:377

Skalpe JO, Amundsen P (1975) Thoracic and cervical myelography with metrizamide. Radiology 116:101–106

Sorgo W (1941) Einführung in die Kontrastmitteldiagnostik cerebraler Erkrankungen. Deuticke, Vienna

Sortland O (1978) X-ray diagnosis of expanding lesions in the cerebello-pontine angle (in Norwegian). Paper read at Congress Nord Soc. Radiol, Oslo, June 1978

Sortland O (1979) Computed tomography combined with gas cisternography for the diagnosis of expanding lesions in the cerebello-pontine angle. Neuroradiology 18: 19–22

Soyka D (1969) Neues auf dem Gebiete der Pneumoencephalographie (1955–1967). Fortschr Neurol Psychiatr 37:1

Spatz H, Stroescu GJ (1934) Zur Anatomie und Pathologie der äußeren Liquorräume des Gehirns (Die Zisternenverquellung beim Hirntumor.) Nervenarzt 7:425–437, 481–498

Steinberg J, Evans JA (1959) A safe and practical intravenous method for abdominal aortography, peripheral arteriography and cerebral angiography. AJR 82:758

Tänzer A (1971) Die direkte Sinugraphie. Radiologe 11:390–394

Takahashi K (1940) Die percutane Arteriographie der Arteria vertebralis und ihrer Versorgungsgebiete. Arch Psychiatr Nervenkr 111:373–379

Takahashi M (1974) Atlas of vertebral angiography. Urban & Schwarzenberg, Munich Berlin Vienna

Takahashi M, Wilson G, Hanafee W (1967) The significance of the petrosal vein in the diagnosis of cerebellopontine angle tumors. Radiology 89:834–840

Talairach J, David M, Fischgold H, Aboulker H (1951) Falcotentoriographie et phlébographie basale. Presse méd 35:724–727

Taveras JM, Wood EH (1976) Diagnostic neuroradiology, 2nd edn. Williams & Wilkins, Baltimore

Tönnis W (1938) Die Hirngeschwülste. Z Gesamte Neurol Psychiatr 161:114–149

Tönnis W (1939a) Anzeigestellung zur Arteriographie und Ventrikulographie bei raumbeengenden intrakraniellen Prozessen. Dtsch Med Wochenschr 65:246

Tönnis W (1939b) Hydrocephalus infolge Liquorzirkulationsstörung. Arch Kinderheilkd 118:65–79

Tönnis W (1959) Pathophysiologie und Klinik der intrakraniellen Drucksteigerung. In: Olivecrona H, Tönnis W (eds) Angewandte Anatomie, Physiologie, Pathophysiologie. Springer, Berlin Göttingen Heidelberg (Handbuch der Neurochirurgie, vol 1/1, pp 304–445)

Tönnis W, Marguth F (1961) Kreislaufstörungen des Zentralnervensystems. Acta Neurochir [Suppl] (Wien) 7

Tönnis W, Schiefer W (1954) Die Bedeutung der Serienangiographie für die Artdiagnose. ROEFO 81:616–828

Tönnis W, Schiefer W (1958) Die Komplikationen bei Angiographie der Hirngefäße. Fortschr Neurol Psychiatr 26:265–300

Tönnis W, Schiefer W (1959) Zirkulationsstörungen des Gehirns im Serienangiogramm. Springer, Berlin Göttingen Heidelberg

Torkildsen A, Penfield W (1933) Ventriculographic interpretation. Arch Neurol 30:1011

Unio Internationalis Contra Cancrum (1965) Illustrated tumor nomenclature. Springer, Berlin Heidelberg New York

Van der Eecken H (1959) The anastomoses between the leptomeningeal arteries of the brain. Thomas, Springfield

Van der Eecken H, Adams RD (1953) The anatomy and functional significance of the meningeal arterial anastomoses of the human brain. J Neuropathol Exp Neurol 12:132–157

Verbiest H (1962) Arterial and arteriovenous aneurysms of the posterior fossa. Psychiat Neurol Neurochir (Amst) 65:329–369

Viallet M, Viallet P, Chevrot L, Sendra L, Combe P, Anbaniac R, Aubry P, Sarrouy J, Keller T (1955) Nouvelle méthode d'angiographie. Algérie Méd 59:135

Vignaud J, Clay C, Aubin ML (1972) Orbital arteriography. Radiol Clin North Am 10:39

Vignaud J, Aubin ML, Clay C (1975) La vascularisation de l'orbite. I. Artériographie normale de l'artère ophthalmique. Ann Radiol (Paris) 18:171–180

Vogelsang H (1969) Die spinale Ossovenographie. de Gruyter, Berlin

Wackenheim A (1971) Some views regarding the diagnostic value of the veins of the posterior fossa. Neuroradiology 3:75–76

Wackenheim A, Braun JP (1970) Angiography of the mesencephalon: normal and pathological findings. Springer, Berlin Heidelberg New York

Weibel J, Fields WS (1963) Direct percutaneous intraclavicular catheterization of the subclavian artery. J Neurosurg 20:233

Weibel J, Fields WS (1969) Atlas of arteriography in occlusive cerebrovascular disease. Thieme, Stuttgart

Wellauer J (1961) Die Myelographie mit positiven Kontrastmitteln. Thieme, Stuttgart

Wende S (1960) Der diagnostische Wert des "Frontalistest" bei der Karotisangiographie. ROEFO 93:185–186

Wende S, Ciba K (1968) Der Wert der Jugularis-Venographie für die Darstellung des Sinus cavernosus. ROEFO 109:56

Wende S, Schulze A (1961) Die zerebrale Angiographie und ihre Komplikationen. Ein Bericht über 2864 Untersuchungen. ROEFO 94:494–505

Wende S, Zieler E, Nakayama N (1974) Cerebral magnification angiography. Springer, Berlin Heidelberg New York

Wende S, Aulich A, Kretzschmar K, Grumme T, Meese W, Lange S, Steinhoff H, Lanksch W (1977) Die Computertomographie der Hirngeschwülste. Eine Sammelstudie über 1658 Tumoren. Radiologe 17:149–156

Werner H (1962) Zur Angiographie der Kopf-Hals-Region. Med Klin 57:531

Wickbom I (1947) Cerebral angiography. A comparative study. Acta Psychiatr Scand 47:337

Wickbom I (1948) Angiography of the carotid artery. Acta Radiol [Suppl] (Stockh) 82

Wickbom I (1950) Angiographic examination of intracranial arterio-venous aneurysms. Acta Radiol (Stockh) 34:385

Wickbom I (1953) Angiographic determination of tumour pathology. Acta Radiol (Stockh) 40:529

Wickbom I, Stattin S (1958) Roentgen examination of intracranial meningiomas. Acta Radiol (Stockh) 50:175–186

Wideröe S (1921) Über die diagnostische Bedeutung der intraspinalen Luftinjektion bei Rückenmarksleiden, besonders bei Geschwülsten. Zentralbl Chir 48:394–397

Wilcke O (1964) Eine einfache Methode zur Bestimmung der Hirndurchblutung mit Radio-Isotopen. Acta Neurochir (Wien) 12:31–39

Witt AN (1950) Praktische Erfahrungen mit der Nukleographie. Z Orthop 80:57

Wolf BS, Huang YP, Newman CM (1963) The lateral anastomotic mesencephalic vein and other variations in drainage of the basal cerebral vein. AJR 89:411–422

Wolff H, Schaltenbrand G (1939) Die percutane Arteriographie der Hirngefäße. Zentralbl Neurochir 4:233–241

Wolff H, Schmidt B (1939) Das Arteriogramm des pulsierenden Exophthalmus. Zentralbl Neurochir 4:241–250, 310–318

Yasargil MG (1957) Die Röntgendiagnostik des Exophthalmus unilateralis. Bibl Ophthalmol [Suppl] 50:10–11

Yasargil MG (1962) Die Vertebralisangiographie: Ihre Bedeutung für die Diagnose der Tumoren. Acta Neurochir [Suppl] (Wien) 9:1–108

Yates PO, Hutchinson EC (1961) Cerebral infarction: the role of stenosis of the extracranial cerebral arteries. Her Majesty's Stationery Office, London (Special report series of the medical research council, vol 300)

Ziedses des Plantes BG (1961) Subtraktion. Thieme, Stuttgart

Zülch KJ (1950) Röntgendiagnostik beim cerebralen Anfall. Verh Dtsch Ges Inn Med 56:24–48

Zülch KJ (1954) Mangeldurchblutung an der Grenzzone zweier Gefäßgebiete als Ursache bisher ungeklärter Rückenmarksschädigungen. Dtsch Z Nervenheilkd 172:81–101

Zülch KJ (1956a) Röntgendiagnostik des Schädelhirntraumas. In: Rehwald E (ed) Das Hirntrauma, Thieme, Stuttgart, pp 283–319

Zülch KJ (1956b) Biologie und Pathologie der Hirngeschwülste. In: Olivecrona H, Tönnis W (eds) Pathologische Anatomie der raumbeengenden intrakraniellen Prozesse. Springer, Berlin Göttingen Heidelberg (Handbuch der Neurochirurgie, vol 3, pp 1–702)

Zülch KJ (1958) Die Hirngeschwülste in biologischer und morphologischer Darstellung. 3rd edn. Barth, Leipzig

Zülch KJ (1959) Störungen des intrakraniellen Druckes. In: Olivecrona H, Tönnis W (eds) Grundlagen I, Angewandte Anatomie – Physiologie – Pathophysiologie. Springer, Berlin Göttingen Heidelberg (Handbuch der Neurochirurgie, pp 208–303)

Zülch KJ (1962) Réflexions sur la physiopathologie des troubles vasculaires médullaires. Rev Neurol (Paris) 106:102–115

Zülch KJ (1964) Neurologische Diagnostik bei endokraniellen Komplikationen von otorhinologischen Erkrankungen. Arch klin Exp Ohren Nasen Kehlkopfheilkd 183:1–85

Zülch KJ (1965) Brain tumors. Their biology and pathology, 2nd edn. Springer, New York (3rd edn in press)

Zülch KJ (1968) The morphologic basis of the abnormal echo-encephalogram. In: Kazner E, Schiefer W, Zülch KJ (eds) Proceedings in echo-encephalography. Springer, Berlin Heidelberg New York, pp 12–24

Zülch KJ (1970) Angiographische Befunde zur Pathogenese der Hirndurchblutungsstörungen. Zentralbl Neurochir 31:1–25

Zülch KJ (1971 a) Some basic patterns of the collateral circulation of the cerebral arteries. In: Zülch KJ (ed) Cerebral circulation and stroke. Springer, Berlin Heidelberg New York, pp 106–122

Zülch KJ (1971 b) Atlas of the histology of brain tumors. Springer, Berlin Heidelberg New York

Zülch KJ (1975) Atlas of gross neurosurgical pathology. Springer, Berlin Heidelberg New York

Zülch KJ (1976) Pathogenetic and clinical observations in spinovascular insufficiency. Zentralbl Neurochir 37:1–13

Zülch KJ (1978) Principles of the new WHO classification of brain tumors. In: Frowein RA, Wilcke O, Karimi-Nejad A, Brock M (eds) Head injuries. Tumors of the cerebellar region. Springer, Berlin Heidelberg New York (Advances in neurosurgery, vol 5, pp 279–284)

Zülch KJ (in collaboration with pathologists in 14 countries) (1979) Histological typing of tumours of the central nervous system, no 21. International histological classification of tumours. World Health Organization, Geneva

Zülch KJ (1981) Cerebrovascular pathology and pathogenesis as a basis of neuroradiological diagnosis. In: Diethelm L, Wende S (eds) Röntgendiagnostik des Zentralnervensystems. – Roentgen diagnosis of the central nervous system. Springer, Berlin Heidelberg New York (Handbuch der medizinischen Radiologie – Encyclopedia of medical radiology, vol 14/1A, pp 1–192)

Zülch KJ, Eschbach O (1965) Die Typen des inneren und äußeren Hydrocephalus bei atrophisierenden Prozessen des Hirns. Radiologe 5:431–435

Zülch KJ, Eschbach O (1972) The interhemisperic steal syndromes. Neuroradiology 4:179–184

Zülch KJ, Mennel HD (1974) The biology of brain tumours. In: Vinken PJ, Bruyn GW (eds) Handbook of clinical neurology, vol 16. North-Holland, Amsterdam, pp 1–55

Zülch KJ, Mennel HD, Zimmermann V (1974a) Intracranial hypertension. In: Vinken PJ, Bruyn GW (eds) Handbook of clinical neurology, vol 16. North-Holland, Amsterdam, pp 89–149

Zülch KJ, Dreesbach HA, Eschbach O (1974b) Occlusion of the middle cerebral artery with the formation of an abnormal arterial collateral system – Moyamoya-Type – 23 months later. Neuroradiology 7:19–24

Subject Index

Abducens nerve palsy 172
acoustic neurilemmoma 248
air bubbles, pneumoencephalography 236
– embolism 195
– myelogram 282
ambient cisterns 213, 247
amipaque, myelography 271, 274, 276
amputation, root sleeve 289
anastomoses 159, 167
–, circular 166
–, extracranial 159
–, Fischer's callosal 161, 166
–, intracranial 161
–, meningeal 161, 163, 164
–, occipitovertebral 160, 165
–, ophthalmic 159
–, over the anterior spinal artery 161
–, posterior cerebral artery 166
–, typical of Moya-Moya disease 168
–, via the ophthalmic artery 160
anesthesia, of the elderly 157
aneurysm(s) 53
–, anterior cerebral artery 128
–, – communicating artery 127, 129, 132
–, basilar artery 127
–, – bifurcation 130
–, fusiform 127
–, giant 126
–, infraclinoid carotid 127
–, internal carotid artery 129
–, middle cerebral artery 127, 129
–, multiple 127
–, posterior communicating artery 127
–, predilections 127
–, vein of Galen, angiogram, pneumoencephalogram 239
–, venous 132
Angiogram, intracranial, pathological 94
angiography 55ff.
–, circulatory standstill 173
–, complications 136, 137
–, –, anesthesia 136
–, head injuries 118
–, history 57
–, indication, contraindication 136, 264, 266

–, internal carotid artery 81
–, jugular vein 178
–, metastases 118
–, ophthalmic artery 174
–, technique 58
–, –, positioning 85
–, ulcerated plaques 136
angioma, vertebral body 309
anomalies, cranial 216
anterior cerebral artery 105, 140
– commissure 200
– pituitary tumors 41
– spinal artery, anastomoses over the 161
– – –, cervical region 299
– – –, thoracolumbar junction 299
apex of frontal horn 198
aplasia of corpus callosum 106, 262
aqueduct 198, 199
–, occlusion 18, 233
aqueductal stenoses 241
arachnoical cysts 261
– hemorrhages 252
– ring anastomoses 161
arterial aneurysms 127
– spasm 169
Arter(y)ies, anatomical variations 139
–, angular 85
–, anterior cerebral, changes 105
–, – – lesions, signs 108, 109
–, – –, parallel displacement 108
–, – –, "stretched" 106
–, – inferior cerebellar 90
–, – spinal 85
–, ascending pharyngeal 84
–, auditory 90
–, basilar 152
– of Bernasconi and Cassinari 76
–, internal carotid, cervical portion 99
–, – occipital 90
–, lateral occipital 90
–, medial occipital 90
–, middle cerebral 104
–, – –, spreading of branches 105
–, – meningeal 118
–, occipital 84
–, posterior auricular 84
–, – cerebral 89, 90, 91, 108
–, – –, occipital ramus 90
–, – choroidal 89
–, – communicating 90

–, – inferior cerebellar 89, 90, 91, 108
–, superficial temporal 84, 85
–, superior cerebellar 89, 91
–, temporo-occipital 90
–, thalamic 89
– of Wallenberg 89
arteriosclerosis 142, 147
arteriovenous fistulas 116
– malformations (AVM) 53, 132, 133, 169
astrocytic tumors 27
astrocytoma, malignant 115
atlanto-occipital membrane 85
atlas, arcuate foramen of 85
atrophic processes 251
– –, mass displacements 20
– –, unilateral 256
autonomic reactions, pneumoencephalography 193
autoregulation 169
avascular space 95
AVM 53, 132, 169
–, blood supply, shape, size 133
axial displacements 10

basal cisterns 209
– ganglia tumors 231
– vein of frontal lobe 82
– – of Rosenthal 82, 112
base of the brain 78
basilar artery bifurcation 90
– –, displacement posteriorly 108
– –, giant fusiform aneurysm 157
– –, "laminar" flow 158
– –, occlusion 167
– –, retrograde filling 141
– –, shifting 157
– –, stenosis 152
– "fork" (basilar artery) 90
– plexus 84
"beaten silver" skull 264
berry aneurysms 127
bihemispheric filling in carotid occlusion 162
bilateral frontal tumors 225
– subdural hematomas 250
– tumors 228
blood lakes 116, 117
"blush", tumor 113
body of frontal horn 198
brain abscess 265
– death 173

brain death, confirmation of, angiography 266
– edema, traumatic 46
– injuries 252
– stem tumors 187
– tumors, classification 25
branch occlusion, middle cerebral artery 153
"brushstroke" vessel in glioblastoma 116
"butterfly" glioma, pneumoencephalogram 229, 230

capsule of abscess 265
carotid angiogram 75
– –, capillary phase 81
– –, external 84
– – in infant 81
– –, venous phases 81
– arteriogram, anteroposterior view 78
– – in early childhood 80
– artery, puncture of 58
– –, stenosis after puncture 149
– bifurcation 99
– –, anterior cerebral artery 99
– –, "covered" 101
– –, "opening" of 101
– –, pars circularis 99
– –, sphenoid wing segment of m.c.a. 99
– cavernous fistula 47, 126, 133, 135
– occlusion, bihemispheric filling in 162
– –, old 255
– sinus, hypersensitive 171
– siphon, cisternal segment 99
– –, narrowing 145
– –, occlusion from an embolus 147
– –, "opened" 99
– –, shifts 8
– –, stenosis 154
catheterization, femoral artery 59
–, superselective 85
cavernous sinus, flattening 178
cavum Vergae cyst 260, 261
cella media 198, 203
central gyri tumors 226
cerebellar arteries 140
– atrophy 254
– cortical (Purkinje cell) atrophies 256
– hemangioblastoma 121
– hemisphere tumors 244
– herniations 196
– –, upward 241
– (olivo-ponto-) atrophies 256
– tumors 187
– vermis tumors 244
cerebellopontine angle 108
– – tumors 247, 248
cerebral angiography 55ff.
– atrophy, generalized 252

– –, unilateral 255
– circulation standstill 172, 173
– hemisphere tumors 219
– veins 81
cervical discography, technique 305
– myelography 276
chiasmatic cistern 212
childhood, carotid arteriogram in 80
children, retrograde angiography in 62
choroid glomus 207
– plexus 198, 205
– – of lateral ventricles 91
circle of Willis 161
circular anastomoses 166
circulation time 139
cisterna magna cerebellomedullaris 208
– medullaris 208
cisternal pneumoencephalography 186
cistern(s) 208, 210, 212
–, ambient 213
–, corpus callosum 213
–, – –, "rabbit-ears" image 243
–, horizontal section 8
–, lamina terminalis 204, 212
–, puncture of 186
–, superior cerebellar 213
–, Sylvian fissures 212
–, velum interpositum 213, 243
classification of brain tumors 25
clivus 108
cock's comb convolutions 255
coiling 149
–, internal carotid artery 146
collateral circulation 159
colloid cyst 251
communicating hydrocephalus 253, 254
complete block, myelography 274, 290
complications, pneumoencephalography 194, 195
–, tonsillar herniation 195
confluence of sinuses 83
congenital malformations of spine 293
contrast cisternogram, positive 249
– medium 58
contusion, cortical 20
convexity meningioma 120, 251
corkscrew vessels 116
corpus callosum, agenesis of 261
– –, aplasia 106, 261
– – cistern, widening 219
– –, displacement 222
– –, radiation of 200
– –, splenium of 90
– – tumors 265
– – –, anterior 229
– – –, posterior 231
craniocerebral trauma, consequences of 48
– –, open or blunt 258

craniopharyngioma, cisternogram 240
"crown of three peaks" 210
crural cisterns 210
– – ("crown of three peaks") 211
CSF changes 194
CVA, neuroradiological investigation 137
"cyclopia", association with arrhinencephalies 261
cyclops ventricle, typical demonstration 262
cysticercosis 251
cyst(s) 113, 260ff.
–, cavum Vergae 260, 261
–, septum pellucidum 261
–, traumatic 46

Dandy-Walker syndrome 246
dementias 252
diastematomyelia 294
direct sinography 175
discography 303ff.
–, complications 306
–, history 305
–, technique 305
displacements, across the midline 220
–, anterior inferior cerebral artery 111
–, axial 10
–, corpus callosum 222
–, deep venous system 94, 111
–, lateral 14
–, parallel 108
–, posterior cerebral artery, downward 109
–, – communicating artery, downward 109
–, vertebral artery 110
dissolution of thrombus and thromboembolus 158
disturbances in venous outflow 171
"double Queckenstedt maneuver", myelography 276
draining veins 122
"dry" cistern 187
dumbbell tumor 245
dural sinus 83

early reactions, pneumoencephalography 193, 194
"early" veins 135, 166
edema 251
EKG changes 195
embolism 149, 151
embolus, "riding saddle" 151
embryonal tumors 36
eminentia collateralis (calcar avis) 207
empty sella 212
encephalitides 252
ependymal and choroid plexus tumors 30
– cysts, foramen of Monro 235

epidermoid (cholesteatoma) 113,
251
epidural empyema, spinal 285
– hematomas 196, 265
– venous plexuses, spinal cord 282,
309
etiology of intracranial pressure 6
expert legal testimony 257
external carotid angiogram 84
– – artery, selective filling of 119
extracranial anastomoses 159
extradural infiltration of contrast,
spinal 286
– neurilemmoma 285
– tumor, complete block 286
extramedullary AVM, embolism
297

femoral artery, catheterization 59
fibrolipoma, spinal 293
fibrosarcoma, vessels of 118
filum terminale, shortened 294
Fischer's callosal anastomosis 161,
166
fish mouth 204
fistula, carotid/cavernous 126
fluid pathways near the midline, obstructions 16
foramen, arcuate of the atlas 85
– of Monro 201
– –, occlusion 235
foramina, costotransverse 85
fourth ventricle, occlusion 18, 233
– –, positive contrast 188
– – tumors 187, 241
"fractional" pneumoencephalography 184
"Frankfurt horizontal" 191
frontal horn 201
– –, radiatio corporis callosi 201
– lobe tumors 265
– tumors 14
– –, general signs 224
– –, pneumoencephalography 224
frontobasal (subfrontal) tumors
225
frontodorsal tumors 224
frontolateral meningioma 119
– tumors 225
frontomedial tumors 225
frontotemporoparietal tumors 228

gas resorption, pneumoencephalography 193
ganglia, basal, tumors 16
ganglion segment, internal carotid
artery 99
germ cell tumors 40
"German horizontal" 191
giant aneurysm 126
glioblastoma, "brushstroke" vessels
in 116
– multiforme 36
– –, vascular picture 116
glomus, choroid plexus 207
– jugulare tumor 118, 122, 178

Gradenigo's syndrome 172
grading of malignancy 39, 44
granulomatous processes 113

head injuries, angiogram 118
headaches, pneumoencephalography 194
hemangioblastomas 118
–, cerebellar 121
hematomas 113, 196
–, bilateral subdural 106
–, extracerebral 118
–, frontal epidural 123
hemispheric processes 14
hemodynamics 137
hemorrhage(s), hypertensive 53
–, predilection 171
–, traumatic 46
herniation 7
–, cerebellar, upward 108
–, intravertebral disc 285
– symptoms 195
– syndromes 9, 196
–, temporal lobe 109
–, tonsillar 10, 108
–, transtentorial (temporal) 9
hippocampal digitations 204
"hour-glass" neurilemmoma, spinal 309
– – tumor 108, 285
hydrocephalus, anterior cerebral artery 107
–, degree of 235
–, internal carotid arteriogram 107
–, thalamostriate vein 107
–, various causes 252
hypersensitivity, reactions 278
hypertensive hemorrhage 53
hypotensive crisis 137
– episode 157

impending herniation, sign of 264
impression, basilar 108
increased intracranial pressure 264
indentation of lateral ventricle 223
indication, myelography 279
– for neuroradiological procedures,
comparison, CT 267
infarcts, pathogenesis of 49
injection techniques, retrograde 60
injuries, after falls 46
–, blunt trauma 46
internal acoustic canal, contrast
249
– carotid arteriogram 78
– carotid artery 99
– – –, coiling 146
– – –, iatrogenic stenosis 144
– – –, occlusion 162
– – –, stenosis 146, 150
– cerebral veins 82
interpeduncular cisterns ("crown of
three peaks") 211
intervertebral disk herniation 287
intoxications 252
intracerebral abscess 259

– hemorrhage 171
– –, "atypical" 171
intracranial anastomoses 161
– anatomy 3
– pressure, etiology 6
– space-occupying processes 25
intramural hemorrhage 144
intrasellar cistern 212
intravenous segment, internal
carotid artery 99
intraventricular epidermoid 232
– meningioma 231
Jirout's technique, myelography
277
jugular venogram, normal 179

kinking 149

lamina terminalis 200
"laminar" flow, basilar artery 158
late reactions, pneumoencephalography 193, 194
lateral disc herniation 288
– ventricle tumors 16, 231
"leakage" of contrast medium 171
leucocytosis 194
lesions, anterior cerebral artery,
signs 108, 109
ligamentum flavum 281
lipoma at craniospinal junction 284
"low pressure" headache 276
– – hematoma 196
lumbar pneumoencephalogram 184
– spine, space-occupying 272
lymphomas, primary malignant 39
–, spinal 285
Lysholm's line 199

magnification angiography 64
main cisterns 8
malformations 260
malformative tumors 40
mamillary bodies 209
mass displacements 3, 6
– –, atrophic processes 20
– –, falx 5
– –, important 9
– –, pathophysiology 4
– –, rules of 4
massa intermedia 189, 200
masses, presellar 95
–, suprasellar 95
–, temporal lobe 95
measurement of ventricular size
218
medulloblastoma 36
megadolichobasilaris 157, 158
megadolichocarotis 157
membrane, atlanto-occipital 85
meningeal adhesions and arachnoiditis, spinal 291
– anastomoses 161, 163, 164
– sarcomas 38
– tissue tumors 37

meningioma(s), avascular 114
–, clivus 110
– en-plaque 227
–, frontolateral 119
–, olfactory groove 105
–, parasagittal 106
–, sphenoid wing 103, 104
–, vessels of 116
meningismus 194
meningocele 293
mesencephalic herniations 196
metabolic disturbances 252
metastases, "early veins" 118
–, multiple 122
metastatic tumors 41
microangioma 135, 171
"middle" anterior cerebral artery
    140
– cerebral artery, occlusion 151,
    163, 165
– – –, retrograde filling 165
– – veins 81
midline disc herniation 287, 290
– tumors 219, 238
migraine, angiography 137
monitoring 195
Moya-Moya disease 164
– – –, typical 168
multiple sclerosis 252
– tumors 250
Murtagh's technique, myelography
    277
"mushroom deformity", carotid
    fork 101
myelocytic leukemia, spinal cord
    286
myelogram, cervical 281
–, normal 280
–, pathological 283
myelography 269 ff.
–, complications and errors 278
–, history 271
–, indication 279
–, negative contrast 276
–, positive contrast 273, 275
–, – –, water-insoluble 272
–, – –, water-soluble 274
–, technique 272
myeloid leukemia, spinal cord 285
myelomeningocele (spina bifida
    cystica) 293

"narrow carotid artery" 149
"near" shift 95
needle-hole leakage, myelography
    274
negative contrast media, myelogra-
    phy 276
nerve root avulsions 292
– sheath cell tumors 37
neurilemmoma, acoustic 111
– (hour-glass) 108
–, third cervical root 110
neuroepithelial tissue, tumors of 27
neuronal tumors 36
neuroradiological examination 139

– investigation (CVA) 137
nuchal rigidity 195

obstructions, third ventricle 17
–, ventricular fluid pathways 16
obstructive hydrocephalus 253
occipital horn 198, 204
– lobe tumors 265
– tumors 16, 228
occipitovertebral anastomoses 160,
    165
occlusion, aqueduct 18, 233, 242
–, basilar artery 167
–, external carotid artery 143
–, internal carotid artery 143, 162,
    167
–, foramen of Magendie 245
–, – –, arachnoid scarring 245
–, – –, high cervical cord tumors
    245
–, – of Monro 235
–, fourth ventricle 18, 233
–, middle cerebral artery 151, 163,
    164, 165
–, posterior cerebral artery 156
–, – – –, four major sites 155
–, predilection site 142
–, right common carotid artery 144
–, sinus 171, 172
–, superior sagittal sinus 177
–, third ventricle 233
–, vertebral artery 167
occlusive hydrocephalus, develop-
    ment 11
– –, various forms 11
olfactory sulci 214, 215
oligodendroglial tumors 28
oligodendroglioma, vessels of 116
ophthalmic anastomosis 159
– venogram, normal 176
opposite hemisphere, impaired circu-
    lation to 169
orbital hemangioma 175
– venography 174
ossovenography 307 ff
–, complications 310
–, history, anatomy, technique,
    results 309
osteophytic spurring 144
"otitic" hydrocephalus 173

Pain, neck and shoulder 194
papilledema 264
paramedian tumors 219
paresthesias in shoulders 195
parietal lobe tumors 265
– tumors 15
– –, pneumoencephalogram 227
parietodorsal tumors 226, 227
parietolateral tumors 228
pathological myelogram 283
– vascularization 113
– venogram, intraorbital 175
pathophysiology, mass displace-
    ment 4

pericallosal artery, stenotic change
    159
Pick's disease 256
"pincer-like" effect 282
pineal cell tumors 31
– region tumors 237
pinealoma 237
pituitary tumor, cisternogram 240
plexus, basilar 84
–, choroid 198
–, –, lateral ventricles 91
–, epidural venous 282
–, pterygoid venous 83
pneumencephaly 47
pneumoencephalogram 197
–, pathological 219
–, septum pellucidum cyst, closed
    230
pneumoencephalography 181 ff.
–, headaches 194
–, history 183
–, indication and contraindication
    264
–, injection technique 184
–, midline tomogram 200
–, parietal tumor 223
–, technique 190
–, 24-hours 193
pontine cistern 208, 211
– glioma 244
– tumors 243
pontocerebellar cisterns 208, 247
porencephalic cyst 256
positioning techniques 85
positive contrast myelogram 273,
    289
– –, third and fourth ventricle 188,
    189
posterior cerebral artery 140
– – –, anastomosis 166
– – –, occlusion, stenosis 152, 156
– – –, supplied by internal carotid
    artery 141
– disc herniation 287
– fossa tumors 242
posttraumatic changes, spinal cord
    292
predilections of space-occupying
    processes 25
pressure cone 196
primary intracranial vascular dis-
    ease, diagnosis 127
– malignant lymphomas 39
– melanotic tumors 39
pseudotumor cerebri 250
"pulsating exophthalmus" 133
puncture, angular vein 174
–, carotid artery 58
–, cistern, direct and indirect meth-
    od 186
– methods 58
–, vertebral artery 59
pupillary changes 195

radiation of corpus callosum 200
ramus, occipital 90

reactive edema 195
"red" veins 166
references 311
regional tumors, local extensions
    41
resorption 194
reticulum cell sarcoma, spinal 285
retrograde angiography in children
    62
– injection 60
reversible ischemic neurological defi-
    cit (RIND) 137
"riding saddle" embolus 151
root pain 272
– sleeves 282

sarcoma, angiographic picture of
    118
seizures 252
"selective" spinal angiography 300
sella, erosion of 264
"senile tumors" 250
septum pellucidum cyst 260
– – –, closed 230
– – –, open 261
serpiginous contrast defects 290
shifts, carotid syphon 8
Sinography, direct 175, 177
sinus(es), cavernous 83, 84
–, confluence of 83
–, dural 83
–, inferior petrosal 83, 84
–, inferior sagittal 83
–, occipital 83
– occlusion 172
– rectus 83
–, sigmoid 83, 84
–, sphenoparietal 82, 83, 84
–, superior petrosal 83, 84
–, – sagittal 83
–, transverse 83
space-occupying lesions 6
– – –, intradural, extramedullary
    284, 285
– – –, intramedullary 283
– – –, site, type 13
– – processes 108, 113, 219
– – –, dorsal group 222
– – –, intracranial and spinal 25
– – –, lateral and basal groups 222
– – –, other than neoplasms 43
– – –, predilections 25
spasm, arterial 132, 138
speckled appearance, intraventricu-
    lar epidermoid 232
sphenoid wing meningioma 103,
    104
– – –, pneumoencephalogram 223
spinal angiography 295ff.
– –, history 297
– arteriovenous malformations
    290, 297, 298
– cord atrophy 292
– – AVM 291, 301
– – vessels, normal/pathological
    anatomy 297

– predilections, space-occupying
    processes 25
– tumors 42
splenium of corpus callosum 90
spreading sutures 264
standstill, cerebral circulatory 172,
    173
–, – –, angiography 173
"steal" syndromes 166
"steer horn" ventricle 261, 262
stenosis 142
–, aqueductal 241
–, basilar artery 152
–, carotid siphon 154
–, degree of 157
–, external carotid artery 162
–, internal carotid artery 143
–, – – –, iatrogenic 144
–, posterior cerebral arteries 152,
    156
–, – – –, four major sites 155
–, predilection sites 142
–, subclavian arteries 162
–, vertebral artery 152
stenotic plaque, basilar artery 155
"stretched" small vessels 113
"string of pearls" deformity 150
subarachnoid hemorrhage 169, 266
– pathways 208
"subclavian steal" 170
subdural air 215
– hematomas 196, 260, 265
– –, angiography 266
– –, avascular halfmoon zone 123
– –, bilateral 250
– –, chronic, lenticular shape 124
– space 214
suboccipital (cisternal) pneumoence-
    phalography 186
subtraction 66
sulci 215
superior cerebellar arteries 210
– – cisterns 213
– ophthalmic vein 135
– sagittal sinus, occlusion 177
supracallosal anastomosis 140
suprapineal recess, third ventricle
    207
supratentorial compartment 5
surrounding sickle of air 251
syringomyelia 292
"systematic atrophies" 256

technique of Jirout, Lindgren,
    Murtagh (myelography) 277
temporal horn 191, 198, 204, 207
– lobe tumors 265
– pole tumors 226
– tumors 15, 226
temporobasal tumors, pneumoence-
    phalogram 223, 226
temporolateral tumors 226
tentorial hiatus 108
tentorium meningioma 245
thalamus tumors 231
third ventricle 200, 203

– –, catheterization 187
– –, obstructions 17
– –, occlusion 233
– –, positive contrast 188, 189
– –, suprapineal recess 207
– – tumors 12, 187, 235, 237
thromboangiitis obliterans 166
thrombosis 149
–, ulcerating plaques 149
–, venous 171
–, "youthful" vessels 149
TIA 137
tilt table, myelography 274
tomography 192
torcular Herophili 172
torn root sleeves 292
tortuosity 148, 149
–, vertebral artery 148, 157
transient ischemic attack (TIA) 137
– paresthesia in shoulders 264
transtentorial (temporal) hernia-
    tions 9
trauma 46
–, craniocerebral 258
–, pathological changes 257
– to skull and brain, testimony
    about 260
trigone 198, 204
tumor(s), acoustic neurilemmoma
    111
–, anterior corpus callosum 229
–, – pituitary 41
–, astrocytic 27
–, basal ganglia 231
–, base of the brain 219
–, – of the skull 41
–, blood vessel origin 39
– blush 118
–, both hemispheres 106
–, in the elderly 106
–, ependymal and choroid plexus
    30
–, fourth ventricle 241, 245
–, frontal 14, 101
–, frontotemporal 103
–, lateral ventricles 16, 231
–, meningeal tissues 37
–, meningioma 110
–, nerve sheath cells 37
–, neurilemmoma 37
–, – (hour-glass) 108
–, neuroepithelial tissue 27
–, neuronal 36
–, occipital 16
–, oligodendroglial 28
–, orbit 176
–, parietal 15, 105
–, poorly differentiated 36
–, posterior corpus callosum 231
–, primary melanotic 39
–, regional local extensions 41
–, temporal 15, 101
–, thalamus 231
–, third ventricle 12
–, various 219, 220
– vessels 113ff., 118

tumor(s) vessels, star-shaped
    pattern 119
–, xanthomatous 39
tumor-like lesions 40
Twining's line 198
– point 243

unclassified tumors 41
unilateral filling, pneumoencepha-
    lography 193
upward herniation, cerebellar 241

vascular malformations 41
– occlusions 136
– – or stenoses, angiography 266
– stenoses 136
vasospasm 169
–, aortography 301
vein(s), anatomical variations 139
–, angular 83
–, –, puncture of 174
–, anterior medullary 82, 92
–, – pontomesencephalic 82, 92, 93,
    112
–, – spinal 82, 92
–, ascending 81
–, – occipital 91
–, basal 82
–, bridging 81
–, choroidal 82
–, cortical 112
– of Dandy, petrosal 112
–, deep cerebral 82
–, – –, displacement 94
–, descending 81
–, dorsal occipital, descending 91

–, "early" 166
– of Galen 82, 112
–, inferior cerebellar 93
–, – ophthalmic 83
–, – retrotonsillar 93
–, – vermian 93
–, internal cerebral 82, 112
–, jugular 178
– of Labbé 82
–, medial occipital, descending 91
–, occipital 83
–, petrosal 93
–, pontomesencephalic 112
–, posterior cranial fossa 92
–, precentral cerebellar 82, 92, 93,
    112
–, "red" 166
– of Rolandi, parietal 81
– of Rosenthal, basal 82, 112
–, septum pellucidum 82, 112
–, superior cerebellar 83, 93
–, superior ophthalmic 83, 135
–, superior retrotonsillar 93
–, temporal occipital 82
–, thalamostriate 82, 112
– of Trolard, precentral 81
velum interpositum cistern, widen-
    ing 219
venogram, intraorbital, pathologi-
    cal 175
venography, epidural 307 ff.
venous anatomy, normal 111
– angle 82
– channels, infratentorial 91
– –, supratentorial 91
– plexus, pterygoid 83

– thrombosis 171
ventricle tumors 16
ventricular displacement 259
– hypoplasia 218
– migration 255
– size, measurements 218
– system, nonfilling 192
ventriculography 187
–, indication and contraindication
    264
vertebral angiogram, anteroposterior
    view 86
– –, arterial phase 85, 108
– –, axial view 89
– –, half-axial sagittal view 88
– –, lateral view 87, 88, 108
– –, venous phase 91
– artery, puncture of 59
– –, tortuosity 148, 157
– –, stenosis 152
vessel changes, extracranial 142
– –, thrombotic 142
visualization of spinal cord AVM
    299
vomiting 264

Wallenberg's artery 89
"watershed areas" 166
water-soluble positive contrast, mye-
    lography 274
worm-like vessels, spinal cord 291

xanthomatous tumors 39

"youthful" vessels, thrombosis 149